Intensive Care in Neurosurgery

American Association of Neurological Surgeons

Thieme

American Association of Neurological Surgeons • Rolling Meadows, Illinois

Intensive Care in Neurosurgery

EDITED BY

BRIAN T. ANDREWS, MD, FACS
Chairman, Division of Neurosurgery
Vice-Chairman, Department of Neuroscience
California Pacific Medical Center

Attending Neurosurgeon
Department of Neurological Surgery
University of California, San Francisco
San Francisco, California

Thieme
New York • Stuttgart

American Association of Neurological Surgeons
Rolling Meadows, Illinois

Thieme New York
333 Seventh Avenue
New York, NY 10002

American Association of Neurological Surgeons
5550 Meadowbrook Drive
Rolling Meadows, IL 60008

Director of Production and Manufacturing: Anne Vinnicombe
Production Editor: Noelle Barrick, Graphic World Publishing Services, St. Louis, Missouri
Marketing Director: Phyllis Gold
Sales Manager: Ross Lumpkin
Chief Financial Officer: Peter van Woerden
President: Brian D. Scanlan
Compositor: Graphic World, Inc.
Printer: Maple–Vail Book Manufacturing Group

Library of Congress Cataloging-in-Publication Data

Intensive care in neurosurgery / edited by Brian T. Andrews.
p. ; cm
Includes bibliographical references and index.
ISBN 1-58890-125-4 (hardcover : alk. paper)
1. Neurological intensive care. 2. Surgical intensive care. I. Andrews, Brian T.
[DNLM: 1. Intensive Care—methods. 2. Nervous System Diseases—surgery. WL 368 I5955 2003]
RC350.N49 I58 2003
616.8′0428—dc21

2002023189

Important note: Medical knowledge is ever-changing. As new research and clinical experience broaden our knowledge, changes in treatment and drug therapy may be required. The authors and the editors of the material herein have consulted sources believed to be reliable in their efforts to provide information that is complete and in accord with the standards accepted at the time of publication. However, in view of the possibility of human error by the authors, editors, or publisher of the work herein, or changes in medical knowledge, neither the authors, editors, publisher, or any other party who has been involved in the preparation of this work warrants that the information contained herein is in every respect accurate or complete, and they are not responsible for any errors or omissions or for the results obtained from use of such information. For example, readers are advised to check the product information sheet included in the package of each drug they plan to administer to be certain that the information contained in this publication is accurate and that changes have not been made in the recommended dose or in the contraindications for administration. This recommendation is of particular importance in connection with new or infrequently used drugs.

Some of the product names, patents, and registered designs referred to in this book are in fact registered trademarks or proprietary names even though specific reference to this fact is not always made in the text. Therefore, the appearance of a name without designation as proprietary is not to be construed as a representation by the publisher that it is in the public domain.

Printed in the United States of America

5 4 3 2 1

ISBN 1-58890-125-4

Contents

Preface vii

Contributors ix

Chapter 1
Pulmonary Physiology, Monitoring, and Management in the Neurosurgical Intensive Care Unit 1
Perry A. Ball

Chapter 2
Cardiovascular Physiology, Monitoring, and Management in the Neurosurgical Intensive Care Unit 11
Martin C. Holland, David C. Bonovich, and Wayne Schmedel

Chapter 3
Neurological Monitoring 21
Brian T. Andrews

Chapter 4
Cerebrovascular Pathophysiology and Monitoring in the Neurosurgical Intensive Care Unit 29
Jamie S. Ullman

Chapter 5
Pathophysiology and Treatment of Intracranial Hypertension 47
Donald W. Marion

Chapter 6
Fluid, Electrolyte, and Acid-Base Balance 55
Joseph M. Darby

Chapter 7
Metabolic, Nutritional, and Endocrine Aspects of Neurosurgical Intensive Care 83
David McKalip

Chapter 8
Infectious Disease 95
L.J.S. Yang and J.T. Hoff

Chapter 9
Head Injury Management 125
Brian T. Andrews

Chapter 10

Spinal Cord Injury Management 137
Ash Singhal, Andrew Baker, and Michael G. Fehlings

Chapter 11

Multisystem Injury Management 145
Robert Mackersie, Andre Campbell, and Brian T. Andrews

Chapter 12

Subarachnoid Hemorrhage 161
Kevin C. Yao and Joshua B. Bederson

Chapter 13

Stroke and Nontraumatic Hemorrhage 173
David C. Bonovich and J. Claude Hemphill, III

Chapter 14

Management of Patients with Epilepsy 191
David King-Stephens and Peter B. Weber

Chapter 15

Management of Patients with Brain Tumors 197
Guy Lin, G. Evren Keles, and Mitchel S. Berger

Chapter 16

The Pediatric Neurosurgical Patient 207
Daniel Falco and Gregory B. Hammer

Chapter 17

Witholding and Withdrawal of Life Support in the Intensive Care Unit 221
John M. Luce

Chapter 18

Declaration of Brain Death 229
Grant E. Gauger

Index 235

Preface

Our understanding of the physiology of head and spinal cord injury, stroke, brain tumors, and other disorders have improved dramatically in recent years. Translation of this knowledge to clinical practice, however, has often not occurred in the operating room. Rather the neurosurgical intensive care unit has more often been the place where physiological understanding has been conceived and applied for practical results. Many advances have been made in bedside monitoring techniques in recent years, and we have entered a time in which specific therapies to reverse, compensate, and control the detrimental physiological results of injury or disease processes are based upon results of such monitoring. Also neurosurgeons and more recently neurologists have become more directly involved in the care of patients in the intensive care unit. In medical centers it has become mandatory that they work closely with critical care specialists so that the intensive care unit can provide the best care to patients. And in some, they are directing overall care of the patient including pulmonary and hemodynamic management.

The goal of this book is to provide neurosurgeons, neurologists, critical care specialists, and all of those who care for neurosurgical patients a reference to assist in further advancing the intensive care of neurosurgical patients.

Acknowledgements

This book is the culmination of efforts by the members of the Joint Section of Neurotrauma and Critical Care of the AANS and CNS. I was proud to be the president of this joint section in 1999 to 2000 and to have worked with many people who have devoted their lives to the study of head injury, spinal cord injury, and the betterment of care for patients suffering from these devastating injuries. Many members of this section contributed chapters to this book and I thank them for their efforts. I would also like to acknowledge the members of the Department of Neurological Surgery at the University of California, San Francisco, and the San Francisco General Hospital. Finally without the encouragement and support of my wife Linda and my children Christopher and Lauren, I would not have been motivated to begin or to complete this book.

Brian T. Andrews, MD, FACS
May 2002

Contributors

Andrew Baker, MD, FRCPC
Medical Director of Trauma and Neurosurgery
Intensive Care Unit
Director of Cara Phelan Center for Trauma Research
St. Michael's Hospital
Professor
University of Toronto
Toronto, Ontario, Canada

Perry A. Ball, MD
Associate Professor of Surgery (Neurosurgery)
Section of Neurosurgery
Dartmouth-Hitchcock Medical Center
Lebanon, NH

Joshua B. Bederson, MD
Professor and Vice-Chairman
Department of Neurosurgery
Director of Cerebrovascular Surgery
Mount Sinai Scool of Medicine
Mount Sinai Medical Center
New York, NY

Mitchel S. Berger, MD
Professor and Chair
Director, Brain Tumor Research Center
Department of Neurological Surgery
University of California, San Francisco
San Francisco, CA

David C. Bonovich, MD
Assistant Clinical Professor of Neurology
Associate Director
Neurocritical Care and Stroke Service
Department of Neurology
San Francisco General Hospital
University of California, San Francisco
San Francisco, CA

Andre Campbell, MD
Director of Surgical Critical Care
San Francisco General Hospital
Associate Professor of Clinical Surgery
Department of Surgery
University of California, San Francisco
San Francisco, CA

Joseph M. Darby, MD
Associate Professor
Department of Critical Care Medicine
University of Pittsburgh School of Medicine
Medical Director Trauma Intensive Care Unit
University of Pittsburgh Medical Center
Presbyterian Hospital
Pittsburgh, PA

Daniel Falco, MD
Pediatric Critical Care
Sutter Memorial Hospital
Sacramento, CA

Michael G. Fehlings, MD, PhD
Senior Scientist
Division of Cellular and Molecular Biology
Toronto Western Research Institute
Toronto Western Hospital
Toronto, Ontario, Canada

Grant E. Gauger, MD
Associate Clinical Professor
Department of Neurological Surgery
University of California, San Francisco
San Francisco, CA

Gregory B. Hammer, MD
Associate Professor
Anesthesiology and Pediatrics
Stanford University School of Medicine
Associate Director
Pediatric Intensive Care Unit
Department of Anesthesiology
Lucile S. Packard Children's Hospital
Stanford, CA

J. Claude Hemphill, III, MD
Director
Neurocritical Care and Stroke Service
Department of Neurology
San Francisco General Hospital
University of California, San Francisco
San Francisco, CA

J.T. Hoff, MD
Professor and Chair
Department of Neurosurgery
The University of Michigan Health Systems
Ann Arbor, MI

Martin C. Holland, MD
Assistant Clinical Professor
Department of Neurological Surgery
San Francisco General Hospital
University of California, San Francisco
San Francisco, CA

G. Evren Keles, MD
Assistant Adjunct Professor
Department of Neurological Surgery
University of California, San Francisco
San Francisco, CA

David King-Stephens, MD
Co-Director of the California Pacific Epilepsy Program
Director of the Neurophysiology Laboratory
Department of Neurology
California Pacific Medical Center
San Francisco, CA

Guy Lin, MD
Resident
University of Pennsylvania Hospital
Department of Otorhinolaryngology
University of Pennsylvania
Philadelphia, PA

John M. Luce, MD
Professor of Clinical Medicine and Anesthesia
University of California, San Francisco
Associate Director
Medical-Surgical Intensive Care Unit
San Francisco General Hospital
San Francisco, CA

Donald W. Marion, MD, FACS
Professor of Neurological Surgery and Director
Brain Trauma Research Center and Center for Injury Research and Control
University of Pittsburgh School of Medicine
Associate Chief of Neurological Surgery
University of Pittsburgh Medical Center
Presbyterian Hospital
Pittsburgh, PA

Robert Mackersie, MD
Director of Trauma
San Francisco General Hospital
Professor of Surgery
Department of Surgery
University of California, San Francisco
San Francisco, CA

David McKalip, MD
Clinical Assistant Professor
Department of Neurological Surgery
University of South Florida
St. Petersburg, FL

Wayne Schmedel
Nurse
San Francisco General Hospital
San Francisco, CA

Ash Singhal, MD
Senior Resident
Neurosurgery Residency Program
University of Toronto
Toronto, Ontario, Canada

Jamie S. Ullman, MD
Director of Neurosurgery
Elmhurst Hospital Center
Assistant Professor
Department of Neurosurgery
Mount Sinai School of Medicine
Mount Sinai Medical Center
New York, NY

Peter B. Weber, MD
Neurosurgeon
Co-Director of California Pacific Epilepsy Program
Department of Neurosciences
California Pacific Medical Center
San Francisco, CA

L.J.S. Yang, MD
Senior Resident
Department of Neurosurgery
The University of Michigan Health Systems
Ann Arbor, MI

Kevin C. Yao, MD
Chief Resident
Department of Neurosurgery
Mount Sinai Medical Center
New York, NY

CHAPTER 1

Pulmonary Physiology, Monitoring, and Management in the Neurosurgical Intensive Care Unit

PERRY A. BALL

INTRODUCTION

The delivery of oxygen to the tissues and the removal of carbon dioxide from the blood depend on the exchange of these gases in the lung. Pulmonary dysfunction is a relatively common complication of the management of neurosurgical patients. An understanding of some of the principles of respiratory physiology can be helpful in the logical management of pulmonary dysfunction.

BACKGROUND

Ventilation

The process of respiration involves moving air into the respiratory tract: The amount of air moved with each respiratory cycle is the *tidal volume* (TV). The usual unit of measurement of respiration is the *minute ventilation* (MV), which is determined by multiplying the tidal volume by the respiratory rate. The normal resting minute ventilation is approximately 4 L/min. Increasing minute ventilation can be achieved by breathing more rapidly, but because of resistance to airflow in the pulmonary system, the energy expended during breathing increases quite markedly at greater than approximately 10 L/min.

Actual gas exchange occurs at the alveolus of the lung, but not all air moved into the respiratory system actually reaches the alveoli. The amount of air that does reach the alveoli is referred to as the *alveolar ventilation* (V_A). The amount of air that does not reach the alveolus is referred to as *dead space ventilation;* under normal conditions, this comprises approximately 30% of the minute ventilation. There are two components of dead space ventilation. The first is the anatomical dead space, which is the approximately 250 ml of air in the conducting airways of the pharynx, trachea, and bronchi. The second is the *physiological dead space,* which refers to the air that does not fully equilibrate with alveolar gas. An increase in the minute ventilation such as what is seen with an increase in the respiratory rate usually results in an increase in the alveolar ventilation, but this is not always the case. For instance, shallow breaths, in which the largest percentage of air only moves in the conducting airways, can result in no increase or even a decrease in the alveolar ventilation.

Gas Exchange

Carbon dioxide is produced by the tissues, and there is a straightforward relationship between the partial pressure of carbon dioxide (PCO_2) in arterial blood and the amount of alveolar ventilation. If alveolar ventilation is increased, the PCO_2 falls; the opposite occurs if alveolar ventilation falls. Under normal circumstances the minute ventilation is constantly adjusted by the respiratory centers of the brainstem to maintain a PCO_2 of approximately 40 mm Hg.

The oxygen content of the blood is determined primarily by the amount of hemoglobin and its degree of saturation. At any given pH, hemoglobin binds increasing amounts of oxygen with increasing partial pressure of oxygen (PO_2) until it is fully saturated. This curve has an approximately sigmoid shape, and hemoglobin becomes fully saturated at a PO_2 of approximately 100 mm Hg. A decrease in pH under conditions of acidosis shifts the curve to the right; an increase in pH shifts the curve to the left (Figure 1-1). Each gram of hemoglobin can carry 1.34 ml of oxygen when it is fully saturated. Oxygen is poorly soluble in the plasma: 0.003 ml for each mm Hg of PO_2. The total

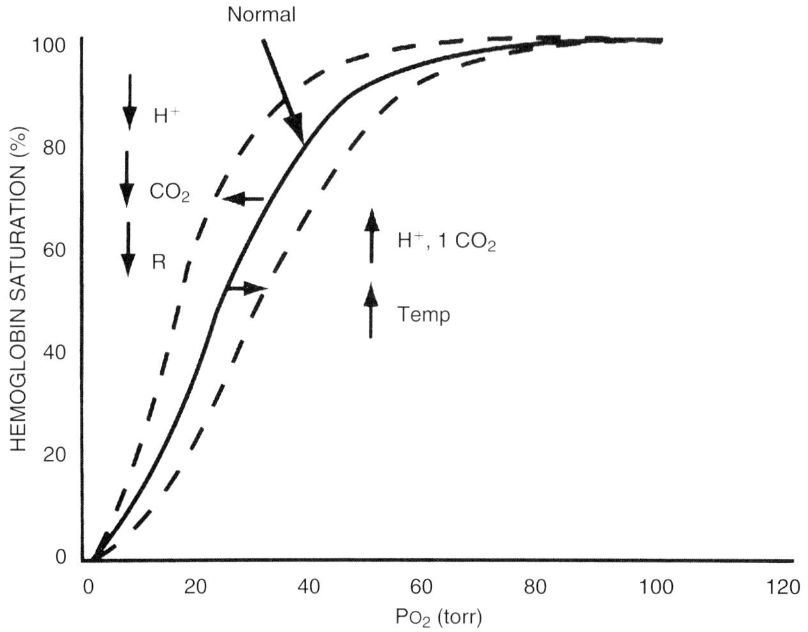

FIGURE 1-1 ■ **The oxyhemoglobin dissociation curve.**

oxygen content of the blood can be determined with the following equation:

Oxygen content = (1.34 × grams hemoglobin × % saturation) + (0.003 × PO_2)

Three things should be apparent at this point. The first is that the degree of saturation of hemoglobin in arterial blood ($S_{ao}2$) is a good indicator of the oxygen content of the blood at any level of hemoglobin. The second is that the shape of the hemoglobin association curve starts to flatten at a saturation of 90%, so increases in saturation above this level have relatively small effects on the oxygen content of the blood. The third is that once hemoglobin is saturated, because of the poor solubility of oxygen in plasma, large increases in the PaO_2 have trivial effects on the oxygen content of the blood; this is why the PaO_2 is a poor indicator of the oxygen content of the blood (Figure 1-2).

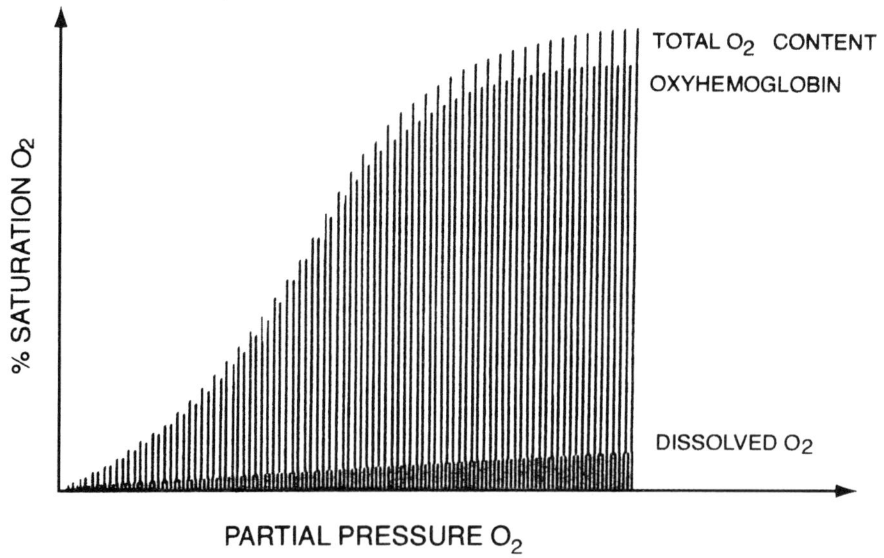

FIGURE 1-2 ■ **A diagram of the oxygen content of the blood.** The large percentage of oxygen is carried on hemoglobin. Once the flat portion of the curve has been saturated, further increases in the PO_2 will not have significant increases in the oxygen content of the blood. Adapted from Shapiro BA, Peruzzi WT, Kozelowski-Templin R: **Clinical Application of Blood Gases (ed 4).** Chicago: Year Book Medical Publishers, 1989.

The PaO_2 is, however, an excellent indicator of the degree of efficiency of gas exchange in the lungs. This can be determined by comparing the partial pressure of oxygen in the alveoli (PAO_2) with the partial pressure of oxygen in arterial blood (PaO_2). This is referred to as the *alveolar-arterial (A-a) gradient.*

The partial pressure of oxygen in the alveolus is determined by the alveolar gas equation:

$$PAO_2 = FiO_2(P_B - PH_{2O)-(PaCO}2/RQ)$$

Therefore, when at sea level breathing room air, where the fractional inspired oxygen concentration (FiO_2) is 21%, the barometric pressure (PB) is 760 mm Hg and the pressure of water vapor (PH_2O) is 47 mm Hg, and the respiratory quotient is 0.8 yields, an expected partial pressure of oxygen in the alveoli is 100 mm Hg. There is a small normal A-a gradient, so healthy subjects breathing room air at sea level are expected to have a PaO_2 of approximately 95 mm Hg.

The efficiency of gas exchange in the lung can thus be determined by comparing the measured partial pressure of oxygen in arterial blood with the expected partial pressure of oxygen in the alveolus for the given level of inspired oxygen. From a practical standpoint, it is not necessary to commit to memory all the components of the alveolar gas equation, but knowledge of the expected PAO_2 at certain levels of inspired oxygen can be useful. For instance, at 50% oxygen the expected value is 320 mm Hg, and at 100% oxygen it is 720 mm Hg. These expected values can then be compared with the measured PaO_2.

There are four pathological processes that result in an increase in the A-a gradient and consequent hypoxemia: ventilation/perfusion (V/Q) mismatch, shunt, diffusion abnormalities, and alveolar hypoventilation. In neurosurgical practice, V/Q mismatch and shunt are the most significant.

V/Q mismatch refers to air in alveoli that is not exposed to the pulmonary blood flow. An example of this is the large bullae that are seen in patients with emphysema. The important issue with V/Q mismatch is that it can be corrected with administration of 100% oxygen.

Shunt refers to that portion of the right-sided heart output that does not equilibrate with air in the alveoli (Figure 1-3). Shunt is the result of conditions that cause blood flow to be directed to alveoli that are not fully aerated. There are two types of situations in which this occurs. The first are those situations in which alveoli are either filled with fluid, such as pneumonia, or situations in which the alveoli are collapsed, such as in atelectasis; in these situations a portion of the right-sided heart output goes to those alveoli that are not

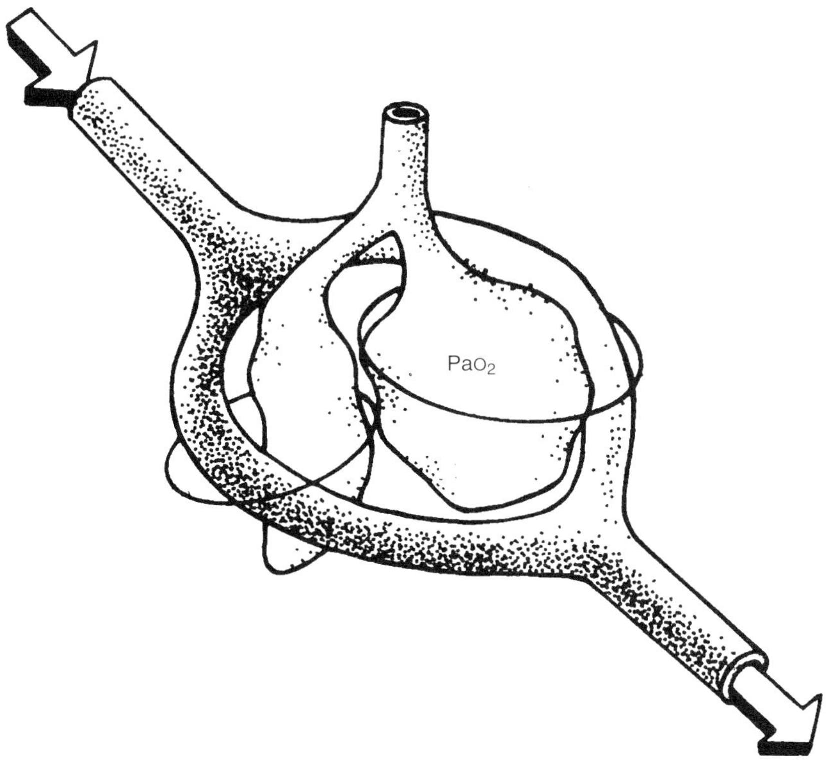

FIGURE 1-3 ■ **Shunt.** Blood that goes to poorly aerated alveoli is mixed with blood that goes to well aerated alveoli. Adapted from Shapiro BA, Peruzzi WT, Kozelowski-Templin R: **Clinical Application of Blood Gases (ed 4).** Chicago: Year Book Medical Publishers, 1989.

exposed to inspired air. In this situation, the chest radiograph is often abnormal. The other situation in which shunt occurs is when alterations in pulmonary blood flow occur in inflammatory conditions such as pancreatitis or in pulmonary embolism. In this situation the chest radiograph may be normal despite severe hypoxemia.

The significant issue of shunt is that the PO_2 increases but A-a gradient is not fully corrected by adding supplemental oxygen. This means that in the presence of shunt there is an A-a gradient even when 100% oxygen is administered. The degree to which the arterial oxygenation increases by raising the fraction of inspired oxygen is determined by the percentage of right-sided heart output that does not see aerated alveoli. This is referred to as the *shunt fraction*. As the shunt fraction becomes larger, there is a smaller increase in the PO_2, with an increase in the FIO_2. When the shunt fraction reaches 50% and half the right-sided heart output does not equilibrate with alveolar air, increasing the inspired oxygen has no effect on PaO_2.

MECHANICAL VENTILATION

Indications

The indications for intubation and mechanical ventilation are an inability to protect the airway, an inability to ventilate, and thus an inadequate alveolar ventilation or an inability to oxygenate with consequent hypoxemia.

An inability to protect the airway is seen in patients with a decreased level of consciousness, as well as in patients with lower facial injuries or injuries to the cranial nerves IX and X. An inability to ventilate may be seen in patients with spinal cord injuries. An inability to oxygenate is usually caused by those conditions that result in shunt.

It is difficult to provide firm guidelines for intubation, but in general, concern about the adequacy of ventilation should be raised when patients have a respiratory rate greater than 25 breaths/min or a PCO_2 greater than 50 mm Hg. The adequacy of oxygenation should be a concern at a PO_2 less than 50 mm Hg or a hemoglobin saturation of less than 90%. The decision can be based on whether the patient's condition is improving or deteriorating, but in general it is preferable and easier to proceed with intubation under controlled circumstances rather than when conditions have progressed to respiratory arrest.

Ventilator Modes

The commonly used ventilator modes are either volume cycled or pressure cycled. With volume-cycled modes, the amount of tidal volume is set and pressure developed within the system depends on the resistance of the lungs and the airways. With pressure-cycled modes, the amount of pressure supplied to the system is set and the tidal volume delivered depends on the resistance of the lungs and airways. Intermittent mandatory ventilation (IMV) delivers a set tidal volume at a set rate. The patient can breathe through the circuit, but not every breath is supported. This is probably the most widely used ventilator mode. Assist control (A/C) delivers a set tidal volume with each respiratory effort the patient attempts. A backup rate is set to deliver a minimal amount of ventilation if the patient does not make enough respiratory effort. The advantage of A/C is that it is useful in situations in which the patient has an abnormal respiratory drive. Pressure control ventilation (PCV) delivers a set level of airway pressure at a set rate. Pressure support ventilation (PSV) delivers a set amount of pressure to the circuit with each effort the patient makes. This can be used as the sole mode of ventilation or it can be used in concert with IMV to support the patient's spontaneous breaths. It is widely used in the process of weaning patients from ventilatory support.

Airway Pressure

As opposed to spontaneous breathing, in which air is drawn into the lungs by negative intrathoracic pressure, mechanical ventilation forces air into the chest with positive pressure. Mechanical ventilators can do this by either delivering a set amount of tidal volume or by supplying a set amount of airway pressure. In either case the lungs are inflated and a level of pressure is developed within the pulmonary system. The peak inspiratory pressure (PIP) is the maximal pressure within the pulmonary system during the inspiratory cycle, whereas the plateau pressure is the pressure within the system at the end of inspiration. These two pressures are usually quite similar, but the plateau pressure is lower because it does not incorporate the pressure caused by the resistance to flow in the airways.

The amount of pressure that is required to inflate the lung to a certain volume is referred to as the *compliance* of the lung. An understanding of lung compliance is crucial to understanding ventilator management. At the end of expiration, some alveoli remain open; the amount of air remaining in the lung is referred to as the *functional residual capacity* (FRC). Lung compliance is maximal (and thus the least amount of pressure is required to inflate the lung) at the normal resting FRC. In situations in which the FRC is decreased and consequently more alveoli are collapsed at the end of expiration, lung compliance is decreased and more pressure is required to inflate the lung (Figure 1-4). Most conditions that result in shunt and the need for mechanical ventilation are associated with a decrease in compli-

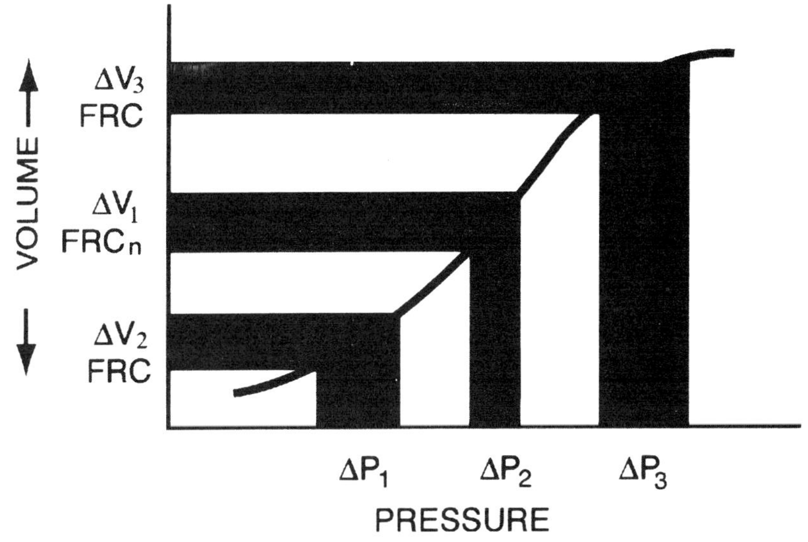

FIGURE 1-4 ■ **An illustration of the effect of FRC on lung compliance.** Adapted from Kandra TG, Rosenthal M: The pathophysiology of respiratory failure, **Int Anesthesiol Clin 31(2):**119-147, 1993.

ance and FRC; these conditions include alveoli that are filled with fluid associated with pulmonary edema or pus when pneumonia is present and mechanical collapse in patients with widespread atelectasis. Some situations, such as bronchospasm, result in overinflation of the lung and excess FRC; this also results in decreased compliance. Much of the management of mechanical ventilation is an attempt to restore the normal FRC and inflate the lung with the least amount of pressure possible. Unfortunately, it is difficult to measure FRC directly at the bedside, so the value must be inferred from the chest radiograph and the airway pressures generated during the ventilatory cycle.

The intrathoracic pressures generated during mechanical ventilation can have adverse effects on the lung, referred to as *barotrauma.* The most apparent forms barotrauma are those in which extraalveolar air can be detected on radiographs: pneumothorax, pneumomediastinum, pneumopericardium, pneumoperitoneum, and subcutaneous emphysema. There appears to be a relationship between high airway pressures and the occurrence of this type of barotrauma.[30] Tension pneumothorax is potentially life threatening and requires prompt treatment, but it is not clear if the occurrence of radiographically apparent barotrauma has an adverse effect on patient outcome.[32]

The other form of barotrauma, ventilator-associated lung injury (VLI), is not necessarily apparent on chest radiographs. There is evidence that high airway pressures can cause lung injury.[34] This has led to recommendations that efforts should be made to limit the pressure across the alveolus (which can be estimated by the plateau pressure) to 35 cm H_2O or less.[33]

It should be apparent that airway pressure and tidal volume are related: For any given lung compliance, a higher inflating pressure is required to achieve a higher tidal volume. It is not clear whether the VLI is due to the elevated pressure itself or to mechanical overdistention of the aerated lung.[10] Airway pressures can be reduced by limiting tidal volume, but as was discussed previously in regard to shallow breathing, even if the total minute ventilation is kept constant by raising the respiratory rate, this can result in lower alveolar ventilation because of the anatomical dead space.

Oxygen

The use of supplemental oxygen raises Pa_{O_2}, and until hemoglobin is fully saturated it also increases the amount of oxygen carried on hemoglobin. In the presence of shunt that results in hypoxemia, the use of supplemental oxygen is vital to deliver adequate oxygen to the tissues. There are, however, clear reasons to attempt to limit the percentage of oxygen employed. Once the hemoglobin saturation is greater than 90%, there is little advantage to a higher Pa_{O_2} in terms of oxygen content of the blood. Furthermore, it should be kept in mind that high fractions of inspired oxygen are toxic to lung tissues. Free radicals that promote lung injury are generated in the presence of high oxygen. It appears that a normal lung can tolerate 60% oxygen,[10] but in the presence of lung injury, damage may begin at 50%.[31] The concern for lung toxicity is part of the balancing of the risks of therapy. If other measures fail to improve the degree of shunting and hypoxemia, a potentially toxic level of inspired oxygen may have to be tolerated to provide adequate systemic oxygenation.

Positive End-Expiratory Pressure

Positive end-expiratory pressure (PEEP) refers to pressure applied to the respiratory system at the end of expiration; it is widely used during mechanical ventilation. PEEP can be added to the ventilator circuit in variable amounts, usually between 5 and 20 cm H_2O.

The optimal or maximal amount of PEEP has been a source of controversy,[2,27] which reflects the fact that PEEP has potential positive and negative effects. The main benefit of PEEP is that it can keep alveoli open at the end of expiration. When PEEP functions in this manner and recruits more open alveoli, it results in an increase in the FRC and often an improvement in lung compliance. In addition, because more alveoli are open, more of the right-sided heart output goes to open alveoli; thus PEEP often reduces the shunt fraction and improves oxygenation.

The potential drawback to PEEP is that it adds pressure to the respiratory system, and this extra pressure can be transmitted to already open alveoli rather than recruiting closed alveoli. This results in the overdistention of already open alveoli. In this situation the lung compliance is often worse and there may be no improvement or even worsening of shunt and oxygenation.[18]

In general, PEEP often is most effective in situations of diffuse lung disease such as acute respiratory distress syndrome (ARDS), when the extra pressure is transmitted throughout the lung, rather than focal lung disease such as pneumonia, when overdistention of open alveoli is more likely to be problematic.[12] This is not always the case, and the amount of PEEP used in any given clinical situation must be individualized. Often, when initiating mechanical ventilation, 5 cm H_2O of PEEP is used as a starting point. Increases in the PEEP are usually made in 2.5 or 5 cm H_2O increments. If the Pa_{O_2} improves as a result, then PEEP is most likely recruiting alveoli and thus decreasing the amount of shunt. Because of the increase in the pressure within the pulmonary system, an increase in the PEEP generally increases the peak inspiratory pressure (PIP). If the PIP increases by less than the amount of the increase in the PEEP, then the compliance of the lung has been improved, but often the increase in the PIP is equal to or more than the amount of increase in the PEEP. The benefit to oxygenation must therefore be balanced against the risk of increased pulmonary pressure.

Auto-PEEP refers to air that is trapped in the alveoli at end expiration. The most common instance of this occurs when there is obstruction to exhalation, such as in bronchospasm. This phenomenon can also occur if the expiratory time is insufficient to allow full expiration. Auto-PEEP has similar effects on intrathoracic pressure and FRC as mechanical PEEP.

MANAGEMENT OF SPECIFIC RESPIRATORY PROBLEMS

Acute Respiratory Distress Syndrome

ARDS is a process that occurs within the lung in response to a direct insult either to the lung itself or to other organ systems. The most common pulmonary processes leading to ARDS are aspiration and pneumonia; and systemic causes include head injury, multiple emergency blood transfusions, sepsis, and trauma.[5,16] Regardless of the inciting event, the pulmonary response, referred to as *diffuse alveolar damage*, has two phases. In the first phase the pulmonary capillaries become increasingly permeable, with resultant leakage of edema fluid into the alveoli. In the second phase there is proliferation of fibroblasts.

The clinical manifestations of ARDS are the result of the pulmonary edema, with consequent shunting and hypoxemia. The symptoms of ARDS usually appear quite rapidly after the inciting event, with the onset within 24 hours in half of patients who develop the syndrome.[16] The most widely used diagnostic criteria for ARDS are those of the American-European Consensus Committee.[3] The chest radiograph demonstrates bilateral diffuse infiltrates consistent with pulmonary edema. The infiltrates are usually patchy and scattered throughout both lung fields, but it should be noted that the radiographic appearance can be quite variable and may resemble pulmonary edema from other causes.[14] There is severe hypoxemia, with a ratio of Pa_{O_2} to Fi_{O_2} of 200 mm Hg or less. The formal definition requires a pulmonary artery wedge pressure of 18 mm Hg or less to exclude cardiogenic pulmonary edema. Although this is logical, there are some problems with the strict use of this definition. The first is that in practice, many patients with ARDS are diagnosed and managed without the use of pulmonary artery catheters. The second is that many patients who develop ARDS have received substantial fluid resuscitation and so may have elevated pulmonary artery pressures in the absence of overt congestive heart failure.

The ventilatory management of patients with ARDS can be challenging because the degree of shunting and hypoxemia is significant and lung compliance is markedly reduced, largely as a result of the increased lung water and widespread alveolar collapse. It is in the management of ARDS that the issues related to inspired oxygen, airway pressures, and tidal volume can become complex. This involves balancing the relative risks of the amount of inspired oxygen used and the level of PEEP employed with the resultant airway pressures. Often it requires trying a considerable number of different ventilator settings to achieve acceptable blood gas measurements. It should be emphasized that there is no clear consensus on the optimal ventilator strategy for ARDS: a 1996 survey of intensivists showed a wide variability in practice patterns regarding levels of PEEP and Fi_{O_2}.[7]

Conventional ventilator strategies have typically used volume-cycled modes, with a starting tidal volume of approximately 10 ml/kg and an inspired oxygen fraction of 100%. The level of PEEP is started at 5 cm H_2O and is increased in increments until the Fi_{O_2} can be titrated to less than 60% with the oxygen saturation in arterial blood at 90% or greater.[19]

Unfortunately, in many cases of ARDS this results in airway pressures that exceed 35 mm Hg. In this situation a decision must be made whether to tolerate the risk of higher airway pressures or the risk of higher levels of FiO_2 or to attempt an alternate ventilator strategy.

One strategy is to change the ratio of inspiratory to expiratory time during the ventilatory cycle. This is referred to as *inverse ratio* ventilation. The conventional ventilator cycle has a ratio of 1:3 of inspiratory time to expiratory time. Lengthening the inspiratory phase so that the ratio is 1:1, 2:1, or 3:1 applies the inspiratory pressure over a longer period. Although this can be done with volume-cycled ventilatory modes, it is more common to use the pressure-cycled mode. As the pressure is applied over a longer period, the peak airway pressure is lower but the mean airway pressure increases; in some patients with ARDS this results in better oxygenation. This strategy does, however, have some drawbacks. The elevated mean airway pressures result in higher intrathoracic pressures, which may compromise venous return and cardiac output. The shortened expiratory phase may not allow for full exhalation, with resultant air trapping and auto-PEEP. Thus although the oxygenation may improve, it is not clear that this strategy results in better survival.

Placing ventilated patients with ARDS in the prone position is another strategy that may improve oxygenation. It has been postulated that this improvement is due to the redistribution of pulmonary blood flow.[29] A randomized trial of supine ventilation compared with prone ventilation showed better oxygenation in the prone group but no difference in survival.[13]

Another strategy is the use of lower tidal volumes in an attempt to limit airway pressures and potential lung injury. A large, multicenter randomized trial of the use of tidal volumes of 6 ml/kg versus 12 ml/kg demonstrated reduced number of ventilator days and reduced mortality in the lower tidal volume group.[1] The results of this important study must be interpreted with caution, however, in its application to neurosurgical practice. The use of reduced tidal volumes even with elevated respiratory rates often result in lower alveolar ventilation because of the presence of the anatomical dead space. As a consequence, there is often a rise in the $PaCO_2$; this has been referred to as *permissive hypercapnea*. In many neurosurgical situations this may not be desirable, and it should be noted that patients with elevated intracranial pressure were specifically excluded from the study.[1]

Patient respiratory efforts that are not well synchronized with the ventilator result in lower oxygenation. Many patients with ARDS have such tenuous oxygenation that it is often beneficial to use sedation and in some cases pharmacological paralysis to minimize asynchrony with the ventilator. The use of corticosteroids in the acute phase of ARDS has been shown to be nonbeneficial.[4,21] As mentioned previously, there is a late phase of ARDS that involves fibroblast proliferation, and the role of corticosteroids in this late phase is uncertain.[24]

The overall mortality rate for patients with ARDS is approximately 30% to 40%.[25,35] The cause of death in most patients is not an inability to provide adequate oxygenation but rather sepsis and multiple organ failure.[26,35] Those patients who survive ARDS have a gradual improvement in respiratory function. The majority of those who survive have nearly normal lung function at 1 year after discontinuation of mechanical ventilation.[22]

Ventilator-Assisted Pneumonia

Patients who are mechanically ventilated are at risk for developing pneumonia, but establishing the diagnosis of ventilator-assisted pneumonia (VAP) can be challenging. Part of the problem is that the methods used to diagnose pneumonia in nonventilated patients, such as the presence of fever, cough, sputum production, rales, and radiographic infiltrates, are often difficult to interpret in ventilated patients. Fever from both infections and noninfectious sources is common in critically ill patients. Radiographic infiltrates in ventilated patients can reflect pulmonary edema of cardiac or noncardiac origin or infection. This has led some to advocate the use of invasive testing diagnostic methods, such as bronchoscopy, as part of the diagnosis of VAP.[11] Others have argued that the diagnosis can be reliably achieved by clinical criteria and the analysis of aspirated sputum.[28] A consensus panel of the American College of Chest Physicians evaluated the published evidence for the reliability of the diagnosis of VAP.[15] The recommendations were that in the presence of two or more clinical criteria—temperature greater than 38Y C or less than 36Y C, leukopenia or leukocytosis, purulent secretions, hypoxemia, or an abnormal chest radiograph—empirical diagnosis of VAP is reasonable. The panel found that there was not sufficient evidence that invasive diagnostic procedures added to the reliability of the diagnosis.

The selection of empiric antibiotics for VAP while awaiting the results of sputum cultures should be based on the Gram's stain of the sputum and the length of intubation. VAP that occurs in the first 4 days of intubation is most commonly caused by *Streptococcus pneumoniae* or *Haemophilus influenzae*. In patients who have been ventilated for longer than 4 days, *Staphylococcus aureus* and enteric gram-negative bacilli such as *Pseudomonas aeruginosa*, *Escherichia coli*, and *Klebsiella pneumoniae* predominate.

Respiratory Failure Associated with Spinal Cord Injury

Approximately one third of patients with spinal cord injury develop respiratory failure and require mechanical ventilation during the acute hospitalization period.[9] This may be due to associated chest or head injuries, but acute cervical and upper thoracic spinal cord injury is associated with a marked compromise in ventilatory function. The negative intrathoracic pressure that drives inspiration is achieved by contraction of the diaphragm and expansion of the chest wall by the intercostal muscles and the accessory muscles of respiration. Expiration is mostly a passive process, but the forced expiration that results in coughing and the clearing of secretions depends on the abdominal muscles. Spinal cord injuries that occur at or above the level of C3 often result in apnea caused by loss of innervation of the diaphragm. In mid- and lower cervical injuries, diaphragm innervation is preserved but the innervation to the intercostal muscles is lost; acutely this results in flaccid paralysis of the intercostal muscles. In this situation, when the diaphragm contracts, the chest wall rather than expanding is drawn inward because of the flaccid tone of the intercostal muscles. Inspiration is substantially less efficient in this situation, and shallow breathing results. This can be demonstrated by measuring the negative inspiratory force and the forced vital capacity, which are typically reduced to approximately 25% of the predicted preinjury levels.[20] The shallow breathing and the decreased ability to cough result in progressive atelectasis and consequently a progressive decrease in the FRC. The result is a progressive worsening of compliance, which in turn increases the work of breathing and consequent fatigue. Therefore many patients with cervical injuries may not need immediate intubation, but develop increasing difficulty over the subsequent 24 to 48 hours.

The ability to wean patients with spinal cord injury from mechanical ventilatory support depends on the transition from flaccid to spastic tone in the intercostal muscles. Once this transition starts to occur, the chest wall no longer collapses with each inspiratory effort and thus there is a gradual improvement in the measured pulmonary mechanics. This improvement is mostly in inspiratory function as a result of the change in chest wall tone.[20] Forced expiration, because it depends on active contraction of the abdominal muscles, shows less improvement.[23] This improvement occurs over a variable period but the mean length of time of mechanical ventilation for patients with acute spinal cord injury is approximately 35 days.[17]

Weaning from Mechanical Ventilation

Before patients can be weaned from mechanical ventilatory support, there needs to be substantial resolution of the process that led to respiratory failure. There are no firm guidelines, but in general the inspired fraction of oxygen should be 50% or less and the PEEP should be 5 cm H_2O while maintaining hemoglobin saturation greater than 90%. The minute ventilation should be 10 L/min or less. Any ongoing pulmonary infection should be resolved, and total secretion production should not be excessive. The patient should be awake enough to protect the airway. The appearance of the chest radiograph, however, often lags behind clinical improvement, and the presence of persistent infiltrates or pleural effusions are not necessarily impediments to proceeding with attempts at weaning.

Numerous indices have been proposed over the years to try to predict successful weaning from mechanical ventilation, but many of these have proven to be of limited predictive value. Recently, attention has been given to the rapid shallow breathing index (RSBI). This is determined by dividing the respiratory rate by the minute ventilation in liters. It appears that a value of less than 80 strongly predicts successful extubation and greater than 100 strongly predicts failure of extubation.[36]

In patients who appear to be ready for extubation but fail an extubation attempt, there are options for weaning them from ventilatory support. The most common modes used for weaning patients from mechanical ventilation are pressure support, IMV, and T-piece trials. The evidence for one method being superior to others is not conclusive.[8] If pressure support or IMV are used, the customary approach is to progressively decrease the level of support as long as the patient tolerates this in terms of respiratory rate, until the patient is breathing on minimal support. The T-piece method involves disconnecting the patient from the ventilator, allowing spontaneous breathing through a T-piece for a set period, and then returning the patient to full ventilatory support. The length of these trials is progressively increased until the patient is able to tolerate several hours of spontaneous breathing.

Tracheostomy is a component of the weaning process in many ventilated patients. This procedure is increasingly performed in the intensive care unit using percutaneous techniques. Tracheostomy has many advantages as part of the weaning process, including greater patient comfort and a reduction in the dead space. The ideal length of time of ventilator dependence before performing a tracheostomy is uncertain, but most clinicians prefer to move toward tracheostomy if more than 2 weeks of intubation is anticipated.

REFERENCES

1. Acute Respiratory Distress Syndrome Network: Ventilation with lower tidal volumes as compared with traditional tidal volumes for acute lung injury and the acute respiratory distress syndrome, **N Engl J Med (342)18:**1301-1308, 2000.
2. Albert RK: Least PEEP: Primum non nocere, **Chest (87)1:**2-4, 1985.

3. Bernard GR, Artigas A, Brigham KL, et al: The American-European consensus conference on ARDS: Definitions, mechanism, relevant outcomes and clinical trial coordination, **Am J Respir Crit Care Med 149(3 Pt 1):**818-824, 1994.
4. Bernard GR, Luce JM, Sprung CL: High-dose corticosteroids in patients with the adult respiratory distress syndrome, **N Engl J Med 317(25):**1565-1570, 1987.
5. Bratton SL, Davis RL: Acute lung injury in isolated traumatic brain injury, **Neurosurgery 40(4):**707-712, 1997.
6. Bryan CL, Jenkinson SG: Oxygen toxicity, **Clin Chest Med 9(1):**141-152, 1988.
7. Carmichael LC, Dorinsky PM, Higgins SB: Diagnosis and therapy of acute respiratory distress syndrome in adults: An international survey, **J Crit Care 11(1):** 9-18, 1996.
8. Chao DC, Scheinhorn DJ: Weaning from mechanical ventilation, **Crit Care Clin 14(4):**799-817, 1998.
9. DeVivo MJ, Rutt RD, Black KJ, et al: Trends in spinal cord injury demographics and treatment outcomes between 1973 and 1986, **Arch Phys Med Rehabil 73(5):**424-430, 1992.
10. Dreyfuss D, Saumon G: Barotrauma is volutrauma, but which volume is the one responsible? **Intensive Care Med 18(3):**139-141, 1992.
11. Fagon JY, Chastre J, Hance AJ, et al: Evaluation of clinical judgment in the identification and treatment of nosocomial pneumonia in ventilated patients, **Chest 103(2):**547-553, 1993.
12. Gattinoni L, Pelosi P. Suter PM, et al: Acute respiratory distress syndrome caused by pulmonary and extrapulmonary disease: Different syndromes? **Am J Respir Crit Care Med 158(1):**3-11, 1998.
13. Gattinoni L, Tognoni G, Pesenti, et al: Effect of prone positioning on the survival of patients with acute respiratory failure, **N Engl J Med 345(8):**568-573, 2001.
14. Goodman PC: Radiographic findings in patients with acute respiratory distress syndrome, **Clin Chest Med 21(3):**419-433, 2000.
15. Grossman RF, Fein A: Evidence-based assessment of diagnostic tests for ventilator-associated pneumonia, **Chest 117(4 Suppl 2):**177S-181S, 2000.
16. Hudson LD, Milbert JA, Anardi D, et al: Clinical risks for development of the acute respiratory distress syndrome, **Am J Respir Crit Care Med 151(2 Pt 1):**293-301, 1995.
17. Jackson AB, Groomes TE: Incidence of respiratory complications following spinal cord injury, **Arch Phys Med Rehabil 75(3):**270-275, 1994.
18. Kanarek DJ, Shannon DC: Adverse effect of positive end-expiratory pressure on pulmonary perfusion and arterial oxygenation, **Am Rev Respir Dis 112(3):** 457-459, 1975.
19. Kollef MH, Schuster DP: The acute respiratory distress syndrome, **N Engl J Med 332(1):**27-37, 1995.
20. Ledsome JR, Sharp JM: Pulmonary function in acute cervical cord injury, **Am Rev Respir Dis 124(1):**41-44, 1981.
21. Luce JM, Montgomery AB, Marks JD, et al: Ineffectiveness of high-dose methylprednisolone in preventing parenchymal lung injury and improving mortality in patients with septic shock, **Am Rev Respir Dis 138(1):**62-68, 1988.
22. McHugh LG, Milberg JA, Whitcomb ME, et al: Recovery of lung function in survivors of acute respiratory distress syndrome, **Am J Respir Crit Care Med 150(1):**90-94, 1994.
23. McMichan JC, Michel L, Westbrook PR: Pulmonary dysfunction following traumatic quadriplegia: Recognition, prevention, and treatment, **JAMA 243(6):**528-531, 1980.
24. Meduri GU, Belenchia JM, Estes RJ, et al: Fibroproliferative phase of ARDS: Clinical findings and effects of corticosteroids, **Chest 100(4):**943-952, 1991.
25. Milberg JA, Davis DR, Steinberg KP, et al: Improved survival of patients with acute respiratory distress syndrome (ARDS): 1983-1993, **JAMA 273(4):**306-309, 1995.
26. Montgomery AB, Stager MA, Carrico CJ, et al: Causes of mortality in patients with adult respiratory distress syndrome, **Am Rev Respir Dis 132(3):**485-489, 1985.
27. Nelson LD: High-inflation pressure and positive end-expiratory pressure on pulmonary perfusion and arterial oxygenation: Injurious to the lungs? No, **Am Rev Respir Dis 12(3):** 603-625, 1996.
28. Niederman MS, Torres A, Summer W: Invasive diagnostic testing is not needed routinely to manage suspected ventilator-associated pneumonia, **Am J Respir Crit Care Med 150(2):**565-569, 1994.
29. Pappert D, Rossaint R, Slama K: Influence of positioning on ventilation-perfusion relationships in severe adult respiratory distress syndrome, **Chest 106(5):**1511-1516, 1994.
30. Parker JC, Hernandez LA, Peevy KJ: Mechanisms of ventilator induced lung injury, **Crit Care Med 21(1):**131-143, 1993.
31. Register SD, Downs JB, Stock MC, et al: Is 50% oxygen harmful? **Crit Care Med 15(6):**598-601, 1987.
32. Schnapp LM, Chin DP, Szarflarski N, et al: Frequency and importance of barotrauma in 100 patients with acute lung injury, **Crit Care Med 23(2):**272-278, 1995.
33. Slutsky AS: Mechanical ventilation, **Chest 104:**1833-1859, 1993.
34. Tobin MJ: Mechanical ventilation, **N Engl J Med 330(15):**1056-1061, 1994.
35. Valta P, Uusaro A, Nunes S: Acute respiratory distress syndrome: Frequency, clinical course, and costs of care, **Crit Care Med 27(11):**2367-2374, 1999.
36. Yang KL, Tobin MJ: A prospective study of indexes predicting the outcome of trials of weaning from mechanical ventilation, **N Engl J Med 324(21):**1445-1450, 1991

CHAPTER 2

Cardiovascular Physiology, Monitoring, and Management in the Neurosurgical Intensive Care Unit

MARTIN C. HOLLAND
DAVID C. BONOVICH
WAYNE SCHMEDEL

Hemodynamic instability in neurosurgical patients may arise from a variety of causes, including ischemic heart disease, sepsis, and hypovolemia. In addition, it may be associated with neurological conditions such as brain and spinal cord injury, subarachnoid hemorrhage, or increased intracranial pressure. Some neurosurgical patients, although hemodynamically stable, may require sustained elevated cardiac output and hypertension to maintain adequate cerebral perfusion, as is needed for the treatment of subarachnoid hemorrhage–associated vasospasm or intracranial hypertension. Because of these issues, an understanding of hemodynamic principles, monitoring, and treatment options is essential to the care and treatment of patients in a neurosurgical intensive care unit (ICU).

The most important concern in neurosurgical patients is maintenance of adequate cerebral blood flow, mainly to prevent secondary injury from ischemia. Because many of these patients also have intracranial pressure monitors, the neurosurgeon is able to institute hemodynamic support tailored to meet the patients' cerebral perfusion requirements.

This chapter addresses the general organization of the cardiovascular system, hemodynamic monitoring options, the rationale for monitoring, and medical management of cardiovascular instability.

ORGANIZATION OF THE CARDIOVASCULAR SYSTEM

Conceptually the cardiovascular system may be looked on as two fluid circuits in series—the pulmonary circulation and the systemic circulation (Figure 2-1). The pulmonary circuit pumps unoxygenated blood from the right side of the heart through the pulmonary vascular beds and returns it, oxygenated, to the left side of the heart. The systemic circuit then pumps oxygenated blood from the left ventricle to the rest of the body, and returns it, unoxygenated, to the right side of the heart, where the cycle repeats. The movement of blood through these pathways is primarily a result of the muscular contractions of the heart.

The dynamics of blood flow closely parallel an electrical circuit within the heart, which functions as a battery (Figure 2-2). As such it can be described with the equation $V = I \times R$, in which voltage *(V)* represents blood pressure (actually, difference between arterial and venous pressure across a vascular bed); current *(I)*, cardiac output (or cardiac index); and resistance *(R)*, vascular resistance. Thus for any given cardiac output, blood pressure increases with increasing vascular resistance. Similarly, given a fixed vascular resistance, blood pressure increases in parallel with cardiac output.

Cardiac output (CO) is the product of two other variables—heart rate (P = pulse) and stroke volume (SV)—and is defined by the equation $CO = P \times SV$. Thus as either pulse or stroke volume increases, so does cardiac output. SV itself depends on three parameters: preload, afterload, and cardiac contractility.

Preload is defined as the "load" or tension placed on a muscle before contraction. In the heart it is equivalent to ventricular end diastolic volume (VEDV). Because VEDV is difficult to measure clinically, end diastolic filling pressure (EDFP) is usually used as a measure of cardiac preload.[6] EDFP, however, is only a relative indicator of the VEDV and only accurately reflects VEDV in normally compliant ventricles. In cases in which the ventricle is less compliant, EDFP may overestimate VEDV. On the right side of the heart, ven-

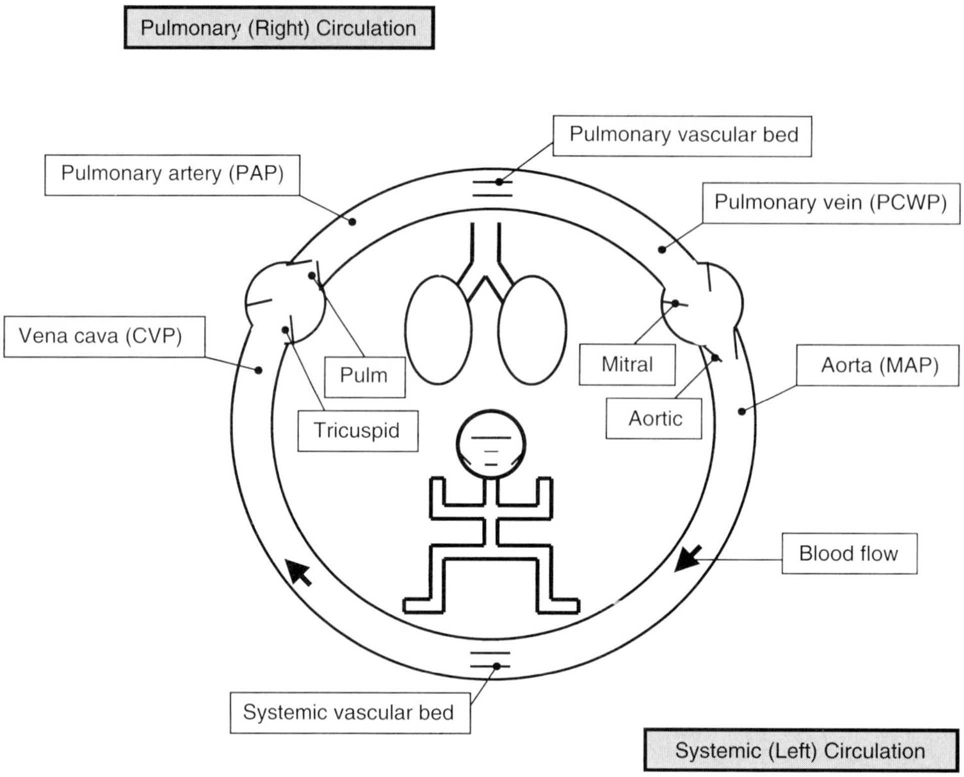

MAP, Mean arterial pressure (systemic);
PAP, pulmonary artery pressure;
CVP, central venous pressure;
PCWP, pulmonary capillary wedge pressure.

FIGURE 2-1 ■ **Cardiac circuit.**

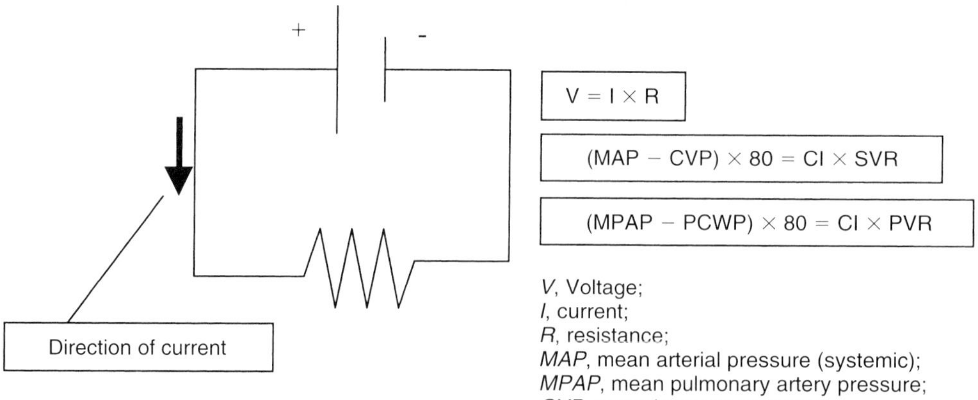

V, Voltage;
I, current;
R, resistance;
MAP, mean arterial pressure (systemic);
MPAP, mean pulmonary artery pressure;
CVP, central venous pressure;
PCWP, pulmonary capillary wedge pressure;
CI, cardiac index;
SVR, systemic vascular resistance;
PVR, pulmonary vascular resistance.

FIGURE 2-2 ■ **Electrical circuit/cardiac circuit parallels.**

tricular filling pressure is essentially equivalent to central venous pressure (CVP), and on the left, to pulmonary capillary wedge pressure (PCWP), assuming the absence of significant mitral or tricuspid stenosis or significant pulmonary vascular resistance.[2,7]

Afterload is the "load" or stress imposed on a muscle during contraction. In the heart it is the tension that develops across the wall of the heart during contraction. This tension is due mainly to the resistance to ventricular outflow in the aorta and the major proximal arteries. In the setting of mitral or tricuspid valvular disease, there may also be a valvular component to afterload. Systolic blood pressure indirectly reflects afterload, although it also varies with cardiac contractility.

Contractility is essentially the force with which a muscle squeezes, or contracts, and is best understood within the context of myocardial cellular structure. Myocardium is composed of striated muscle fibers arranged in bundles, with each fiber consisting of functional units, called sarcomeres, joined end to end to form the fiber itself (Figure 2-3). Each sarcomere contains actin and myosin strands held in a highly organized fashion. Bounding the sarcomere are the Z-lines, which define the anchor point of individual actin filaments.[4]

Midway between the Z-lines is the M-line, which defines the anchor point for myosin. Actin filaments run parallel to one another from either Z-line toward the center of the sarcomere, whereas myosin strands extend laterally and parallel to one another from the M-line toward the Z-line. This arrangement places the free ends of both actin and myosin filaments parallel to one another and overlapping to some degree. Muscle contraction results from interaction between myosin and actin filaments, which causes them to slide past one another, bringing adjacent Z-lines closer to one another and shortening the muscle fiber (see Figure 2-3).

The force of contraction depends on a number of factors, including myocardial fiber length and cardiac inotropic tone.[5] As fiber length increases, so does contractility.[1] Thus increasing preload not only affects CO by increasing end diastolic ventricular volume, it also increases contractility by increasing myocardial fiber length. The presence of factors such as increased sympathetic tone or of inotropic drugs such as epinephrine also increases force of contraction. Thus CO depends on stroke volume and heart rate, whereas stroke volume depends on preload, afterload, and contractility.

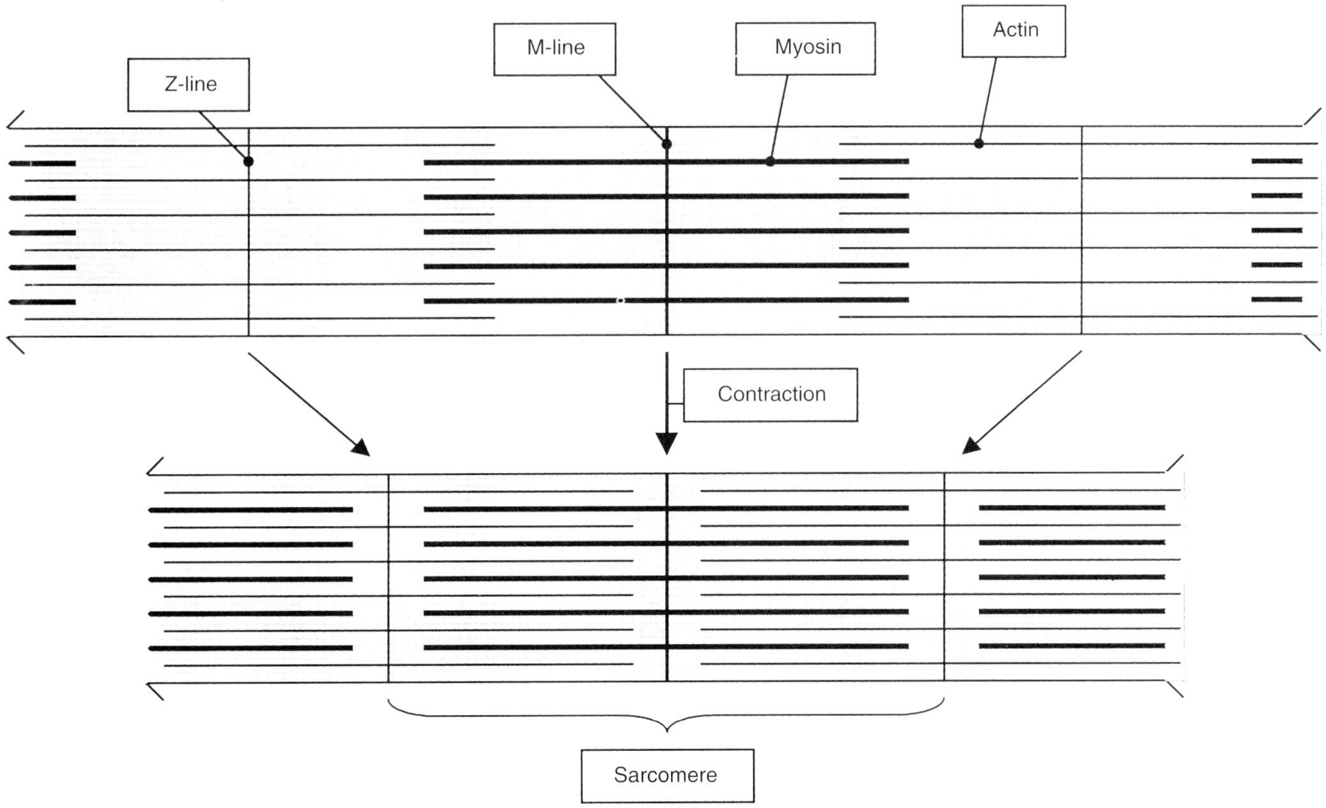

FIGURE 2-3 ■ **Sarcomere contraction.**

HEMODYNAMIC MONITORING

The purpose of hemodynamic monitoring is to establish and maintain optimal tissue perfusion. As such, the most important parameters influencing this goal are intravascular volume status, blood pressure, and cardiac output.

Because CO depends on pulse and stroke volume ($CO = P \times SV$) and SV on preload (ventricular filling pressure), afterload (vascular resistance), and contractility, the ability to optimize CO depends on the ability to measure and manipulate these factors. In the ICU setting, the range of available invasive and noninvasive monitoring techniques is somewhat limited. Noninvasive techniques include cuff sphygmomanometry and transthoracic and transesophageal echocardiography (TTE and TEE, respectively), and invasive techniques are limited to monitoring through intravascular catheters.

Preload

Right ventricular preload can be assessed from right ventricular filling pressure or right ventricular end diastolic volume. In the absence of significant tricuspid valve stenosis, right ventricular EDFP is equal to right atrial pressure, which is equal to CVP. This is usually measured via a central venous catheter introduced through an external jugular (EJ) or subclavian approach. CVP measurement is most accurate when the tip of the central line is adjacent to the right atrium. Subclavian lines are preferable to EJ lines because they are significantly easier to maintain and can be placed easily in patients with cervical collars, such as trauma patients with suspected or confirmed cervical spine injuries.

Left ventricular preload is usually measured via pulmonary artery (PA) catheter and is reflected in PCWP. The PA catheter is long (100 cm or more) with two access ports. One of the ports is located at the very end of the catheter; the other is approximately 30 cm from the tip. In addition, there is a small inflatable balloon just proximal to the tip and a thermistor located near the end of the catheter.

This catheter is usually placed through a large central venous access line or introducer and directed across the right atrium and ventricle and into the pulmonary artery. The tip thus rests in a medium-sized pulmonary artery such that inflation of the balloon can temporarily occlude this artery.

During balloon occlusion, pressure equilibrates across the pulmonary vascular bed and the left atrium. Thus the pressure noted during balloon occlusion is reflective of the left atrial pressure (Figure 2-4). This is the PCWP. Just as CVP reflects the right ventricular filling pressure, so too PCWP reflects the left ventricular filling pressure; in the absence of significant mitral or tricuspid valvular stenosis, both are measures of preload.

Both right and left VEDV can be estimated using TTE or TEE,[9] but because of the heart's geometry, left VEDV is more accurate.

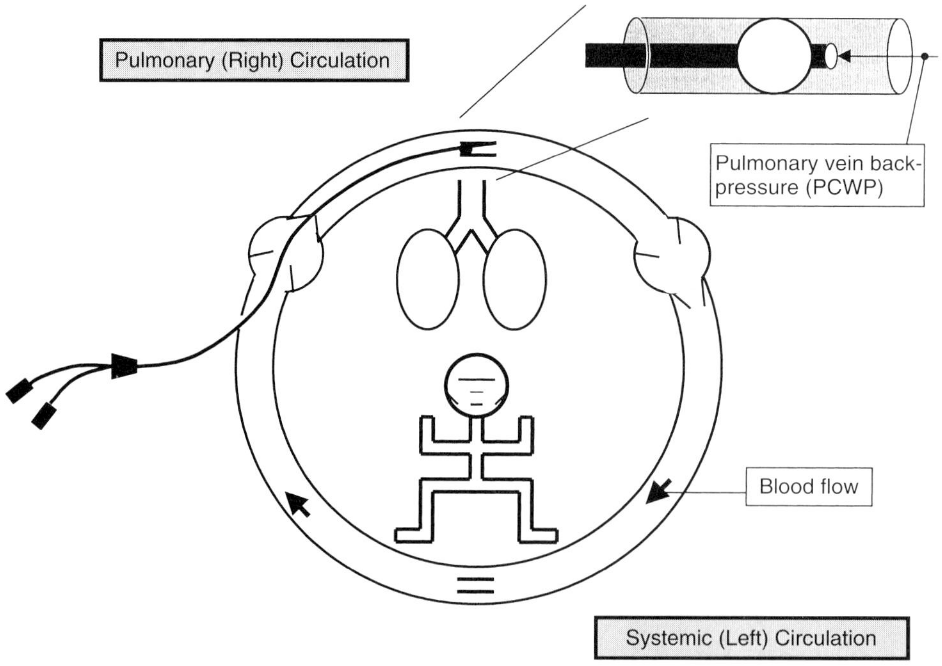

FIGURE 2-4 ■ **Pulmonary artery catheter.**

Afterload

Afterload itself cannot be measured directly. It must be calculated using the formula SVR = 80 (MAP − CVP)/CI or PVR = 80 (MAP − PCWP)/CI, in which *MAP* is mean arterial pressure, *SVR* is systemic vascular resistance, and *PVR* is pulmonary vascular resistance. In the absence of a PA catheter, both blood pressure (systemic or pulmonary) and pulse pressure (the difference between systolic and diastolic pressures) may be used as indirect measures of vascular resistance and thus of afterload.

Systemic blood pressure can be measured either with cuff (usually brachial) sphygmomanometry or invasive arterial (usually radial) catheters. Although cuff sphygmomanometry readings are thought to be interchangeable with arterial catheter (A-line) readings, they do not always coincide. In as-yet-unpublished data, the authors have found a predictable relationship between arterial and cuff MAP (Figure 2-5). Whereas an A-line MAP of 70 mm Hg corresponds roughly to a cuff reading of 70 mm Hg, an A-line MAP of 100 corresponds to a cuff reading of roughly 90 mm Hg. This relationship is linear throughout a wide range of pressures, and a similar relationship also holds for both systolic and diastolic blood pressures.

In contrast to the left side of the heart, right ventricular afterload (as reflected in PA pressures) can only be measured invasively using a PA catheter.

Cardiac Output

CO can be measured directly with the aid of a PA catheter. The most common method of measuring CO is via the thermodilution method whereby approximately 10 ml of ice-cold saline are infused as a bolus through the proximal port of the PA line. The thermistor distal to the injection port registers the transient change in temperature. CO can then be calculated based on temperature change over time. Some catheters have the ability to calculate CO based on venous oxygen saturation. Regardless of how CO is measured, it is usually "normalized" by dividing CO by body surface area (in m^2) to obtain the patient's cardiac index (CI). Normal CI is between 2.8 and 3.6 L/min (m^2) (Table 2-1).

Contractility

This parameter cannot be measured directly. Instead, blood pressure, pulse pressure, and TEE/TTE-derived qualitative and calculated parameters must be used as indirect measures of contractility. Generally, normal or high blood and pulse pressures indicate good cardiac contractility. Low pressures, on the other hand, can indicate either poor contractility or low intravascular volume.

MANAGEMENT

Hemodynamic management of the neurosurgical patient aims at maintaining adequate cerebral perfusion. In some instances this involves preventing or reversing cardiovascular instability; in other instances it involves increasing CO, blood pressure, or both above normal values. In either case it is important to understand how to manipulate CO and cardiac contractility through the manipulation of preload and afterload or through the use of inotropic or chronotropic agents.

Although the right and left sides of the heart support different pressures (the right is a low pressure system, whereas the left is a high pressure system), op-

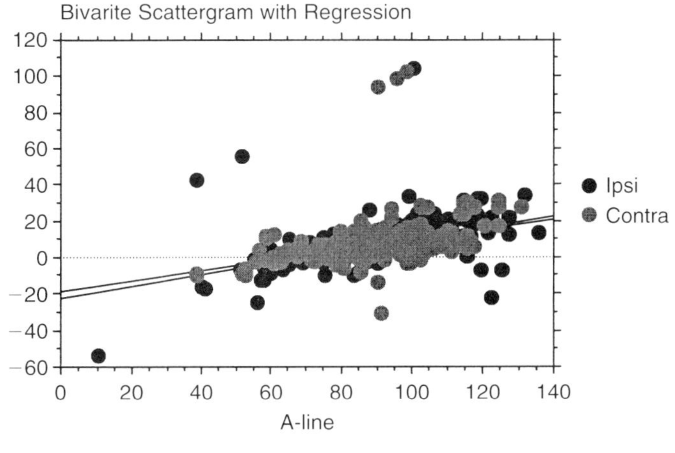

A-line, MAP of A-line (in mm Hg);
Delta MAP, difference between A-line and cuff MAP (in mm Hg);
Ipsi, cuff ipsilateral to A-line;
Contra, cuff contralateral to A-line.

FIGURE 2-5 ■ **Comparison between sphygmomanometer and A-line MAP.**

TABLE 2-1 ■ **Cardiorespiratory Variables**

Variable	Abbreviation	Unit	Calculation	Normal Value
Right & Left Pressures				
Mean arterial pressure	MAP	mm Hg	Direct measurement	70-105
Mean pulmonary artery pressure	MPAP	mm Hg	Direct measurement	10-15
Central venous pressure	CVP	cm H_2O	Direct measurement	1-9
Pulmonary capillary wedge pressure	PCWP	mm Hg	Direct measurement	5-15
Cardiac Outflow				
Cardiac output	CO	L/min	Direct measurement	4.0-8.0
Cardiac index	CI	L/min(m^2)	CO/BSA*	2.8-3.6
Stroke volume	SV	ml	CO/P	60-100
Stroke index	SI	ml/m^2	SV/BSA	40-50
Afterload				
Systemic vascular resistance	SVR	Dyne(s)/cm^5(m^2)	SVR = 79.92(MAP − CVP)/CI	1760-2600
Pulmonary vascular resistance	PVR	Dyne(s)/cm^5(m^2)	PVR = 79.92(MAP − WP)/CI	45-225

*BSA, Body surface area.

timal cardiac function requires that $CO_{right} = CO_{left}$. The heart's own self-regulatory mechanisms take care of much of that. For example, if right-sided filling pressures suddenly increase, the increase in right VEDV results in increased right-sided contractility and thus right-sided stroke volume and CO_{right}. This increase in right-sided output results in increased left-sided ventricular filling pressures and left VEDV, with a subsequent increase in left-sided contractility, stroke volume, and CO_{left}. This autoregulatory system can be taken advantage of to optimize cardiac output by manipulating preload, afterload, and contractility. Table 2-1 indicates the normal range of right- and left-sided cardiac preload and afterload values.

Preload

Management of preload essentially involves manipulating CVP and PCWP. This is most easily accomplished by manipulating central venous and pulmonary venous volumes. Because we can gain direct access to the central venous circulation, right-sided volumes are the easiest to both monitor and manipulate. Normal CVP is approximately 5 mm Hg, with a range of 1 to 9 mm Hg (see Table 2-1).

Increasing CVP simply requires intravenous infusion of either crystalloid or colloid solutions, although evidence suggests that crystalloid infusions are preferable to colloid in most circumstances.[8,10] The two most common crystalloid solutions are 0.9% sodium chloride (NaCl) and lactated Ringer's solution (LR). Occasionally, NaCl solutions with 5% dextrose (e.g., D_5 0.9% NaCl) are used, but rarely in the acute post-injury period, because this may result in hyperglycemia. The advantage of 0.9% NaCl is its ability to raise serum sodium concentrations and thus help manage intracranial hypertension. Serum sodium greater than 145 mmol/L has been found to be ideal for accomplishing this goal. However, chronic infusion of 0.9% NaCl can induce a severe hyperchloremia, which may result in a metabolic acidosis. LR infusion is useful for treating hyperchloremic metabolic acidosis, although it may also result in lower serum sodium concentrations.

Decreasing CVP usually involves the administration of a diuretic. Furosemide (Lasix) is often used for this purpose because it is quick acting, reliable, and fairly predictable. Its main disadvantage is its tendency to excrete K^+ through the kidneys, resulting in hypokalemia. Table 2-2 lists various diuretic agents that can be used to decrease central venous volume. Optimal CVP in the neurosurgical patient is 5 to 10 mm Hg. Such pressure maximizes right VEDV without overloading the heart with fluid. In any case, there is little evidence to suggest that increasing CVP beyond these levels improves cerebral perfusion. The presence of significant tricuspid stenosis, however, may require a slightly higher CVP to overcome valvular resistance and optimize right VEDV.

Left ventricular preload (PCWP) responds to volume resuscitation in much the same way as CVP. The main difference is that fluid cannot be infused directly into the pulmonary vein. Normal PCWP is approximately 10 mm Hg with a range of 5 to 15 mm Hg (see Table 2-1). When pulmonary vascular resistance is nor-

TABLE 2-2 ■ Intravenous Diuretic Agents

Medication	Onset	Peak	Duration	Adverse Effects	Relative Contraindications
Furosemide	5 min	30 min	2 hr	Hypokalemia, hyponatremia, hyperglycemia, hypovolemia, ototoxicity	Anuria, metabolic alkalosis, sulfonamide sensitivity
Ethacrynic acid	15 min	25 min	3 hr	Same as above (ototoxicity more significant)	Anuria, metabolic alkalosis

mal, PCWP can be manipulated simply by increasing CO_{right}. However, when pulmonary vascular resistance is elevated (e.g., from pneumonia, acute respiratory distress syndrome, acute lung injury), left ventricular preload may drop because of decreased blood flow through the pulmonary vascular bed. This situation requires treatment of underlying lung conditions or the use of pulmonary afterload–reducing agents. Doing so allows blood to flow more freely across the pulmonary vasculature, improving both left-sided heart filling pressure and CO_{left}. The presence of significant mitral stenosis may require increasing left ventricular filling pressure to optimize left VEDV. Alternatively, decreasing the pulse may help by allowing the ventricle more time to fill, thus increasing left VEDV before systole.

Afterload

Afterload management is considerably trickier than preload management. On the one hand, there is the need to decrease afterload (vascular resistance) to maximize CO. On the other hand, blood pressure (a measure of vascular resistance) must be maintained high enough to overcome tissue vascular resistance and allow tissue perfusion.

Left ventricular afterload is the main focus of treatment because it is the left side of the heart that determines cerebral perfusion. The goal is to maintain an adequate perfusion pressure without compromising CO. To that aim, cerebral perfusion pressure (CPP) should be kept above 70 mm Hg, with CPP defined as MAP minus intracranial pressure (ICP; CPP = MAP − ICP).

In the absence of significant aortic valve stenosis, left-sided cardiac afterload management essentially involves the infusion of either pressor or hypotensive medications (Tables 2-3 and 2-4). Pressors with primarily α_1 receptor selectivity (e.g., phenylephrine) are preferred because cerebral vasculature is thought to lack significant α_1 receptors.[3] As such, blood pressure can be increased without inducing significant cerebral vasoconstriction. Medications such as dopamine, dobutamine, and epinephrine are also useful pressors, especially in patients with poor response to phenylephrine or in patients who develop severe bradycardia in response to it. Intravenous afterload–reducing agents such as sodium nitroprusside, nitroglycerine, and labetalol are used to decrease peripheral vascular resistance. Sodium nitroprusside, although an effective afterload reducing agent, should be used with some caution because it may result in cerebral venous hypertension and may interfere with cerebral autoregulation. Other medications, such as sublingual nifedipine, topical clonidine, and captopril, may also be used to decrease afterload.

Afterload reduction is necessary only when either CO or tissue perfusion is compromised as a result of severe vasoconstriction. When PVR becomes elevated and right-sided heart failure develops, treating the underlying pulmonary process is usually sufficient.

TABLE 2-3 ■ Pressor Agents

	Receptor Affinity				
Medication	α_1	α_2	β_1	β_2	Dopamine
Phenylephrine	High	x	x	x	x
Dopamine					
Low dose		x		x	High
Moderate dose		x	High	x	
High dose	High	x		x	
Dobutamine	Low	x	High	Low	x
Epinephrine					
Low dose			Moderate	High	x
Moderate dose	Low		High	High	x
High dose	High	High	High	High	x
Norepinephrine	High	High	Moderate	x	x

TABLE 2-4 ■ Hypotensive Agents

Medication	Action	Onset	Peak	Duration	Side Effects
Intravenous					
Sodium nitroprusside	Arteriolar and venous vasodilator	Seconds	1 min	1-3 min	Cerebral hypertension and cerebral dysautoregulation
Labetalol	α-adrenergic and β-adrenergic blocker	5 min	10 min	3-6 hr	
Nitroglycerin	Venous >> arteriolar vasodilator	1 min	1 min	1-3 min	
Hydralazine	Arteriolar vasodilator	10 min	30 min	3-6 hr	Cerebral dysautoregulation
Oral					
Nifedipine	Calcium channel blocker	5 min	15 min	3-5 hr	
Clonidine	Central α-adrenergic agonist	30 min	2 hr	3-8 hr	
Captopril	Angiotensin-converting enzyme (ACE) inhibitor	15 min	60 min	4-6 hr	

Occasionally, direct measures against pulmonary hypertension—such as infusion of prostaglandins or low-dose dopamine—can also be instituted. Left-sided heart failure—which may lead to elevated PCWP, pulmonary edema, oxygen desaturation, or a low CO_{left}—can result from myocardial ischemia, severe valvular disease, or volume overload. These must be distinguished from pump failure caused by high afterload and treated appropriately.

Contractility

Cardiac contractility can be manipulated in one of two ways: by adjusting preload or by infusing inotropic medications. The first is discussed earlier in this chapter; the second involves infusing medications such as epinephrine, dopamine, or dobutamine (see Table 2-4). Although these medications increase cardiac contractility, they also increase heart rate and cardiac metabolic rate. Therefore they can precipitate myocardial ischemia and must be used with caution in the elderly and in patients with a history of hypertension, smoking, diabetes, or atherosclerotic vascular disease.

SUMMARY

Cardiovascular support is extremely important for the optimal treatment of critically ill neurosurgical patients.

The need to induce and maintain high CO and elevated blood pressure to optimize cerebral perfusion makes thorough understanding of the cardiovascular system imperative. That CO is a function of pulse, preload, afterload, and cardiac contractility allows for many avenues of treatment. Preload is essentially a function of the patient's volume status and may be manipulated by infusion of crystalloid or colloid solutions or infusion of diuretic medications. Afterload is predominately a function of vascular resistance. As such it represents not only the force against which the heart must pump but also the blood pressure with which to perfuse tissue. Afterload management essentially involves infusion of pressor or hypotensive medications. Contractility is a function of both extrinsic factors, such as preload, and intrinsic factors, such as inotropic tone. Manipulation of contractility therefore relies on our ability to optimize preload and maximize cardiac inotropic tone.

To take advantage of our ability to manipulate these cardiovascular parameters, hemodynamic monitoring techniques must allow us to accurately measure right and left circulatory pressures and CO and to calculate SVR and PVR. A full understanding of the indications and appropriate use of both noninvasive and invasive hemodynamic monitoring are essential for taking care of critically ill neurosurgical patients. In addition, a thorough understanding of the mechanism of action and the benefits and risks of hemodynamically active medications is required for optimal care in the neurosurgical ICU.

REFERENCES

1. De Tombe PP, Little WC: Inotropic effects of ejection are myocardial properties, **Am J Physiol 266(3 Pt 2):**H1202-1213, 1994.
2. Downes TR, Hackshaw BT, Kahl FR, et al: Frequency of large V waves in the pulmonary artery wedge pressure in ventricular septal defect of acquired (during acute myocardial infarction) or congenital origin, **Am J Cardiol 60(4):**415-417, 1987.
3. Harik SI, Sharma VK, Wetherbee JR, et al: Adrenergic and cholinergic receptors of cerebral microvessels, **J Cereb Blood Flow Metab 1(3):**329-338, 1981.

4. Huxley HE: The structural basis of muscular contraction, **Proc R Soc Lond B Biol Sci 178(51):**131-149, 1971.
5. Kass DA, Yamazaki T, Burkhoff D, et al: Determination of left ventricular end-systolic pressure-volume relationships by the conductance (volume) catheter technique, **Circulation 73(3):**586-595, 1986.
6. Little WC, Downes TR: Clinical evaluation of left ventricular diastolic performance, **Prog Cardiovasc Dis 32(4):**273-290, 1990.
7. Snyder RW II, Glamann DB, Lange RA, et al: Predictive value of prominent pulmonary arterial wedge V waves in assessing the presence and severity of mitral regurgitation, **Am J Cardiol 73(8):**568-570, 1994.
8. Tonnesen AS: Hemodynamic management of brain-injured patients, **New Horiz 3(3):**499-505, 1995.
9. Wynne J, Green LH, Mann T, et al: Estimation of left ventricular volumes in man from biplane cineangiograms filmed in oblique projections, **Am J Cardiol 41(4):**726-732, 1978.
10. Zornow MH, Prough DS: Fluid management in patients with traumatic brain injury, **New Horiz 3(3):**488-498, 1995.

CHAPTER 3

Neurological Monitoring

BRIAN T. ANDREWS

The neurological examination is the most important method of assisting patients in the neurosurgical intensive care unit (NICU). The initial neurological examination should include a complete medical history, vital signs, a general physical evaluation, and a detailed neurological evaluation. Other useful data include any initial measurements of intracranial pressure (ICP) and the results of brain imaging studies if available. It is important to assess neurological function as soon after admission to the hospital as possible, and thereafter at regular intervals throughout the hospital course. Accurate documentation of findings are critical because it is the change in findings over time that allows early detection of neurological deterioration. Using a systematic approach to the examination and regular documentation help to avoid significant omissions.

HISTORY

Knowledge of the history of present illness, past medical history, and recent hospital or prehospital course of treatment are valuable for understanding the patient's current neurological status. A comprehensive medical history should be obtained, if not directly from the patient, then from the patient's family or from the family's primary medical care providers. In cases of traumatic head injury it is important to attempt to determine the circumstances surrounding the accident. For example, the sudden onset of a headache or chest pain before the accident may indicate that an underlying intracranial or cardiac insult was causal to the trauma. The mechanism of injury may alert the neurosurgeon to the possibilities of certain types of injuries; for example, a fall may place the patient at risk for a spinal cord injury, and major blunt trauma may lead to intrathoracic or abdominal injury. The documentation by paramedics of apnea or airway obstruction places the patient at risk for a secondary hypoxic insult, which is known to have a profound impact on prognosis.[19,20,22] The initial neurological status of the patient, as documented by the paramedics or other observers at the initial scene, is also important. Deteriorating neurological function usually means the presence of an ongoing insult, such as an expanding intracranial mass lesion, which may be amenable to treatment; a stable, severe dysfunction often portends a severe parenchymal injury to the brain, which is less directly treatable.

Knowledge of the mechanism of disease allows the neurosurgeon to focus on particular aspects of care. Patients with traumatic head injury should be monitored for cerebrospinal fluid leakage, signs of elevated ICP, diffuse brain edema, and the evolution of contusions into intracranial hematomas. Patients with aneurysmal subarachnoid hemorrhage should be observed for recurrent hemorrhage, hydrocephalus, and vasospasm. Patients with prior or recent surgery for brain tumors are at risk for seizures, cerebral edema, and postoperative hemorrhage in the tumor bed. Those who have had surgery in the region of the pituitary gland or hypothalamus are at risk for diabetes insipidus, hypernatremia, and hyponatremia.

The presence of prior medical problems or other acute insults may make the physical examination and neurological assessment more difficult. For example, prior orthopedic insults may limit the patient's ability to perform physical examination tasks; a spinal cord injury may make the assessment for chest or abdominal injury more difficult because response to pain may be masked.

VITAL SIGNS

Core body temperature, blood pressure, pulse, and respiratory rate and pattern are important aspects of the general neurological examination.

Core Body Temperature

Although currently in use at mild to moderate levels as a therapeutic measure for elevated ICP after head injury,[17,18] hypothermia, defined as a core body temperature below 32° C, can significantly alter the findings of a neurological examination.[26] The most common causes of spontaneous hypothermia are alcohol or drug intoxication in patients exposed to the cold and, less frequently, adrenal insufficiency, hypothalamic dysfunction, hypopituitarism, and hypoglycemia. Postoperative patients arriving in the NICU after prolonged general anesthesia are also often hypothermic.

Patients with a core body temperature over 32.2° C are usually conscious unless there is another reason for stupor or coma.[26] Those with a core temperature below this level may appear obtunded, comatose, or even brain dead.[26] In patients with an underlying brain lesion, the neurological examination may be more profoundly altered by hypothermia than those with normal brain function. For instance, a patient with severe head injury and induced hypothermia may have a more depressed examination than the same patient examined in a normothermic state. Dehydration, lactic acidosis, and cardiac arrhythmias are the primary systemic complications of profound hypothermia. In general, patients should be managed in a way that maintains body temperature at normal levels unless a specific attempt is being made to provide mild or moderate hypothermia for therapeutic purposes.[17,18]

A core body temperature greater than 42° C will also cause coma.[26] Lesser elevations in temperature may cause lethargy or delirium, particularly in patients with underlying brain dysfunction. In the NICU the most common causes of hyperthermia are infections and hypothalamic dysfunction. Hyperthermia without an infectious cause is common after a variety of brain insults and often is ascribed to "central fever." Unlike the variable temperature of a fever caused by sepsis, central fevers are often persistent for days and may approach 40° C. Fever increases cerebral blood flow, CO_2 production, Pa_{CO_2}, and cerebral metabolic rate of lactate and may elevate ICP. All efforts should be made to lower temperature to normal levels, including the use of cooling blankets and antipyretics as needed. When core temperature has been lowered to normal, neurological dysfunction should resolve, although if the temperature has climbed to more than 42° C, permanent sequelae may occur, such as encephalopathy, hemiparesis, and cerebellar ataxia.[26]

Blood Pressure

Blood pressure measurement can provide important information. Extreme variations can significantly reduce the reliability of the neurological examination. Continuous monitoring of blood pressure may provide an early indicator of ICP elevation or direct brainstem compression.

Hypertension and bradycardia in a neurosurgical patient with cerebral injury should alert the clinician to the likelihood of an expanding mass lesion and increased ICP. As ICP rises there is a compensatory vasomotor response manifested by an increase in mean arterial blood pressure and usually bradycardia. In 1902, Cushing reported that this response was graded and occurred when ICP exceeded systolic blood pressure (SBP); he postulated that it was stimulated by brainstem ischemia.[9] This vasomotor response became known as Cushing's reflex. In classic feline experimental studies aimed at localizing the receptive areas that mediate Cushing's reflex, Hoff and Reis[13] found that the pressor response was due to stimulation of pressure-sensitive regions in the dorsal brainstem extending paramedially along the floor of the fourth ventricle from the obex and rostrally to the level of the facial colliculus. Pressor responses were also elicited in the cervicothoracic spinal cord. Pressure on neural tissue appeared to be an adequate stimulus.

In the author's experience, ICU patients with progressive increases in ICP may have both hypertension and bradycardia, but often have only blood pressure elevation without a change in heart rate; a few patients have bradycardia without hypertension. In deeply comatose patients, these clinical signs often precede further neurological deterioration as a result of elevated ICP. The presence of hypertension or bradycardia should prompt a careful assessment of the patient and repeated computed tomography (CT) scanning or institution of ICP monitoring.

An SBP of less than 60 mm Hg or cardiac arrest of any duration has been shown to render inaccurate the neurological examination in severely head-injured patients.[3,4] In a series of 100 head-injured patients with brainstem dysfunction, Andrews and colleagues[5] reported that 38% of patients were in cardiac arrest or had systemic hypotension with SBP less than 90 mm Hg on admission. They subsequently reviewed 36 head-injured patients who presented with brainstem dysfunction and cardiac arrest, an SBP less than 60 mm Hg, or an SBP of 60 to 90 mm Hg. In patients with cardiac arrest or SBP less than 60 mm Hg, the neurological findings of brainstem dysfunction did not reliably indicate mechanical brainstem compression from a mass lesion but rather diffuse brain ischemia, whereas in those with an initial SBP greater than 60 mm Hg, such findings accurately reflected brainstem compression.[3]

If SBP remains above 60 mm Hg, cerebral autoregulation maintains adequate cerebral blood flow. Below this level, cerebral ischemia occurs as blood flow to the brain decreases linearly with decreasing blood pressure. Cerebral ischemia caused by compressive lesions or increased ICP is exacerbated by systemic hypotension, which decreases cerebral perfusion pressure. The result is worsening neurological function and increased morbidity and mortality. In patients with severe head injury, cerebral autoregulation may fail at less severe levels of hypotension. The most common cause of hypotension in head-injured patients is hemorrhagic shock soon after injury; hypotension may also occur as a result of dehydration from the use of mannitol or diuretics or from unrecognized diabetes insipidus. Systematic hypotension and high fevers may also occur in patients with sepsis; thus great care must be taken to avoid systemic hypotension in neurosurgical patients. In patients with SBP less than 60 mm Hg, the neurological examination may be both abnormal and misleading.[3]

Heart Rate

Heart rate monitoring, combined with other cardiopulmonary findings, provides useful information about central nervous system (CNS) status. Sinus tachycardia may indicate sympathetic stimulation, such as pain, fever, or early hemorrhage shock, even if hypotension is not yet present. Bradycardia, when associated with increased SBP and decreased mental status, suggests severely increased ICP (Cushing's reflex). In contrast, the presence of bradycardia and hypotension in a trauma patient should quickly alert the clinician to the possibility of a cervical or upper thoracic spinal cord injury. It is important to realize that this cardiovascular compromise is due to decreased sympathetic tone and should be treated with atropine and/or a-adrenergic agonists rather than with large amounts of intravascular volume expanders unless there has also been significant blood loss. In patients with spinal cord injuries, close monitoring of heart rate and blood pressure is critical.

Respirations

The rate and pattern of respirations can be important indicators of underlying neurological dysfunction. Patients in stupor or coma and those with upper cervical cord injuries or airway compromise commonly require ventilatory support, but most patients in a NICU are not intubated. Therefore it is important to understand the implication of, and promptly identify, abnormal breathing patterns such as posthyperventilation apnea, Cheyne-Stokes apneustic breathing, and ataxic breathing.

Posthyperventilation apnea is defined as respirations that stop when deep breathing has lowered Pa_{CO_2} below its usual resting level. This is seen in patients with bihemispheric lesions.[26] Rhythmic breathing resumes when endogenous CO_2 production raises Pa_{CO_2} to normal. Normal persons whose Pa_{CO_2} is lowered by hyperventilation generally continue to breath regularly with reduced tidal volume until the Pa_{CO_2} returns to normal range.

Cheyne-Stokes respirations are characterized by escalating hyperventilation followed by decremental hypoventilation and finally apnea. Hyperpnea alternates smoothly and regularly with apnea. Arterial blood gases show a rise in pH and a falling Pa_{CO_2}, which becomes maximal when breathing ceases and never returns to normal.[30] Patients with Cheyne-Stokes ventilations have an abnormally increased ventilatory response to rising Pa_{CO_2}, which caused hyperpnea, and an abnormally decreased forebrain ventilatory stimulus, which allows apnea to occur.[6,23,26] This breathing pattern is usually caused by bilateral cerebral or diencephalic dysfunction resulting from structural lesions such as severe head trauma[6,23] and has been described in patients with incipient transtentorial herniation.[26] It is also seen in patients with metabolic disorders and hypertensive encephalopathy.[26,30] Care must be taken to monitor patients with Cheyne-Stokes respiration for prolonged apnea, as occurs with posthyperventilation apnea. In addition, level of consciousness, pupillary size and responsiveness, muscular tone, and cardiac rhythms may change cyclically in patients with Cheyne-Stokes respirations.[10]

Apneustic respirations are characterized by prolonged end-inspiratory pauses,[26,30] reflecting a failure of normal respiratory off-switching. The breathing pattern reflects dysfunction of the pneumotaxic centers, which are located in the middle or lower pons, or at the level of the nucleus parabrachialis.[26,29] Apneustic respirations are common in patients with pontine infarctions caused by basilar artery occlusion[25] and occasionally occur in patients with transtentorial herniation.

Ataxic breathing is completely irregular, characterized by deep alternating with shallow breaths, random pauses, and apnea.[26] This pattern reflects dysfunction in the region of the reticular formation, located in the dorsolateral medulla and extending down to the obex; these areas are responsible for respiratory rhythm.[26] In patients with ataxic breathing, the respiratory center is hypersensitive to depressant drugs, and even mild sedations can cause apnea to occur. Importantly, ataxic breathing may indicate an expanding mass in the posterior fossa, which can rapidly lead to complete respiratory arrest.

PHYSICAL EXAMINATION

A general physical examination should be performed on admission and, based on clinical changes, at intervals throughout the patient's hospital stay. Common medical illnesses that complicate the NICU course include pulmonary and genitourinary infections, sepsis, cardiopulmonary compromise, hematological abnormalities, gastrointestinal disorders, and renal dysfunction. The occurrence of such complications, particularly febrile disorders, can significantly alter the patient's neurological status.

NEUROLOGICAL EXAMINATION

To be useful in a critical care setting, the neurological examination must be performed frequently and without variation. In head-injured patients and those with other brain insults treated in the NICU, the Glasgow Coma Scale (GCS)[31] is most often used to assess hemispheric function on admission and repeatedly thereafter (Table 3-1). This scale has proven to be useful for guiding initial and subsequent patient evaluation[24] and management[2] and in predicting the prognosis for recovery after head injury.[7,14] Some controversy exists as to the timing of GCS measurement, in that earlier scoring (e.g., before cardiopulmonary resuscitation) can reduce the predictive value of the GCS. There are also distinct limitations to the application of the GCS, such as alterations in the score as a result of the presence of sedative-hypnotics such as alcohol; pharmacological sedation; or paralysis of the patient by hospital personnel for intubation (when best verbal performance cannot be assessed). In addition, orbital swelling can make assessment of eye opening difficult, and there are questions regarding the applicability of the GCS to the pediatric population.

In most NICUs a standardized form is completed for all head-injured patients at the time of admission; this form incorporates the GCS as well as other pertinent data such as vital signs and lateralizing neurological deficits. It facilitates rapid and complete neurological evaluation, documents the findings, and enables comparisons to be made with subsequent examinations.

TABLE 3-1 ■ Glasgow Coma Score

		Score
Eye Opening:	None	1
	To pain	2
	To voice	3
	Spontaneously	4
Vocalization:	None	1
	Incomprehensible sounds	2
	Incomprehensible words	3
	Confused speech	4
	Normal speech	5
Motor Exam:	Flaccid bilaterally	1
	Extensor posturing	2
	Flexion posturing	3
	Withdrawal from pain	4
	Localizes pain	5
	Follows commands	6

Similarly, to minimize variations in the hourly neurological assessment, which is usually performed by the NICU nurses, a standard neurological flow sheet is used to evaluate the level of consciousness, brainstem function, and motor responses. Repeated sensory examination is usually performed only in patients with spinal cord injuries. Using the flow sheet maximizes objective portions of the neurological examination and minimizes subjective responses and interobserver variability.

Level of Consciousness and Mental Status

A change in the level of consciousness may be the first indication of neurological decline. The usual terms used to describe level of consciousness are *awake and alert, lethargic, stuporous, obtunded,* and *comatose.* The level of consciousness reflects both level of arousal and the presence of cognitive or conscious behavior. Arousal is dependent on proper functioning of the reticular activating system (RAS), whereas conscious behavior is dependent on proper function of the cerebral hemispheres.[4,26]

The reticular activating system is a diffuse network of neurons located in the brainstem, from the midbrain, where it forms part of the tegmentum, into the thalamus and subthalamic structures.[4,26] The neurons of the RAS are extensively interconnected and receive collateral input from every major somatic and special sensory pathway. Numerous axons ascend from the RAS through the central tegmental fasciculus of the midbrain into the thalamus, hypothalamus, basal forebrain, limbic system, and diffusely into the neocortex. Stimulation of the RAS results in generalized nonspecific activation of the cerebral cortex.[4,26] This activity appears to occur in part because of abolition of tonic inhibitory input from the thalamic reticular nucleus and through modulation of the limbic system by the hypothalamus. An injury or insult that interrupts or reduces rostral input from the RAS will decrease alertness and cortical arousal, even in the absence of significant cortical injury. For example, it has recently been shown that acute pupillary dilation in patients with severe head injury may be associated with a marked decrease in brainstem blood flow (BBF).[28] Such a decrease in BBF with ischemia of the RAS would also explain the concurrent decrease in alertness that typifies severe head injury.

Conscious behavior depends on arousal of the cerebral cortex in many localized areas that participate in specific cognitive functions.[4,26] Of special importance are cortical association areas important for motivation, such as the basifrontal forebrain, but the entire cortex is important. Intact cognitive function requires continuous stimulation among all parts of the neocortex through corticothalamic and direct intercortical connections. Cortical lesions of increasing size cause a progressive decline in alertness and cognitive function regardless of their location. Earlier and more prominent deficits may be noted if the dominant hemisphere is involved. When cortical function diffusely ceases, the patient loses all alertness, even if the RAS remains intact. Damage to connections between cortical regions probably explains the influence of a lesion on uninjured areas.

Orientation and mentation are assessed as a part of the routine neurological examination. Changes in conscious behavior may signify the development of an intracranial lesion. However, it is also important to check for other systemic abnormalities that may contribute to a change in the level of consciousness. These may include fever, hypothermia, seizures, systemic hypotension, severe hypertension leading to encephalopathy, hypoxia, hypercapnia, sepsis, metabolic changes such as severe hyponatremia, and the use of sedatives such as phenytoin, propofol, benzodiazepines, or other medications.

Brainstem Function

Brainstem function should be evaluated systematically, beginning from the midbrain and extending down to the medulla oblongata. Olfaction and visual acuity or visual fields are often difficult to assess in NICU patients with altered mental status; thus the brainstem reflexes are tested to evaluate brainstem function.

Afferent defects in optic nerve function can be detected by testing the consensual pupillary response to light. For example, the Marcus Gunn pupillary test is performed by swinging a flashlight from the normal eye to the other at 3-second intervals. Normally each pupil will respond by constriction to the directed light; in the case of an eye with impaired optic nerve function, the pupil will dilate along with the opposite side. In such instances the direct light stimulus is not sufficient to maintain the previously evoked consensual pupillary constriction.

Pupillary symmetry and reactivity are among the most important parts of the brainstem examination in patients at risk for expanding intracranial mass lesions. Unilateral pupillary dilation was previously thought to represent transtentorial herniation, with compression of the third cranial nerve; the third nerve nuclei in the brainstem, including the Edinger-Westphal nucleus; and the superior colliculus.[4,24] More recently Ritter and colleagues[28] have shown that such a clinical finding in head injury patients occurs in the presence of midbrain ischemia, rather than resulting from direct compression alone. The clinical finding still represents a critical dysfunction of the upper brainstem, often caused by the expansion of an intracranial mass lesion. Ischemia or direct compression of the midbrain results in dysfunction of the parasympathetic output from the Edinger-Westphal nucleus of the third cranial nerve; with unopposed sympathetic input from the carotid plexus, the involved pupil dilates, often in an irregular manner.[4,24] As midbrain compression or ischemia progresses, both parasympathetic and sympathetic output to the pupils are lost, resulting in fixed, 4- to 5-mm midposition pupils bilaterally. The progression of pupillary dysfunction to bilateral represents a grave prognostic sign.[28] The key point is that pupillary asymmetry in a patient who may harbor an intracranial mass lesion signifies an acute crisis involving the upper brainstem, requiring prompt neurosurgical attention.[4,5,24,26]

Unilateral pupillary dilation does not always signify a mass lesion compressing the Edinger-Westphal nucleus or represent upper brainstem ischemia. A patient who has undergone clipping of a basilar artery or posterior communicating artery aneurysm may have an oculomotor palsy as a result of surgical manipulation or aneurysmal compression of the third cranial nerve. Direct trauma to the eye may also cause traumatic iridoplegia. In such cases, other methods of assessing intracranial physiology and function may be needed, such as ICP monitoring.[4]

With lesions of the midbrain tegmentum, the pupils are usually midposition and unreactive. Pontine lesions usually cause the pupils to be pinpoint and minimally reactive because of loss of descending sympathetic output to the sympathetic plexus. With hemorrhage into and around the third ventricle, the pupils are also small and poorly reactive.

Many pharmacological agents can affect pupillary function. Barbiturates and atropine are drugs commonly used in the NICU setting. Barbiturates at lower doses usually cause pupillary constriction and at higher doses result in loss of pupillary function. Atropine is a parasympathetic agent most commonly used to treat bradycardia, which also results in pupillary dilation. Any asymmetry in patients receiving these sort of drugs must be presumed to harbor a mass lesion until proven otherwise.

The corneal reflex reflects the integrity of afferent fifth cranial nerve input and seventh cranial nerve motor output, as well as their interconnection in the pons. The absence of a corneal reflex indicates pontine dysfunction; in head injury patients, such a finding is a grave prognostic sign.[1]

If there is no contraindication to manipulation of the cervical spine, the oculocephalic reflex should be tested by performing the doll's eye maneuver. This tests the integrity of the midbrain and the pons, specifically the preservation of the prepontine gaze centers, the third and sixth cranial nerve nuclei, and their interconnections via the medial longitudinal fasciculus. If cervical movement is contraindicated, the oculovestibular reflex can still be evaluated by performing ice-water caloric testing of the middle ear.[26] This test is performed by the instillation of 100 ml of ice water onto the tympanic membrane; if the reflex is intact, the ice water produces a tonic deviation of the eyes *toward* the side of the test.

The gag response evaluates the functioning of the ninth and tenth cranial nerves, the nuclei of which are located in the medulla oblongata. Finally, respiratory rate and pattern reflect the integrity of the pontomedullary respiratory centers, as detailed earlier in this chapter. Such function is of importance when determination of brain death is needed.

Motor Function

Asymmetric findings on the motor examination indicate dysfunction of the motor cortex or descending fibers of the corticospinal tracts. In patients with a depressed level of consciousness and unilateral pupillary dilation, a hemiparesis completes the clinical triad for making the diagnosis of transtentorial herniation.[4] Usually the hemiparesis is contralateral to the pupillary abnormality and the mass lesion, but in up to 25% of patients the hemiparesis is ipsilateral to the dilated pupil as a result of displacement of the brainstem away from the mass lesion and compression of the contralateral fibers of the cerebral peduncle against the adjacent edge of the tentorium (Kernohan's notch phenomenon).[16]

In the awake patient, motor function can be graded from 0 to 5, with 5/5 normal; 4/5, decreased strength to resistance; 3/5, able to lift against gravity; 2/5, able to move with gravity eliminated; 1/5, muscle contraction without joint movement; and 0/5, no contraction whatsoever. The notations <#+> and <#−> may be used to suggest more subtle connotations.

In patients with an abnormal level of consciousness, motor function may be tested by determining the best motor response to voice or, if necessary, to a painful stimulus. These movements can be recorded as normal, abnormal, or absent altogether. The Glasgow Coma Scale score[31] further characterizes motor function in terms of cerebral hemispheric integrity. Normal motor function is the ability to follow commands. Decreasing motor scores include localization to painful stimulation; normal flexion, usually noted as brisk withdrawal to pain; abnormal flexion posturing (usually to deep supraorbital pain); and abnormal extension posturing.[26] A flaccid response to deep, painful stimulus is the most abnormal response possible.

Although the exact level of injury within the brainstem is not clear in human subjects, abnormal flexion probably represents a diffuse injury to the cerebral hemispheres with preserved brainstem function, and abnormal extension indicates an additional injury to the midbrain and upper pons.[4,24,26] Severe metabolic disorders may also combine with parenchymal tissue injuries to the brain to result in such abnormal motor responses. Flaccidity usually corresponds to dysfunction at the level of the medullopontine reticular formation.[26] Bilateral flaccidity is an ominous sign in patients with severe head injury or intracranial mass lesions. It should be recalled that a flaccid motor examination may also occur in a patient with a spinal cord injury.

Myoclonus is common after hypoxic insults or cardiac arrest. Asterixis or tremors suggest metabolic abnormalities such as severe hepatic dysfunction or respiratory failure.[11]

Other Factors Associated with Neurological Examination and Monitoring

Arterial Blood Gases

In the NICU the most common abnormalities in arterial blood gases are those reflecting respiratory failure. A PaO_2 of less than 60 mm Hg or a $PaCO_2$ greater than 50 mm Hg unequivocally intensifies respiratory failure.[11] Patients with neurological disease rarely complain of dyspnea. The more common neurological signs of respiratory failure are confusion, restlessness, agitation, and headache.[11] As respiratory failure advances, there may be pupillary constriction, tremors, or asterixis. Coma with associated papilledema are the end-stage findings of severe hypoxia and hypercarbia.

The effect of systemic hypoxia on the neurological examination has most often been evaluated in cases of acute airway obstruction, suffocation, and drowning. Systemic hypotension usually develops with acute hypoxia caused by reflex depression of cardiac function[8]; thus the adverse effects of hypoxia on the brain are in part caused by hypoperfusion.[30] Cerebral ischemia often results from the combined effects of both hypoxia and hypotension.

If systemic hypotension is adequately treated, humans can tolerate extremely low PaO_2 without obvious neurological sequelae. In a study of a series of 22 patients with a PaO_2 of less than 20 mm Hg, Gray and Horner[12] reported that eight were alert, seven were somnolent, and seven were comatose. When systemic hypoxia is combined with hypercapnia, however, neurological function is invariably poor and recovery much less frequent.[27]

Severe hypoxia may cause clinical signs of a metabolic encephalopathy, which may include progressive change in level of consciousness, leading to coma, tremors, asterixis, myoclonus, and, at a later state, flexor or extensor posturing and alterations in respiratory patterns.[23,26,27] Pupillary constriction occurs with acute anoxia, followed by dilation combined with loss of oculocephalic reflex function at the time of severe, persistent anoxia.[4,26]

Systemic hypoxia is a frequent complication of severe head injury. In a series of patients in coma after head injury, Katsurada and colleagues[15] showed that 43% of patients had a Po_2 of less than 70 mm Hg and 14% had a $Paco_2$ of more than 45 mm Hg; 20% had respiratory acidosis. Similar results have been reported by others.[19,20] Hypoxia may result from the immediate onset of apnea after the injury,[19,20] subsequent abnormal central breathing patterns,[6,23,30] associated airway obstruction or trauma to the chest wall or lungs, fat emboli to the lungs from long-bone fractures, or spinal cord injury with loss of thoracic motor enervation.

In patients with severe systemic hypoxia, the findings of a neurological examination should never be the sole basis for determining treatment of a potential prognosis for recovery; rather the examination should be repeated as hypoxia and any associated metabolic abnormalities such as acidosis are corrected. Other data, such as the results of CT scanning and ICP monitoring, are important additional information.

Hypercapnia ($Paco_2$ 55 mm Hg) is often accompanied by elevated ICP.[4,19,20] The cause of hypercapnia is usually airway obstruction, neuromuscular disease, or depression of central respiratory centers. Neurological dysfunction caused by hypercapnia is dependent on the rate of increase in $Paco_2$; a rapid elevation may be more detrimental than a slow rise.[30] Indeed, with slow and chronic elevation in $Paco_2$ in neurologically normal patients, a rise to 75 and as high as 110 mm Hg may be tolerated without neurological alterations.[21]

ELECTROCARDIOGRAM

Neurogenic cardiac arrhythmias, including supraventricular and ventricular tachycardias, are common after such insults as severe head injury and acute subarachnoid hemorrhage. This may reflect central effects on the conducting system of the heart or myocardial ischemia caused by intense sympathetic and parasympathetic stimulation, with elevated levels of circulating catecholamines.

Thus continuous electrocardiography (ECG) monitoring is a vital element of NICU monitoring. All abnormalities of the ECG should be thoroughly investigated to rule out new neurological problems or a myocardial insult.

REFERENCES

1. Le Roux PD, Choudri H, Andrews BT: Cerebral concussion and diffuse brain injury. In Cooper PR and Golfinos JG (Editors). **Head Injury** (4th ed.). New York: McGraw-Hill, 2000, pp. 175-200.
2. Andrews BT: The intensive care management of patients with head injury, in Andrews BT (ed): **Neurosurgical Intensive Care.** New York: McGraw-Hill, 1993, pp 227-242.
3. Andrews BT, Levy ML, Pitts LH: The implications of systemic hypotension for the neurological examination in patients with severe head injury, **Surg Neurol 28:**419, 1987.
4. Andrews BT, Pitts LH: **Traumatic Transtentorial Herniation.** New York: Futura Press, 1991.
5. Andrews BT, Pitts LH, Lovely MP, et al: Is computed tomographic scanning necessary in patients with tentorial herniation? Results of immediate surgical exploration without computed tomography in 100 patients, **Neurosurgery 19:**408, 1986.
6. Brown HW, Plum F: The neurologic basis of Cheyne-Stokes respirations, **Am J Med 30:**849, 1961.
7. Choi SC, Narayan RK, Anderson RL, et al: Enhanced specificity of prognosis in severe head injury, **J Neurosurg 69:**381-385, 1988.
8. Cross CE, Rieben PA, Barron CI, et al: Effects of arterial hypoxia on the heart and circulation: an integrative study, **Am J Physiol 205:**963, 1963.
9. Cushing H: Some experimental and clinical observations concerning states of increased intracranial tension, **Am J Med Sci 124:**375, 1902.
10. Dowell AR, Buckley CE, Cohen R, et al: Cheyne-Stokes respirations, **Arch Intern Med 127:**712, 1971.
11. Fink ME: Respiratory care: diagnosis and management, in Rowland LP (ed): **Merrit's Textbook of Neurology.** Philadelphia: Lea and Febiger, 1989, pp 871-876.
12. Gray FD, Horner GJ: Survival following extreme hypoxemia, **JAMA 211:**1815, 1970.
13. Hoff JT, Reis DJ: Localization of regions mediating the Cushings response in CNS of cats, **Arch Neurol 23:**228, 1970.
14. Jennett B, Teasdale G, Braakman R, et al: Prognosis of patients with severe head injury, **Neurosurgery 4:**282-289, 1979.
15. Katsurada K, Yamada R, Sugimoto T: Respiratory insufficiency in patients with severe head injury, **Surgery 73:**191, 1973.
16. Kernohan JW, Woltman HE: Incisura of the crus due to contralateral brain tumor, **Arch Neurol Psychiatry 21:**274, 1929.
17. Marion DW, Obrist WD, Carlier PM, et al: The use of moderate therapeutic hypothermia for patients with severe head injuries: a preliminary report, **J Neurosurg 79:**354-362, 1993.
18. Marion DW, Penrod LE, Kelsey SF, et al: Treatment of traumatic brain injury with moderate hypothermia, **N Engl J Med 336:**540-546, 1997.
19. Miller JD: Head injury and brain ischaemia—implications for therapy, **Br J Anaesth 547:**120, 1985.

20. Miller JD, Sweet RC, Narayan R, et al: Early insults to the injured brain, **JAMA 240:**439, 1978.
21. Neff TA, Petty TL: Tolerance and survival in severe chronic hypercapnia, **Arch Intern Med 129:**591, 1972.
22. Newfield P, Pitts LH, Katkis J, et al: The influence of shock on mortality after head injury, **Crit Care Med 8:**254, 1980.
23. North JB, Jennet B: Abnormal breathing patterns associated with acute brain damage, **Arch Neurol 31:**338, 1974.
24. Obana WG, Andrews BT: The neurological examination and neurologic monitoring in the intensive care unit, in Andrews BT (ed): **Neurosurgical Intensive Care.** New York: McGraw-Hill, 1993, pp 31-42.
25. Plum F, Alvord EC: Apneustic breathing in man, **Arch Neurol 10:**101, 1964.
26. Plum F, Posner JB: **The Diagnosis of Stupor and Coma.** Philadelphia: F.A. Davis, 1980.
27. Refsum HE: Relationship between state of consciousness and arterial hypoxemia and hypercapnia in patient with pulmonary insufficiency breathing air, **Clin Sci 25:**361, 1963.
28. Ritter AM, Muiizelaar JP, Barnes T, et al: Brain stem blood flow, pupillary response and outcome in patients with severe head injury, **Neurosurgery 44:**941-948, 1999.
29. Sears TA: The respiratory motor neuron and apneusis, **Fed Proc 36:**2412, 1977.
30. Simon RP: Breathing and the nervous system, in Aminoff MJ (ed): **Neurology and General Medicine.** New York: Churchill Livingston, 1989, pp 1-22.
31. Teasdale G, Jennett B: Assessment of coma and impaired consciousness: a practical scale, **Lancet 2:**81, 1974.

CHAPTER 4

Cerebrovascular Pathophysiology and Monitoring in the Neurosurgical Intensive Care Unit

JAMIE S. ULLMAN

The brain uses approximately 20% of the total body oxygen consumption, receiving 15% of the total cardiac output. As with other major organ systems, the brain is subject to autoregulatory influences and adjusts for environmental changes to prevent oxygen deprivation. Such oxygen deprivation can lead to devastating physical and cognitive dysfunction.

Knowledge of cerebral blood flow and metabolism is essential to understanding the effect of ischemic insults on the brain. In all ischemic conditions, neuronal damage can extend far beyond the initial insult if attention is not paid to maximizing oxygen delivery to threatened areas. Therefore a working knowledge of cerebrovascular physiology can help the physician apply appropriate treatments during ischemic insults with the ultimate goal of preserving and promoting good functional outcomes.

CEREBRAL BLOOD FLOW

Cerebral blood flow (CBF) is defined as the velocity of blood through the cerebral circulation. CBF is expressed as milliliters per 100 g of brain tissue per minute. Once CBF is determined, other metabolic parameters can be calculated, such as the cerebral metabolic rate of oxygen consumption ($CMRO_2$) and oxygen delivery. A summary of pertinent physiological formulas is listed in Table 4-1.

Global CBF is approximately 50 ml/100g/min. Gray matter blood flow is approximately 3 to 4 times greater than white matter.[25] Newborn blood flow is approximately 40 ml/100g/min.[18,90] In infants and children, CBF is generally higher, increasing to 108 ml/100 g/min by 2 to 4 years of age,[64,90] and can remain above 100 into adolescence.[37] "Hyperemia" occurring in children after head injury may actually be a relative state of ischemia given the higher normative values (Table 4-2).

According to Ohm's law, flow is directly related to perfusion pressure (inflow minus outflow) and inversely related to cerebrovascular resistance. The main resistance vessels are the small arteries and pial arterioles, the smallest of which are capable of dilating to up to 300% of their original diameters. These vessels may account for up to 85% of the total cerebrovascular resistance.[76]

CBF is maintained according to Poiseuille's law, which relates flow to physiological and anatomical variables within the cerebrovascular system.

$$Q = \frac{\Delta P \pi r^4}{81\eta}$$

Flow (Q) is directly proportional to the pressure gradient, or differential (ΔP), which is synonymous with the cerebral perfusion pressure (CPP), and the fourth power of the vessel radius (r^4). Flow is also inversely proportional to the length of the vascular tree (l), a constant, and the blood viscosity (η), which can vary under certain circumstances.

Autoregulation is the maintenance of constant CBF in the face of physiological changes, mainly brain perfusion. Altering elements of Poiseuille's law can help improve blood flow in ischemic states such as head injury or vasospasm.

TABLE 4-1 ■ Blood Flow and Metabolic Parameters—Calculations and Values

Parameters (Units)*	Formula	Conversion Factor	Normal Values: Reference[38] (n = 14)	Normal Values: Reference[77] (n = 50)	Normal Values: Reference[30] (n = 8)	Head Injury Values (n = 282)
CBF (ml/100 g/min)			54 ± 12		52 ± 12	51 ± 23
CaO_2 (ml/dl)	$1.34 \cdot Hb \cdot SaO_2 + .0031 \cdot PaO2$	$\frac{CaO_2\ (ml/dl)}{2.24} = CaO_2\ (\mu mol/ml)$		19.6 ± 1.2	16.9 ± 1.5	14.1 ± 2.4
$CjvO_2$ (ml/dl)	$1.34 \cdot Hb \cdot SjvO_2 + .0031 \cdot Pjvo2$	$\frac{CjvO_2\ (ml/dl)}{2.24} = CjvO_2\ (\mu mol/ml)$		12.9 ± 1.3		9.7 ± 2.3
$AVDO_2$ (ml/dl)	CaO_2 (ml/dl) − $CjvO_2$ (ml/dl)	$\frac{AVDO_2\ (ml/dl)}{2.24} = AVDO_2\ (\mu mol/ml)$	6.3 ± 1.2	6.7 ± 0.8	6.5 ± 1.8	4.4 ± 1.6
$CMRO_2$ (ml/100 g/min)	$\frac{AVDO_2\ (ml/dl) \cdot CBF\ (ml/100\ g/min)}{100}$	$\frac{CMRO_2\ (ml/100\ g/min)}{2.24} = CMRO_2\ (\mu mol/110\ g/min)$	3.3 ± 0.4		3.3 ± 0.6	2.1 ± 1.2
O_2ER (%)†	$\frac{AVDO_2\ (ml/dl) \cdot 100\%)}{CaO_2}$			34 ± 4		31 ± 10
AVDG (ml/dl)	ArtGluc (ml/dl) − JVGluc (ml/dl)	$\frac{AVDG\ (ml/dl)}{18} = AVDG\ (\mu mol/ml)$		9.6 ± 1.7	11.0 ± 2.3	7.2 ± 3.6
CMRG (ml/100 g/min)	$\frac{AVDG\ (ml/dl) \cdot CBF\ (ml/100\ g/min)}{100}$	$\frac{CMRG\ (ml/100\ g/min)}{18} = CMRG\ (\mu mol/g/min)$			5.5 ± 1.1	3.5 ± 2.4
AVDL (ml/dl)	ArtLact (ml/dl) − JVLact (ml/dl)	$\frac{AVDL\ (ml/dl)}{9} = AVDL\ (\mu mol/ml)$		−1.70 ± .9	−0.5 ± 0.9	−0.5 ± 1.2
CMRL (ml/100 g/min)	$\frac{AVDL\ (ml/dl) \cdot CBF\ (ml/100\ g/min)}{100}$	$\frac{CMRL\ (ml/100\ g/min)}{9} = CMRL\ (\mu mol/g/min)$			−0.23 ± 0.37	−0.25 ± 0.73
LOI	$\frac{-AVDL\ (\mu mol/ml)}{AVDO_2\ (\mu mol/ml)}$				0.06 ± 0.03	0.02 ± 0.05

From Robertson CS: Nitrous oxide technique for CBF measurement, in Narayan RK, Wilberger J, Povlishock JT (eds): **Neurotrauma**. New York: McGraw-Hill, 1996.
*All average values are given in the units used in the first column.

†O_2ER can also be calculated by the formula $1 - \frac{SjvO_2}{SaO_2}$ or $\frac{SaO_2 - SjvO_2}{SaO_2} \cdot 100\%$.

CaO_2, Arterial oxygen content; *$CjvO_2$*, jugular venous oxygen content; *SaO_2*, arterial oxygen saturation; *$SjvO_2$*, jugular venous oxygen saturation; *Hb*, hemoglobin concentration; *PaO_2*, arterial PO_2; *$PjvO_2$*, jugular venous PO_2; *$AVDO_2$*, arterial venous oxygen difference; *O_2ER*, oxygen extraction ratio; *ArtGluc*, arterial glucose concentration; *JVGluc*, jugular venous glucose concentration; *AVDG*, arterial venous glucose difference; *CMRG*, cerebral metabolic rate of glucose; *ArtLact*, arterial lactate concentration; *JVLact*, jugular venous lactate concentration; *AVDL*, arterial venous lactate difference; *CMRL*, cerebral metabolic rate of lactate; *LOI*, lactate oxygen index.

TABLE 4-2 ■ Normal CBF Values According to Age[18,64,90]

Age	CBF (ml/100g/min)
Newborn	40
6 months	65
1 year	80
2-4 years	108
8 years	85
14 years	70
Adult	50

Components of Poiseuille's Law

Cerebral Perfusion Pressure (ΔP)

Cerebral perfusion pressure is also referred to as the transmural pressure gradient. CPP is the differential pressure of arterial inflow and venous outflow, the latter usually equaling the intracranial pressure (ICP). CPP can also be defined as the differential mean pressure within the arterial vessel (MAP) and the pressure surrounding the vessel wall (ICP).

Dewey and colleagues[23] further defined CPP as the MAP minus the critical closing pressure, which is determined by ICP and vascular smooth muscle tone. When ischemia results in maximal vessel dilation, the smooth muscles are maximally relaxed (zero tone). When the ICP approaches MAP, the vessel collapses at CPP less than 10 mm Hg, resulting in blood flow cessation (Figure 4-1, *bottom panel*).[76]

CPP is the primary stimulus for autoregulatory changes.[23] In low-flow states, increasing CPP raises CBF. MAP manipulation is used most often in ischemic conditions such as cerebral vasospasm[23,93,101] and head injury.[76] Reducing ICP through ventricular drainage, evacuation of mass lesion, and pharmacological therapy also improves CPP. Normal CPP is above 50 mm Hg but may be higher in pathological states such as head injury or chronic hypertension.

Vascular Radius (r^4)

As stated previously, small arteries and arterioles are capable of dilating and constricting in response to altered blood flow. As CPP decreases below 50 mm Hg, vascular smooth muscle begins to relax and vessels dilate to increase the volume of blood traveling within them, improving oxygen delivery. If CPP is raised above 50, vessels begin to constrict to decrease blood volume to match the decreasing oxygen demand until a steady-state diameter is reached (Figure 4-1, *top and middle panels*).[76] The adjustment of vessel diameter regulates the inflow according to metabolic demands. Other environmental factors can affect vascular muscle tone such as sympathetic and parasympathetic innervation, nitric oxide, adenosine, hypoxia, anemia, and hypercarbia/hypocarbia.

Blood Viscosity (η)

Cerebral blood flow is inversely proportional to whole blood viscosity. However, blood is a nonnewtonian fluid, containing proteinaceous elements that are capable of aggregating in low-flow states.[36] Therefore the relationship of blood flow and viscosity is not strictly linear under all conditions.

Viscosity, expressed in centipoise units, measures a liquid's resistance to flow. Blood traveling through vessels is subject to laminar flow, meaning the velocity is faster in the periphery than in the center. Shear rate (sec^{-1}) is the velocity gradient within the vessel and is directly proportional to velocity and inversely proportional to the radius. At higher blood velocities/shear rates, the viscosity is less, thus defining the inverse relationship between shear rate and viscosity.[36] At relatively high shear rates ($<10\ sec^{-1}$), viscosity is incumbent on the hematocrit.[36] At low shear rates, erythrocyte aggregation occurs, which is reversible at elevated shear rates.

Manipulating blood viscosity is an integral part of hypertensive, hypervolemic, hemodilution (triple-H) therapy of cerebral vasospasm and subarachnoid hemorrhage. This therapy uses decreased hematocrit to improve blood rheology, which optimizes flow and deformation of blood elements through different diameter blood vessels.[36] Increasing blood flow with pressors in addition to hemodilution can help push blood through the microvasculature more efficiently.

Pharmacological agents such as mannitol, dextran, albumin, and hetastarch help improve hemorheology by promoting intravascular volume expansion, or hemodilution. These agents, especially dextran,[103,104] can prevent red blood cell (RBC) aggregation while traveling through the microvasculature.[12] It is in these small vessels where viscosity contributes the most to Poiseuille's CBF equation, especially in ischemic states.[36]

CEREBRAL AUTOREGULATION

According to a landmark review by Lassen in 1959,[44] "cerebral perfusion is controlled very efficiently by homeostatic regulation of the perfusion pressure and the so-called cerebral vascular resistance." *Autoregulation* therefore refers to the maintenance of a relatively constant CBF during fluctuations in CPP. Constant CBF is maintained over a MAP range of 60 to 160 mm Hg.[25] Cellular metabolism also influences vascular radius and consequently autoregulation. Through autoregulation the brain protects itself from ischemia. At the extreme, Cushing's response provides a physiological attempt to improve CBF during times of critical ischemia.

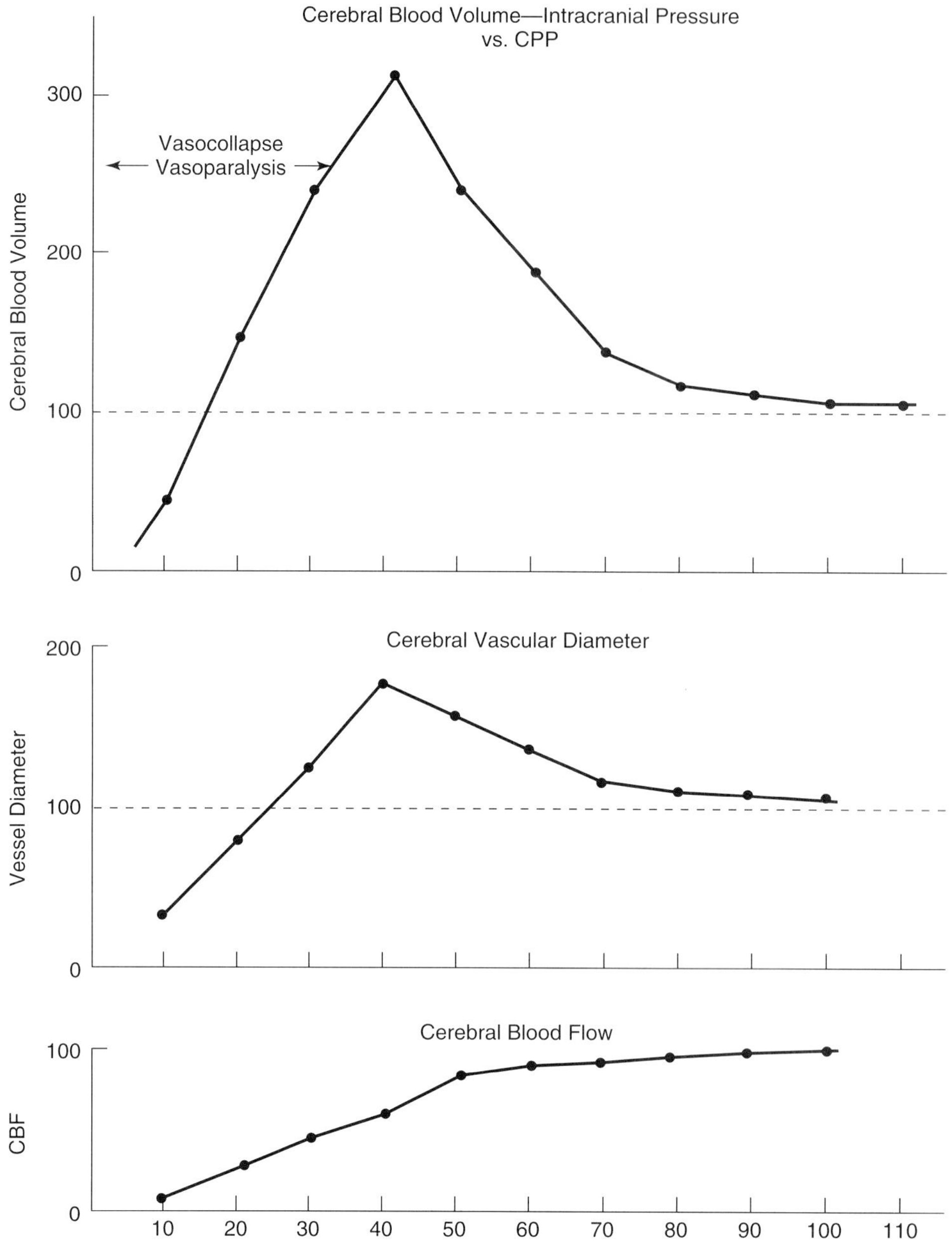

FIGURE 4-1 ■ **Cerebral blood volume *(top panel)*, 40-50 μm bed pial arteriolar diameter *(middle panel)*, and cerebral blood flow versus cerebral perfusion pressure.** (From Rosner MJ: Pathophysiology and management of increased intracranial hypertension, in Andrew BT (ed): **Neurosurgical Intensive Care.** New York: McGraw-Hill, 1993, pp 57-112.)

Limits of Autoregulation

Figure 4-1 *(bottom panel)* demonstrates a small decrease in CBF as the CPP values fall to 50 mm Hg, which can be considered the lower limit of autoregulation.[40,76] As CPP declines, vascular radius reaches its peak, the point of maximal dilation (Figure 4-1, *middle panel*). Below this threshold, vessels collapse and cerebral blood flow declines. Below this lower limit of autoregulation, cerebral blood volume (CBV) decreases proportionately with the blood pressure. As perfusion is restored, CBV increases until smooth muscle responsivity is restored and constricts to maintain constant blood flow. CBV thus decreases. Therefore CBV does not increase proportionately with increased blood flow within the autoregulatory range, but in fact decreases until a steady state is reached (Figure 4-1, *top panel*).[76]

Increasing perfusion at the upper limit of autoregulation results in passive dilation of many of the autoregulatory pial arterioles, leading to increased CBF and decreased CVR.[42,43] Kontos[43] demonstrated that smaller vessels dilate more than larger ones. Fusiform microaneurysms were found in smaller vessels in cats subjected to induced hypertension to greater than 200 mm Hg. Above this level, dilatory responses were largely irreversible. Such responses can lead to blood brain barrier disruption, cerebral edema, or intracranial bleeding.

Vasoresponsivity

Vasoresponsivity is the ability of blood vessels to dilate or constrict in response to environmental influences. Such factors include CPP fluctuations, hypoxia, and hypocarbia/hypercarbia. By determining the CBF response to such stimuli, assessment of the brain's ability to autoregulate can be made. The brain may lose this ability if subject to critical, irreversible ischemia. Such loss can occur either regionally or globally.[53]

Blood vessel diameter does change in the face of CPP alterations. Normal latency is approximately 5 to 10 seconds. In pathological states such as head injury, responsivity is delayed. Manipulation of CPP may result in an initial rise in ICP as blood volume transiently increases proportionately, then decreases as vessels vasoconstrict.[76]

Carbon dioxide vasoresponsivity is defined by a 3% change in CBF per 1 mm Hg change in P_{CO_2}. By using induced hypocarbia, responsivity can be assessed both globally and regionally during various tests for CBF determination.[9,53] Acetazolamide is also used for this purpose. In dosages greater than 10 mg/kg, acetazolamide inhibits carbonic anhydrase in the erythrocyte. Vorstrup and colleagues[97] demonstrated a 53% to 75% increase in CBF in patients given acetazolamide. Although the exact mechanism is uncertain, RBC carbonic anhydrase inhibition results in a decrease in brain pH by impeding CO_2 removal through the circulation. Acetazolamide has been found to be equal or superior to CO_2-induced vasomotor reactivity.[72]

Vasoresponsivity may still be present despite autoregulatory impairment. Impaired autoregulation can be seen in head injury, subarachnoid hemorrhage, and other global ischemic insults. In severe head injury, focal and global autoregulation may still be intact.[9,53] Global, severe, and persistent autoregulation eventually leads to autoregulatory loss. This loss is evidenced by passive changes in ICP with blood pressure caused by passive increases in CBV.

Theories of Autoregulation

Although the above discussion assumes that autoregulation is largely incumbent on vascular smooth muscle tone and the response to pressure changes, various theories have been proposed for the autoregulatory mechanism, such as myogenic, neurogenic, and metabolic.

The myogenic theory proposes that vascular smooth muscle reacts to changes in stretch forces, or the transmural pressure.[24,42] The metabolic theory, as defined by Krontos,[42] states that cell metabolites arising from blood flow changes alter vascular diameter. Hydrogen, potassium, and adenosine have been shown to have vasoactive properties under conditions of hypoxia, ischemia, or cortical activation.[98]

The endothelial cell may have a strong influence on vessel caliber. Reduced CBF stimulates endothelium-derived relaxing factor (EDRF) release, identified as the vasodilator nitric oxide (NO) or an NO-containing compound.[41,98,99] Prostaglandins are also vasodilators. Endothelin and thromboxane A_2 are vasoconstrictors.[98] Arguments against the metabolic theory are primarily based on the longer delay in activation compared with the normal autoregulatory latency.[25]

In neurogenic theory, perivascular sympathetic and parasympathetic nerves may have autoregulatory effects. Evidence suggests that these factors are not essential for autoregulation.[25,42] It is likely that all three mechanisms work in concert to regulate blood flow. Certainly, although pressure change is the primary factor in vasoactivity, chemical and molecular contributions as a consequence of pressure changes are also very important.

Ischemic Penumbra and Ischemic Thresholds

The *ischemic penumbra* refers to the ischemic zone of brain tissue surrounding a core area of infarction or severe ischemia. As CBF decreases, less oxygen is carried to neurons, resulting in a decrease in mitochondrial adenosine triphosphate (ATP) production and ATP depletion. This depletion leads to lactic acid, free radical, lipid peroxidase, and other toxic metabolites production. Sodium and calcium influx and potassium efflux are also noted, eventually resulting in membrane breakdown and cell death. Just before this point, slowing and eventual cessation of synaptic transmission occurs without cell breakdown. This phenomenon occurs at 8 to 23 ml/100g/min.[16,35,45] Cortical potentials cease at 16 to 18 ml/100 g/min.[3,45]

In the penumbral range, lactic acid accumulates, ATP production remains normal, and the Na^+/K^+ pump is intact. Blood flow restoration in this ischemic range can result in neuronal recovery as evidenced by the return of cortical evoked responses.[3] After suffering an ischemic stroke, optimal cerebral perfusion can help limit the extent of functional impairment.[35]

Return of function also depends on the duration of ischemia at various levels of CBF.[105] For example, flows ranging from 18 to 23 ml/100g/min can be tolerated for up to 2 weeks, 10 to 12 ml/100g/min for less than 3 hours, and 8 ml/100 g/min for about 1 hour until neuronal death occurs.[16] The ischemic threshold can be raised by hyperglycemia, chronic hypertension, head injury, and vasospasm and lowered by certain anesthetic agents (isoflurane) and other neuroprotective drugs.[16]

Cushing's Response

The classic Cushing's triad—hypertension, bradycardia, and respiratory depression—can occur with significant intracranial hypertension.[21] As ICP rises to significant levels, nearing the MAP (with a concomitant dangerous decrease in CPP), the systemic blood pressure (BP) becomes elevated to a systolic BP greater than 200 mm Hg. This hypertension results from peripheral vasoconstriction and catecholamine release.[47] Brainstem/medullary ischemia results in bradycardia.[78-81]

In a series of animal experiments, Schrader and colleagues[78,80] demonstrated that expanding infra- and supratentorial masses resulted in progressive brainstem ischemia. Supratentorial mass expansion led to ischemia traveling in a rostral-caudal direction. Cushing's response resulted from ischemia extending to the lower pons.[78] The hypertensive response increased the ability of the brain to tolerate the expanding mass.[79] During Cushing's response, there is decreased blood flow to peripheral tissues but increased flow to the myocardium and adrenals.[33,80,95] Harris and colleagues[33] found that blood levels of epinephrine, norepinephrine, and arginine vasopressin were increased in fetal sheep. Blood flow increased in organs vital for sustaining and increasing blood pressure. As a result, Cushing's response helped to maintain adequate blood flow and tissue oxygenation during periods of ischemia.[5,51,80]

Cushing's response is the physiological response to life-threatening cerebral ischemia and is the body's attempt to preserve neuronal function through CBF improvement. Failure to recognize this critical need often leads to inappropriate antihypertensive therapy, which may precipitate irreversible neuronal damage.

METHODS OF CBF MEASUREMENT

Bedside Measurements

Kety-Schmidt/Nitrous Oxide Technique

The Kety-Schmidt technique, first described in 1945,[38] uses nitrous oxide (N_2O), a diffusible gas, for global CBF measurement. This examination is based on the Fick principle, which states that the amount of inert substance taken up by the brain is equal to the difference between substance delivery through the arterial system and removal by the venous system. After inhalation, N_2O reaches equilibrium between arterial blood, venous blood, and brain; arterial and jugular venous samples are obtained and analyzed for N_2O concentration over time. The integral of the arteriovenous difference is used to calculate CBF. $CMRO_2$ can also be calculated given the knowledge of arteriovenous oxygen difference ($AVDO_2$) and CBF.[25,74]

The Kety-Schmidt method is inexpensive and can be repeated multiple times. However, this method does not allow for regional CBF measurement or change detection, which may exist in disease processes such as traumatic brain injury, infarction, and vasospasm.

Xenon-133

Bedside regional CBF monitoring has been performed for many years using radioactive Xenon-133 (Xe-133), a low gamma emitter. Xe-133 has a half-life of approximately 5 days and is freely diffusible throughout the brain. Approximately 90% is cleared by first pass through the lungs, preventing recirculation in the brain. Bedside collimated scintillators are used to gather data about Xe-133 washout. The washout curve is approximately 15 minutes and is composed of two major compartments—fast (gray matter) and slow (white matter).[25] The two compartments can be analyzed separately. Regional CBF is calculated via several methods, a more detailed review of which can be found in Anderson.[1] Xe-133 can be administered invasively (intraarterially) or noninvasively (inhaled gas).[68] The gas form is soluble in normal saline. Given the small doses used, radiation exposure risk to the patient and medical staff is small.

Bedside Xe-133 CBF monitoring provides regional CBF measurements, allowing the clinician to evaluate several areas in both hemispheres simultaneously. Spacial resolution, however, is poor. The "look-through" phenomenon overestimates areas of low or no flow as a result of uptake in the immediately surrounding tissues.[1] CBF in deep hemisphere structures, brainstem, and cerebellum are obscured by surface uptake detection.[25] Despite various artifactual interferences, regional CBF changes can be easily recognized, making this technique useful in the clinical setting.

CBF Imaging

MR Diffusion and Perfusion[108]

Magnetic resonance (MR) diffusion imaging uses the apparent diffusion coefficient (ADC) of water to qualitatively evaluate areas of low blood flow. Diffusion imaging has been used in patients with ischemic stroke. Areas with low ADC values are bright (Figure 4-2). Such changes can be seen as early as 10 minutes after the occlusive event and as late as 1 week, recovering to baseline in 5 to 10 days.

MR perfusion imaging uses intravenous contrast such as gadolinium-diethylenetriamine pentaacetic acid (Gd-DTPA). Such imaging provides a map of

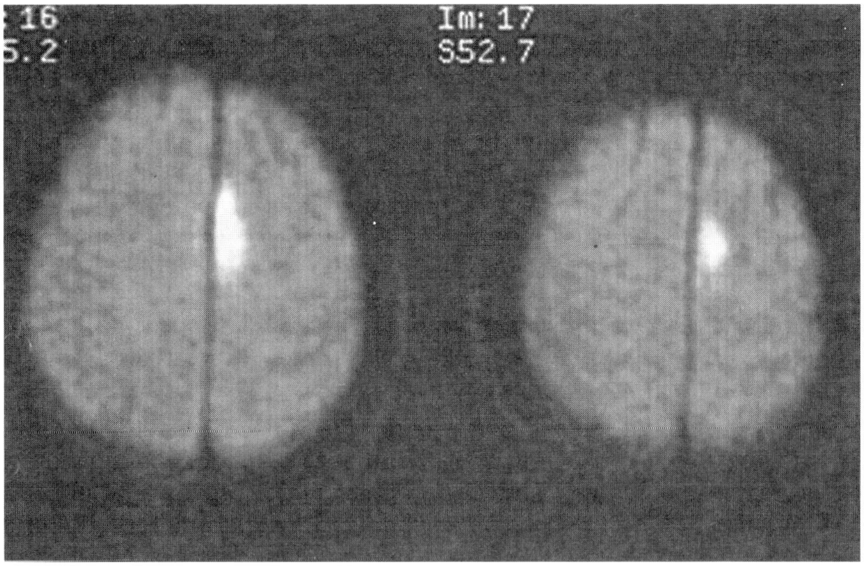

FIGURE 4-2 ■ **Diffusion MR image.** This patient developed a right hemiplegia as a result of a stroke in the supplementary motor area *(bright signal).* (Courtesy J. Bederson.)

cerebral blood volume by measuring the magnetic field gradient between the blood vessel lumen and surrounding tissue over time on the first pass of contrast agent. Low areas of CBV indicate poor perfusion.

Combined diffusion and perfusion imaging may allow for ischemic penumbra visualization as areas of perfusion-diffusion mismatch. This is because perfusion cannot distinguish between reversible and irreversible ischemia, whereas acute diffusion imaging might underestimate the ultimate infarct volume.

Xenon-CT

Stable xenon computed tomography (Xe-CT) involves inhalation of 28% to 33% stable xenon gas. Xenon, a general anesthetic in high concentrations, crosses the blood-brain barrier easily because of its lipid solubility. Combining CT with the radiodense Xe allows for a cross-sectional view of Xe concentration in various regions within the brain, as well as globally. The 33% concentration is a safe, nonanesthetic concentration. Xenon washout takes 20 minutes, after which the test can be repeated. Using a region of interest (ROI), the exact CBF can be calculated by computer. Because the test is repeatable within a relatively short period, vasoresponsivity can be assessed by methods such as hypercarbia or acetazolamide. Care must be taken to avoid motion artifact and Xe gas leakage around the mask. Spiral CT scanning has improved Xe-CT images.[7,107]

Xe-CT is commercially available (Diversified Diagnostic Products, Houston, Tex.). This technology is particularly useful in conditions in which regional CBF quantification is useful in directing management. Such conditions include cerebrovascular surgery, head injury, stroke, and subarachnoid hemorrhage.*

SPECT

Single photo emission tomography (SPECT)[65] employs radioactive tracers to measure CBF using tomographic images (Figure 4-3, *A-C*) through the detection of scattered photons. Regional and global CBF can be visualized. Various agents have been used, including Xe-133 gas, I-123, and various compounds of technecium-99m. Of these, only Xe-133 gas provides *quantitative* CBF measurements. Xe-133 also allows for multiple rapid measurements. I-123 must be imaged rapidly because of its quick redistribution within the brain. The brain retention half-life is 60 minute to 6 hours, depending on the compound.

Tc-99m compounds are the most widely used because of their availability and lower expense. Redistribution is slower, and brain retention half-life can be up to 24 to 28 hours, limiting the temporal resolution of each study. Tests for cerebrovascular reserve can also be done using SPECT technology. However, only qualitative blood flow assessments can be made. Stroke, brain death determination, and epilepsy are among the applications for SPECT blood flow studies.

PET

Positron emission tomography (PET) uses gamma ray (positron)–emitting nuclides, which produce two photons when captured by electrons. PET provides quantitative evaluation of the flowing parameters: CBF, CBV, $CMRO_2$, oxygen extraction fraction (OEF), cerebrovascular mean transit time (t-CBV/CBF), and cerebral metabolic rate of glucose consumption (CMRG). PET thus uniquely gives dynamic information in blood flow and metabolism. ^{15}O-labeled gases, carbon dioxide, oxygen, and carbon monoxide are used for CBF, CBV, $CMRO_2$, OEF, and mean transit time. 18-F-fluoro-2-decoxy-D-glucose (18FDG) is used for CMRG. Non–steady-state ^{15}O-labeled water can also be used to measure CBF.

*References 7, 9, 15, 29, 53, 106, 107.

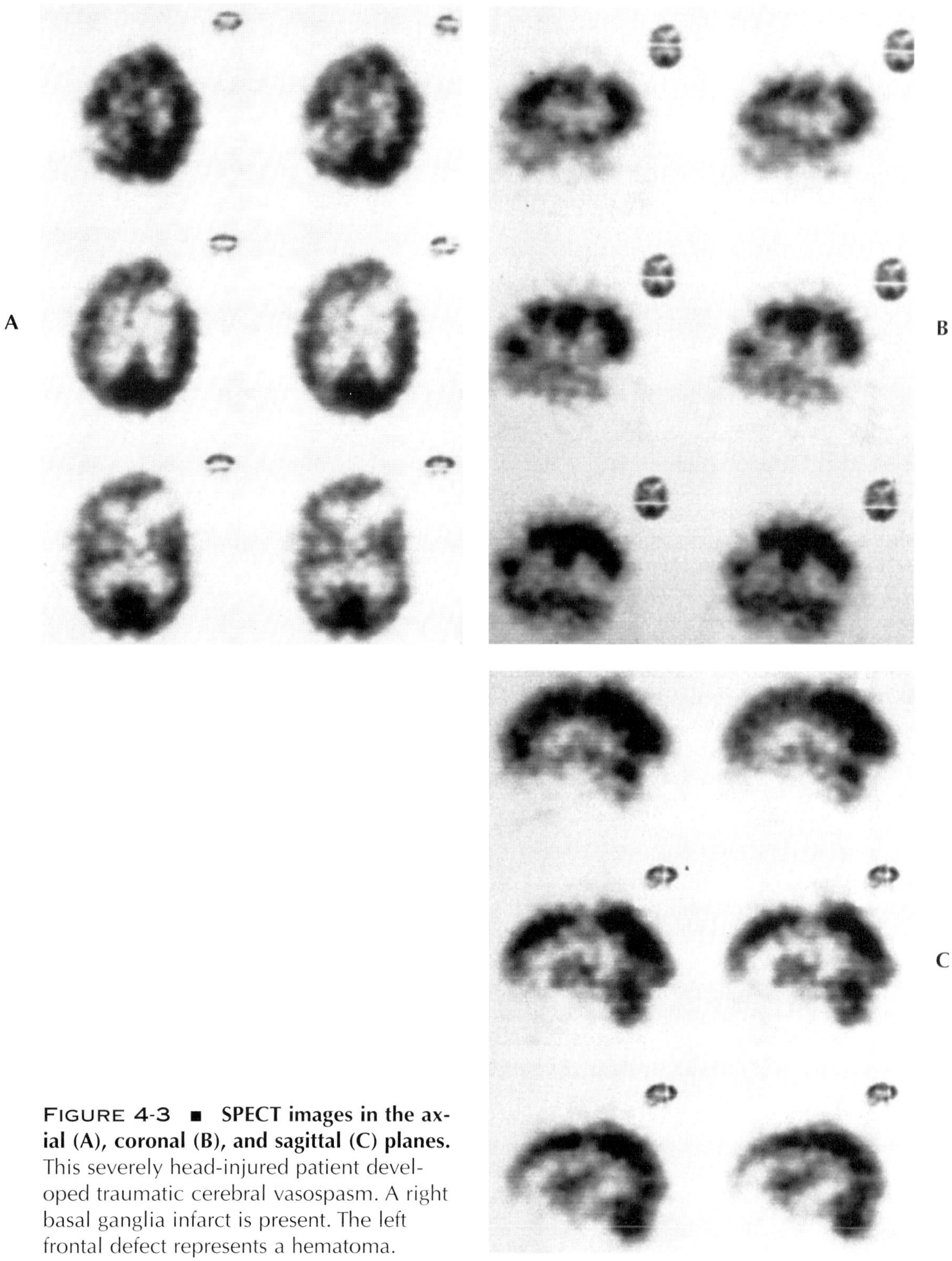

FIGURE 4-3 ■ **SPECT images in the axial (A), coronal (B), and sagittal (C) planes.** This severely head-injured patient developed traumatic cerebral vasospasm. A right basal ganglia infarct is present. The left frontal defect represents a hematoma.

PET measurements of CBF, OEF, and $CMRO_2$ can demonstrate ischemic penumbral areas and be used to augment flow. Although PET is a well-rounded, multifaceted technique for evaluating cerebral hemodynamics and metabolism, limited availability and expense restrict its usage in routine clinical practice.

Continuous CBF Monitoring

Continuous regional CBF monitoring can be adapted for bedside monitoring. Applications include head injury, intraoperative aneurysm/arteriovenous malformation (AVM) resection, subarachnoid hemorrhage, and epilepsy. Such monitoring can alert the clinician to changes in regional CBF and allow for minute-to-minute hemodynamic alterations.

Thermal Diffusion Flowmetry

Thermal diffusion flowmetry[24,50] uses a temperature gradient on the sensor to calculate the cerebral blood flow. The sensor contains two gold plates, one heated, one neutral. The heat dissipates to the neutral plate and this temperature difference (dT) is converted to flow in ml/100g/min. Blood flow is inversely proportional to dT. Therefore the higher the blood flow, the lower the temperature difference between the heated and neutral plates. Although correlating with global CBF as measured by N_2O technique,[13] this method does not correlate well with Xe-CT regional or global values.[82]

The sensor comes as a flat silicone plate for intraoperative or postoperative monitoring. A "trauma bolt" has been developed for placement inside a standard burrhole (Flowtronics, Inc., Phoenix, Ariz.). Each plate must touch relatively normal cortex, avoiding large surface vessels. The confidence factor helps determine whether both plates are in contact with the cortical surface. Once the heater is turned off, both plates should be at the same temperature. A confidence factor of 0.8[13] and above is considered reliable for use. Sioutos and colleagues[87] found that in 56 severely head-injured patients, 66% had reliable data with a confidence factor greater than or equal to 0.75.

Laser Doppler Flowmetry

Laser Doppler flowmetry estimates regional cerebral blood flow by using low-power laser light through cerebral tissue. Photons are randomly scattered by moving blood cells in capillary-sized vessels and are Doppler shifted. The proportion of Doppler-shifted light, which scatters back to the photo sensor, gives information regarding the blood cell velocity and blood volume in "arbitrary units."[32] These values poorly correlate with absolute CBF.[2]

The laser Doppler probes can be placed on the cortical surface or within the brain parenchyma. As in thermal diffusion, avoidance of macroscopic vessels is key. The special resolution is 1 mm^3, the smallest of all regional CBF methods, which may be a significant disadvantage. Other problems include the susceptibility to motion artifact, reducing reliability; fluctuation of signal without obvious cause[88]; and tissue and capillary density.[2] However, because of the high temporal resolution, allowing for a high frequency of data collection during continuous monitoring, changes in blood flow can be ascertained and treated quickly.

Indirect CBF Measurements

Transcranial Doppler Sonography

Transcranial Doppler sonography (TCD) is a useful, noninvasive bedside method for inferring blood flow. TCD measures blood flow velocity in intracranial vessels. Depending on the clinical circumstances, increased or decreased velocity can indicate low or compromised blood flow.

Cerebral blood flow can be mathematically calculated if certain parameters are known and constant. Such parameters include vessel cross-sectional area and the angle of incidence between arterial blood flow and the ultrasonic beam.[8] However, in pathological states, such parameters may vary over time and with environmental conditions, rendering CBF calculations unreliable.

TCD uses the Doppler principle to measure blood flow velocity via ultrasonic waves, which reflect off moving red blood cells. The transducer emits these waves at a known frequency, usually 2 MHz.[92] A wave form is generated with a systolic peak, dicrotic notch, and diastole. Mean velocities are used and are determined as the area under the curve.

Intracranial vessels are insonated through three "windows" (Table 4-3). The *transtemporal* window lies within the temporal squama just above the zygoma,

TABLE 4-3 ■ Guide to Identifying Cerebral Conducting Vessels by Transcranial Doppler Sonography

Window	Vessel	Depth (mm)	Normal Vm (cm/sec)	Direction of flow*
Transtemporal	MCA	45-55	60 ± 12	Toward
	ACA	55-75	50 ± 12	Away
	PCA	65-80	40 ± 11	Toward/away
Transorbital	OA	30-55	20 ± 10	Toward
	ICA	55-70	50 ± 15	Toward/away
Transforamental	VA	65-85	40 ± 10	Away
	BA	>85	40 ± 10	Away

From McCartney JP, Thomas-Lukes KM, Gomez CR: **Handbook of Transcranial Doppler.** New York, Springer-Verlag, 1997.

*In relation to transducer.

Vm, Mean velocity; *MCA*, middle cerebral artery; *ACA*, anterior cerebral artery; *PCA*, posterior cerebral artery; *OA*, ophthalmic artery; *ICA*, internal carotid artery; *VA*, vertebral artery; *BA*, basilar artery.

the thinnest portion of the temporal bone, and allows for anterior circulation insonation. The *suboccipital/foramen magnum* window studies the vertebrobasilar system. The *orbital* approach insonates the ophthalmic and cavernous carotid arteries. This window is especially useful in diagnosing proximal carotid occlusions, which, as a result of external carotid collateralization, demonstrate flow reversal in the ophthalmic artery.

Blood flow velocity is inversely related to the vessel radius. Velocities can therefore be increased in vasospasm (Figure 4-4). Other factors, such as fever, anemia, hypoxia, dominant vessels, and vasopressor therapy, can also result in increased blood velocity. Blood flow and velocities are higher in young patients and lower in the elderly. Cessation of cerebral blood flow, or brain death, can be identified as small spikes with reversal of diastole in intracranial vessels and high-spiked systolic flow with reversal of diastolic flow in the extracranial carotid artery, indicating high-flow resistance (Figure 4-5). The pulsatility index (PI) is an indicator of flow resistance and is calculated as the systolic minus the diastolic velocities divided by the mean. Normal PI is 0.7 to 1.1.[92] High PI may indicate atherosclerosis, intracranial hypertension, or brain death.

The Lindegaard ratio can help discern between elevated flow velocities caused by high-flow states and vasospasm. This ratio is calculated as the mean middle cerebral artery divided by the mean extracranial internal carotid artery velocities. Ratios greater than 3 correlate with angiographic spasm, whereas 6 and above indicate severe spasm.[49,92,94] Mean velocities of 200 cm/sec are consistent with severe vasospasm. Severely compromised blood flow is usually indicated by clinical deficits.

TCD can provide continuous, real-time blood flow velocities intraoperatively during carotid endarterectomies to detect altered middle cerebral artery blood flow during cross clamping or from emboli. AVM flow velocities and collateral flow patterns in patients with

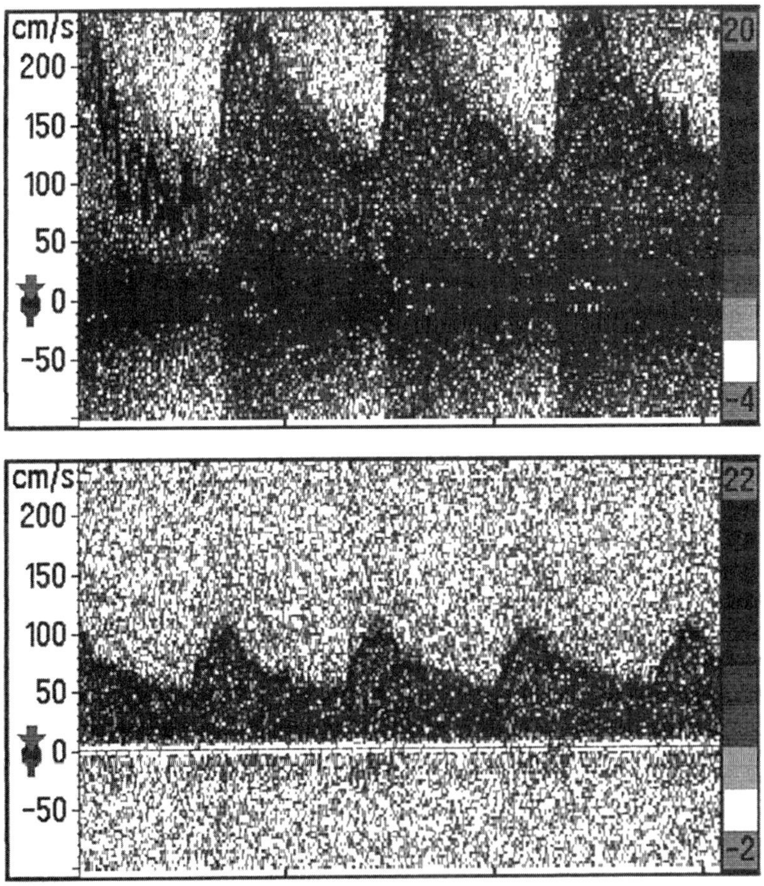

FIGURE 4-4 ■ **Transcranial Doppler tracing of a patient with middle cerebral artery spasm *(top panel).*** The mean velocity is 160 cm/sec, representing moderate vasospasm. A later study *(bottom panel)* demonstrated resolution of the middle cerebral spasm (mean velocity, 66 cm/sec).

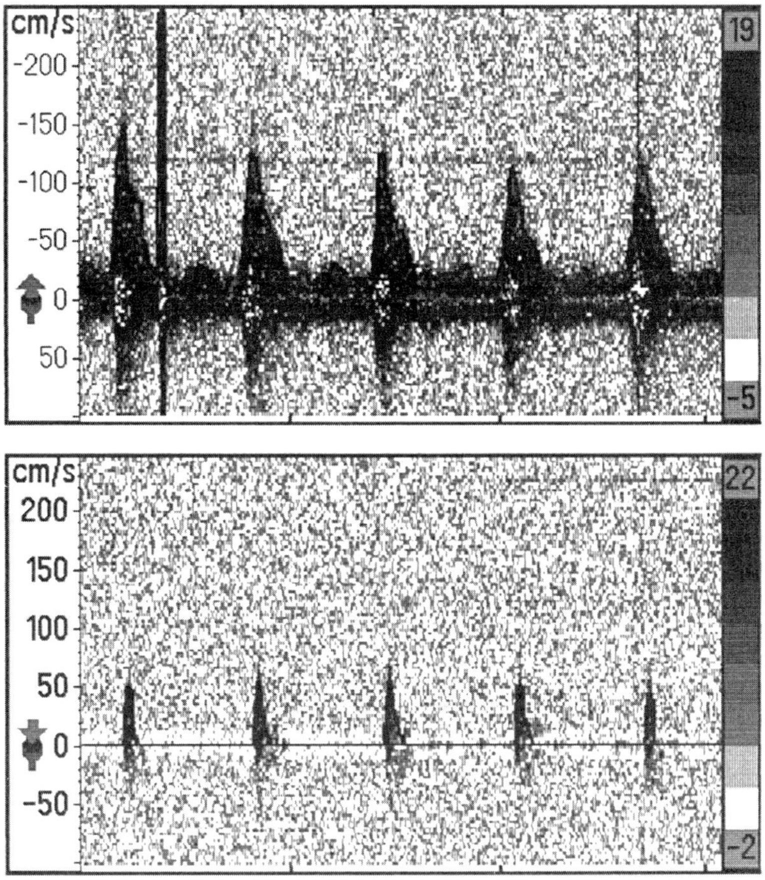

FIGURE 4-5 ■ **Transcranial Doppler tracing in brain death.** Extracranial internal carotid signal *(top panel)* reveals a pulsatility index of 2.58. Note the sharp systolic peak and reversal of diastole. The middle cerebral artery signal *(bottom panel)* is barely extant.

stenotic or occlusive vascular disease can also be determined. Noting velocity changes over time is helpful. Recently, transcranial color duplex sonography has been available for greater anatomical viewing of blood vessels, their diameter, and flow velocities.

Inaccuracies in TCD arise when the angle of insonation is greater than 15 degrees.[92] By catching the edge of the blood vessel, as opposed to the center, the velocity can be underestimated. It has been observed that the resistance index (V_s- V_d/V_s) often remains constant through each vessel when the angle of insonation is correct. Turbulence at branch points can overestimate velocities. Thick temporal squamae make insonation difficult. Vertebrobasilar ectasia can create difficulty finding wave forms at certain depths.

Brain Oxymetry

Brain oxymetry measures oxygen delivery to the brain, which is an indirect measure of cerebral blood flow. Oxymetry best reflects the balance between brain oxygen supply and demand, or metabolism, and is discussed in further detail later in this chapter.

CEREBRAL METABOLISM

As stated previously, the brain uses 20% to 25% of the total body oxygen consumption.[44,73] During aerobic metabolism, 1 mole of glucose plus 2 moles of oxygen combine through a series of well-known pathways (glycolytic, citric acid cycle, electron transport chain) to ultimately yield 38 moles of ATP. ATP provides energy for cellular metabolism, including maintenance of membrane integrity and protein synthesis. Under normal circumstances, less than 10% of glycolysis occurs under aerobic conditions, converting 1 mole of glucose into 2 moles of ATP plus 2 moles of lactic acid. Such metabolism results in less energy production and lactate accumulation, ultimately leading to acidosis and cellular breakdown if allowed to become the predominant pathway.[69] For the neuron, 55% of the energy metabolism is used for nerve conduction and synaptic transmission, whereas 45% is for cellular maintenance. Gray matter consumes nearly twice as much glucose and oxygen as white matter.[73]

Knowledge of CBF is critical to assessing the state of cerebral metabolism. The metabolic parameters include the cerebral oxygen delivery (DO_2), $CMRO_2$, CMRG, and cerebral metabolic rate of lactate consumption (CMRL). Oxygen delivery is the product of the arterial oxygen content, which takes hemoglobin levels into account, and the CBF. Determination of the metabolic rates of consumption or production requires comparison of the cerebral arterial and venous substrate content. Jugular bulb sampling is the most common method of obtaining the venous blood.

The arteriovenous oxygen difference compares the oxygen content of the arterial and venous blood. The normal value is approximately 6.5 ml/dl[74,75] because the jugular oxygen content is usually less than arterial. The brain extracts oxygen from the arterial supply as the metabolic demand dictates. The oxygen extraction ration (O_2ER) indicates the state of cerebral metabolism independent of the hemoglobin by using the ratio of arterial and venous oxygen saturation. Normal O_2ER is approximately 35%. This parameter may arguably be more "stable," or reliable, than the $AVDO_2$ in assessing cerebral metabolism supply and demand.[19,20] In ischemic states the brain extracts as much oxygen as needed for metabolism, resulting in an increase in $AVDO_2$ and O_2ER, at least initially. Metabolic activity (demand) therefore exceeds the oxygen supply (CBF). When blood flow and oxygen delivery exceed the metabolic demand, $AVDO_2$ and O_2ER are decreased, resulting in hyperemia, or luxury perfusion. As is apparent, these parameters ($AVDO_2$ and O_2ER) do not require CBF and can be performed inexpensively and frequently.

$CMRO_2$ is calculated from the product of CBF and $AVDO_2$. The $CMRO_2$ is 3.4 ml/100g/min, or 1.5 μmole/g/min. $CMRO_2$ can be increased by 10% per 1° C temperature elevation and decreased by 5% per 1° C temperature decrease.[73] CMRG and CMRL are calculated in a similar fashion as $CMRO_2$, using the arterial and venous contents of glucose and lactate, respectively. Normal average CMRG is 5.5 ml/100g/min. Normal average CMRL is -0.23 ml/100g/min, indicating a small degree of baseline lactate production. An increase in lactate production (more negative) indicates possible ischemia. An increase in the lactate/oxygen index (LOI), determined by the ratio of AVDLactate (AVDL) to $AVDO_2$ to greater than 0.8 is an indicator of increased anaerobic metabolism.[73,75] This parameter can be easily obtained without knowledge of CBF.

Robertson and colleagues[75] identified a pattern relating O_2 consumption to blood flow in severely head-injured patients. Two states were identified when ischemia was present. The first, "compensated hypoperfusion," related low CBF to an increase in $AVDO_2$, while $CMRO_2$ remained unchanged and CMRL was normal. An increase in brain O_2 extraction, demonstrated by an increased $AVDO_2$, allowed the total O_2 consumption to remain constant. With persistently low CBF (the "ischemic/infarct" state) the brain is no longer able to extract enough oxygen to maintain normal metabolic function. Therefore, lactate production increases and $AVDO_2$ decreases, possibly because of the decreased total volume of brain able to extract O_2. The authors concluded that as long as the lactate/oxygen index remains normal, $AVDO_2$ can predict the status of cerebral blood flow through an inverse relationship. When ischemia/infarction sets in, the relationship is not reliable and direct CBF measurements are required.

Hypoglycemia/Hyperglycemia

Experimental and clinical evidence suggest that preexisting hyperglycemia exacerbates neuronal injury in ischemia states.[67,70,71,102] Diabetics and nondiabetics with elevated glucose levels may have worse outcomes after stroke.[70,102] Lactic acid production had long been postulated as the mechanism.[71] Nakai and colleagues[67] found that significantly decreased tissue pH is ischemic hemisphere in hyperglycemic rates. Other possible causes are reduction in regional cerebral blood flow[27,67] and increased glutamate levels.[48]

Not all experimental studies have shown a negative effect of hyperglycemia, especially in focal, permanent ischemic damage.[31,109] Schurr and colleagues[83] found that glucose loading 15 minutes before experimental ischemia resulted in increased neuronal damage. However, preloading with glucose 120 minutes before the ischemia decreased delayed neuronal damage over the 15-minute subjects and control animals. Both groups exhibited similar lactate levels despite their different outcomes.

Hypoglycemia is usually well tolerated in normal brain metabolism.[69] Mild hypoglycemia may offer some neuronal protection during ischemia.[70,89] There has been recent interest in using insulin as a neuroprotective agent.[4,89] The glucose insulin in stroke trial (GIST) is currently underway.[84]

CBF/METABOLIC COUPLING

CBF/metabolic coupling refers to the matching of oxygen and glucose supply (CBF) with utilization (metabolism/consumption). Normally these functions are closely related and change proportionately. During cortical activation, increase in glucose and oxygen consumption is matched with a concomitant increase in blood flow. The reverse is true during hypothermia, anesthesia, or when using high-dose barbiturates.

Several mediators for coupling have been postulated.[25] Among these are vasodilators: hydrogen ion and lactic acid produced by anaerobic metabolism; increased extracellular potassium concentration: prostacyclin; adenosine from ATP breakdown; and nitric oxide. Arachidonic acid derivatives such as thromboxane A_2 are vasoconstrictors.

Neuronally derived nitric oxide may contribute to physiologic coupling. Nitric oxide is a vasodilator produced by nitric oxide synthase, whose action is stimulated by *N*-methyl-D-aspartate (NMDA) receptor activation by the excitatory amino acid glutamate.[91] The latter is released in increased amounts during ischemia.

Adenosine has been identified as a potentially significant mediator of physiological coupling. Adenosine is a purine derivative formed by ATP breakdown and a potent vasodilator. Adenosine production is increased in ischemia, hypoxia, seizures, and states of hypermetabolism.[17,25] During carotid endarterectomy, jugular adenosine concentrations increased in patients experiencing ischemia during carotid cross-clamping.[100] Adenosine may play a key role in hyperemia and uncoupling during the later phases of head injury.[39] After release, adenosine acts on the A_2 vascular smooth muscle receptor. A neuroprotective role has also been identified because adenosine may attenuate ischemic brain injury through A_1 receptor activation.[14,39,69] This activation may inhibit excitatory amino acid release, thereby preventing calcium influx.

Hypothermia in severe head injury provides an example of the decoupling of CBF and metabolism in pathological states. Early CBF decrease and increases in $CMRO_2$, CMRG, and CMRL have been demonstrated.[9,53,54,63] Hypothermia lowers $CMRO_2$, thereby promoting improved CBF/metabolic coupling.[55,66] Early prophylactic hypothermia has been shown in some studies to improve outcomes from severe head injury (SHI).[55]

METABOLIC MONITORING TECHNIQUES

Brain Oxymetry

Near-Infrared Spectroscopy

Near-infrared spectroscopy (NIRS) is a continuous, noninvasive method, having been used during carotid endarterectomies, head injury, cerebral embolic events, and seizures to detect changes in brain oxygen supply and demand.[56] Hemoglobin and cytochrome oxidase, which carry oxygen, have well-developed absorption spectra. Oxyhemoglobin concentration can be used as a "tracer" to determine CBF. Information can be mathematically applied to calculate CBF and CBV.[28] NIRS does not require pulsatile flow.

Near-infrared light (650 to 1000 nm) emanates from emitters placed on the scalp, penetrating to a depth of 2.5 cm. This light is reflected back to a sensor.[56,65] The temporal resolution is approximately 0.5 seconds. Scalp ischemia can influence measurements, although the significance of bone blood flow is uncertain.[56] NIRS was found to correlate well with jugular venous oxygen measurements.[60]

Tissue PO_2

Partial oxygen pressure in tissue (TPO_2) is measured through a sensor coupled with an oxygen pressure measuring instrument, which can be intraparenchymal, on the cortical surface [61] or in the CSF.[51] Using such monitors, differences in TPO_2 have been noted in pathological (edematous) brain tissue and normal cortex.[61] Mass and colleagues[51] found that Cushing's response resulted in good TPO_2 maintenance in experimental intracranial hypertension. Such devices may be useful and minimally invasive for monitoring for cerebral ischemia.

Multi-Modality Monitoring

Currently, monitoring systems such as Neurotrend (Diametrics, Inc., Codman, Raynham, Mass.) measure multiple parameters including PO_2, PCO_2, pH, and temperature to infer blood flow and metabolic status. This technology combines optical fibers with indicators, such as fluorescent ruthenium (PO_2), phenol red (pH), and phenol red plus carbonate (PCO_2). Temperature is measured through a copper thermocoupled system (personal communication, Codman, Raynham, Mass.).

Multimodality monitoring has been applied to head injury[62,110] and aneurysm and hematoma surgery.[26] Zauner and colleagues[100] found that severely head-injured patients who died or remained vegetative had statistically significant decreases in tissue PO_2, increased PCO_2, and decreased pH compared with patients who had favorable outcomes.

Jugular Bulb Oxymetry

Assessing cerebral metabolism is incumbent on knowledge of venous oxygen content, which retrograde jugular bulb sampling can provide. Although such sampling cannot give direct information about blood flow, it provides knowledge of the delicate balance between supply and demand. Measuring jugular venous oxygen saturation ($SjvO_2$) provides a quick, easy estimate of the brain's metabolic needs at any point.

Technique The apex of the triangle formed by the two heads of the sternocleidomastoid muscle forms the landmark for jugular bulb catheter insertion. The carotid artery, lying medial to the internal jugular vein, is palpated and gently displaced. Under sterile conditions, a 23-gauge needle finds the internal jugular vein, aiming cephalad, toward the mastoid process. A large-bore needle then cannulates the vein at a 30-degree angle, and, using the Seldinger technique, a 20-gauge single-lumen central venous pressure catheter is inserted in a retrograde fashion until light resistance is felt. This resistance occurs approximately 12 to 16 cm from the insertion site and represents the jugular bulb at the foramen jugulare. It is helpful to estimate the distance between the insertion site and the mastoid process a priori. Once resistance is felt, the catheter is withdrawn 0.5 cm. This is especially important when using a fiberoptic catheter, because the $SjvO_2$ reading is inaccurate if the light source abuts the wall of the foramen. The catheter must lie within 2 cm of the jugular bulb or the extracerebral circulation will contaminate the venous blood.[34] An anteroposterior skull and neck radiograph confirms the catheter tip location medial to the mastoid process. Complications include catheter malposition, carotid artery puncture, infection, or thrombosis.

Usually 80% to 90% of venous blood drains through the superior sagittal sinus to the dominant (usually right) transverse sinus and internal jugular vein.[22,34] There is little difference between the O_2 content of the left and right jugular veins. Perhaps with focal hemispheric lesions, the ipsilateral jugular might be most representative. In general, most practitioners place the catheter within the right jugular unless there is clearly lateralizing pathology. When in doubt, manual jugular compression can be performed while observing for intracranial hypertension. The dominant jugular usually causes a greater ICP rise.[22]

$SjvO_2$ Information $SjvO_2$ monitoring at the jugular bulb is an indication of global cerebral metabolism and does not demonstrate regional changes. The normal $SjvO_2$ range is 60% to 80%.[52,58] A low oxygen saturation (<50%) indicates a critically ischemic or hypoxic state, resulting in increased cerebral oxygen extraction, usually before cell death sets in.[58] Also, a low $SjvO_2$ represents either decreased supply from hyperventilation, anemia, or intracranial hypertension or increased metabolic demand such as hyperthermia, agitation, or seizures.[44,52,58]

High $SjvO_2$ (>85% to 90%) indicates a hyperemic state in which oxygen delivery exceeds cellular metabolic needs. Increased $SjvO_2$ may also result from vasodilation (e.g., sepsis, acetazolamide challenge), hypercarbia, increased PaO_2, late ischemia, and cerebral blood flow cessation (brain death). Decreased metabolic need resulting from hypothermia; agents such as propofol, barbiturates, and anesthetic gases; and paralysis can also raise $SjvO_2$.[44,52,58]

Continuous $SjvO_2$ Monitoring Continuous fiberoptic $SjvO_2$ monitoring is helpful during situations in which critical global ischemic is anticipated. Such situations include severe head injury,[85] especially in those patients experiencing intracranial hypertension[10,75]; subarachnoid hemorrhage[96]; cardiac bypass; and cerebrovascular, tumor, or hematoma surgery.[58]

A specially designed fiberoptic catheter or pediatric pulmonary artery catheter has been used for the above purpose. The optical fiber transmits two or three wavelengths at 1-ms intervals, reflecting along a receiving fiber to a photosensor.[22] The catheters are precalibrated and may also be calibrated in vivo using co-oximeter data obtained from a jugular bulb sample. Anything that decreases fiberoptic light intensity, such as abutting the jugular foramen, decreases the apparent $SjvO_2$ reading. Therefore most abnormal readings are confirmed with simultaneous blood sampling. An increase in O_2 saturation might indicate catheter pull-out proximal to the jugular bulb, resulting in extracranial venous contamination. Withdrawing blood slowly from the catheter, when properly positioned, also reduces such contamination. Fiberoptic catheter maintenance is labor intensive. Alternatively, intermittent sampling can be performed at regular intervals or during crises to assess the metabolic state. However, improved time resolution with continuous monitoring affords quicker assessment and the ability to perform hemodynamic or metabolic alterations to optimize the balance between supply and demand.

Sheinberg and colleagues[85] used continuous $SjvO_2$ monitoring in 45 patients with severe head injury. The authors noted an excellent correlation between jugular venous samples and fiberoptic catheter values ($r = 0.87$, $p \leq 0.01$) when light intensity was sufficient. Oxygen desaturations were due to intracranial hypertension, hyperventilation/hypocarbia, hypotension, and vasospasm. Increasing $PaCO_2$ in hyperventilated patients improved $SjvO_2$.

Therapeutic maneuvers for intracranial hypertension, such as CPP therapy and hyperventilation, can be more safely performed with $SjvO_2$ monitoring. Improving low CBF through CPP increase may result in positive changes in $SjvO_2$ when global ischemia is present. This information can also help identify the lower CPP limit required to restore adequate oxygen supply. An algorithm for treating jugular oxygen desaturation is provided in Figure 4-6.

Microdialysis

Microdialysis analyzes the concentration of metabolic byproducts in the extracellular space. Such byproducts include lactate, glutamate, pyruvate, aspartate, Na^+, and K^+. This technique uses a small probe and membrane continuously perfused with a physiological solution. At various intervals, dialysate is collected in aliquots and frozen for analysis. High-performance liquid chromatography (HPLC) is used for the final

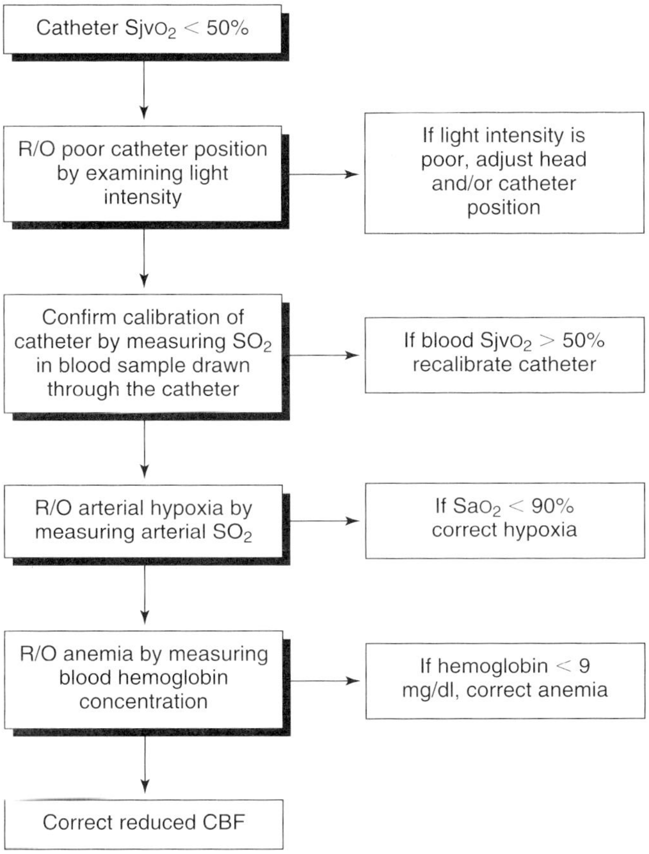

FIGURE 4-6 ■ **Algorithm for diagnosing and treating jugular desaturation.** *SaO_2*, arterial oxygen saturation; *R/O*, rule out (exclude). (From Sheinberg M, Kanter MJ, Robertson CS, et al: Continuous monitoring of jugular venous oxygen saturation in head-injured patients, **J Neurosurg 76:**212-217, 1992.)

analysis. Microdialysis has been used in experimental and clinical head injury and subarachnoid hemorrhage to determine the effects of ischemic insults on brain metabolism.[6,11,57] Knowledge of lactate production and glutamate release may help in thwarting the ischemic process through intervention. However, at present, high cost and maintenance prohibit its use in general clinical practice.

MRI Spectroscopy/PET

Magnetic resonance spectroscopy analyzes regional metabolism. This technology depends on the magnetic spin moment of nuclei such as 1H. Within a specified area of interest, metabolites such as glutamate, aspartate, choline, and lactate can be measured.[86] The aforementioned PET demonstrates and quantifies cerebral metabolism, which is useful in patients with epilepsy and tumors, among other applications. Cortical activation representing increased metabolism can also be visualized with new functional MRI techniques.[46,86]

REFERENCES

1. Anderson RE: Cerebral blood flow xenon-133, **Neurosurg Clin N Am 7:**703-708, 1996.
2. Arbit E, DiResta G: Application of laser Doppler flowmetry in neurosurgery, **Neurosurg Clin N Am 7:**741-748. 1996.
3. Astrup J, Symon L, Branston NM, et al: Cortical evoked potential and extracellular K+ and H+ at critical levels of brain ischemia. **Stroke 8:**51-57, 1977.
4. Auter RN: Insulin, blood glucose levels, and ischemic brain damage, **Neurology 51(Suppl 3):**S39-S43, 1998.
5. Beiner JM, Ogilvy CS, DuBois AB: Cerebral blood flow changes in response to elevated intracranial pressure in rabbits and bluefish: a comparative study, **Comp Biochem Physiol 116A:**245-252, 2000.
6. Bentzer P, Davidsson H, Grande P: Microdialysis-based long term measurements of energy-related metabolites in the rat brain following fluid-percussion trauma, **J Neurotrauma 17:**441-447, 2000.
7. Beristain X, Dujovny M, Gaviria M: Xenon/CT quantitative local cerebral blood flow, **Surg Neurol 46:**437-440, 1996.
8. Beere J, Melot C, Moraine JJ: Bedside estimation of cerebral blood flow, in Vincent JL (ed): **Yearbook of Intensive Care and Emergency Medicine 1994.** Berlin: Springer-Verlag, 1994, pp 646-654.
9. Bouma GJ, Muizelaar JP, Stringer WA, et al: Ultra-early evaluation of regional cerebral blood flow in severely head injury patients using xenon-enhanced computerized tomography, **J Neurosurg 77:**360-368, 1992.
10. Bullock R, Steward L, Rafferty C, et al: Continuous monitoring of jugular bulb oxygen saturation and the effect of drugs acting on cerebral metabolism, **Acta Neurochir Suppl (Wien) 59:**113-118, 1993.
11. Bullock R, Zauner A, Myseros JS, et al: Evidence for prolonged release of excitatory amino acids in severe human head trauma, **Ann N Y Acad Sci 765:**290-298, 1995.
12. Burke AM, Chien S, McMurtry JG, et al: Effects of low molecular weight dextran on blood viscosity after craniotomy for intracranial aneurysms, **Surg Gynecol Obst 148:**9-15, 1979.
13. Carter LP: Thermal diffusion flowmetry, **Neurosurg Clin N Am 7:**749-754, 1996.
14. Chen J, Huang Z, Ma J, et al: A_{2a} adenosine receptor deficiency attenuates brain injury induced by transient focal ischemia in mice, **J Neurosci 19:**9192-9200, 1999.
15. Clyde BL, Firlik AD, Kaufmann AM, et al: Paradoxical aggravation of vasospasm with infusion following aneurysmal subarachnoid hemorrhage, **J Neurosurg 84:**690-695, 1996.
16. Cold E: Cerebral blood flow in acute head injury: the regulation of cerebral blood flow and metabolism during the acute phase of head injury, and its significance of therapy, **Acta Neurochir Suppl (Wien) 49:**2-64, 1990.
17. Coney AM, Marshall JM: Role of adenosine and its receptors in the vasodilation induced in the cerebral cortex of the rat by systemic hypoxia, **J Physiol 1998:**507-518, 1998.

18. Cross KW, Dear PRF, Hathorn MKS, et al: An estimation of intracranial blood flow in the new-born infant, **J Physiol 289:**629-345, 1979.
19. Cruz J: Cerebral oxygenation: monitoring and management, **Acta Neurochir Suppl (Wien) 59:**86-90, 1993.
20. Cruz J, Jaggi JL, Hoffstad OJ: Cerebral blood flow and oxygen consumption in acute brain injury with anemia: an alternative for the cerebral metabolic rate of oxygen consumption? **Crit Care Med 21:**1218-1224, 1993.
21. Cushing H: Concerning a definite regulatory mechanism of the vaso-motor center which controls blood pressure during cerebral compression, **Johns Hopkins Hosp Bull 126:**290-292, 1901.
22. Dearden NM, Midgley S: Technical considerations in continuous jugular venous oxygen saturation measurement, **Acta Neurochir Suppl (Wien) 59:**91-97, 1993.
23. Dewey RC, Pieper HP, Hunt WE: Experimental hemodynamics: vasomotor tone, critical closing pressure, and vascular bed resistance, **J Neurosurg 41:**597-606, 1974.
24. Dickman CA, Carter LP, Baldwin HZ, et al: Continuous regional cerebral blood flow monitoring in acute craniocerebral trauma, **Neurosurgery 28:**264-272, 1991.
25. Doberstein C, Martin NA: Cerebral blood flow in clinical neurosurgery, in Youmans JR (ed): **Neurological Surgery.** Philadelphia: WB Saunders, 1996, pp 519-569.
26. Doppenberg EM, Watson JC, Broaddus WC, et al: Intraoperative monitoring of substrate delivery during aneurysm and hematoma surgery: initial experience in 16 patients, **J Neurosurg 87:**809-816, 1997.
27. Duckrow RB, Beard DC, Brennan RW: Regional cerebral blood flow decreases during hyperglycemia, **Ann Neurol 17:**267-272, 1985.
28. Elwel CE, Owen-Reece H, Cope M, et al: Measurement of adult cerebral hemodynamics using near infrared spectroscopy, **Acta Neurochir Suppl (Wien) 59:**74-80, 1993.
29. Firlik AD, Kaufman AM, Jungreis CA, et al: Effect of transluminal angioplasty on cerebral blood flow in the management of symptomatic vasospasm following aneurysmal subarachnoid hemorrhage, **J Neurosurg 86:**830-839, 1997.
30. Gibbs EL, Lennox WG, Nims LF, et al: Arterial and cerebral venous blood: arterial-venous differences in man, **J Biol Chem 144:**325-332, 1942.
31. Ginsberg MD, Prado R, Dietrich WD, et al: Hyperglycemia reduces the extent of cerebral infarction in rates, **Stroke 18:**570-574, 1987.
32. Haberl RL, Villringer A, Dirnagle U: Applicability of laser-Doppler flowmetry for cerebral blood flow monitoring in neurological intensive care, **Acta Neurochir Suppl (Wien) 59:**64-68, 1993.
33. Harris AP, Koehler RC, Gleason CA, et al: Cerebral and peripheral circulatory responses to intracranial hypertension in fetal sheep, **Circ Res 64:**991-1000, 1989.
34. Jakobsen M, Enevolden E: Retrograde catheterization of the right internal jugular vein for serial measurements of cerebral venous oxygen content, **J Cereb Blood Flow Metab 9:**717-720, 1989.
35. Jones TH, Morawetz RB, Crowell RM, et al: Thresholds of focal cerebral ischemia in awake monkeys, **J Neurosurg 54:**771-782, 1981.
36. Kee DB, Wood JH: Influence of blood rheology on cerebral circulation, in Wood JH (ed): **Cerebral Blood Flow: Physiologic and Clinical Aspects**. New York: McGraw-Hill, 1987, pp 173-185.
37. Kennedy C, Sokoloff L: An adaptation of the nitrous oxide method to the study of the cerebral circulation in children: normal values for cerebral blood flow and cerebral metabolic rate in childhood, **J Clin Invest 36:**1130-1137, 1957.
38. Kety S, Schmidt CF: The determination of cerebral blood flow in man by the use of nitrous oxide in low concentrations, **Am J Physiol 143:**53-55, 1945.
39. Kochanek PM, Clark RSB, Obrist WD, et al: The role of adenosine during the period of delayed cerebral swelling after severe traumatic brain injury in humans, **Acta Neurochir Cuppl (Wien) 70:**109-111, 1997.
40. Koehler RC, Backofen JE, McPherson RW, et al: Cerebral blood flow and evoked potentials during Cushing response in sheep, **Am J Physiol 256:**H779-788, 1989.
41. Kontos HA: Nitric oxide and nitrosothiols in cerebrovascular and neuronal regulation, **Stroke 24 (suppl I):**I-155-I-158, 1993.
42. Kontos HA: Regulation of the cerebral circulation, **Ann Rev Physio 43:**397-407, 1981.
43. Kontos HA, Wei EP, Navari R, et al: Responses of cerebral arteries and arterioles to acute hypotension and hypertension, **Am J Physiol 234:**H371-383, 1978.
44. Lassen NA: Cerebral blood flow and oxygen consumption in man, **Physio Rev 39:**183-238, 1959.
45. Lassen NA, Astrup J: Ischemic penumbra, in Wood JH (ed): **Cerebral Blood Flow: Physiologic and Clinical Aspects**. New York: McGraw-Hill, 1987, pp 458-466.
46. Lee C, Jack CR, Riederer SJ: Use of functional magnetic resonance imaging, **Neurosurg Clin N Am 7:**665-683, 1996.
47. Lee KR, Hoff JT: Intracranial pressure, in Youmans JR (ed): **Neurological Surgery.** Philadelphia: WB Saunders, 1996, pp 491-518.
48. Li P, Shuaib A, Miyashita H, et al: Hyperglycemia enhances extracellular glutamate accumulation in rates subjected to forebrain ischemia, **Stroke 31:**183-192, 2000.
49. Lindegaard KF, Nornes H, Bakke SJ, et al: Cerebral vasospasm diagnosis by means of angiography and blood velocity measurements, **Acta Neurochir 100:**12-24, 1989.
50. Lucke KT, Kerr ME, Chovanes GI: Continuous bedside cerebral blood flow monitoring, **J Neurosci Nurs 27:**164-173, 164.
51. Maas AIR, Fleckenstein W, deJong DA, et al: Monitoring cerebral oxygenation: experimental studies and preliminary clinical results of continuous monitoring of cerebrospinal fluid and brain tissue oxygen tension, **Acta Neurochir Suppl (Wien) 59:**50-57, 1993.
52. March K: Retrograde jugular catheter: monitoring SjO_2, **J Neurosci Nurs 26:**48-51, 1994.
53. Marion DW, Darby J, Yonas H: Acute regional cerebral blood flow changes caused by severe head injuries, **J Neurosurg 74:**407-414, 1991.
54. Marion DW, Obrist WD, Carlier PM, et al: The use of moderate hypothermia in patients with severe head injury: a preliminary report, **J Neurosurg 79:**354-362, 1993.

55. Marion DW, Penrod LE, Kelsey SF, et al: Treatment of traumatic brain injury with moderate hypothermia, **N Engl J Med 336:**540-546, 1997.
56. Masden PL, Secher NH: Near-infrared oxymetry of the brain, **Prog Neurobiol 58:**541-560, 1999.
57. Matz PG, Pitts L: Monitoring in traumatic brain injury, **Clin Neurosurg 44:**267-294, 1994.
58. Mayberg TS, Lam AM: Jugular bulb oxymetry for the monitoring of cerebral blood flow and metabolism, **Neurosurg Clin N Am 7:**755-765, 1996.
59. McCartney JP, Thomas-Lukes KM, Gomez CR: **Handbook of Transcranial Doppler.** New York, Springer-Verlag, 1997.
60. McCormick PW, Stewart M, Goetting MG, et al: Regional cerebrovascular oxygen saturation measured by optical spectroscopy in humans, **Stroke 22:**596-602, 1991.
61. Meixensberger J, Dings J, Kuhnigk H, et al: Studies of tissue PO_2 in normal and pathological human brain cortex, **Acta Neurochir Suppl (Wien) 59:**58-63, 1993.
62. Menxel M, Doppenberg EMR, Zauner A, et al: Cerebral oxygenation in patients after severe head injury, **J Neurosurg Anesthesiol 11:**240-251, 1999.
63. Metz C, Holzschuh M, Bein T, et al: Moderate hypothermia in patients with severe head injury: cerebral and extracerebral effects, **J Neurosurg 85:**533-541, 1996.
64. Muizelaar JP: CBF and management of the head-injured patient, in Narayan RD, Wilberger J, Povlishock JT (eds): **Neurotrauma.** New York: McGraw-Hill, 1996, pp 531-561.
65. Mullan BP, O'Connor MK, Hung JC: Single photon emission computed tomography brain imaging, **Neurosurg Clin N Am 7:**617-645, 1996.
66. Myseros JS, Bullock R: The rational for glutamate antagonists in the treatment of traumatic brain injury, **Ann N Y Acad Sci 765:**262-271, 1995.
67. Naki H, Yamamoto YL, Diksic M, et al: Triple-tracer autoradiography demonstrates effects of hyperglycemia on cerebral blood flow, pH, and glucose utilization in cerebral ischemia of rats, **Stoke 19:**764-772, 1988.
68. Obrist WD, Thompson HK, King CH, et al: Determination of regional cerebral blood flow by inhalation of 133-Xenon, **Circ Res 20:**124-135, 1967.
69. Pasqualin A: Cerebral metabolism, in Youmans JR (ed): **Neurological Surgery.** Philadelphia: WB Saunders, 1996, pp 455-481.
70. Pulsinelli WA, Levy DE, Sigsbee B, et al: Increased damage after ischemic stroke in patients with hyperglycemia with or without established diabetes mellitus, **Am J Med 74:**540-544, 1983.
71. Pulsinelli WA, Waldman S, Rawlinson D, et al: Moderate hyperglycemia augments ischemic brain damage: a neuropathologic study in the rat, **Neurology 32:**1239-1246, 1982.
72. Ringelstein EB, Otis SM: Physiological testing of vasomotor reserve, in Newell DW AR (eds): **Transcranial Doppler.** New York: Raven Press, 1992, pp 83-99.
73. Ritter AM, Robertson CS: Cerebral metabolism, **Neurosurg Clin N Am 5:**633-645, 1994.
74. Robertson CS: Nitrous oxide technique for CBF measurement, in Narayan RD, Wilberger J, Povlishock JT (eds): **Neurotrauma.** New York: McGraw-Hill, 1996, pp 487-501.
75. Robertson CS, Narayan RK, Gokaslan ZL, et al: Cerebral arteriovenous oxygen difference as an estimate of cerebral blood flow in comatose patients, **J Neurosurg 70:**222-230, 1989.
76. Rosner MJ: Pathophysiology and management of increased intracranial hypertension, in Andrew BT (ed): **Neurosurgical Intensive Care.** New York: McGraw-Hill, 1993, pp 57-112.
77. Rowe GG, Maxwell GM, Castillo CA, et al: A study in man of cerebral blood flow and cerebral glucose, lactate, and pyruvate metabolism before and after eating, **J Clin Invest 38:**2154-2158, 1959.
78. Schrader H, Hall C, Zwetnow NN: Effects of prolonged supratentorial mass expansion on regional blood flow and cardiovascular parameters during the Cushing response, **Acta Neurol Scan 72:**283-294, 1985.
79. Schrader H, Lofgren J, Swetnow NN: Influence of blood pressure on tolerance to an intracranial expanding mass, **Acat Neurol Scand 71:**114-126s, 1985.
80. Schrader H, Lofgren J, Swetnow NN: Regional cerebral blood flow and SCF pressures during the Cushing response induced by an infratentorial expanding mass, **Acta Neurol Scand 72:**273-282, 1985.
81. Schrader H, Zwetnow NN, Morkrid L: Regional cerebral blood flow and CSF pressures during Cushing response induced by a supratentorial mass, **Acta Neurol Scand 71:**453-463, 1985.
82. Schroder ML, Muizelaar JP: Monitoring of regional cerebral blood flow (CBF) in acute head injury by thermal diffusion, **Acta Neurochir 59:**47-49, 1993.
83. Schurr A, Payne RS, Tseng MT, et al: The glucose paradox in cerebral ischemia: new insights, **Ann N Y Acad Sci 893:**386-390, 1999.
84. Scott JF, Robinson GM, French JM, et al: Glucose potassium insulin infusions in the treatment of acute stroke patients with mild to moderate hyperglycemia: the glucose insulin in stroke trial (GIST), **Stroke 30:**793-799, 1999.
85. Sheinberg M, Kanter MJ, Robertson CS, et al: Continuous monitoring of jugular venous oxygen saturation in head-injured patients, **J Neurosurg 76:**212-217, 1992.
86. Shulman RG, Balmire AM, Rothman DL, et al: Nuclear magnetic resonance imaging and spectroscopy of human brain function, **Proc Natl Acad Sci 90:**3127-3133, 1993.
87. Sioutos PJ, Orozco JA, Carter LP, et al: Continuous regional cerebral cortical blood flow monitoring in head-injured patients, **Neurosurgery 36:**943-950, 1995.
88. Steimeier R, Bondar I, Bauhuf C: Assessment of cerebral hemodynamics in comatose patients by laser Doppler flowmetry—preliminary observations, **Acta Neurochir Suppl (Wien) 59:**69-73, 1993.
89. Strong AJ, Fairfield JE, Monteiro E, et al: Insulin protects cognitive function in experimental stroke, **J Neurol Neurosurg Psychiatry 53:**847-853, 1990.
90. Susuki K: The changes of regional cerebral blood flow with advancing age in normal children, **Nogoya Med J 34:**159-170, 1990.

91. Szabo C: Physiological and pathophysiological roles of nitric oxide in the central nervous system, **Brain Res Bull 41:**131-141, 1996.
92. Taormina MA, Nichols FT: Use of transcranial Doppler sonography to evaluate patients with cerebrovascular disease, **Neurosurg Clin N Am 7:**589-603, 1996.
93. Ullman JS, Bederson JB: Hypertensive, hypervolemic, hemodilutional therapy for aneurysmal subarachnoid hemorrhage: is it efficacious? Yes, **Crit Care Clin 12:**697-707, 1996.
94. Ullman JS, Morgan BC, Eisenberg HM: Traumatic subarachnoid hemorrhage, in Bederson HB (ed): **Subarachnoid Hemorrhage: Pathophysiology and Management.** Park Ridge, IL: American Association of Neurological Surgeons, 1997, pp 225-237.
95. van Wylen DGL, D'Alecy LG: Regional blood flow distribution during the Cushing response: alterations with adrenergic blockade, **Am J Physiol** 248(1 Pt 2):H98-H108, 1985.
96. von Helden A, Schneider GH, Unterberg A, et al: Monitoring of jugular venous oxygen saturation in comatose patients with subarachnoid hemorrhage and intracerebral hematomas, **Acta Neurochir Suppl (Wien) 59:**102-106, 1993.
97. Vorstrup S, Henriksen L, Paulson OB: Effect of acetazolamide on cerebral blood flow and cerebral metabolic rate for oxygen, **J Clin Invest 74:**1634-1639, 1984.
98. Wahl M, Schilling L: Regulation of cerebral blood flow—a brief perspective, **Acta Neurochir Suppl (Wien) 59:**3-10, 1993.
99. Wei EP, Kukreja R, Kontos HA: Effects in cats of inhibition of nitric oxide synthesis on cerebral vasodilation and endothelium-derived relaxing factor from acetylcholine, **Stroke 23:**1623-1629.
100. Weigand MA, Michel A, Eckstien H, et al: Adenosine: a sensitive indicator of cerebral ischemia during carotid endarterectomy, **Anesthesiology 91:**414-421, 1999.
101. Wilkins RH: Cerebral vasospasm: prevention and treatment, in Wood JH (ed): **Cerebral Blood Flow: Physiologic and Clinical Aspects.** New York: McGraw-Hill, 1987, pp 613-650.
102. Woo W, Chan YW, Yu YL, et al: Admission glucose level in relation to mortality and morbidity outcome in 252 stroke patients, **Stroke 19:**185-191, 1988.
103. Wood JH, Simeone FA, Fink EA, et al: Correlative aspects of hypervolemic hemodilution: low molecular weight dextran infusions after experimental cerebral artery occlusion, **Neurology 34:**24-34, 1984.
104. Wood JH, Simeone FA, Kron RE, et al: Rheological aspects of experimental hypervolemic hemodilution with low molecular weight dextran: relationships of cortical blood flow, cardiac output, and intracranial pressure to fresh blood viscosity and plasma volume, **Neurosurgery 11:**739-753, 1982.
105. Yamagata S, Carter LP, Erspamer R: Cortical ischemia: effect upon direct cortical response, **Stroke 13:**680-1982.
106. Yonas H, Gur D, Claasen D, et al: Stable xenon enhanced computed tomography in the study of clinical and pathological correlates of focal ischemia in baboons, **Stroke 19:**228-238, 1988.
107. Yonas H, Pindzola R, Johnson DW: Xenon/computed tomography cerebral blood flow and its use in clinical management, **Neurosurg Clin N Am 7:**605-616, 1996.
108. Yoshiura T, Wu O, Sorensen AG: Advanced MR techniques: diffusion MR imaging, perfusion MR imaging, and spectroscopy, **Neuroimag Clin N Am 9:**439-453, 1999.
109. Zasslow MA, Pearl RG, Shuer LM, et al: Hyperglycemia decreases acute neuronal ischemic changes after middle cerebral artery occlusion in cats, **Stroke 20:**519-523, 1989.
110. Zauner A, Doppenbert EMR, Woodward JJ, et al: Continuous monitoring of cerebral substrate delivery and clearance: initial experience in 24 patients with severe acute brain injuries, **Neurosurgery 41:**1082-1093, 1997.

CHAPTER 5

Pathophysiology and Treatment of Intracranial Hypertension

DONALD W. MARION

INTRODUCTION

Severe intracranial hypertension is the proximate cause of death for most patients who die of central nervous system diseases. This is particularly true for traumatic brain injury (TBI) and stroke. However, the successful treatment of intracranial hypertension remains a challenge, and for nearly 40 years no new and effective treatment has been identified, presumably because of an inadequate understanding of the pathophysiology of brain swelling and edema formation.

This chapter describes several critical aspects of the pathophysiology of brain swelling and intracranial hypertension and concludes with a discussion of the clinical treatment of elevated intracranial pressure (ICP).

PATHOPHYSIOLOGY

The intracranial contents include cerebrospinal fluid (CSF), blood, and brain. The brain weighs approximately 1400 g, of which 80% is water. Twenty percent of brain water is extracellular. Normally there is approximately 75 ml of CSF, most of which is located in the ventricles. There is an additional 75 ml of blood, most of which is contained in the postcapillary venous circulation. The intracranial contents are enclosed in a rigid skull that is nonexpansile. Therefore, the appearance of a new mass lesion (e.g., tumor or blood clot) or enlargement of an existing component of the intracranial contents (e.g., brain swelling or hydrocephalus) can occur only if there is displacement of CSF, blood, or brain, or if there is an increase in ICP. This is classically known as the Monro-Kellie doctrine. In fact, the intracranial contents do have the capacity to absorb up to 100–150 ml of new intracranial volume without a significant increase in ICP by displacing blood in the venous circulation and ventricular CSF out of the cranial vault (Fig. 5-1). This ability to accommodate a new or expanding mass lesion is also dependent on age and the time over which the mass expands. Thus a 5-year-old child is least able to accommodate an intracranial mass lesion that appears suddenly, such as a traumatic subdural hematoma, whereas an elderly individual may be found to have a large, slow-growing asymptomatic meningioma occupying one third of the cranial vault. With old age the brain may shrink by as much as 20% to 30%.

Hydrocephalus

CSF is produced within the ventricles by the choroid plexus at a rate of approximately 0.4 ml per minute or 400–500 ml per day. It is produced through active

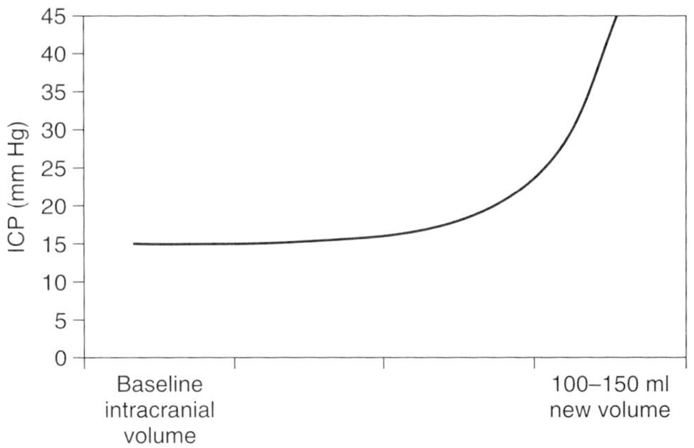

FIGURE 5-1 ■ Intracranial pressure volume curve.

transport and thus under some pressure. CSF normally circulates through the lateral ventricles, the foramen of Monro, the third ventricle, the aqueduct of Sylvius, the fourth ventricle, and out the foramina of Luschka and Magendie. It then circulates over the spinal cord and brain and is eventually absorbed by passive transport into the arachnoid granulations and superior sagittal sinus. In trauma or aneurysmal subarachnoid hemorrhage, it is not uncommon for the breakdown products of blood to disturb the passive absorption of CSF at the arachnoid granulations and lead to communicating hydrocephalus. Lesions of the fourth ventricle (e.g., tumors), or lesions in the brainstem that obstruct the aqueduct of Sylvius can cause obstructive hydrocephalus. This condition is suspected when the lateral and third ventricles are disproportionately larger than the fourth ventricle.

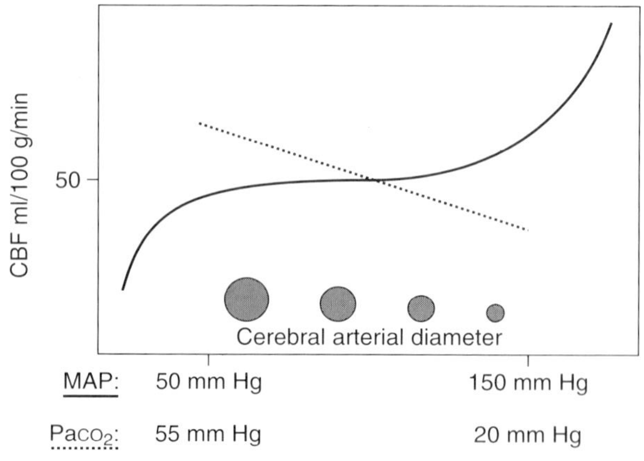

FIGURE 5-2 ■ Normal pressure and chemical autoregulation of cerebral blood flow.

Cerebral Blood Flow and Blood Volume

Abnormalities of cerebral blood flow (CBF) also can contribute to intracranial hypertension. Although cerebral blood flow is not directly related to ICP, in healthy individuals it is directly related to the cerebral blood volume. Normally there is a 2% change in cerebral blood volume with each unit change in CBF. But this relationship may be lost, either regionally or globally, following traumatic brain injury (TBI), stroke, or aneurysmal subarachnoid hemorrhage. In one study of patients with severe TBI, elevation of the mean arterial blood pressure by 30 mm Hg led to a 30% increase in CBF in some patients, but the ICP actually decreased in those same patients.[9] Obviously there could not have been an increase in blood volume associated with the increase in CBF.

Abnormalities in the normal reflexive response of cerebral arteries to changes in the mean arterial blood pressure (pressure autoregulation) or to changes in the arterial $P\text{CO}_2$ and pH (chemical autoregulation) also are common soon after TBI and stroke[10] (Fig. 5-2). Diminished or supranormal pressure or chemical autoregulation usually occurs within and surrounding contusions and infarcts but may be present throughout most of the brain in cases of severe diffuse injury.[9,16,28,35] Because of the loss of autoregulation, prolonged hypotension or aggressive hyperventilation therapy can cause or exacerbate ischemia and subsequent brain swelling in vulnerable regions of the brain following trauma or stroke.

Cerebral Edema

During the first few days after severe TBI or stroke, intracranial hypertension is most likely the result of brain swelling, assuming that hematomas have been surgically removed. Although either cerebral edema or hyperemia can cause brain swelling, edema is the most prominent cause soon after the insult. Damage to or infarction of brain tissue causes cytotoxic and vasogenic edema. Cytotoxic edema results from a disturbance of the energy-dependant, cell membrane–associated systems that are responsible for maintaining normal intracellular and extracellular ionic and fluid balance. Vasogenic edema results from disruption of the blood-brain barrier, a common accompaniment of both stroke and TBI, but probably lasting less than 24 hours before spontaneous reconstitution or death of the brain tissue. Vasogenic edema causes an increase in interstitial brain water, and cytotoxic edema refers to swelling of the cells.

Brain Compliance/Elastance

The physiologic relationship between the ICP and brain volume can be referred to as the compliance of the brain. Compliance reflects the stiffness of the brain and is defined as the change in volume divided by the change in pressure ($C = \Delta v/\Delta p$). Elasticity is defined as the change in pressure divided by the change in volume, or the inverse of compliance. If one were to eliminate the effect of ICP on brain compliance by plotting the ICP on a logarithmic axis against volume, a straight line would result. The logarithmic shape of the pressure volume curve is considered to be due to the fact that as the ICP increases, the brain compliance decreases. The slope of this line represents the intrinsic compliance of the brain with the effects of ICP removed. Marmarou and colleagues have referred to the slope as the "pressure volume index," signifying the volume required to increase the ICP tenfold[33] (Fig. 5-3).

In the intensive care unit, a crude measure of compliance can be observed by studying the waveform of the continuous ICP monitor, particularly if a ventricu-

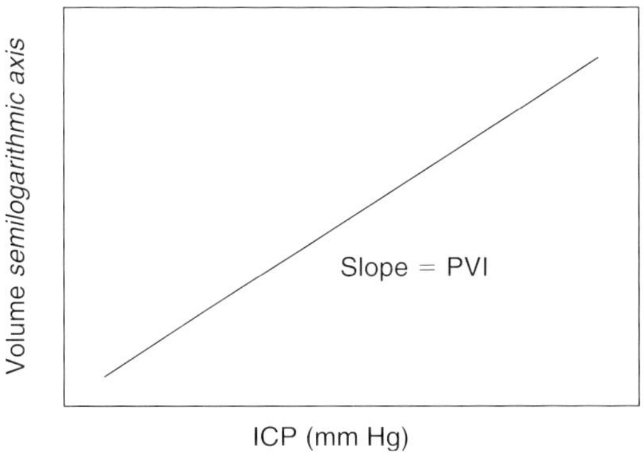

FIGURE 5-3 ■ Pressure volume index. The effect of ICP on brain compliance is eliminated by plotting the ICP on a logarithmic axis.

lostomy catheter is used as the monitor. A high amplitude of the waveform, or wide pulse pressure, indicates a poorly compliant brain. Such patients will tolerate very little or no increase in the intracranial volume before ICP severely rises. Conversely, if the amplitude or pulse pressure of the ICP wave is narrow, an increase in ICP would not be anticipated with a mild increase in intracranial volume.

In summary, the successful treatment of elevated ICP must take into account the Monro-Kellie doctrine. All large intracranial mass lesions must be surgically removed. Hydrocephalus must be treated by CSF diversion, and brain swelling must be successfully treated. Ideally the treatment of brain swelling would be directed by the relative components of hyperemia versus edema, both at a global and regional level. Unfortunately, noninvasive clinical monitoring technology does not yet exist that allows for the accurate distinction between hyperemia and edema at a regional level. The problem is further confounded by the fact that the relative contribution of edema and hyperemia to brain swelling changes over time.

TREATMENT OF INTRACRANIAL HYPERTENSION

Goals of Therapy

It is not entirely clear for any given patient or any given disease state what the critical threshold of ICP is above which there will be irreversible cerebral ischemia or brain death. It is obvious that if intracranial hypertension exceeds the mean arterial blood pressure there will be a hydrostatic block to CBF and brain death will occur within minutes. For patients with severe TBI there is evidence that far less extreme elevations of ICP may also be deleterious. Analysis of ICP data from the Traumatic Coma Data Bank suggests that brain-injured patients who had ICPs greater than 20 mm Hg, particularly if sustained and refractory to treatment, had significantly worse outcomes than those who did not.[32] Numerous other investigators have reported similar findings, as well as an association between ICPs greater than 20–25 mm Hg and an increased incidence of herniation.[20,34,42] Recently several investigators have found that brain tissue oxygenation and metabolism are worsened if the cerebral perfusion pressure (CPP) falls below 60–70 mm Hg.[4,51,53] Because the normal adult mean arterial pressure (MAP) is 90–100 mm Hg and CPP is the difference between ICP and MAP, maintenance of ICP below 20–25 mm Hg also appears to be physiologically desirable.

Clinical Monitoring

Continuous monitoring of ICP is indicated for any patient at risk for intracranial hypertension (Table 5-1). A ventriculostomy fluid coupled to an external strain-gauge transducer is the oldest, least expensive, and many believe the most reliable monitoring technique. Catheters or probes with the transducer contained in their tip also are popular and relatively accurate. It is not possible to obtain accurate or absolute ICP measurements noninvasively. Monitors placed in the ventricles or brain parenchyma provide more accurate information than those placed in the subdural or epidural space.[5,12,18] Monitoring systems that include a ventriculostomy allow not only for the measurement of ICP, but also for CSF drainage as a means of treatment of intracranial hypertension.

For critically ill neurosurgical patients, particularly those with large infarctions or those with severe TBI, continuous monitoring of systemic temperature and hemodynamics also is strongly recommended. Specifically, the MAP and the central venous pressure or pulmonary artery pressure should be monitored with appropriate

TABLE 5-1 ■ **CNS Diseases Likely to Cause Intracranial Hypertension**

Severe Traumatic Brain Injury
Glasgow Coma Scale score 3–8 after cardiopulmonary resuscitation
Abnormal CT scan of the head with hematoma, contusion, edema, or compressed basilar cisterns
Age over 40
Unilateral or bilateral motor posturing
Severe Hypoxic or Ischemic Brain Injury
Prolonged hypotension, hypoxia, or anoxia
Large Middle Cerebral Artery Infarction
Acute Hydrocephalus

indwelling catheters. The core body temperature is ideally monitored with a bladder or pulmonary artery probe, because rectal temperatures have been shown not to change very quickly with changes in systemic temperature. In both laboratory and clinical studies, hypotension, hypovolemia, and hyperthermia have been associated with worsened neurologic outcomes after TBI, stroke, and subarachnoid hemorrhage.[2,15,23,55] Therefore, optimal critical care of these patients should include maintenance of normotension (MAP > 90–100 mm Hg in adults), normovolemia (CVP > 6 cm H_2O) and normothermia (T < 38°C). The simultaneous monitoring of the ICP and MAP allows for the calculation of the CPP (CPP = MAP minus ICP). This measure of the adequacy of cerebral perfusion is perhaps more relevant than the ICP or MAP alone.[45,46] However, the critical threshold of the CPP is somewhat controversial and most likely lies between 60–70 mm Hg based on current physiologic and clinical studies.[13] The restoration and/or maintenance of a normal intravascular volume is particularly important because therapies commonly used to improve CPP (e.g., vasopressor agents to elevate MAP, barbiturates or hypothermia to reduce ICP) can cause vasoconstriction and worsen regional cerebral ischemia if used when the patient is hypovolemic.

Treatment of Intracranial Hypertension

Sedation and Paralysis

The use of sedatives, such as narcotics, benzodiazepines, or propofol, as well as the use of systemic neuromuscular paralytic agents for the sole purpose of lowering elevated ICP, is controversial. In the absence of agitation or anxiety, there is no clear evidence that paralysis and sedation are of benefit. A study that reviewed data from the Traumatic Coma Data Bank found that the general use of these medications did not appear to be associated with improved outcomes.[24] The study also suggested that those patients who received sedatives and paralytic medications for prolonged periods had significantly longer stays in the intensive care unit and more medical complications compared with those who did not receive those medications.

However, agitation, anxiety, or spontaneous posturing can contribute to intracranial hypertension. For such patients, morphine sulfate at a dose of 2–5 mg/kg/hr together with vecuronium bromide (Norcuron) 10 mg/hr is usually effective in providing optimal sedation and neuromuscular paralysis in adults. Alternatively, a propofol drip may be used to provide adequate sedation without the need for systemic neuromuscular paralysis.[1,8] Propofol may be more easily titrated to the needs of the patient and has a relatively short duration of action, so that within minutes of discontinuing the drip the patient can be examined. Table 5-2 lists commonly used narcotics, sedatives, and neuromuscular paralytic agents together with their usual doses and relative advantages or disadvantages.

CSF Drainage

Drainage of even a small amount of CSF can be very effective in reducing elevated ICP as predicted by the pressure volume curve (see Fig. 5-1). An additional theoretical advantage of CSF drainage is the evacuation of neurotoxic compounds released into the CSF as a result of stroke or TBI. For example, frequent drainage of CSF may help to clear the high levels of ventricular glutamate known to be present after TBI.[3,43] Because these small molecules have been shown to diffuse into the ventricular CSF from damaged brain tissue, a favorable diffusion gradient could thereby be achieved for clearance of the extracellular load of these and other toxic neurochemicals. Intermittent rather than continuous drainage is recommended for two reasons: If the stop cock is open to the atmosphere most of the time, continuous ICP measurements that accurately reflect the pressure in the cranium are not being obtained, and there is evidence that continuous drainage is associated with a greater likelihood of the ventricular walls collapsing around the ports of the ventriculostomy catheter, causing it to malfunction.

Unfortunately, the ease of insertion of transducer-tipped parenchymal ICP monitors has made ventriculostomy catheters relatively less popular and infrequently used in recent years, in favor of the white matter probes.[31]

Diuretics

The intravenous administration of osmotic diuretics, specifically urea, was found to be effective in reducing elevated ICP more than 40 years ago; however, it also was observed that within 90 minutes or more the ICP often returned to its pretreatment level. Since that time, mannitol has replaced urea as the osmotic diuretic of choice for management of ICP because it is associated with fewer side effects. Bolus doses of mannitol (25–50 g/kg) are recommended rather than a continuous infusion because a continuous infusion appears to be more likely to lead to uptake of the mannitol into edematous brain tissue, which causes an unfavorable reversal of the osmotic gradient.[25,37] When first introduced, mannitol was thought to effect a reduction in brain swelling solely by providing a favorable intravascular/extravascular osmotic gradient. Subsequent studies have confirmed this effect.[37] However, when the time course of maximal ICP reduction after administration of the drug is compared with the time needed for diffusion of water from the brain into the intravascular space, it is found that the reduction in ICP often occurs more rapidly than would be expected.[6] Investigators have subsequently shown that mannitol also causes a decrease in blood viscosity,

TABLE 5-2 ■ Sedative and Paralytic Agents Commonly Used for Control of Intracranial Hypertension

Category	Drug	Usual Dose	Duration of Effect	Comments
Sedatives	Diazepam	0.1–0.2 mg/kg	>60 min	Sedation
	Lorazepam	0.04 mg/kg	>60 min	Somewhat
	Midazolam	0.025–0.35 mg/kg	>60 min	Unpredictable
	Propofol	5–50 _g/kg/min	8 min	Expensive
	Etomidate	0.3–0.4 mg/kg/hr	30–60 min	Adrenal suppression
	Pentobarbital	60–120 mg/hr	Hours	Absorbed in fat, long duration
Narcotics	Morphine	2–5 mg/hr	>60 min	
	Fentanyl	50–100 _g/hr	>60 min	Can be easily reversed with (naloxone
	Sufentanil	0.01–0.05 _g/kg/hr	>60 min	Narcan)
Neuromuscular paralytic agents	Succinylcholine	1 mg/kg	5–10 min	Dose can be titrated with twitch monitor
	Vecuronium	4–10 mg/hr	45–60 min	
	Pancuronium	4–8 mg/hr	>2 hrs	

probably by enhancing red blood cell deformability.[41] Studies have shown that mannitol increases CBF by as much as 20% and decreases cerebral blood volume.[39] These seemingly contradictory effects occur because mannitol leads to a decrease in the mean transit time of blood passing through the brain and may also reduce the volume of blood in the venous circulation. So the early reduction in ICP caused by mannitol is most likely because of a reduction in blood viscosity, and later effects are because of diffusion of water from the edematous brain into the blood.

There is some evidence that deterioration of renal function (acute tubular necrosis) is likely to occur if serum osmolarity exceeds 320 mOsm,[21] and most believe that mannitol should not be used if serum osmolarity exceeds this threshold. Likewise, hypernatremia will likely be aggravated by mannitol, and the drug is not recommended if the serum sodium is greater than 155 or 160 mg/dl. In fact, the data supporting these critical thresholds are not strong.

Loop diuretics such as furosemide are sometimes used either alone or in combination with mannitol. The usual dose is 20–40 mg IV. They are thought to be effective by increasing the serum osmolarity, and as with mannitol they are not recommended if serum osmolarity exceeds 320 mOsm or the sodium exceeds 155 mg/dl.

Hyperventilation

Hyperventilation therapy for the treatment of intracranial hypertension was first introduced by Lundburg in the late 1950s.[27] He found a significant decrease in ICP in many patients with severe TBI or brain tumors when the arterial P_{CO_2} was reduced from 40 to 25 mm Hg. He also found that ICP increased if the arterial P_{CO_2} was then normalized. Subsequent investigators showed that in a normal individual, one could expect a 3% to 4% reduction in cerebral blood flow per torr reduction in arterial P_{CO_2}, at least down to an arterial P_{CO_2} of 22–23 mm Hg.[44] They found that there was a fairly predictable relationship between the change in CBF and cerebral blood volume of an approximate 1% reduction in cerebral blood volume per torr change in P_{CO_2}. They concluded that hyperventilation caused a reduction in ICP by causing vasoconstriction, leading to a decrease in CBF and an associated decrease in the cerebral blood volume.

Unfortunately, when hyperventilation therapy was first introduced, there was little or no understanding of the blood flow abnormalities and the abnormalities of autoregulation often associated with severe TBI, stroke, and subarachnoid hemorrhage. Subsequent studies have clearly demonstrated that CBF is often reduced by 50% soon after these insults.[11,29] Indeed, in trauma in particular, CBF surrounding a contusion is typically very near the threshold for irreversible ischemia.[35] Thus the further reduction of CBF caused by hyperventilation therapy could theoretically lead to irreversible ischemia in a vulnerable region of the brain with preexisting low flows. In addition, stroke and TBI can cause loss of chemical autoregulation of the cerebral vasculature soon after the insult.[35] As a result, the response of the regional circulation to changes in arterial Pa_{CO_2} may be quite unpredictable and result in steal of blood flow from vulnerable brain tissue.[17]

The clinical evidence suggesting that aggressive prophylactic hyperventilation therapy worsens outcome for TBI patients is relatively weak.[40] However, there is a large amount of physiologic evidence to support this notion. Several investigators have found that hyperventilation therapy is one of the most common causes of jugular venous oxygen desaturation and reductions in brain tissue Po_2.[22,26,47] Xenon CT/CBF studies have demonstrated a 20% to 30% reduction in CBF following hyperventilation, particularly in the brain tissue surrounding contusions or infarcts.[35]

Our current understanding of the potential deleterious effects of hyperventilation therapy lead to the recommendation that the arterial $Paco_2$ be kept at 35 ± 2 mm Hg whenever possible following severe TBI, subarachnoid hemorrhage, or stroke. Hyperventilation to a $Paco_2$ below this level should only be considered when absolutely necessary to treat intracranial hypertension. Ideally, the patient is hyperventilated only while diagnostic tests are obtained (e.g., computed tomography [CT] scan of the head) to define the cause of the elevated ICP. Surgical causes are immediately treated, and alternative medical treatment for nonsurgical swelling is attempted so that normal arterial $Paco_2$ can be restored as soon as possible.

Barbiturates

The use of barbiturates, particularly pentobarbital, as a means to reduce elevated ICP after all other therapy has failed, has been reported by several investigators during the past three decades. Several prospective randomized clinical trials of this therapy were completed, but none clearly demonstrated efficacy of barbiturates.[20,49,54] However, one of these studies did suggest improved outcomes with barbiturate treatment if the drug was effective in reducing elevated ICP.[20] In addition, some of the studies found that if patients were hypovolemic while receiving barbiturates, their outcomes were actually worse than control subjects, and some have argued that this therapy may have been found to be beneficial if the treated patients were kept normovolemic. Current recommendations are that pentobarbital be considered for the treatment of intracranial hypertension that is refractory to all other medical or surgical therapy. Before initiating treatment, central venous or pulmonary arterial pressure monitoring should be instituted and normal or high-normal intravascular volume achieved. We use a loading dose of pentobarbital administered as 200 mg boluses over the course of 20 to 30 minutes, up to a maximum of 1 g or less if there is a reduction in ICP or reduction in the MAP suggesting cardiotoxicity. The patient is then started on an intravenous infusion of 60 mg/hr, which may be increased to 120 mg/hr or more in adults. Continuous EEG monitoring can be used to help guide the most appropriate dose, because little or no benefit should be expected from further increases in the dose once burst suppression has been achieved. The most common toxic effect of barbiturates is suppression of myocardial contractility and reduced cardiac output. This can be minimized by maintaining a normal intravascular volume.

Attempts should be made to wean the patient from barbiturate therapy as soon as possible because a relatively high risk of infection, particularly pneumonia, is associated with long-term barbiturate use.

Novel Therapies

Increasing clinical evidence suggests that moderate hypothermia (32–33° C) can be effective in reducing elevated ICP.[14,19,30,36,50] The use of hypothermia as a last resort after barbiturate therapy and other conventional treatments have failed has been reported,[50] as has its use as an initial treatment to help reduce the mediators of secondary brain injury that are most prominent soon after TBI.[30] Although virtually all clinical trials have shown that hypothermia leads to a significant decrease in ICP, only one trial has demonstrated improved outcomes for a subgroup of TBI patients who received this treatment.[30] Schwab et al recently reported the use of hypothermia for patients with middle cerebral artery infarctions.[48] The patients were cooled to a core body temperature of 33–34° C for 48 to 72 hours, with treatment initiated at a mean of 14 hours after onset of symptoms. Although this was not a randomized clinical trial, the mortality rate was nearly half of what might have been expected based on historical controls for this group of patients.

Unfortunately, therapeutic moderate hypothermia is the only new treatment that has been shown to be of benefit. Numerous drug trials of different N-methyl-D-aspartate (NMDA) receptor antagonists, calcium channel antagonists, antioxidants, systemic alkalizing agents, and blockers of other critical pathways thought to be responsible for secondary brain injury have been completed, and none have found a beneficial effect of the drugs being tested.

Based on these and other investigations, it is increasingly apparent that new therapies that are effective in reducing elevated ICP and improving neurologic outcome following TBI, stroke, or subarachnoid hemorrhage will have to block more than one, and probably multiple, mechanisms responsible for secondary brain injury.

Targeted Versus Stepwise Therapy

The traditional approach to the treatment of intracranial hypertension is to begin with therapies that are least toxic and progress to more toxic therapies only after the less toxic therapies are no longer effective for reducing the ICP. With this "stepwise" or "staircase" approach one might begin the treatment of intracranial hypertension with intermittent CSF drainage, then add narcotics and neuromuscular paralysis, then intermittent boluses of mannitol, and finally barbiturates, each new therapy being added only if the previous therapies were ineffective.

Some 20 years ago, J. Douglas Miller argued that we should be able to identify a predominant pathophysiologic or hemodynamic cause of intracranial hypertension in individual patients and target our therapy to treat that cause.[38] For example, he suggested that some patients had intracranial hypertension primarily as a result of hyperemia. For those patients the most rational initial treatment would be hyperventilation therapy. In other patients edema was the predominant cause, and they would best respond to osmotic diuretics rather than a reduction of CBF. Based on Miller's philosophy, a number of neurotrauma units have adopted various protocols for the targeted therapy of intracranial hypertension; however, this approach relies on the availability of physiologic monitoring techniques that can define the cause of brain swelling. The technology for monitoring blood flow at a global and regional level remains relatively crude. Continuous measures of jugular venous oxygen saturation represent global averages that ignore significant regional heterogeneity. Brain tissue PO_2 or microdialysis samples only a very small area of the brain. Xenon CT/CBF studies provide regional CBF information but can only be obtained once a day or less because of the need to transport the patient. Therefore, we believe that it is premature to recommend targeted therapy for intracranial hypertension, particularly if it includes the use of hyperventilation.

CONCLUSION

During the next several years, it is likely that more effective therapies for elevated ICP will be discovered. Because uncontrollable intracranial hypertension is the single most common cause of neurologic death and disability following stroke and TBI, the identification of such therapies should be a research priority. Recent research already has provided a much better understanding of the compounds and metabolic cascades responsible for secondary brain injury and suggested several potential therapeutic strategies. For example, recent investigations suggest that the IL-6/IL-10 ratio in CSF is very closely associated with outcome[7] and therapies that suppress the IL-1–levels in the CSF have been shown in at least one study to be associated with improved outcomes.[30] Verifying the linkage between these molecular mediators of secondary brain injury and subsequent brain swelling should help to define new therapies that can improve outcomes for patients who suffer a TBI, stroke, or aneurysmal subarachnoid hemorrhage.

REFERENCES

1. Albrecht S, Frenkel C, Ihmsen H, et al: A rational approach to the control of sedation in intensive care unit patients based on closed-loop control. **Eur J Anaesthesiol 16:**678–687, 1999.
2. Azzimindi G, Bassein L, Nonino F, et al: Fever in acute stroke worsens prognosis: a prospective study. **Stroke 26:**2043–2050, 1995.
3. Baker AJ, Moulton RJ, MacMillan VH, et al: Excitatory amino acids in cerebrospinal fluid following traumatic brain injury in humans. **J Neurosurg 79:**369–372, 1993.
4. Bardt TF, Unterberg AW, Hartl R, et al: Monitoring of brain tissue PO_2 in traumatic brain injury: effect of cerebral hypoxia on outcome. **Acta Neurochir Suppl (Wien) 71:**153-6:153-156, 1998.
5. Barlow P, Mendelow AD, Lawrence AE, et al: Clinical evaluation of two methods of subdural pressure monitoring. **J Neurosurg 63:**578-582, 1985.
6. Barry KG, Berman AR: Mannitol infusion. Part III. The acute effect of the intravenous infusion of mannitol on blood and plasma volume. **N Engl J Med 264:**1085-1088, 1961.
7. Bell MJ, Kochanek PM, Doughty LA, et al: Interleukin-6 and interleukin-10 in cerebrospinal fluid after severe traumatic brain injury in children. **J Neurotrauma 14:**451-457, 1997.
8. Birka A: New perspectives on the use of propofol [letter]. **Crit Care Nurse 19:**18-19, 1999.
9. Bouma GJ, Muizelaar JP: Relationship between cardiac output and cerebral blood flow in patients with intact and with impaired autoregulation. **J Neurosurg 73:**368-374, 1990.
10. Bouma GJ, Muizelaar JP: Cerebral blood flow, cerebral blood volume, and cerebrovascular reactivity after severe head injury. **J Neurotrauma 9:**S333-S3481992.
11. Bouma GJ, Muizelaar JP, Choi SC, et al: Cerebral circulation and metabolism after severe traumatic brain injury: the elusive role of ischemia. **J Neurosurg 75:**685-693, 1991.
12. Bruder N, N'Zoghe P, Graziani N, et al: A comparison of extradural and intraparenchymatous intracranial pressure in head injured patients. **Intensive Care Med 21:**850-852, 1995.
13. Bullock R, Chesnut RM, Clifton G, et al: Guidelines for the management of severe head injury. **J Neurotrauma 13:**639-731, 1996.
14. Burger R, Vince H, Meixensberger J, et al: Hypothermia influences time course of intracranial pressure, brain temperature, EEG and microcirculation during ischemia-reperfusion. **Neurol Res (20 Suppl) 1:**S52-60, 1998.
15. Chesnut RM, Marshall SB, Piek J, et al: Early and late systemic hypotension as a frequent and fundamental source of cerebral ischemia following severe brain injury in the Traumatic Coma Data Bank. **Acta Neurochir Suppl (Wien) 59:**121-125, 1993.
16. Cold G, Jensen FT, Malmros R: The effects of Pa_{CO_2} reduction on regional cerebral blood flow in the acute phase of brain injury. **Acta Anaesthesio Scand 21:** 359-367, 1977.
17. Darby JM, Yonas H, Marion DW, et al: Local "inverse steal" induced by hyperventilation in head injury. **Neurosurgery 23:**84-88, 1988.
18. Dearden NM, McDowall DG, Gibson RM: Assessment of Leeds device for monitoring intracranial pressure. **J Neurosurg 60:**123-129, 1984.
19. Dempsey RJ, Combs DJ, Maley EM, et al: Moderate hypothermia reduces postischemic edema development and leukotriene production. **Neurosurgery 21:**177-181, 1987.

20. Eisenberg HM, Frankowski RF, Contant CF, et al: High-dose barbiturate control of elevated intracranial pressure in patients with severe head injury. **J Neurosurg 69:**15-23, 1988.
21. Feig PU, McCurdy DK: The hypertonic state. **N Engl J Med 297:**1449–1977.
22. Gopinath SP, Robertson CS, Contant CF, et al: Jugular venous desaturation and outcome after head injury. **J Neurol Neurosurg Psychiatry 57:**717-723, 1994.
23. Hindfelt B: The prognostic significance of subfebrility and fever in ischemic cerebral infarction. **Acta Neurol Scand 53:**72-79, 1976.
24. Hsiang JK, Chesnut RM, Crisp CB, et al: Early, routine paralysis for intracranial pressure control in severe head injury: is it necessary? [see comments]. **Crit Care Med 22:**1471-1476, 1994.
25. Kaufman AM, Cardozo E: Aggravation of vasogenic edema by multiple dose mannitol. **J Neurosurg 77:**584-589, 1992.
26. Kiening KL, Hartl R, Unterberg AW, et al: Brain tissue pO2-monitoring in comatose patients: implications for therapy. **Neurol Res 19:**233-240, 1997.
27. Lundberg N, Kjallquist A, Bien C: Reduction of increased intracranial pressure by hyperventilation. **Acta Psychiatr Scand 34:**4-64, 1959.
28. Marion DW, Bouma GJ: The use of stable xenon-enhanced computed tomographic studies of cerebral blood flow to define changes in cerebral carbon dioxide vasoresponsivity caused by a severe head injury. **Neurosurgery 29:**869-873, 1991.
29. Marion DW, Darby J, Yonas H: Acute regional cerebral blood flow changes caused by severe head injuries. **J Neurosurg 74:**407-414, 1991.
30. Marion DW, Penrod LE, Kelsey SF, et al: Treatment of traumatic brain injury with moderate hypothermia. **N Engl J Med 336:**540-546, 1997.
31. Marion DW, Spiegel TP: Changes in the management of severe traumatic brain injury: 1991-1997. **Crit Care Med 28:**16-18, 2000.
32. Marmarou A, Anderson RL, Ward JD, et al: Impact of ICP instability and hypotension on outcome in patients with severe head trauma. **J Neurosurg 75:** S59-S661991.
33. Marmarou A, Shulman K, Rosende RM: A nonlinear analysis of the cerebrospinal fluid system and intracranial pressure dynamics. **J Neurosurg 48:**332-338, 1978.
34. Marshall LF, Barba D, Toole BM, et al: The oval pupil: clinical significance and relationship to intracranial hypertension. **J Neurosug 58:**566-568, 1983.
35. McLaughlin MR, Marion DW: Cerebral blood flow and vasoresponsivity within and around cerebral contusions [see comments]. **J Neurosurg 85:**871-876, 1996.
36. Metz C, Holzschuh M, Bein T, et al: Moderate hypothermia in patients with severe head injury: cerebral and extracerebral effects [see comments]. **J Neurosurg 85:**533-541, 1996.
37. Miller JD: Clinical management of cerebral edema. **Brit J Hosp Med 20:**152-166, 1979.
38. Miller JD, Piper IR, Dearden NM: Management of intracranial hypertension in head injury: matching treatment with cause. **Acta Neurochir Suppl (Wien) 57:**152—9:152-159, 1993.
39. Muizelaar JP, Lutz H, Becker DP: Effect of mannitol on ICP and CBF and correlation with pressure autoregulation in severely head injured patients. **J Neurosurg 61:**700-706, 1984.
40. Muizelaar JP, Marmarou A, Ward JD, et al: Adverse effects of prolonged hyperventilation in patients with severe head injury: a randomized clinical trial. **J Neurosurg 75:**731-739, 1991.
41. Muizelaar JP, Wei EP, Kontos HA, et al: Mannitol causes compensatory cerebral vasoconstriction and vasodilation in response to blood viscosity changes. **J Neurosurg 59:**822-828, 1983.
42. Narayan RK, Kishore PR, Becker DP, et al: Intracranial pressure: to monitor or not to monitor? A review of our experience with severe head injury. **J Neurosurg 56:**650-659, 1982.
43. Palmer AM, Marion DW, Botscheller ML, et al: Increased transmitter amino acid concentration in human ventricular CSF posttrauma. **Neuro Report 6:**153-156, 1994.
44. Raichle ME, Posner JB, Plum F: Cerebral blood flow during and after hyperventilation. **Arch Neurol 23:**394-403, 1970.
45. Rosner MJ, Becker DP: Origin and evolution of plateau waves: experimental observations and a theoretical model. **J Neurosurg 60:**312-324, 1984.
46. Rosner MJ, Rosner SD, Johnson AH: Cerebral perfusion pressure: management protocol and clinical results [see comments]. **J Neurosurg 83:**949-962, 1995.
47. Schneider GH, von Helden A, Lanksch WR, et al: Continuous monitoring of jugular bulb oxygen saturation in comatose patients—therapeutic implications. **Acta Neurochir (Wien) 134:**71-75, 1995.
48. Schwab S, Schwarz S, Spranger M, et al: Moderate hypothermia in the treatment of patients with severe middle cerebral artery infarction. **Stroke 29:**2461-2466, 1998.
49. Schwartz ML, Tator C, Towed D, et al: The University of Toronto head injury treatment study: a prospective randomized comparison of pentobarbital and mannitol. **Can J Neurol Sci 11:**434-440, 1984.
50. Shiozaki T, Sugimoto H, Taneda M, et al: Effect of mild hypothermia on uncontrollable intracranial hypertension after severe head injury [see comments]. **J Neurosurg 79:**363-368, 1995.
51. Unterberg AW, Kiening KL, Hartl R, et al: Multimodal monitoring in patients with head injury: evaluation of the effects of treatment on cerebral oxygenation. **J Trauma 42:**S32-37, 1997.
52. Valadka AB, Goodman JC, Gopinath SP, et al: Comparison of brain tissue oxygen tension to microdialysis-based measures of cerebral ischemia in fatally head-injured humans. **J Neurotrauma 15:**509-519, 1998.
53. Vespa P, Prins M, Ronne-Engstrom E, et al: Increase in extracellular glutamate caused by reduced cerebral perfusion pressure and seizures after human traumatic brain injury: a microdialysis study. **J Neurosurg 89:**971-982, 1998.
54. Ward JD, Becker DP, Miller JD, et al: Failure of prophylactic barbiturate coma in the treatment of severe head injury. **J Neurosurg 62:**383-388, 1985.
55. Yamamoto M, Marmarou CR, Stiefel MF, et al: Neuroprotective effect of hypothermia on neuronal injury in diffuse traumatic brain injury coupled with hypoxia and hypotension. **J Neurotrauma 16:**487-500, 1999.

CHAPTER 6

Fluid, Electrolyte, and Acid-Base Balance

JOSEPH M. DARBY

GENERAL CONSIDERATIONS

The central nervous system (CNS) plays a vital role in fluid, electrolyte, and acid-base homeostasis. Critically ill neurosurgical patients are uniquely predisposed to perturbations in this homeostasis due to the combined effects of CNS dysfunction, associated systemic problems, and routine therapeutic interventions employed in treatment. Moreover, the potential consequences of such disorders on brain function may be profound. Altered consciousness, impaired cerebral autoregulation, the presence of brain edema, and intracranial hypertension are all factors that present unique challenges in management. Early recognition and treatment of these disorders should favorably affect secondary brain injury in the neurosurgical intensive care unit.

Body Compartments, Water, and Electrolyte Distributions

Under normal circumstances, total body water (TBW) in the adult is approximately 60% of body weight and varies with age and body fat content. Newborns and children have higher body water content than adults, while women and the obese have lower body water contents because of the lower percentage of water in adipose tissue. Roughly two thirds of TBW is intracellular fluid (ICF), with the remaining one third distributed to the extracellular fluid (ECF). Approximately one fourth of the ECF is in the intravascular compartment, with the remaining three fourths in the interstitial space (Fig. 6-1). Included in the extracellular fluid is the transcellular space, which includes water formed by active transport of extracellular water across epithelial cells into such spaces as the gastrointestinal (GI) tract, cerebrospinal fluid (CSF), biliary tract, and lymphatics.[204] The term *third space* is commonly used to refer to fluid accumulating in tissue as a result of direct injury or inflammation that is functionally excluded from the ECF for a variable period. Examples include fluid accumulation in burned or traumatized tissue, or in operative beds.

Total body potassium is approximately 50 mEq/kg, 98% of which is intracellular and 2% of which is extracellular. The intracellular [K^+] ranges from 140 to 150 mEq/L, while the extracellular concentration ranges from 3.5 to 5.0 mEq/L. The high intracellular to extracellular concentration gradient is maintained primarily by the Na-K ATPase pump and is essential for the maintenance of a normal resting membrane potential. Total body sodium is approximately 40 mEq/kg with a concentration gradient that is similar to K^+ but in the opposite direction. Extracellular [Na^+] ranges from 138 to 142 mEq/L, while the intracellular concentration ranges from 5 to 15 mEq/L.

Osmolality and Tonicity

Osmolality is the sum total of particles in solution and is expressed as the molal concentration of all solutes in water (mOsm/kg). Although the relative solute concentrations between the ICF and ECF differ, most cell membranes are freely permeable to water, permitting osmotic equilibrium to occur. Thus osmolality is a major determinant of water distribution between the ICF and ECF. Osmotic pressure is the force for water movement that is generated by differences in osmolality across membranes. Oncotic pressure is the osmotic pressure that is due solely to differences in protein concentration.

Extracellular fluid osmolarity is determined principally by Na^+ and its associated anion, Cl^-, glucose, and urea. Normal serum osmolality is 286±4 mOsm/kg and can be estimated by the following equation[80]:

$$\text{Osmolality (mOsm/kg)} = 2 \times [Na^+] + [\text{glucose}]/18 + \text{BUN}/2.8$$

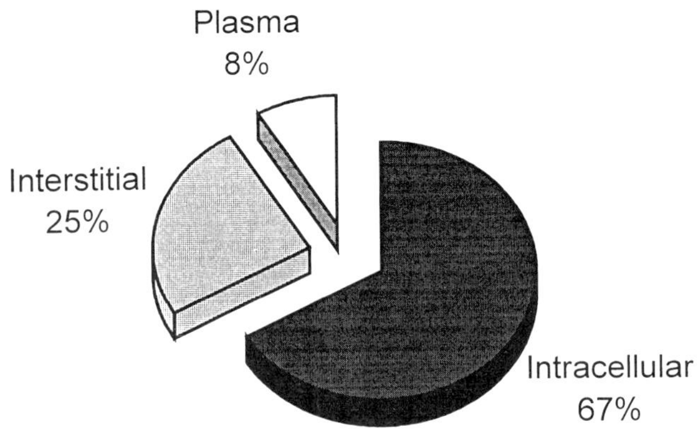

FIGURE 6-1 ■ Compartmental distribution of total body water as a percent of total body water

The measured osmolality is about 10 mOsm/kg greater than the calculated osmolality because of other minor solutes, including calcium, magnesium, protein, and amino acids. This "osmolal gap" can be increased by unmeasured solutes such as alcohol and mannitol or when there is pseudohyponatremia, secondary hyperlipidemia, or hyperproteinemia.

For the purposes of determining the relative state of hydration, the concept of tonicity or effective osmolality is useful, especially in regard to the CNS. *Effective osmolality* refers to osmolality as it relates to solutes that are capable of creating an osmotic gradient. Highly permeable solutes such alcohol and urea do not generally contribute to the development of an osmotic gradient and therefore have little influence on the distribution of water between compartments.

$$\text{Effective osmolality (mOsm/kg)} = 2 \times [Na^+] + [\text{glucose}]/18$$

To this equation, the osmolal concentration of any other osmotically active solute (e.g., mannitol) can be added to calculate effective osmolality. As has been noted, urea is freely permeable to most cell membranes; however, it is only partially permeable to capillaries of the blood-brain barrier (BBB). Therefore, urea contributes to effective osmolality and water flux across the brain when plasma urea concentration is acutely changed, such as therapeutic administration of urea.

In the neurosurgical patient, hypo- or hyperosmolar states are common clinical problems caused mainly by disturbances in water balance (e.g., syndrome of inappropriate secretion of antidiuretic hormone [SIADH], diabetes insipidis) or by osmotherapy. Nonetheless, routine serum osmolality measurements are of limited value in the intensive care unit for the evaluation of fluid and electrolyte disorders because effective osmolality can easily be estimated using plasma sodium and glucose. Monitoring serum osmolarity, however, may be of value in patients receiving mannitol for the control of brain swelling or intracranial hypertension to minimize the potential for exacerbation of brain edema[224] and for the prevention of mannitol-induced renal failure,[54] especially when patients are receiving very high doses or prolonged therapy. The generally recommended upper limits of plasma osmolality during mannitol therapy range from 320 to 350 mOsm/kg.[86,136] Limited data in patients with head injuries indicate that prolonged elevations in plasma osmolality greater than 320 mOsm/kg are associated with high mortality.[14,238] These clinical and other data relating to disruption of the blood-brain barrier[223] reasonably support an upper therapeutic osmolality threshold of 320 mOsm/kg. Calculation and monitoring of the osmolal gap is also useful during mannitol therapy, especially when there is coexistent hyponatremia. The osmolal gap is an indirect measure of plasma mannitol concentration and should be kept at less than 55 mOsm/kg to prevent renal failure.

REGULATION OF BODY FLUIDS

Regulation of Body Water and Osmolality

The regulation body water and tonicity is of extreme importance for proper cellular function, especially within the CNS. Hypoosmolality and cellular swelling within the CNS not only have deleterious effects on cellular function but when unchecked may lead to increases in brain volume and intracranial pressure (ICP). Hyperosmolality and cellular dehydration may also impair CNS function and cause intracranial hemorrhage.

In healthy adults, plasma Na^+ and osmolality are maintained within a markedly narrow range. This stability is achieved primarily by adjusting total body water to keep it in balance with sodium. The posterior pituitary hormone, arginine vasopressin (AVP) or antidiuretic hormone (ADH), is largely responsible for the control of water balance. AVP is a small peptide made in the supraoptic and paraventricular nuclei of the anterior hypothalamus. It is carried down the hypothalamo-hypophyseal tract to the posterior lobe of the pituitary gland from which it is secreted. AVP acts on the collecting duct of the renal tubule, increasing water reabsorption. Osmoreceptors are located in the anterior hypothalamus in the area of the organum vasculosum laminae terminalis (OVLT), a structure that is excluded from the BBB. Changes in osmoreceptor cell volume due to changes in effective plasma osmolarity provide the stimulus for osmotically induced AVP release.[179] The osmotic threshold for

AVP release in humans is approximately 280 mOsm/kg, with AVP levels increasing linearly with osmolality.[193] Under maximal stimulation by AVP the kidney can concentrate urine to achieve a urinary osmolality well over 1000 mOsm/kg, thus conserving water. For example, if solute intake is 600 mOsm/day, renal concentrating mechanisms can raise urine osmolality to 1200 mOsm/kg, necessitating a daily urine output of only 500 ml to eliminate the solute load:

$$\frac{600 \text{ mOsm/day}}{1200 \text{ mOsm/kg}} = 500 \text{ ml/day}$$

Under hyperosmolar conditions, thirst and drinking behavior also contribute importantly to the maintenance of water balance. Even in the absence of AVP, plasma osmolality can generally be maintained as long as water is available and the patient's level of consciousness permits thirst perception.

Suppression of AVP release is the major mechanism controlling water balance under hypoosmolar conditions, permitting the excretion of maximally diluted urine (50–100 mOsm/kg); however, renal water excretion is not only dependent on circulating levels of AVP, but also dependent on solute intake. For example, if solute intake is 900 mOsm/day and urine can be diluted to 50 mOsm/kg, 18 L of urine can be excreted:

$$\frac{900 \text{ mOsm/day}}{50 \text{ mOsm/kg}} - 18 \text{ L/day}$$

Conceptually, 3 L of this fluid is near isotonic and 15 L is solute free or free water. If solute intake decreases to 450 mOsm/day, maximum urinary water excretion is only 9 L and free water excretion is reduced to 7.5 L. In addition, it can be seen that if AVP levels are also increased (reducing urinary dilution), free water excretion will be further impaired. Thus under conditions of reduced solute intake and/or increased AVP, water intake in excess of renal capacity to excrete a free water load will result in hyponatremia and hypoosmolarity.

Although the main stimulus for AVP release is an increase in plasma osmolality, AVP can also be released by a variety of nonosmotic stimuli, including drugs commonly used in neurointensive care (narcotics, barbiturates, carbamazepine), nausea, and conditions associated with an increase in sympathetic tone (pain, hemorrhage, and hypovolemia).[193] One of the most potent nonosmotic stimuli to AVP release is hypovolemia. Baroreceptors in the atria, aortic arch, and carotid sinus are sensitive to decreases in pressure, resulting in AVP release. Hypovolemia is such a potent stimulus to AVP release that AVP will continue to be released even in the presence of plasma hypoosmolality.[77] Renal diluting capacity therefore can be impaired under hypovolemic conditions and may, in part, explain the development hyponatremia and excess circulating AVP in some postoperative patients who are receiving hypotonic fluids.[7,24] Intracranial hypertension has been shown in animal studies to result in nonsuppressible increases in AVP, and in humans increases in both plasma and CSF AVP.[78215,216] It has been suggested that AVP release under such circumstances may be an adaptive response to maintain brain perfusion under ischemic or near ischemic conditions.

Regulation of Intracellular Volume

Many cells have been shown to possess mechanisms for control of cellular volume that balance changes in plasma osmolality with changes in intracellular solute concentration. These adaptive solute changes are operative in the CNS and appear to be important in controlling brain volume under both hypoosmolar or hyperosmolar conditions.[33,212,232,233,249] Under hypoosmolar conditions, intracellular solute concentration decreases by a variety of mechanisms, including increased intracellular binding and extrusion of Na^+, K^+, and Cl^-, preventing cellular swelling. Under hyperosmolar conditions, intracellular solute content increases by an influx of electrolytes, decreased intracellular binding, and increases in amino acid concentration, preventing cellular dehydration.

Transcapillary Water Flux

Water movement between the extracellular and intracellular space is driven mainly by osmotic forces; however, water flux from the intravascular to the interstitial space is more complex and is of concern in the critically ill patient, especially as it relates to the formation of edema fluid in the lung and brain. The forces operative in the bulk transport of water across the capillary membrane are hydrostatic and osmotic. The Starling equation generally describes the factors determining the transcapillary filtration rate (Q_f).

$$Q_f = K_f\,[(P_c - P_i) - \delta(\pi^c - \pi^i)]$$

K_f is the hydraulic conductivity or filtration coefficient of the membrane and is a measure of the relative permeability of the membrane to water under osmotic or hydrostatic stress. P_c is the capillary hydrostatic pressure, and P_i is the interstitial hydrostatic pressure. The relative permeability of a given solute to the membrane is given by its reflection coefficient (δ) and is a measure of its osmotic effectiveness. The higher the reflection coefficient, the more impermeable the solute. Capillary osmotic pressure is π^c and π^i is the interstitial osmotic pressure. Because most capillaries are relatively permeable to salts (e.g., Na^+) and impermeable to proteins, osmotic pressure is determined by oncotic pressure in the steady state. Differences in oncotic pressure between plasma and the interstitium result in a net force favoring fluid movement from the interstitium to the vascular compartment, while hydrostatic pressure forces favor fluid movement out of the vascular space. The net effect in most capillary beds is a slight positive fluid movement out of the vascular space into the interstitium. The lymphatics remove interstitial fluid until their capacity is exceeded, at which point edema occurs.

Unlike most other organ systems, the brain does not have a lymphatic system, nor is there a wide margin of safety in regard to the accumulation of edema fluid, given the fact that it is rigidly encased within the intracranial compartment. CNS capillaries, with their tight junctions, are well adapted to prevent and buffer water movement across the capillary membrane and are an integral component of the BBB.[63,172] Capillaries within the CNS have a very low hydraulic conductivity for water, resulting in relatively less water flux for a given hydrostatic or osmotic gradient. Furthermore, the BBB has very high reflection coefficients for almost all solutes, including sodium. Consequently, any water flux across the intact BBB into the brain interstitium tends to be solute free, setting up an opposing osmotic gradient and buffering further water flux. Under normal conditions, these membrane characteristics minimize water flux between the plasma and brain interstitium. When the BBB is disrupted, hydraulic conductivity and solute permeability increase, resulting in an increase in water flux across the capillary membrane via hydrostatic forces (vasogenic edema) and by reducing the normally high osmotic buffering capacity as salts become freely permeable and proteins leak into the brain interstitium. Excess interstitial fluid may be accommodated in the brain via the Virchow-Robin spaces or by bulk flow through white matter to the ventricular CSF.

Regulation of Body Sodium

Sodium salts are the predominant osmotically active solutes in the ECF and thus are important in determining ECF volume. Body Na^+ balance is controlled by a variety of mechanisms affecting renal Na^+ excretion, which have been described in detail elsewhere.[173,192] Briefly, the relative fullness of the ECF is detected by receptors located in low (intrathoracic) and high (intraarterial) pressure areas of the cardiovascular system. Once changes in ECF volume are detected, renal, neural, and hormonal mechanisms modulate renal Na^+ excretion, decreasing renal Na^+ and water excretion when absolute or relative ECF volume is low and increasing excretion when ECF volume is high. One of the principal renal mechanisms influencing Na^+ excretion in response to changes in ECF volume is physical factors in the peritubular capillary environment, such as hydrostatic and oncotic pressure. Accordingly, when renal perfusion pressure is decreased or oncotic pressure is increased in the peritubular capillary, the balance of Starling forces will favor net Na^+ and water reabsorption in the proximal tubule. Similarly, increases in hydrostatic pressure in the peritubular capillary will favor Na^+ excretion. Independent of changes in renal perfusion pressure or oncotic pressure, changes in the resistance of the glomerular afferent or efferent arteriole can also affect renal Na^+ reabsorption. Vasodilation will tend to increase capillary hydrostatic pressure and renal Na^+ excretion (e.g., low-dose dopamine), while vasoconstriction (e.g., heart failure) reduces hydrostatic pressure and Na^+ excretion. Adrenergic nerve fibers innervate the renal tubules and can also influence renal Na^+ excretion independent of changes in renal hemodynamics. Adrenergic stimulation enhances renal Na^+ reabsorption, while denervation reduces reabsorption of Na^+.

The main hormonal mechanism influencing renal Na^+ excretion is the renin-angiotensin-aldosterone system. Reductions in effective circulating blood volume are detected by the juxtaglomerular apparatus, increasing renin release from the kidney, resulting in increased angiotensin II and aldosterone levels. Aldosterone increases distal tubular Na^+ reabsorption and K^+ excretion. Angiotensin also increases proximal tubular Na^+ reabsorption.

Atrial natriuretic peptide (ANP) is another hormone that is increasingly recognized as an important regulator of Na^+ and water balance. ANP is produced both in atrial myocytes and within the CNS.[153,188] Its overall actions generally oppose those of AVP and angiotensin and plays an important role in the regulation of systemic fluid and electrolyte balance and hemodynamics. Detailed discussions of the role of atrial natriuretic peptides and their role in control of body fluid homeostasis can be found elsewhere.[88,126] Evidence is now accumulating that ANP is involved with local control of brain volume and water and electrolyte content as well.[217,228]

ANP is released into the systemic circulation from the atria under conditions of increased intravascular volume, increased atrial pressure independent of intravascular volume, and under salt-loading conditions. In addition to causing a decrease in renal vascular resistance, an increase in glomerular filtration rate, natriuresis, and diuresis, it also is an inhibitor of the renin-angiotensin-aldosterone axis and reduces salt and water intake. ANP also reduces systemic vascular resistance and blood pressure.

ANP found in the central nervous system is of lower molecular weight than the 28 amino acid peptides that circulates in the periphery. ANP-containing cell bodies and receptor sites are widely distributed throughout the CNS, with their locations and physiologic effects suggesting an important role in cardiovascular and endocrine homeostasis.[10,107,188,242] ANP-containing neurons are concentrated in the anteroventral periventricular region of the third ventricle, the lateral hypothalamus, and visceral centers in the brainstem. Projections of these neurons and ANP receptors are found in such areas as the median eminence, hypothalamus, spinal cord, mesencephalon, and choroid plexus. In concert with its systemic actions, ANP released locally in the CNS inhibits AVP release and blocks angiotensin II–mediated increases in blood pressure and dipsogenesis. Angiotensin II also appears to be locally produced in the brain, with binding sites or local effects in regions that are also involved in the control of fluid balance and hemodynamics (e.g., OVLT, subfornical area, nucleus tractus solitarius, and area postrema).[93,175,242] It is highly likely that neural pathways involving vagal and glossopharyngeal afferents from peripheral baroreceptors control the release of ANP from the heart via ANP-containing neurons in the hypothalamus.[88] Other peptides produced locally in the brain (brain natriuretic peptide and C-type natriuretic peptide) have recently been discovered and appear to have actions similar to ANP.

ANP locally released in the CNS also appears to play an important role in the control of intracellular volume of the brain.[49,50,51,149] ANP opposes AVP-mediated increases in brain capillary permeability, reduces brain water after ischemic insult, and prevents water accumulation under systemic hypoosmolar conditions. These protective effects may occur through ANP-mediated alterations in capillary permeability for both Na^+ and water. ANP also decreases CSF production, contributing to overall volume homeostasis of the brain.[217,228]

FLUID MANAGMENT

Fluid and electrolyte therapy is an essential but often complicated therapeutic intervention in the critically ill patient. Its complexity derives from a variety of neurohumoral responses to critical illness, variable degrees of organ system dysfunction, and commonly used therapeutic interventions such as mechanical ventilation, diuretics, and parenteral nutrition, all of which may affect fluid and electrolyte balance. While proper water and sodium balance are essential in preventing or minimizing brain edema, the restoration and maintenance of an adequate circulating blood volume and tissue oxygenation is essential to prevent multiple systems organ failure and secondary ischemic neuronal injury in the neurosurgical patient.

Fluid and Electrolyte Shifts

Fluid and electrolyte changes associated with critical illness, injury, or surgical stress are generally characterized by salt and water retention. Under such conditions, neurohumoral and renal mechanisms act in concert with compensatory cardiovascular reflexes to preserve intravascular volume and maintain vital organ perfusion. Reduced renal perfusion results in enhanced proximal tubular reabsorption of Na^+, while reductions in effective circulating blood volume activate the renin-angiotensin-aldosterone system, further reducing renal sodium excretion. Water accompanies retained sodium, and baroreceptor-mediated AVP release decreases renal free water excretion, promoting further water retention. Another mechanism acting to preserve intravascular volume in patients with hemorrhage involves the translocation of interstitial fluid to the intravascular compartment.[270]

As a consequence of changes in salt and water balance, critically ill patients often become edematous, gain weight, and occasionally develop hyponatremia with fluid therapy. Increases in vascular permeability associated with sepsis or severe third space fluid losses with multiple trauma further increase fluid requirements, aggravating fluid retention and weight gain. Sodium and water retention are usually maximal during the first several days after insult but may last longer, especially if the patient remains on positive pressure ventilation, which may cause continued AVP release.[211] Resolution is heralded by mobilization of retained salt and water with a spontaneous diuresis and weight loss. Mobilization of retained fluid into the intravascular space can be associated with the development of pulmonary vascular congestion and edema, especially in patients with impaired ventricular function. Tissue trauma or prolonged impaired tissue underperfusion causes cellular K^+ release and a transient increase in plasma K^+. If renal function is intact, increased filtered and excreted K^+ combined with elevated aldosterone levels may cause depletion of total body K^+, predisposing the patient to hypokalemia.

Assessment of Requirements

Among variables to be considered in the assessment of daily fluid and electrolyte requirements are body weight, prior fluid intake and output, serum electrolytes, arterial blood gases, hemodynamics, renal function, and the radiographic appearance of the lungs. Time-related changes in the distribution of fluids as a result of injury, sepsis, or prior fluid resuscitation must also be anticipated and taken into consideration. Fluid administration must be frequently reevaluated in clinical context using basic principles to restore and maintain normal water and electrolyte balance and tissue oxygenation while avoiding complications of therapy.

Fluid requirements can be broken down into three basic components, including maintenance needs, ongoing losses, and deficits. Maintenance water requirements in the uncomplicated surgical patient average

30 to 35 ml/kg/day to balance urinary (800–1500 ml/day), GI (0–250 ml/day) and insensible losses through the lungs and skin (600–900 ml/day). Fever increases insensible water loss by approximately 250 to 300 ml/day per degree Celsius. In the critically ill patient, maintenance water requirements may be reduced variably. For example, patients receiving mechanical ventilation will have insensible water loss through the lung reduced to near zero as a result of breathing fully warmed and saturated gas. In addition, water normally produced via the oxidation of foodstuffs (100–200 ml/day) can be increased to as much as 1000 ml/day in highly stressed patients as a result of tissue catabolism.[204] These factors, combined with increased circulating levels of AVP occurring in response to hemorrhage, hypovolemia, and intracranial disease, may notably reduce maintenance water requirements, perhaps to as low as 20 to 25 ml/kg/day in some patients. Minimum maintenance electrolyte requirements are approximately 75 mEq of sodium and 40 mEq of potassium.

Until the patient resumes a normal dietary intake or nutritional support is instituted, routine maintenance intravenous (IV) fluids are generally given as 5% dextrose in 0.21% to 0.45% saline solutions with supplemental potassium unless intravascular volume deficits dictate the need to use fluids with better intravascular retention (e.g., 0.9% saline or Ringer's lactate). The choice of maintenance fluids becomes problematic in neurosurgical patients given their somewhat unique predisposition to impaired water excretion and the potential consequences of hyponatremia. Cerebral or spinal cord autoregulation may also be impaired soon after injury, necessitating the maintenance of intravascular volumes higher than would normally be necessary in the routine postoperative patient.

Another important consideration in fluid management of the neurosurgical patient is the administration of glucose. Animal data clearly indicate that the presence of hyperglycemia prior to or during ischemic brain injury has a negative impact on neurologic outcome. Hyperglycemia also has also been shown to adversely impact outcome in experimental spinal cord injury.[55] Hyperglycemia probably exerts a negative effect by providing additional substrate to marginally perfused tissue, resulting in anaerobic metabolism, lactic acidosis, and cellular injury.[250] Clinical studies in patients soon after stroke,[15,20,102] cardiac arrest,[131] and head injury[120,142,177,262] corroborate the negative impact on outcome although absolute proof of effect is still lacking. In clinical studies, glucose levels greater than 200 to 250 mg appear to be in the range in which adverse outcomes increase.

With these considerations, early maintenance fluid therapy in critically ill neurosurgical patients at risk for further brain ischemia or edema should be isotonic to plasma (0.9% saline) and dextrose free for at least the first 24 hours after insult. Beyond the early phase of insult, maintenance fluid and electrolyte therapy is tailored after reassessing the clinical condition, fluid and electrolyte balance, and response to therapy. When severe hyperglycemia is present, glucose should be lowered no more than 75 to 100 mg/dl/hr to avoid brain edema brought about by rapid reduction in plasma osmolality. Nutritional support is usually instituted within 48 to 72 hours when possible to meet energy and protein requirements and minimize catabolism, as reviewed in Chapter 7.

Ongoing fluid and electrolyte losses in the neurosurgical patient occur commonly as a result of nasogastric suction, diarrhea, osmotic diuretic use, and third space fluid losses in patients who are multiply traumatized or septic. Accurate replacement requires measurement of the electrolyte composition and volume of lost fluids. Ongoing third space fluid losses cannot be directly measured but are usually manifested by evidence of volume contraction, hemodynamic instability, or impaired organ perfusion. These losses are usually replaced with isotonic crystalloids with or without supplemental colloid.

Volume Resuscitation

Intravascular volume deficits and volume resuscitation are discussed later, separate from common water and electrolyte deficits. Absolute deficits in intravascular volume usually are the result of hemorrhage, third space losses from trauma or sepsis, or overaggressive diuretic use. Relative reduction in intravascular volume may occur in patients who are receiving positive pressure ventilation or in those who are vasodilated from sepsis or spinal cord injury.

Typically, hypovolemia is manifested by one or more signs, including hypotension, tachycardia, oliguria, and lactic acidosis. In such patients, the indications and therapeutic endpoints for volume resuscitation will usually be clear. Often, however, clinical estimates of volume status may be inaccurate because of coexisting organ dysfunction, inexperience, or misinterpretation of available data.[28,29,57,240] In addition, the volume status and appropriate hemodynamic endpoints in neurosurgical patients may be uncertain or require a therapeutic trial to optimize cerebral or spinal cord O_2 delivery under conditions in which autoregulation may be impaired.

Empiric volume resuscitation using crystalloid, colloid, and/or blood are appropriate in acute shock or when there is obvious hypovolemia. Invasive hemodynamic monitoring using either central venous or pulmonary artery catheterization should be considered when empiric volume resuscitation fails to respond as anticipated or when hemodynamic status remains in question. As is reviewed in Chapter 12 reductions in circulating blood volume probably occur more commonly than appreciated in patients after subarachnoid hemorrhage and may increase the risk of delayed cerebral ischemia from vasospasm.[119,155,213,256] Benefit from volume expansion in these patients may derive from improvement in cerebral O_2 delivery by augmentation of low cardiac output or blood pressure or by independent mechanisms such as hemodilution and improved microcirculatory flow. Patients at risk for vasospasm should at a minimum have CVP monitored. Pulmonary artery catheterization may provide the best guide to therapy in those who develop clinical vasospasm.

Multiply traumatized patients with head or spinal cord injury or other neurosurgical patients, particularly those requiring high-dose barbiturate therapy, should also be strongly considered for invasive hemodynamic monitoring to guide volume resuscitation. In the multiply traumatized patient with head injury, volume resuscitation to restore arterial blood pressure is essential to prevent secondary ischemic injury.[135] Although it is widely recommended that mean arterial pressure be maintained at least 80 to 90 mm Hg to maintain continuous positive pressure (CPP) of at least 70 mm Hg, this endpoint is not scientifically established; however, when there are problems with intracranial hypertension, maintaining a cerebral perfusion pressure of at least 70 to 80 mm Hg may be valuable in preventing sudden rises in ICP (plateau waves).[182,183] Patients with acute spinal cord injury and spinal shock should be volume resuscitated to normotensive blood pressure ranges with the goal of minimizing secondary ischemic injury.[230] Caution should be exercised, however, because they are at risk for fluid overload and pulmonary edema due in part to impaired ventricular function, especially when pulmonary capillary wedge pressure (PCWP) exceeds 18 mm Hg.[134] Volume resuscitation in other neurosurgical patients with septic shock, adult respiratory distress syndrome (ARDS), or preexisting cardiopulmonary disease may also be most appropriately guided using the pulmonary artery catheter.

Titration of volume resuscitation to absolute central pressure values (central venous pressure [CVP] and PCWP) may unreliably reflect cardiac filling volumes, especially when there is coexisting cardiac or lung disease or when high levels of airway pressure are required in ventilated patients. Under such conditions, timed fluid boluses guided by baseline pressures and their response to the fluid challenge may be helpful in assessing the limits of volume resuscitation[251] (Table 6-1). Typical empiric fluid challenges in the ICU are usually in the range of 500 ml; however, such challenges often have minimal effect on hemodynamics.[9] Therefore, when hypovolemia is obvious and pulmonary edema is not at issue, a 1 L fluid challenge may effect a better hemodynamic response.

Concern over increasing ICP by fluid resuscitation may temper the vigor with which the hypotensive neurosurgical patient is resuscitated; however, there are no human data indicating that elevation of the CVP alone with fluid resuscitation is sufficient to cause clinically important increases in ICP. In an animal model of head injury and hemorrhagic shock, resuscitation with Ringer's lactate was associated with an increased ICP and reduced brain compliance with increasing CVP.[94] However, because Ringer's lactate is hypotonic and is known to increase ICP and worsen brain edema, it cannot be concluded that the elevation in CVP worsened intracranial dynamics. The endpoints of fluid resuscitation in the brain injured should not be limited by arbitrary CVP or PCWP endpoints.

Resuscitation Fluids

Once the need for volume resuscitation or expansion has been established, the type of fluid employed (i.e., crystalloid versus colloid) must be chosen. Character-

TABLE 6-1 ■ Fluid Challenge Protocol

	Pressures (mm Hg) CVP	PCWP	Volume Challenge (ml/10 min)
Baseline observations	< 6	<12	200
	<10	<16	100
	≥10	≥16	50
Increase during infusion	> 4	> 7	Stop
Increase after infusion	≤ 2	≤ 3	Continue infusion
	>2 >4	>3 >7	Wait 10 min
Increase after 10 minute wait	> 2	> 3	Stop challenge
	≤ 2	≤ 3	Repeat challenge

Modified from reference 67.

istics of commonly available crystalloids and colloids are shown in Table 6-2. Crystalloid solutions such as Ringer's lactate (RL) and 0.9% NaCl are the least expensive and most commonly used for fluids for acute volume resuscitation. Under normal conditions, these crystalloids are evenly distributed to the ECF, with only one fourth or less of the administered volume remaining in the intravascular space in critically ill patients.[91,97] Volumetric replacement of acute blood losses with crystalloid therefore requires at least 3 to 4 times the estimated blood loss and is associated with an expansion of the interstitial space.

Colloid volume expanders are solutions of high-molecular-weight compounds with low vascular permeability. The colloids have longer intravascular retention, resulting in a more rapid and sustained volume expanding effect compared with crystalloids.[91,203] Intravascular retention times of the available colloids are variably quoted, with albumin preparations having relatively shorter intravascular retention than other available colloids. Hyperoncotic colloids (e.g., 6% hydroxyethylstarch, dextran 70) may result in an acute expansion of the intravascular space that transiently exceeds the administered volume. In addition to their added expense, all colloids share common problems, including the potential for volume overload, dilutional coagulopathy, anaphylactoid reactions, and interstitial edema when capillary permeability is increased.[152] Human albumin has a molecular weight of approximately 69,000 and is available in hyperoncotic (25%) and isooncotic (5%) preparations. Five percent purified protein fraction (PPF), containing 83% to 90% albumin, is also available; however, it has no physiologic advantage over 5% albumin and has occasionally been reported to cause hypotension related to impurities. Human albumin has been a favored colloid in neurosurgical practice, perhaps because of reports suggesting that albumin might have a favorable effect on brain edema and ICP[76,105,241,261] and because of a potential beneficial effect on microcirculatory flow.[129] Although there are no prospective controlled trials assessing efficacy of albumin as a volume expander in neurosurgical patients, a review of randomized studies comparing crystalloid with albumin indicates that crystalloids are as effective as albumin when titrated to hemodynamic stabilization.[59]

Dextrans are polymers of glucose that are available as low molecular weight (dextran 40) and high molecular weight (dextran 70) preparations. The higher molecular weight dextrans have been preferred to the lower molecular weight preparation because of better vascular retention. The total dosage is limited to 20 ml/kg within the first 24 hours of use. Interference with platelet function limits the utility of dextrans in the neurosurgical population.

Hydroxethylstarch (HES), or Hetastarch, is a synthetic starch polymer composed mainly of amylopectin, with an average molecular weight of 450,000. Similar to dextrans, infusion volumes have been limited to no greater than 20 to 30 ml/kg because of interference with hemostatic function. Reports of bleeding problems in neurosurgical patients[34,227] argue strongly

TABLE 6-2 ■ Characteristics of Commonly Available Crystalloids and Colloids

Type	[Na$^+$] (mEq/L)	Osmolality (mOsm/kg)	Oncotic Pressure (mm Hg)
CRYSTALLOIDS			
Hypotonic			
5% Dextrose	—	252	—
0.21% NaCl	34	68	—
0.45% NaCl	77	154	—
Isotonic			
0.9% NaCl	154	308	—
Ringer's lactate	130	273*	—
Hypertonic			
3% NaCl	513	1026	—
5% NaCl	856	1712	—
7.5% NaCl	1280	2560	—
COLLOIDS			
5% Albumin	130–160	300	20
5% PPF	130–160	290	20
6% HES	154	310	30
6% Dextran 70	154	310	40–60

*Calculated osmolality. Measured osmolality is lower (see text).
PPF, purified protein fraction; *HES,* hydroxyethylstarch.

against its use as a volume expander in such patients if there is any risk of intracranial hemorrhage.

Colloids versus Crystalloids

The choice of crystalloids over colloids in acute fluid resuscitation has been a subject of longstanding controversy. Until recently, attention has focused on the effect of the type of resuscitation fluid on the development of or exacerbation of pulmonary edema. Although this issue is not entirely resolved, there do not appear to be major differences in the degree of pulmonary dysfunction.[132,147,248] Furthermore, the weight of the available data suggests that colloids are no better in regard to survival and are less cost effective than crystalloids.[17,26,190,245] Mortality rates may actually be higher with colloid-based fluid resuscitation regimens. Interestingly, a recent review of randomized studies has suggested that crystalloid resuscitation is associated with a lower mortality in trauma patients.[23] When colloids are chosen for volume expansion in the neurosurgical patient, albumin is probably the safest in regard to the potential for bleeding complications.

Although there are other aspects to this controversy (e.g., wound healing, gut edema), the effects of fluid type on intracranial dynamics are especially important. It is well recognized that volume expansion with hypotonic crystalloid promotes brain edema in both normal and injured brain. Hemodilution by high-volume isotonic crystalloid resuscitation has also been of concern in regard to the potential for generation or exacerbation of brain edema and intracranial hypertension by lowering oncotic pressure. Although controlled clinical data in this regard are lacking, isovolemic hemodilution studies in uninjured animals suggest that crystalloids increase brain water and ICP only when they result in hypoosmolality.[236,273] Furthermore, studies in animals with cryogenic brain injury and hemorrhagic shock with and without epidural brain compression have shown no important benefit of colloidal solutions over isotonic crystalloids in regard to ICP and brain water[87,110,272] or cerebral hemodynamics.[166] Tranmer[237] did show that ICP and electrical function were worse in animals receiving 0.9% saline compared with 6% HES after cryogenic brain injury; however, this study was heavily criticized on both methodologic and statistical grounds.[234]

In summary, the available data suggest that any detrimental effects of fluid resuscitation on brain edema or ICP are largely dependent on changes in osmolality rather than oncotic pressure. Thus high-volume resuscitation with isotonic crystalloids appears to be safe. Although it has been difficult to show clear benefit of colloids over isotonic crystalloids in regard to brain edema or ICP, they do provide a measure of greater effectiveness in the rapidity and duration of hemodynamic response and should be considered when these effects are desirable. When large volume resuscitations are required in neurosurgical patients combined use of isotonic crystalloid and colloid in a proportion of 3:1 to 4:1 may provide a cost-effective regimen. It should be noted that Ringer's lactate (RL), a common "isotonic" crystalloid used in acute volume resuscitation, has a measured osmolality that is less than its calculated osmolality. Therefore, large-volume crystalloid resuscitations in neurosurgical patients should employ 0.9% saline rather than RL to minimize the potential for the production of hypoosmolality.

Hypertonic-Hyperoncotic Fluid Resuscitation

Over the past decade, interest has grown in hypertonic saline (HTS) for resuscitation of patients in hypovolemic shock. Intravascular administration of HTS creates an osmolar gradient resulting in fluid transfer from the intracellular space into the intravascular space. The addition of colloid to HTS solutions improves vascular retention. Hypertonic-hyperoncotic fluids have potential advantages in acute resuscitation in that small volumes are more effective than isotonic crystalloids in raising blood pressure and cardiac output.[243] Furthermore, experimental studies[87,168,191,235,271] and clinical reports[65,169,189,225,260] indicate a beneficial effect on ICP and brain edema, suggesting that patients with head injuries might derive additional benefit. Animal models of hemorrhagic shock and head injury have demonstrated both reduced resuscitation volumes and ICP compared with Ringer's lactate.[4,12,171,199] Similarly, beneficial effects of HTS have been found in models of spinal cord injury.[264]

Despite these encouraging animal data, small clinical trials in the prehospital phase of care have shown no significant impact of HTS resuscitation on patients with head injury[244] or multiply traumatized patients with hypotension.[138] The use of HTS has also been extended into early hospital management of patients with head injuries. No significant differences in ICP were evident in a small study of adults when HTS was used to treat periodic hemodynamic instability of reduction in urine output for the first 5 days after injury.[197] When HTS was used as a maintenance fluid in pediatric patients with head injury, treatment intensity for raised ICP was reduced, but there were no differences in mean ICP or survival compared with Ringer's lactate.[209]

Aside from its use in the management of acute intracranial hypertension, the role of HTS in the resuscitation of patients with head or spinal cord injuries remains undefined.

Red Cell Transfusion

Red blood cell transfusion is indicated for volume resuscitation when there is ongoing blood loss caused by hemorrhage or when serial laboratory studies show a reduction in hematocrit. Although the maintenance of a hematocrit in the range of 30% to 35% has been advocated as being optimal for the maintenance of systemic and brain oxygen delivery,[35,103] an analysis of cerebral blood flow studies in humans has suggested that the hematocrit that maximizes cerebral O_2 delivery in the normal brain is in the range of 40%[75] (Fig. 6-2). With brain injury, however, cerebral autoregulation may be impaired, with the potential for a reduction in cerebral oxygen delivery under anemic conditions. Recent animal data suggest that a hematocrit of approximately 30% minimizes infarct size in focal ischemia[124] and maximizes cerebral oxygen transport and consumption in global brain ischemia.[239] Transfusion of red cells to maintain hematocrit in the range of 30% seems reasonable in patients with or who are at risk for cerebral ischemia.

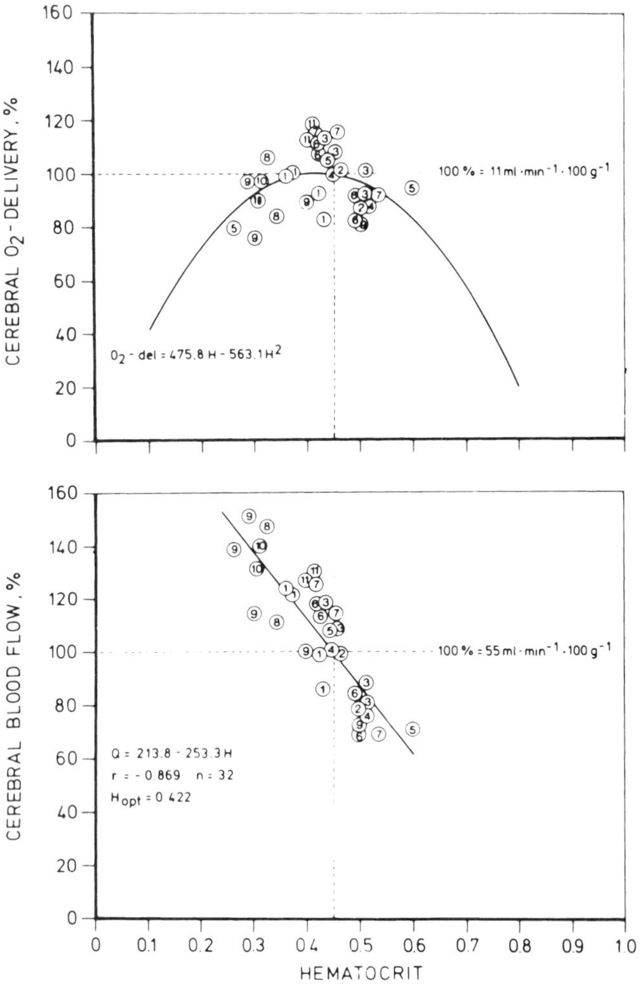

FIGURE 6-2 ■ Summary of human data on the relationship between hematocrit and cerebral O_2 delivery (*top panel*) and cerebral blood flow (*bottom panel*). The hematocrit optimizing O_2 delivery is approximately 42%.[119] (Reproduced with permission.)

DISORDERS OF WATER AND ELECTROLYTE BALANCE

Hyponatremia

Hyponatremia (plasma $Na^+ < 135$ mEq/L) occurs frequently in neurosurgical patients and is of special importance because the osmotic buffering capacity of the brain may be impaired. Hyponatremia occurs in association with various states of body fluid tonicity. Hyponatremia with hyperosmolality may occur with hyperglycemia or mannitol use, while pseudohyponatremia caused by hyperlipidemia or hyperproteinemia is associated with normal plasma osmolality. Hyponatremia observed in critically ill neurosurgical patients is usually associated with reduced osmolarity. Even small decreases in plasma sodium and osmolality may cause cellular swelling, impair brain function, or promote edema formation or raised intracranial pressure.

Neurosurgical patients with subarachnoid hemorrhage and closed head injury are most likely to develop hyponatremia. The incidence of hyponatremia after aneurysmal subarachnoid hemorrhage has been variably reported, with most studies indicating an incidence of approximately 30% to 35%[70,96,202,255]; however, in the International Cooperative Study involving more than 3500 patients the incidence of hyponatremia was only 3.6%.[111] Patients at increased risk for hyponatremia include those with anterior communicating artery aneurysms[121,229] and those who develop third ventricular enlargement.[254] The onset of hyponatremia coincides closely with the time of greatest risk of vasospasm and is associated with an increased incidence of ischemia and infarction.[96,255] In head-injured adults the incidence of hyponatremia is reported in the range of 5% to 12%[53,58,218] and as high as 25% in pediatric patients.[163] The risk of hyponatremia appears to be greater in those with more severe head injuries and those with chronic subdural hematoma and basilar skull fracture.[53,218] Patients with chronic spinal cord injury have been reported to have a prevalence of hyponatremia of 10% to 15% that is related to both renal factors and postural ADH release.[125,206,207,258] Deterioration in level of consciousness, new focal deficits, myoclonus, seizures, or increasing intracranial pressure should raise the suspicion of hyponatremia and hypoosmolality in the acutely brain-injured patient.

SIADH and Cerebral Salt Wasting Syndrome

There are many potential causes of hyponatremia to consider in critically ill patients. In the neurosurgical patient, however, the differential diagnosis of hyponatremia is usually limited to the syndrome of inappropriate ADH (SIADH) and cerebral salt wasting syndrome (CSWS).

Traditionally, hyponatremia occurring in patients with disorders of the central nervous system has been attributed to SIADH.[70,81,92,99,218] SIADH was described in the late 1950s[194] and is defined as the continuous secretion of ADH despite hyponatremia and hypoosmolality with normal or expanded extracellular volume. Other well-recognized causes of hyponatremia such as hypothyroidism, adrenal insufficiency, heart failure, and cirrhosis or nonosmotic causes for increased ADH should be absent. Studies showing increased ADH levels in plasma, CSF, and urine[16,106,137,163,202] tended to support SIADH as the principal cause of hyponatremia in patients with central nervous system disorders. Putative mechanisms for the unregulated ADH release in such patients include a reset hypothalamic osmostat or nonsuppressible "leakage" of ADH from the pituitary gland.[178] The laboratory diagnosis of SIADH in the hyponatremic patient is based largely on an evaluation of urine chemistry, which is inappropriately concentrated (Uosm > Posm) with high urinary Na^+ (>25–30 mEq/L). Although more sophisticated testing can be done, the diagnosis can be presumptively confirmed when simple restriction of fluids results in reduction of urinary sodium losses and correction of hyponatremia. Measurement of uric acid may also be helpful, because uric acid levels are low in SIADH and normal or increased in hypovolemia. A clinical picture similar to SIADH can also be seen in patients with hypopituitarism.[161] ADH levels are increased, but the hyponatremia in these patients is responsive to glucocorticoids.

The "cerebral salt wasting syndrome" (CSWS), was described in the early 1950s[30,164] as hyponatremia occurring in patients with CNS disease with renal salt wasting and volume depletion. Because of the later description of SIADH, CSWS appears to have fallen into obscurity and ultimately led to the widespread and probably incorrect practice of restricting fluid in many neurosurgical patients who developed acute hyponatremia. The weight of current evidence now supports CSWS as the most common cause of hyponatremia in the neurosurgical population.* The evidence favoring salt wasting rather than SIADH includes the poor correlation of ADH levels and plasma sodium, blood volume measurements demonstrating volume depletion, the presence of negative salt balance, and favorable responses to volume expansion and salt repletion.

The pathophysiology of CSWS is not completely understood. The salt wasting is generally thought to be due to a disturbance in central neurohumoral control over the systemic release and regulation of atrial natriuretic peptide. Experimental studies in monkeys with (SAH) lend support to clinical reports in that natriuresis and hyponatremia can occur without increases in ADH.[154] Plasma and CSF ANP levels have been found to be elevated in both eunatremic and hyponatremic patients with subarachnoid hemorrhage and nonaneurysmal intracranial hemorrhage.[46–48,52,181,202] In those with SAH, plasma ANP levels appear to be higher in patients with suprasellar and intraventricular blood.[48] CSF ANP levels have also been found to be significantly increased in SAH patients with increased ICP.[52]

Increased ADH levels may be present soon after brain insult in response to a variety of nonosmotic stimuli (e.g., pain, hypovolemia, narcotics) and is thought to be the main mechanism for hyponatremia when it occurs within the first few days after the ictus. When the onset of hyponatremia occurs several days to a week after insult, it is more likely due to CSWS. ADH levels may also be elevated at this time but are probably an appropriate response to volume depletion. Features distinguishing CSWS from SIADH are shown in Table 6-3.

Firm laboratory criteria differentiating SIADH from CSWS are not yet established. The urinary findings in CSWS are similar to those in SIADH in that urinary osmolarity and sodium are increased. A negative calculated salt balance, increased urinary fractional excretion of sodium (NL = 0.004–0.012), and hypovolemia in an appropriate clinical context usually will be sufficient to establish the diagnosis of CSWS.[130] In contrast to SIADH, an increased urine output may also be present (solute diuresis) in CSWS. The failure of fluid restriction to correct hyponatremia and urinary salt loss in cases of presumed SIADH also is supportive.

Treatment of Hyponatremia

Treatment of critically ill neurosurgical patients with hyponatremia can be complex. The clinical approach to management of hyponatremia requires an evaluation of clinical symptoms, the severity and rate of development and progression, volume status, and the presence of brain edema or intracranial hypertension. Regardless of the mechanism of hyponatremia, excess free water administration will tend to exacerbate hyponatremia or reduce the efficacy of treatment. As a first step, therefore, sources of free water intake (hypotonic IV fluids, parenteral nutrition, and drug carrier solutions) must be eliminated or adjustments made to increase tonicity.

TABLE 6-3 ■ Features of Cerebral Salt Wasting Syndrome

- Late onset
- Volume depletion present
- Hyponatremia responsive to volume and salt loading
- Negative salt balance
- Increased fractional excretion of sodium
- Normal uric acid

*References 37, 95, 106, 108, 130, 155, 210, 247, 253, 256.

In mild, asymptomatic cases of hyponatremia with obvious evidence of hypovolemia (CSWS), isotonic saline is administered and titrated to restore circulating blood volume and normalize serum sodium. In one series of neurosurgical patients with hyponatremia, volume expansion (50 ml/kg/day) in combination with salt loading (12 g/day) was shown to be effective in normalizing serum sodium within 72 hours.[37] When urinary sodium is high and volume status is judged to be normal or increased (SIADH), standard treatment of uncomplicated cases consists of fluid restriction of approximately 800 ml/day. In patients at risk for vasospasm or patients with acute head injury, fluids should not be restricted. Rather, plasma volume should be maintained with volume expanders, and a negative water balance can be effected by employing loop diuretics such as furosemide to correct hyponatremia. This approach requires the use of invasive monitoring and frequent titration of fluids to maintain appropriate volume status.

The rate at which severe symptomatic hyponatremia (<120 mEq/L) is corrected has been of considerable concern and controversy. In this regard, rapid correction of hyponatremia has been linked to the development of neurologic complications such as central pontine myelinolysis or, more generally, osmotic demyelination syndrome.[141,156,221] Experimental studies[220] and a review of clinical studies[25] suggest that neurologic complications that result from correction of severe hyponatremia depend not only on the rate of correction but also on the rate of development of hyponatremia. Cellular adaptation over time to hypoosmolar conditions with the associated loss of intracellular electrolytes probably predisposes to cellular dehydration and injury when challenged by an acute hyperosmolar stress, as would occur when slowly developing hyponatremia is rapidly corrected. It appears that patients who develop hyponatremia at a rate of less than 0.5 mEq/L/hr (chronic) are more prone to develop neurologic complications when their rate of correction is greater than 0.5 mEq/L/hr. On the other hand, hyponatremia that develops at a faster rate can probably be corrected to mildly hyponatremic levels (130–134 mEq/L) at rates of correction in the range of 1 to 2 mEq/L/hr. Most neurosurgical patients developing severe hyponatremia in the ICU will fall into the acute category and should be rapidly corrected when there are seizures, an abrupt deterioration in level of consciousness, or evidence of progressive brain swelling or intracranial hypertension. General principles guiding management in the correction of chronic hyponatremia are shown in Table 6-4.

Most cases of severe symptomatic hyponatremia will be due to SIADH or the administration or absorption of excess free water in the presence of elevated ADH levels. Rapid correction of severe symptomatic hyponatremia is usually accomplished with hypertonic saline and a loop diuretic such as furosemide. It should be remembered that in SIADH the primary problem is usually not salt depletion but excess water. Therefore, treatment is aimed at the reduction of body water, with the goal of restoring osmolality toward normal. The main effect of hypertonic saline is to facilitate a solute diuresis rather than raise serum Na^+, primarily because most of the administered salt is excreted in the urine in SIADH. The use of a loop diuretic enhances free water excretion and contracts intravascular volume, ultimately reducing renal sodium loss. In most cases, 3% saline at an infusion rate of 1 to 2 ml/kg/hr is sufficient to result in a serum Na^+ increase of 1 to 2 mEq/hr.[222] Hypertonic saline is discontinued when signs or symptoms have resolved or when mildly hyponatremic levels have been achieved. In patients with acute intracranial hypertension or mass effect from brain edema, bolus hypertonic saline, mannitol (12.5–25 g), or 30% urea (40–80 g) infused over 6 to 8 hours[41,174] in combination with isotonic saline to maintain intravascular volume should be considered.

TABLE 6-4 ■ General Principles for Correction of Chronic Hyponatremia

- Hourly correction no greater than 0.5 mEq/hr
- Maximum correction not to exceed 20 mEq/L within first 48 hours
- Initial correction not to exceed plasma Na^+ of 128–130 mEq/L
- Delay complete normalization of plasma Na^+ for 1–2 days after initial correction

Modified from reference 274.

Demeclocycline hydrochloride (1200 mg/day in divided doses) can be used in treating the patient with chronic SIADH but has little value in the rapid correction of hyponatremia.[40,69] Demeclocycline should be used cautiously in patients with impairment in renal function. A V_2 (vasopressin) antagonist may soon be available for the treatment of SIADH.[195] For patients with refractory salt wasting and hyponatremia (CSWS), the administration of the mineralocorticoid fludrocortisone (0.1–0.4 mg/day) with increased salt intakes may be effective in reducing renal salt losses and correcting hyponatremia.[106]

Hypernatremia and Hyperosmolarity

Hyperosmolar states in the neurosurgical patient are usually caused by hypernatremia (Na^+ >145 mEq/L). Severe hyperglycemia occasionally contributes to hyperosmolarity in states of insulin resistance, such as sepsis, or as a result of inadequate insulin administration with parenteral nutrition. As has been noted, hyperosmolarity without hypertonicity can occur with alcohol intoxication or renal failure.

In general, hypernatremia can be caused by excessive salt administration (e.g., hypertonic saline resuscitation, $NaHCO_3$) or, more commonly, by excessive water losses. Causes of mild hypernatremia and hyperosmolarity in the neurosurgical ICU include the use of osmotic and loop diuretics, increased evaporative water losses in patients with fever, diaphoresis, or hyperventilation. A solute diuresis caused by enteral feedings in fluid-restricted patients can also cause excessive water losses. More profound degrees of hypernatremia are seen in patients who develop diabetes insipidus.

Clinical signs of isolated hypernatremia and hyperosmolarity are generally seen when serum Na^+ exceeds 160 mEq/L and osmolality is greater than 320 to 340 mOsm/kg. Mortality is increased in head-injured patients who develop hypernatremia and hyperosmolarity.[195,238] Symptoms arising from hypernatremia and hyperosmolarity are generally referable to the central nervous system. A graded impairment of consciousness that depends on the severity of hyperosmolality is the main manifestation of hypernatremia.[184] Seizures are reported; however, these may be related to rapid correction of hypernatremia.[109] Acute hypernatremia may also cause severe brain dehydration and result in subdural, subarachnoid, and intraparenchymal hemorrhage. Venous thrombosis and venous infarction may also occur. The development of intracranial hypotension may also predispose the patient to the development of subdural hygromas. When hypernatremia occurs over a more prolonged period, an adaptive increase in intracellular electrolytes and solute occurs, predisposing the patient to the development of cerebral edema when hypernatremia is corrected rapidly.

In cases of simple dehydration, the free water deficit is calculated using the following formula.

$$\text{Free water deficit} = [0.6 - \text{wt(kg)}] - [1 - (140/\text{current Na}^+)]$$

For example, a 70-kg patient with a plasma sodium of 165 mEq/L would have an estimated free water deficit of approximately 6.4 L.

$$(0.6\ 70\ \text{kg})\ [1 - (140/165)] = 6.4\ \text{kg (L) of water}$$

In general, half the free water deficit can be replaced acutely with the remainder replaced over the next 24 to 36 hours.[79] In patients receiving osmotic diuretics, or in those with prolonged hyperglycemia, hypernatremia may be accompanied by solute loss and depletion of intravascular volume. In such cases, intravascular volume should be replete with volume expanders followed by correction of free water deficits.

Diabetes Insipidus

Diabetes insipidus (DI) is a disorder of excessive renal loss of water, usually caused by a deficiency in secretion of AVP (central DI), and occurs most commonly in the neurosurgical population as a whole. Patients with tumors of pituitary origin as well as head-injured patients account for most of the cases.[27,146] Overall, the incidence of DI in critically ill neurosurgical patients is relatively small and dependent on overall case mix. In one study evaluating the incidence of DI in post-craniotomy patients, the majority of whom were operated on for brain tumors, the incidence was only 6.7%.[11] All cases occurred in patients who had undergone treatment for pituitary tumor. The incidence of DI in patients undergoing aneurysm surgery has been reported at approximately 4%[121,200] and in patients with severe head injury at 2%.[58] Head-injured patients with temporal-parietal injuries and those with fractures that involve the skull base and sella turcica appear to be at increased risk for DI.[32,42,56] Diabetes insipidus can also be expected with high frequency in those patients who develop brain death while receiving somatic life support.[64,162]

In most cases encountered in the ICU, the onset of DI will be heralded by the onset of polyuria (urine output >30 ml/kg/hr), hypernatremia, and plasma hyperosmolality as early as 12 to 24 hours after trauma[158] or in postop patients 1 to 3 days after surgery.[11,205] If damage is limited to the pituitary or lower pituitary stalk, DI may only be transient. On the other hand, high stalk lesions or injury to the hypothalamus usually results in permanent DI. After complete stalk section, a triphasic response may be seen.[198] Polyuria and hypernatremia occur during the first phase, which may last for 2 to 5 days. A second phase of antidiuresis with decreased urinary output and lower serum sodium may last for 5 to 14 days and is eventually followed by permanent DI. Because of associated hypopituitarism, head-injured patients developing DI should have a formal endocrine work up once the patient's clinical condition has stabilized.[56]

Patients with complete DI usually have urinary volumes that range from 10–15 L/day or more, with low urinary osmolality (50–200 mOsm/kg) and specific gravity (1.001–1.005). Characteristically, these patients do not increase urinary osmolality when fluid is restricted, but they remain sensitive to exogenous vasopressin. Because most critically ill neurosurgical patients will not be able to control their own water intake, hemodynamic instability with hypotension is likely in patients with untreated complete DI. Patients with partial DI have urinary volumes well below those with complete DI. Urinary osmolality is in the range of 290 to 600 mOsm/kg and increases with exogenous vasopressin.[145] Several other causes of polyuria must be considered in the neurosurgical patient and include osmotic diuretics (mannitol, iodinated contrast), severe hyperglycemia, and fluid overload. In contrast to DI, a solute diuresis is usually associated with a higher specific gravity (1.009–1.0035) with urinary osmolality usually between 250–320 mOsm/kg.[205] In most cases the diagnosis of DI will be obvious when a patient at risk begins to excrete dilute urine in volumes that exceed fluid intake. Plasma Na^+ and osmolality may be normal at the onset of polyuria; however, the patient will eventually develop hypernatremia and hyperosmolality on repeated measurements. The diagnosis can be confirmed when the administration of vasopressin or the synthetic analog DDAVP causes urine output to decrease and urine osmolality to increase. Patients who have received excessive fluid resuscitations will have concentrated urine and maintain eunatremia when fluid intake is reduced. Examination of the relationship of plasma to urine osmolality may be helpful in evaluating the cause of polyuria (Fig. 6-3). When there are confounding factors such as overhydration or a solute diuresis that coexist with DI, polyuria may persist after vasopressin administration and may create confusion. If salt intake is inadequate or free water administration excessive under these circumstances, hyponatremia may develop rapidly.[122]

Fluid balance is usually in flux during the first few days of ICU admission, complicating management of patients who develop DI. Nonetheless, once the diagnosis is considered, fluid intake, urinary output, and specific gravity must be monitored at least every 1 to 2 hours until the patient has been adequately fluid resuscitated, electrolytes corrected, and a stable regimen of vasopressin established. Standard regimens for acute management have included the use of aqueous vasopressin administered subcutaneously or intramuscularly in doses of 5 to 10 units every 4 to 6 hours. Preexisting expansion of the extracellular volume with resultant edema may result in variable and unpredictable absorption when these routes are used, creating unnecessary difficulty in management. Aqueous vasopressin can also be administered intravenously; however, it has a very short half life and should be given as a continuous infusion starting at 2.5 units/hr and titrated to a urine output in the range of 100 ml/hr.[127] A simpler approach is to use intermittent doses of DDAVP intravenously in doses of 0.5 to 2.0 g. The duration of effect is dose dependent and usually ranges from 8 to 12 hours. Overtreatment can be problematic in patients who have a triphasic response or who develop only transient DI. Therefore, the risk of hyponatremia and brain swelling can be minimized in the ICU phase of care by initiating therapy at lower doses and by redosing when breakthrough polyuria and urinary hypoosmolality occur. The rapidity and degree to which hypernatremia is corrected depends in large part on the severity of hypernatremia and the clinical context. For example, in patients with severe head injury, a slower rate of correction might be preferable to avoid worsening brain edema or intracranial hypertension. Therefore, concomitant with the initiation of vasopressin

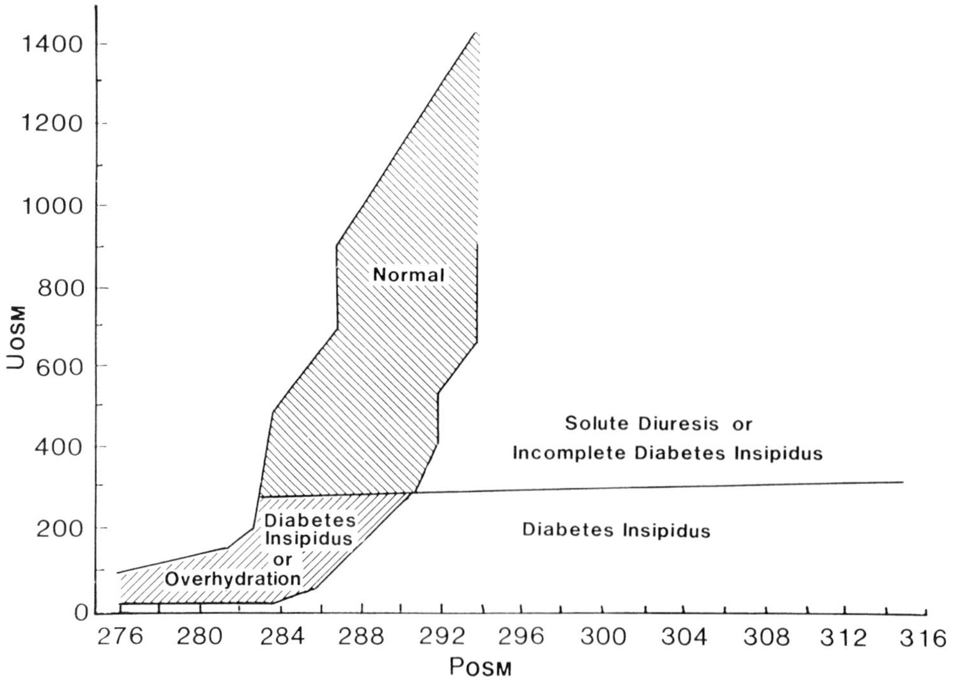

FIGURE 6-3 ■ Relationship of plasma to urinary osmolarity under normal and polyuric conditions.[189] (Modified with permission.)

therapy, the free water deficit is estimated and free water supplemented with 5% dextrose in water or hypotonic saline. The amount of the free water deficit that is replaced acutely depends on clinical circumstances; however, a reasonable goal would be one that results in a plasma sodium of 150 to 155 mEq/L within the first 24 hours of treatment. Similarly, ongoing excess urinary water losses (e.g., >100 ml/hr) are replaced intravenously on an hourly basis with a crystalloid solution approximating that of the urinary loss until polyuria is controlled with vasopressin or DDAVP. Although saline solutions are not recommended for urinary replacement because of associated water loss,[205] salt-containing volume expanders should be used in critically ill patients who are hypotensive and severely volume-depleted to restore blood pressure. Because of the dynamic nature of critically ill patients, serum sodium should be monitored very closely to properly titrate therapy.

Once the patient's condition has stabilized and the patient has left the ICU, a formal dehydration test can be carried out if there is any question of whether the patient has partial or complete DI.[144] Patients with complete DI can be transitioned to intranasal DDAVP, while those with incomplete DI may respond to one of several oral agents, including carbamazepine (200–600 mg/day), chlorpropamide (100–500 mg/day), or clofibrate (500 mg/6 hr).[180]

Other Electrolyte Disorders

Hypokalemia

Hypokalemia (K^+ <3.5 mEq/L) is probably the most commonly recognized and treated electrolyte abnormality in the ICU. As is the case in many other electrolyte disturbances to be discussed later, hypokalemia generally occurs as a result of decreased dietary intake, excessive renal or GI losses, or by intracellular shift from the extracellular space. In most critically ill patients, hypokalemia is likely to be multifactorial in origin and associated with some deficit in total body potassium. Although there are few systematic studies in the neurosurgical population, hypokalemia has been reported to occur in the majority of severely head-injured patients on initial presentation[165] and in approximately 26% of patients within 48 hours of subarachnoid hemorrhage.[5] Despite the limited data, the critically ill neurosurgical population is obviously at high risk for hypokalemia. For example, excessive renal losses of potassium occur as a result of diagnostic and therapeutic use of osmotic diuretics, diabetes insipidus, high doses of glucocorticoids (e.g., methylprednisolone in spinal cord injury), catabolic losses in trauma, and high aldosterone levels in patients who are hypovolemic. Excessive renal potassium loss can also be expected in the presence of alkalemia and hypomagnesemia. Gastrointestinal potassium losses frequently are the result of vomiting, nasogastric suction, and diarrhea. Intracellular shift of K^+ occurs through a variety of mechanisms. Respiratory or metabolic alkalosis, exogenous insulin, or increased insulin stimulated by glucose infusion can all cause intracellular K^+ shift. Adrenergic stimulation by endogenous (or exogenous) catecholamines also causes intracellular K^+ shift and may be the principal mechanism for hypokalemia seen early after severe head injury. Induced hypothermia may also be associated with transcellular shift in potassium and hypokalemia.

Clinical manifestations of hypokalemia may include ventricular and supraventricular arrhythmias, enhancement of digitalis toxicity, reduced gastric and intestinal motility, and impaired renal water conservation, resulting in polyuria when hypokalemia is severe and prolonged. Neuromuscular manifestations include hyporreflexia, weakness, and even paralysis when potassium depletion is severe.

Treatment of hypokalemia is generally initiated when K^+ is less than 3.5 mEq/L. Although there is a linear relationship between serum K^+ and total body K^+ in uncomplicated cases of hypokalemia,[219] acid-base disturbances and other causes of intracellular K^+ shift make estimates of total body potassium difficult to predict in the critically ill patient. Therefore, potassium therapy must be monitored by frequent determinations of serum K^+, especially when hypokalemia is severe, large doses of K^+ are being administered, and there are severe acid-base disturbances or renal insufficiency, or therapeutic hypothermia is being used. Mild asymptomatic hypokalemia is usually treated with 10 to 20 mEq of KCl administered in saline over 1 hour into a large peripheral vein or the central circulation and repeated as necessary. Larger doses (30–40 mEq/hr) can be safely infused in critically ill patients with moderate hypokalemia.[90] The maximum increase in K^+ after such infusions usually occurs at the end of the 1 hour infusion. Profound, symptomatic hypokalemia ($K^+ \leq 2$ mEq/L) can be treated with higher doses of KCl. In fact, doses as high as 80 to 100 mEq/hr have been given.[43] However, when doses larger than 20 mEq/hr are administered, the total dose should be split and administered in aliquots to minimize the risk of inadvertant rapid infusion of a large dose. On the rare occasion when more than 40 mEq/hr is necessary, the dose should be split and administered through separate sites, preferably in large veins away from central veins entering the heart to avoid local cardiac hyperkalemia. Persistent potassium deficits can be treated by adding KCl, or potassium phosphate in phosphate deficient patients, to maintenance IV fluids in a concentration no greater than 40 mEq/L. Alternatively, potassium can be supplemented via the enteric route if NG suction is not being employed. A serum magnesium level should be measured in patients with refractory hypokalemia because these electrolyte disturbances often occur together. In addition, hypokalemia will be difficult to correct without correction of hypomagnesemia. Finally, hypokalemia protects against tetany related to hypocalcemia; therefore, hypocalcemia should be corrected before or concomitant with correction of hypokalemia.

Hypocalcemia

Hypocalcemia occurs in up to 70% of critically ill surgical and medical patients.[45,266] Systematic evaluations of hypocalcemia in critically ill neurosurgical patients have not been done. Hypocalcemia is only clinically important when the physiologically active, ionized fraction (40% of total) is reduced. The remainder is bound to albumin (50%) or chelated (10%). Although hypoalbuminemia can lower total calcium, ionized calcium can be reduced by a variety of factors, including alkalosis, high-circulating free fatty acids (e.g., sepsis, pancreatitis), and agents that chelate calcium such as with albumin infusions, bicarbonate administration, and with high citrate loads administered with massive transfusion.[267] Although citrate received with massive transfusion will lower ionized calcium, this effect is usually transient unless there is a concomitant impairment in citrate metabolism as may occur in patients with hepatic and renal failure or hypothermia. Ionized hypocalcemia occurs in up to 15% to 20% of critically ill patients[269] but cannot be predicted by either total calcium measurements or calculations of ionized calcium corrected for pH and serum albumin concentration.[266]

Common etiologies of hypocalcemia that might be expected to occur in the neurosurgical patient include hypomagnesemia, respiratory alkalosis, sepsis, or, in the multiply traumatized patient, rhabdomyolysis. Hypomagnesemia impairs both parathyroid hormone (PTH) release and action. Alkalosis increases protein binding of calcium; thus patients with marginal calcium levels may develop evidence of frank hypocalcemia when therapeutic hyperventilation is employed. Patients with sepsis or those critically ill patients with unexplained ionized hypocalcemia may be vitamin D deficient, have an impairment in vitamin D metabolism or action, or have impaired release of PTH.[44,265,266] Hyperphosphatemia in severe rhabdomolysis causes hypocalcemia by calcium precipitation or impaired vitamin D metabolism. Patients with renal insufficiency may also develop hypocalcemia secondary to impaired vitamin D metabolism.

Clinical manifestations of ionized hypocalcemia are generally not evident until ionized calcium is less than 0.7 mmol/L (nl = 1.0−1.25 mmol/L) and include hypotension, impaired ventricular function, bradycardia, bronchospasm, and laryngospasm. Neuromuscular manifestations have been described mainly in patients with hypoparathyroidism and include weakness, tetany, paresthesias, hyperreflexia, agitation, confusion, and seizures.[68,82,226] The response to catecholamines and digoxin may be impaired in patients with hypocalcemia.

Before specific treatment for hypocalcemia is initiated, hypomagnesemia should be excluded, because hypomagnesemic patients respond poorly to calcium without correction of magnesium deficiency. Severe symptomatic hypocalcemia is treated with intravenous calcium chloride or calcium gluconate as a bolus of 100 to 200 mg of elemental calcium over 10 minutes (1 g calcium chloride = 272 mg Ca^{+2}, 1 g calcium gluconate = 93 mg Ca^{+2}). Subsequently, a continuous infusion of 1 to 2 mg/kg/hr is initiated and titrated to normalize calcium.[267] Correction usually requires 6 to 12 hours with this regimen. Calcium administration in hyperphosphatemic patients should be done cautiously and concomitant with attempts to lower phosphate to minimize the risk of calcium precipitation in tissues. Rapid infusions of calcium may cause hypertension, bradycardia, A-V nodal blockade, and precipitate digitalis toxicity; thus patients must be monitored closely during infusion. Emergent treatment with IV calcium is generally unnecessary in asymptomatic patients with ionized calcium levels greater than 0.8 mmol/L. In such cases, calcium supplementation in TPN or by the enteric route should be sufficient. Unexplained and persistent hypocalcemia should be further evaluated to exclude hypoparathyroidism and vitamin D deficiency.

Hypophosphatemia

Hypophosphatemia is defined as a serum phosphate level less than 2.7 mg/dl. Clinical manifestations of hypophosphatemia are usually not evident unless levels are severely reduced (<1 mg/dl). Overall, severe hypophosphatemia occurs in more than 0.5% of all hospitalized patients,[19,89,115] but a higher frequency can be expected in critically ill patients, those with multiple trauma,[36] and brain-injured patients who are being hyperventilated.[74] Patients who are malnourished, alcoholic, septic, or who have diabetic ketoacidosis are at increased risk for the development of severe hypophosphatemia. Decreased dietary intake, transcellular shift, or excessive losses through the GI tract or kidney are the main mechanisms by which hypophosphatemia occurs. Transcellular shift of phosphate from the extracellular to the intracellular space occurs by insulin-mediated intracellular transport of phosphate with glucose when carbohydrates are administered parenterally or enterally[98] and has been referred to as "refeeding syndrome."[214] Respiratory alkalosis causes intracellular shift of phosphate by stimulating glycolysis and intracellular phosphate trapping. Hypophosphatemia caused by transcellular shift is associated with hypophosphaturia and the maintenance of normal body stores of phosphate. Drugs such as phosphate-binding antacids, diuretics, and steroids are also commonly implicated as causing or contributing to the development of severe hypophosphatemia. Hypokalemia and hypomagnesemia may also promote hypophosphatemia by impairing renal phosphate reabsorption.[246,252]

A number of complications of severe hypophosphatemia are relevant to the ICU population, including diaphragmatic weakness,[8,84] ventricular dysfunction,[39,159] impaired white cell function,[31] and increased affinity of hemoglobin for oxygen as a result of decreased red cell 2,3-DPG.[123] Neurologic manifestations of hypophosphatemia have been reported to include confusion, seizures, and coma.[123,208,263] Other reported complications include hemolytic anemia, impaired platelet function, and rhabdomyolysis.

Treatment of severe hypophosphatemia has been an issue of some debate. Because most patients developing complications of severe hypophosphatemia have had preexisting illness, alcoholism, or malnutrition and likely have had severe total body phosphate depletion,[118] aggressive treatment in previously healthy but acutely ill patients may not be indicated, especially when the hypophosphatemia is related to transient intracellular shifts. Nonetheless, patients with severe hypophosphatemia who appear to be at risk for complications and those patients with impaired organ function (e.g., respiratory or cardiac failure) should be treated with IV phosphate salts when serum phosphate is less than 1 mg/dl. Infusion of 10 to 15 mmole of phosphate more than 4 hours successfully and safely raises serum phosphate over 1 mg/dl in critically ill patients.[116] Potential complications associated with IV phosphate administration include hypocalcemia and hypotension. Patients without severe hypophosphatemia can be supplemented with a variety of enteric preparations or by adding phosphate to standard TPN formulations as necessary.

Hypomagnesemia

Magnesium is an important ion essential for a variety of cellular processes including enzymatic reactions, protein synthesis, glucose utilization, energy metabolism, and maintenance of membrane integrity. As such, the recognition and treatment of hypomagnesemia, a common problem in the critically ill,[21,186,268] is important. There is little available data in neurosurgical ICU populations; however, in critically ill general surgical patients the frequency of hypomagnesemia (<1.5 mg/dl) has been reported to be as high as 61% and is associated with increased mortality.[21] Similar to hypophosphatemia, decreased dietary intake, excessive renal GI losses, and transcellular shift are general causes of hypomagnesemia and also commonly seen in alcoholic and malnourished patients. Detailed reviews of the pathophysiology and specific etiologies of hypomagnesemia are presented elsewhere.[22,185] Common etiologies to be expected in the neurosurgical patient include osmotic and nonosmotic diuretic use, diabetes insipidus, respiratory alkalosis, sepsis, and drugs such as aminoglycosides.

The clinical diagnosis of magnesium depletion is difficult because only 1% of total body magnesium is represented in plasma and because total plasma magnesium does not accurately reflect the ionized fraction (55% of total), which is the physiologically active form.[268] The remainder of plasma magnesium is bound to protein (33%) or chelated. Although methods are available for estimating magnesium stores, they are neither practical nor routinely available for clinical use in the ICU. Measurement of ionized magnesium is also not available; however, measurement of the fraction unbound to protein shows promise for routine estimation of ionized magnesium.[268] Despite its limitations, total plasma magnesium levels lower than 1 mEq/L are associated with hypokalemia and increased mortality[21] and thus serve as a practical threshold for initiating aggressive therapy.

A variety of complications of hypomagnesemia have been described and include hypocalcemia, refractory hypokalemia, peripheral and diaphragmatic muscle weakness, tetany, cardiac arrhythmias, and enhancement of digitalis-induced arrhythmias. Neurologic manifestations include tremor, hyperreflexia, agitation confusion, and seizures.[66,201] Some of these clinical manifestations may in fact be related to hypocalcemia, which is commonly associated with hypomagnesemia.[117]

Magnesium has received a great deal of attention within the realm of neuroprotective agents because it appears that reductions in intracellular magnesium are found in experimental brain and spinal cord injury and may contribute to secondary neuronal injury.[101,139] In addition, low magnesium may play a role in the pathophysiology of vasospasm after subarchnoid hemorrhage.[2,3,170] In experimental models, the administration of magnesium has been shown to be neuroprotective.[61,101] Possible mechanisms whereby magnesium might be neuroprotective include blockade of NMDA receptors, inhibition of excitatory amino acid release, and inhibition of intracellular calcium entry. At present there are no clinical data in humans to assess the role of magnesium supplementation in the neurosurgical population; however, a single study in patients with acute head injury demonstrating low ionized magnesium levels soon after injury[140] suggests that routine magnesium supplementation may be warranted even when total plasma magnesium levels are normal. Limited clinical data in patients after cardiac arrest have shown no benefit of magnesium supplementation.[60,231]

Given the role that low magnesium may play in promoting secondary brain injury and vasospasm, magnesium levels should be obtained routinely in the neurosurgical patient and hypomagnesemia treated aggressively. Severe hypomagnesemia is treated with intravenous magnesium salts.[18,187] Patients with normal renal function can excrete at least 50% of the administered dose; thus large doses of magnesium can be given to deficient patients without causing hypermagnesemia.[67] Symptomatic hypomagnesemia, such as refractory cardiac arrhythmias or seizures, can be treated with 2 to 3 g of 10% to 25% magnesium sulfate (1 g = 8 mEq Mg^{+2}) administered slowly over 2 to 3 minutes while arterial blood pressure and heart rhythm are monitored. Following the initial bolus, a continuous infusion of 2 g/hr for 5 hours followed by 1 g/hr for 10 hours has been successfully employed.[18] For patients with asymptomatic but severe hypomagnesemia, 6 g of $MgSO_4$ is administered over 3 hours followed by 10 g administered continuously over the remainder of the day. Additional doses of 6 g/day for the next 2 to 5 days can be given as necessary to correct residual deficits. Less severe degrees of hypomagnesemia can be treated as indicated by supplements added to TPN or by enteric administration of magnesium oxide.

ACID-BASE DISORDERS

Acid-base disorders occurring in the critically ill are usually acute, commonly mixed, may cause or contribute to electrolyte imbalance, and may adversely affect organ function, including the central nervous system. In-depth reviews of the evaluation and treatment of acid-base disorders is presented elsewhere.[62,151] The following discussion will focus on disorders than can be expected to occur in the neurosurgical ICU with emphasis on their effect on the CNS.

Respiratory Disorders

Of all common acid-base disorders, acute respiratory disturbances most profoundly affect CNS function. Because of the rapid diffusion of CO_2 across the blood-brain barrier and the limited acute buffering capacity of the CNS, brain extracellular and intracellular pH tracks the systemic pH in acute respiratory alkalosis or acidosis.[6,112,196] Functional disturbances that occur may be related to both changes in intracellular pH or cerebral blood flow (CBF). CBF decreases approximately 3% to 4% per mm Hg decrease in $Paco_2$, with an associated 1% reduction in cerebral blood volume. Similar changes in the opposite direction occur under hypercapnic conditions. Changes in perivascular pH caused by changes in $Paco_2$ modulate changes in CBF. Compensatory mechanisms do exist that return CSF and brain pH to normal in a matter of hours by increased lactate production and decreased bicarbonate in the case of respiratory alkalosis or by the generation of bicarbonate in the case of respiratory acidosis. These compensatory mechanisms help explain why CBF returns to near normal values in as little as 4 to 6 hours after acute hyperventilation-induced hypocapnia and why chronic hypercarbia may be tolerated with minimal symptoms unless there is coexistent hypoxia.

Respiratory Alkalosis

Respiratory alkalosis ($Paco_2 < 35$ mm Hg) is present with or without alkalemia ($pH > 7.44$) in many neurosurgical patients as a result of the primary brain insult,[253] associated pulmonary complications (e.g., pneumonia, aspiration),[73] fever, pulmonary embolism, inappropriate ventilator settings, and when therapeutic hyperventilation is being employed to control ICP. Systemic pH may be normal or lower than expected when there is superimposed metabolic acidosis or it may be inappropriately high when treatments such as diuretics, nasogastric suction, or corticosteroids are being employed concurrently. Acute hypocapnia may cause paresthesias, altered sensorium, and seizures.[72,114] Extreme degrees of hypocapnia can also impair brain tissue oxygenation[1,113,160,167] either by a reduction in CBF or as a result of increased affinity of hemoglobin for oxygen (Bohr effect). Acute respiratory alkalosis also predisposes to a variety of electrolyte disorders and myocardial ischemia and may also reduce cardiac output in patients on mechanical ventilation. Other potentially detrimental effects of respiratory alkalosis include increases in plasma lactic acid concentrations and diminished lactate clearance.

Severe hypocapnia ($Paco_2 < 20-25$ mm Hg) and alkalemia ($pH > 7.55$) should generally be avoided. Treatment is directed at the underlying cause or by adjusting minute ventilation downward in mechanically ventilated patients. Changing the mode of mechanical ventilation (e.g., from assist control to intermittent mandatory ventilation [IMV]) in patients with driven respiration (i.e., sepsis or brain injury) does not usually affect blood gas abnormalities. Therefore, judicious use of narcotics to suppress respiratory drive or the addition or dead space to the ventilator circuit are often required to correct the alkalosis. Narcotics are preferred to minimize ventilatory work. If extreme degrees of hypocapnia are being used to control ICP, consideration should be given to measuring CBF or sampling venous blood from the jugular bulb to ensure adequate CBF and brain oxygenation.

Respiratory Acidosis

Respiratory acidosis ($Paco_2 > 45$ mm Hg) with acidemia ($pH < 7.36$) is an early complication in some neurosurgical patients after acute intracranial insults as a result of airway obstruction and/or hypoventilation. Patients with high cervical spine injury are also at risk for hypoventilation and hypercapnia as a result of loss of motor control over the muscles of respiration, inadequate ventilatory reserve, retained secretions, and impaired coughing.[148] In the brain-injured patient, hypercapnia may increase intracranial pressure and contribute to secondary brain ischemia and poor outcome.[13,143] While in the intensive care unit, metabolic alkalosis, inadequate ventilation, or excessive use of sedatives may also cause or contribute to hypoventilation and hypercapnia. Superimposed metabolic acid-base disorders may cause arterial pH to be greater or less than what would be expected for a simple respiratory acidosis. In addition to its effect on the central nervous system, severe respiratory acidosis may impair cardiac function and result in hypotension.

Treatment of respiratory acidosis is usually straightforward and requires definitive airway control and mechanical ventilation adjusted to normalize systemic pH. Withholding or reversal of narcotic sedatives and correction of metabolic alkalosis is indicated when they may be contributory. Patients with intracranial hypertension or nonintubated patients with spinal cord injury should be monitored closely for hypercapnia with frequent blood gases or by capnography.

Metabolic Disorders

Isolated acute metabolic alkalosis and acidosis have little effect on central nervous system acid-base balance or function because of the relative impermeability of H^+ and HCO_3^- to the blood-brain barrier. Paradoxically, CSF pH can shift in a direction opposite to systemic pH when respiratory compensation for these acute disorders results either in hyperventilation in the case of metabolic acidosis or hypoventilation in the case of metabolic alkalosis. Acute administration of bicarbonate or inorganic acids can produce also produce paradoxic decreases in CSF pH.[112,150]

Metabolic Alkalosis

Metabolic alkalosis (serum HCO_3^- or total $CO_2 > 30$ mEq/L) is the most common acid-base disturbance noted in hospitalized patients.[104,259] Metabolic alkaloses are divided into chloride-responsive and chloride-resistant types.[71,176] In chloride responsive alkaloses, chloride loss stimulates renal HCO_3^- reabsorption. In the neurosurgical patient, common causes of chloride-responsive alkaloses include vomiting, nasogastric suction, and diuretics. Chloride-responsive alkaloses are commonly associated with volume contraction, which may compound the alkalosis as the kidney responds by increasing reabsorption of HCO_3^- and secretion of acid. There are a variety of causes for chloride-resistant alkaloses. In the neurosurgical patient, the use of glucocorticoids with mineralocorticoid activity (e.g., hydrocortisone, methylprednisolone) is usually the most common cause. The mineralocorticoids cause sodium retention and renal H^+ and K^+ loss. Hypokalemia can perpetuate or contribute to metabolic alkalosis by increasing renal tubular acid secretion.

The main complications of metabolic alkalosis that are of concern include hypokalemia, hypoventilation, and the possibility of impaired oxygen delivery because of increased affinity of hemoglobin for oxygen under alkalemic conditions. Neurologic manifestations of severe metabolic alkalosis have been reported to include altered sensorium and seizures[83,133] but are difficult to separate from associated electrolyte and blood gas abnormalities.

Treatment of metabolic alkalosis is generally directed at the underlying cause when possible. The chloride-responsive alkaloses respond to the administration of saline and potassium. In patients with large volumes of nasogastric drainage, H_2 blockers can be used to minimize chloride loss. Glucocorticoid-related alkalosis are treated by either discontinuing steroids or by repleting potassium. Acetazolamide in doses of 250 to 1000 mg/day in divided doses has been used in selected patients with diuretic-induced alkaloses or in hypercapnic patients to correct metabolic alkalosis; however, this agent should not be used in neurosurgical patients with elevated intracranial pressure, because it may cause acute cerebral acidosis and increased cerebral blood flow and volume. Although seldom required, patients with severe metabolic alkaloses and those in whom saline therapy is contraindicated can be treated using intravenous HCl administered through a central vein.[71]

Metabolic Acidosis

Metabolic acidoses ($HCO_3^- < 25$ mEq/L) are divided into anion gap and non−anion gap types. The anion gap ($Na^+ - [Cl^- + HCO_3^-]$) represents the sum of all unmeasured anions in plasma, including negatively charged albumin, sulfate, phosphate, and organic anions. The anion gap is normally 10 to 14 mEq/L. In critically ill patients it must be further recognized that the anion gap can be artifactually lowered when there is coexistent hypoalbuminemia. Lactic acidosis as a result of impaired systemic tissue perfusion or secondary to respiratory alkalosis can be expected to be the most common causes of an increased anion gap in the neurosurgical patient in the ICU. Less common causes of an increased anion gap in these patients include diabetic ketoacidosis and inorganic acidoses caused by acute renal failure. The non-anion gap acidoses are characterized by an increased chloride concentration and a normal anion gap. Hyperchloremic acidoses are commonly seen in neurosurgical patients after prolonged hypocapnia. Other potential causes in this population include large-volume saline administration, diarrhea, and the administration of chloride salts of amino acids used in TPN formulations. Hyperchloremic and anion gap acidoses can coexist or be found in association with other acid-base disorders and are suggested when the serum bicarbonate is decreased or increased to a greater degree than would be expected by the calculated anion gap.

Treatment of metabolic acidoses is, as is the case with other disorders, first directed at the underlying pathophysiology. Patients with severe systemic acidemia (pH <7.1−7.2) are at risk for myocardial depression and hypotension[38,133] and consideration should be given to the administration of $NaHCO_3$ when lactic acidosis is associated with impaired hemodynamics. When used to treat severe lactic acidosis, the immediate goal is to raise systemic pH to non−life-threatening levels (7.25−7.30), which may minimize the risk of overcorrection, paradoxic CSF acidosis, and alkali-related electrolyte problems such as hypokalemia, hypocalcemia, hypernatremia, and hyperosmolality. Estimation of bicarbonate requirements by classical formulas may either overestimate or underestimate bicarbonate requirements. A simple formula that appears to raise pH to acceptable ranges while avoiding overcorrection is as follows[100]:

$$\text{Dose(mEq)} = (-\text{Pa}CO_2^{-}\ [HCO_3^{-}]) - 0.5\ (\text{wt in kg})$$

Treatment is subsequently modified according to repeated measurements of arterial blood gases. Post-hypocapnic hyperchloremic acidosis requires no specific therapy because renal mechanisms will normalize bicarbonate concentration in 12 to 36 hours. TPN-associated hyperchloremic acidosis can be corrected by discontinuation of the TPN or minimized by using sodium or potassium acetate as electrolyte supplements rather than the usual chloride salts.

REFERENCES

1. Alexander SC, Smith TC, Strobel G, et al: Cerebral carbohydrate metabolism of man during respiratory and metabolic alkalosis, **J Appl Physiol 24(1):**66, 1968.
2. Altura BT, Altura BM: The role of magnesium in etiology of strokes and cerebrovasospasm, **Magnesium 1:**277, 1982.
3. Altura BT, Altura BM: Withdrawal of magnesium causes vasospasm while elevated magnesium produces relaxation of tone in cerebral arteries, **Neurosci Lett 20:**323, 1980.
4. Anderson JT, Wisner DH, Sullivan PE, et al: Initial small-volume hypertonic resuscitation of shock and brain injury: short- and long-term effects, **J Trauma 42:**592, 1997.
5. Andreoli A, di Pasquale G, Pinelli G, et al: Subarachnoid hemorrhage: frequency and severity of cardiac arrhythmias, **Stroke 18:**558, 1987.
6. Arieff AI, Kerian A, Massry SG, et al: Intracellular pH of brain: alterations in acute respiratory acidosis and alkalosis, **Am J Physiol 230(3):**804, 1976.
7. Arieff AI: Hyponatremia, convulsions, repsiratory arrest, and permanent brain damage after elective surgery in healthy women, **N Engl J Med 314:**1529, 1986.
8. Aubier M, Murcian D, Lecocguic Y, et al: Effect of hypophosphatemia on diaphragmatic contractility in patients with acute respiratory failure, **N Engl J Med 313:** 420, 1985.
9. Axler O, Tousignant C, Thompson CR, et al: Small hemodynamic effect of typical rapid volume infusions in critically ill patients, **Crit Care Med 25:**965, 1997.
10. Bahner U, Geiger H, Palkovits M, et al: Atrial natriuretic peptides in brain nuclei of rats with inherited diabetes insipidus (Brattleboro rats), **Neuroendocrinology 51:**721, 1990.
11. Balestrieri FJ, Chernow B, Rainey TG: Postcraniotomy diabetes insipidus: who's at risk? **Crit Care Med 10:**108, 1982.
12. Battistella FD, Wisner DH: Combined hemorrhagic shock and head injury: effects of hypertonic saline (7.5%) resuscitation, **J Trauma 31:**182, 1991.
13. Becker DP, Miller JD, Ward JD: The outcome from severe head injury with early diagnosis and intensive management, **J Neurosurg 47:**491, 1977.
14. Becker DP, Vries JK: The alleviation of increased intracranial pressure by the chronic administration of osmotic agents, in Brock M, Dietz H, (eds): **Intracranial pressure, experimental and clinical aspects.** Berlin: Springer-Verlag, 1972, p 309.
15. Berger L, Hakim AM: The association of hyperglycemia with cerebral edema in stroke, **Stroke 17:**865, 1986.
16. Bingham WF: The limits of cerebral dehydration in the treatment of head injury, **Surg Neurol 25:**340, 1986.
17. Bisonni RS, Holtgrave DR, Lawler F, et al: Colloids versus crystalloids in fluid resuscitation: an analysis of randomized controlled trials, **J Fam Pract 32:**387, 1991.
18. Boriss MN, Papa L: Magnesium: a discussion of its role in the treatment of ventricular dysrhythmia, **Crit Care Med 16(3):**292, 1988.
19. Camp MA, Allon M: Severe hypophosphatemia in hospitalized patients, **Miner Electrolyte Metab 16:**365, 1990.
20. Candelise L, Landi G, Orazio EN, et al: Prognostic significance of hyperglycemia in acute stroke, **Arch Neurol 42:**661, 1985.
21. Chernow B, Bamberger S, Stoiko M, et al: Hypomagnesemia in patients in postoperative intensive care, **Chest 95:**391, 1989.
22. Chernow B, Smith J, Rainey TG, et al: Hypomagnemia: implications for the critical care specialist**, Crit Care Med 10(3):**193, 1982.
23. Choi PT, Yip G, Quinonez LG, et al: Crystalloids vs. colloids in fluid resuscitation: a systematic review, **Crit Care Med 27:**200, 1999.
24. Chung HM, Kluge R, Schrier RW et al: Postoperative hyponatremia: a prospective study, **Arch Intern Med 146:**333, 1986.
25. Cluitmans FHM, Meinders AE: Management of severe hyponatremia: rapid or slow correction, **Am J Med 88:** 161, 1990.

26. Cochrane Injuries Group Albumin Reviewers: Human albumin administration in critically ill patients: systematic review of randomised controlled trials, **Br Med J 317:** 235, 1998.
27. Coculescu M, Dumitrescu C: Etiology of cranial diabetes insipidus in 164 adults, **Endocrinology 22:**135, 1984.
28. Connors AF, Dawson NV, McCaffree R, et al: Assessing hemodynamic status in critically ill patients: Do physicians use clinical information optimally? **J Crit Care 2:** 174, 1987.
29. Connors AF, McCaffree DR, Gray BA: Evaluation of right heart catheterization in the critically ill patient without acute myocardial infarction, **N Engl J Med 308:** 263, 1983.
30. Cort JH: Cerebral salt wasting, **Lancet 752,** 1954.
31. Craddock PR, Yawata Y, Vansanten L: Acquired phagocyte dysfunction: a complication of the hypophosphatemia of parenteral hyperalimentation, **N Engl J Med 290(25):**1403, 1974.
32. Crompton MR: Hypothalamic lesions following closed head injury, **Brain 94:**165, 1971.
33. Cserr HF, dePasquale M, Patlak CS: Volume regulatory influx of electrolytes from plasma to brain during acute hyperosmolality, **Am J Physiol 253:**F530, 1987.
34. Cully MD, Larson CP, Silverberg GD: Hetastarch coagulopathy in a neurosurgical patient, **Anesthesiology 66:** 706, 1987.
35. Czer LSC, Shoemaker WC: Optimal hematocrit value in critically ill postoperative patients, **Surg Gynecol Obstet 147:**363, 1978.
36. Daily WH, Tonnesen A, Allen SA: Hypophosphatemia incidence, etiology, and prevention in the trauma patient, **Crit Care Med 18:**1210, 1990.
37. Damaraju SC, Rajshekhar V, Chandy MJ: Validation study of a central venous pressure-based protocol for the management of neurosurgical patients with hyponatremia and natriuresis, **Neurosurgery 40:**312, 1997.
38. Darby TD, Aldinger EE, Gadsden RH: Effects of metabolic acidosis on ventricular isometric systolic tension and the response to epinephrine and levarterenol, **Circ Res 8:**1242, 1960.
39. Davis SV, Olichwier KK, Chakko SC: Reversible depression of myocardial performance in hypophosphatemia, **Am J Med Sci 295(3):**183, 1988.
40. De Troyer A: Demeclocycline, **JAMA 237:**2723, 1977,
41. Decaux G, Unger J, Brimioulle S, et al: Hyponatremia in the syndrome of inappropriate secretion of antidiuretic hormone. Rapid correction with urea, sodium chloride and water restriction therapy, **JAMA 247(4):**471, 1982.
42. Defoer F, Mahler C, Dua G, et al: Posttraumatic diabetes insipidus, **Acta Anaesthesiol Belg 38:**297, 1987.
43. DeFronzo RA, Bia M: Intravenous potassium chloride therapy, **JAMA 245:**2446, 1981.
44. Desai TK, Carlson RW, Gehab MA: Parathyroid-vitamin D axis in critically ill patients with unexplained hypocalcemia, **Kidney Int 32(22):**S225, 1987.
45. Desai TK, Carlson RW, Gehab MA: Prevalence and clinical implications of hypocalcemia in acutely ill patients in a medical intensive care setting, **Am J Med 84:**209, 1988.
46. Diringer M, Ladenson PW, Stern B, et al: Plasma atrial natriuretic factor and subarachnoid hemorrhage, **Stroke 19:**1119, 1988.
47. Diringer MN, Kirsch JR, Ladenson PW, et al: Cerebrospinal fluid atrial natriuretic factor in intracranial disease, **Stroke 21:**1550, 1990.
48. Diringer MN, Lim JS, Kirsch JR, et al: Suprasellar and intraventricular blood predict elevated plasma atrial natriuretic factor in subarachnoid hemorrhage, **Stroke 22:**577, 1991.
49. Doczi T, Joo F, Bodosi M: Central neuroendochrine control of the brain water, electrolyte, and volume homeostasis, **Acta Neurochir Suppl 47:**122, 1990.
50. Doczi T, Joo F, Szerdahelyi P, et al: Regulation of brain water and electrolyte contents: the opposite actions of central vasopressin and atrial natriuretic factor, **Acta Neurochir Suppl 43:**186, 1988.
51. Doczi T, Joo F, Szerdahelyi P, et al: Regulation of brain water and electrolyte content: the possible involvement of central atrial natiruretic factor, **Neurosurgery 21:**454, 1987.
52. Doczi T, Joo F, Vecsernyes M, et al: Increased concentration of atrial natriuretic factor in the cerebrospinal fluid of patients with aneurysmal subarachnoid hemorrhage and raised intracranial pressure, **Neurosurgery 23:**16, 1988.
53. Doczi T, Tarjanyi J, Huszka E, et al: Syndrome of inappropriate secretion of antidiuretic hormone (SIADH) after head injury, **Neurosurgery 10:**685, 1982.
54. Dorman HR, Sondheimer JH, Cadnapaphornchai P: Mannitol-induced acute renal failure, **Medicine (Baltimore) 69:**153, 1990.
55. Drummond JC, Moore SS: The influence of dextrose administration on neurologic outcome after temporary spinal cord ischemia in the rabbit, **Anesthesiology 70:** 64, 1989.
56. Edwards OM, Clark JDA: Post-traumatic hypopituitarism, **Medicine (Baltimore) 65:**281, 1986.
57. Eisenberg PR, Joffe AS, Schuster DP: Clinical evaluation compared to pulmonary artery catheterization in the hemodynamic assessment of critically ill patients, **Crit Care Med 12:**549, 1984.
58. Epstein M, Ward JD, Becker DP: Medical complications of head injury, in Cooper PR, (ed): **Head injury, 2nd ed,** Boston: Williams and Wilkins, pp 390-421.
59. Erstad BL, Gaels BL, Rappaport WD: The use of albumin in clinical practice, **Arch Intern Med 151:**901, 1991.
60. Fatovich DM, Prentice DA, Dobb GJ: Magnesium in cardiac arrest (the magic trial), **Resuscitation 35:**237, 1997.
61. Feldman Z, Gurevitch B, Artru AA, et al: Effect of magnesium given 1 hour after head trauma on brain edema and neurological outcome, **J Neurosurg 85:**131, 1996.
62. Fencl V, Rossing TH: Acid-base disorders in critical care medicine, **Ann Rev Med 40:**17, 1989.
63. Fenstermacher JD: Volume regulation of the central nervous system, in Staub NC, Taylor AE, (eds): **Edema,** New York, Raven Press, pp 383-403.
64. Fiser DH, Jimenez JF, Wrape V, et al: Diabetes insipidus in children with brain death, **Crit Care Med 15:**551, 1987.

65. Fisher B, Thomas D, Peterson B: Hypertonic saline lowers raised intracranial pressure in children after head trauma, **J Neurosurg Anesthesiol 4:**4, 1992.
66. Fishman RA: Neurological aspects of magnesium metabolism, **Arch Neurol 12:**562, 1965.
67. Flink EB: Therapy of magnesium deficiency, **Ann NY Acad Sci 162:**901, 1969.
68. Fonseca OA, Calverly JR: Neurological manifestations of hypoparathyroidism, **Arch Intern Med 120:**202, 1967.
69. Forrest JN, Cox M, Hong C, et al: Superiority of demeclocycline over lithium in the treatment of chronic syndrome of inappropriate secretion of antidiuretic hormone, **N Engl J Med 298:**173, 1978.
70. Fox JL, Falik JL, Shalhoub RJ: Neurosurgical hyponatremia: the role of inappropriate antidiuresis, **J Neurosurg 34:**506, 1971.
71. Friedman BS, Lumb PD: Prevention and management of metabolic alkalosis, **J Intensive Care Med 5(suppl):** S22, 1990.
72. Froman C: Adverse effects of low carbon dioxide tensions during mechanical over-ventilation of patients with combined head and chest injuries, **Br J Anaesth 40:**383, 1968.
73. Frost EAM: The physiopathology of respiration in neurosurgical patients**, J Neurosurg 50:**699, 1979.
74. Gadisseux P, Sica DA, Ward JD, et al: Severe hypophosphatemia after head injury, **Neurosurgery 17:**35, 1985.
75. Gaehtgens P, Marx P: Hemorheological aspects of the pathophysiology of cerebral ischemia, **J Cereb Blood Flow Metab 7:**259, 1987.
76. Gates EM, Graig WM: The use of serum albumin in cases of cerebral edema: preliminary report, **Mayo Clin Proc 23:**89, 1948.
77. Gauer OH: Osmocontrol versus volume control, **Fed Proc 27:**1132, 1968.
78. Gaufin L, Skowsky WR, Goodman SJ: Release of antidiuretic hormone during mass-induced elevation of intracranial pressure, **J Neurosurg 46:**627, 1977.
79. Geheb MA: Clinical approach to the hyperosmolar patient, in Geheb M, Carlson R, (eds): **Critical care clinics,** Philadelphia: W.B. Saunders, pp 797-815.
80. Gennari FJ: Current concepts: serum osmolality, uses and limitations, **N Engl J Med 310:**102, 1984.
81. Goldberg M, Handler JS: Hyponatremia and renal wasting of sodium in patients with malfunction of the central nervous system, **N Engl J Med 263:**1037, 1960.
82. Gotta H: Tetany and epilepsy, **Arch Neurol Psychiatry 66:**714, 1951.
83. Grace WJ, Barr DP: Complications of alkalosis, **Am J Med 4:**331, 1948.
84. Gravelyn TR, Brophy N, Siegart C: Hypophosphatemia-associated respiratory muscle weakness in a general inpatient population, **Am J Med 84:**870, 1988.
85. Gross P, Reimann D, Neidel J, et al.: The treatment of severe hyponatremia, **Kidney Int Suppl 53:**S-6, 1998.
86. Grotta JC: Current medical and surgical therapy for cerebrovascular diseses, **N Engl J Med 317:**1505, 1987.
87. Gunnar W, Jonasson O, Merlotti G, et al: Head injury and hemorrhagic shock: studies of the blood brain barrier and intracranial pressure after resuscitation with normal saline solution, 3% saline solution, and dextran-40, **Surgery 103:**398, 1988.
88. Gutakowska J, Antunes-Rodrigues J, McCann SM: Atrial natriuretic peptide in brain and pituitary gland, **Physiol Rev 77:**465, 1997.
89. Halevy J, Bulvik S: Severe hypophosphatemia in hospitalized patients, **Arch Intern Med 148:**153, 1988.
90. Hamill RJ, Robinson LM, Wexler HR, et al: Efficacy and safety of potassium infusion therapy in hypokalemic critically ill patients, **Crit Care Med 19(5):**694, 1991.
91. Hankeln K, Radel C, Beez M, et al: Comparison of hydroxyethyl starch and lactated Ringer's solution on hemodynamics and oxygen trasport of critically ill patients in prospective crossover studies, **Crit Care Med 17:**133, 1989.
92. Hantman D, Rossier B, Zohlman R, et al: Rapid correction hyponatremia in the syndrome of inappropriate secretion of antidiuretic hormone, **Ann Intern Med 78:** 870, 1973.
93. Harding JW, Jensen LL, Quirk WS, et al: Brain angiotensin: critical role in the ongoing regulation of body fluid homeostasis and cardiovascular function, **Peptides 10:**261, 1989.
94. Hariri RJ, Firlick AD, Shepard SR, et al: Traumatic brain injury, hemorrhagic shock, and fluid resuscitation: effects on intracranial pressure and brain compliance, **J Neurosurg 79:**421, 1993.
95. Harrigan MR: Cerebral salt wasting syndrome: a review, **Neurosurgery 38:**152, 1996.
96. Hasan D, Wijdicks EF, Vermeulen M: Hyponatremia is associated with cerebral ischemia in patients with aneurysmal subarachnoid hemorrhage, **Ann Neurol 27:**106, 1990.
97. Hauser CJ, Shoemaker WC, Turpin I, et al: Oxygen transport responses to colloids and crystalloids in critically ill surgical patients, **Surg Gynecol Oncol 150:**811, 1980.
98. Hayek ME, Eisenberg PG: Severe hypophosphatemia following the institution of enteral feedings, **Arch Surg 124:**1325, 1989.
99. Hayes RM: Antidiuretic hormone, **N Engl J Med 295:** 659, 1976
100. Hazard PB, Griffin JP: Calculation of sodium bicarbonate requirement in metabolic acidosis, **Am J Med Sci 283(1):**18, 1982.
101. Heath DL, Vink R: Neuroprotective effects of $MgSO_4$ and $MgCl_2$ in closed head injury: a comparative phosphorus NMR study, **J Neurotrauma 15:**183, 1998.
102. Helgason C: Blood glucose and stroke, **Stroke 19:**1049, 1988.
103. Hint H: The pharmacology of dextran and the physiological background for the clinical use of rheomacrodex and macrodex, **Acta Anesthesiol Belg 19:**119, 1968.
104. Hodgkin JE, Soeprono EF, Chan DM: Incidence of metabolic alkalemia in hospitalized patients, **Intensive Care Med 8:**725, 1980.
105. Hughes J, Mudd S, Strecker EA: Reduction of increased intracranial pressure by concentrated solutions of human lyophile serum, **Arch Neurol Psychiatry 39:**1277, 1938.

106. Ishikawa SE, Saito T, Aneko K, et al: Hyponatremia responsive to fludrocortisone acetate in elderly patients after head injury, **Ann Intern Med 106:**187, 1987.
107. Itoh H, Nakao K, Yamada T, et al: Brain renin-angiotensin, central control of secretion of atrial natriuresis factor from the heart, **Hypertension 11:**157, 1988.
108. Jackowski A: Disordered sodium and water in neurosurgery, **Br J Neurosurg 6:**173, 1992.
109. Kahn A, Brachet E, Blum D: Controlled fall in natremia and risk of seizures in hypertonic dehydration, **Intensive Care Med 5:**27, 1979.
110. Kaieda R, Todd MM, Cook LN, et al: Acute effects of changing plasma osmolality and colloid oncotic pressure on the formation of brain edema after cryogenic injury, **Neurosurgery 24:**671, 1989.
111. Kassell NF, Torner JC, Haely EC, et al: The international cooperative study on the timing of aneurysm surgery, **J Neurosurg 73:**18, 1990.
112. Katzman R, Pappius HM: **Brain electrolytes and fluid metabolism,** Baltimore: Williams and Wilkins, 1973.
113. Kennealy JA, McLennan JE, Loudon RG, et al: Hyperventilation-induced cerebral hypoxia, **Am Rev Respir Dis 122:**407, 1980.
114. Kilburn KH: Shock, seizures and coma with alkalosis during mechanical ventilation, **Ann Intern Med 65:**977, 1966.
115. King AL, Sica DA, Miller G, et al: Severe hypophosphatemia in a general hospital population, **South Med J 80:**831, 1987.
116. Kingston M, Al Siba MB: Treatment of severe hypophosphatemia, **Crit Care Med 13:**16, 1985.
117. Kingston ME, Al-siba 'I MB, Skooge WC: Clinical manifestations of hypomagnesia, **Crit Care Med 14:**950, 1986.
118. Knochel JP: The clinical status of hypophosphatemia, **N Engl J Med 313:**447, 1985.
119. Kudo T, Suzuki S, Iawbuchi T: Importance of monitoring the circulating blood volume in patients with cerebral vasospasm after subarachnoid hemorrhage, **Neurosurgery 9:**514, 1981.
120. Lam AM, Winn HR, Cullen BF, et al: Hyperglycemia and neurological outcome in patients with head injury, **J Neurosurg 75:**545, 1991.
121. Landolt AM, Yasargil MG, Krayenbuhl H: Disturbances of the serum electrolytes after surgery of intracranial arterial aneurysms, **J Neurosurg 37:**210, 1972.
122. Laredo S, Yuen K, Sonnenberg B, et al: Coexistence of central diabetes insipidus and salt wasting: the difficulties in diagnosis, changes in natremia, and treatment, **J Am Soc Nephrology 7:**2527, 1996.
123. Lee JL, Sibbald WJ, Holliday RL, et al: Hypophosphatemia associated with coma, **Can Med Assoc J 119:** 143, 1978.
124. Lee SH, Heros RC, Mullan JC, et al: Optimum degree of hemodilution for brain protection in a canine model of focal cerebral ischemia, **Neurosurgery 80:**469, 1994.
125. Leehey DJ, Picache AA, Robertson GL. Hyponatremia in quadriplegic patients, **Clin Sci 75:**441, 1988.
126. Levin ER, Gardner DG, Samson WK: Natriuretic peptides, **N Engl J Med 339:**321, 1998.
127. Levitt MA, Fleischer AS, Meislin HW: Acute post-traumatic diabetes insipidus: treatment with continuous intravenous vasopressin, **J Trauma 24:**532, 1984.
128. Lichtman MA, Miller DR, Cohen J: Reduced red cell glycolysis, 2,3-diphosphglycerate and adenosine triphosphate concentration, and increased hemoglobin-oxygen affinity by hypophosphatemia, **Ann Intern Med 74:**562, 1971.
129. Little JR, Lugg RM, Latchaw JP, et al: Treatment of acute focal cerebral ischemia with concentrated albumin, **Neurosurgery 9:**552, 1981.
130. Lolin Y, Jackowski A: Hyponatremia in neurosurgical patients: a diagnosis using derived parameters of sodium and water homeostasis, **Br J Neurosurg 6:**457, 1992.
131. Longstreth WT Jr, Inui TS: High blood glucose level in hospital admission and poor neurologic recovery after cardiac arrest, **Ann Neurol 15:**59, 1984.
132. Lowe RJ, Moss GS, Jilek J, et al: Crystalloid versus colloid in the etiology of pulmonary failure after trauma-a randomized trial in man, **Crit Care Med 7:**107, 1979.
133. Lubash GD, Coehn BD, Young CW: Severe metabolic alkalosis with neurologic abnormalities, **N Engl J Med 258:**1050, 1958.
134. Mackenzie CF, Shin B, Krishnaprasad D, et al: Assessment of cardiac and respiratory function during surgery on patients with acute quadriplegia, **J Neurosurg 62:**843, 1985.
135. Marmarou A, Anderson RL, Ward JD, et al: Impact of ICP instability and hypotension on outcome in patients with severe head trauma, **J Neurosurg 75:**S59, 1991.
136. Marsh ML, Marshall LF, Shapiro HM: Neurosurgical intensive care, **Anesthesiology 47:**149, 1977.
137. Mather H, Ang V, Jenkins JS: Vasopressin in plasma and CSF of patients with subarachnoid hemorrhage, **J Neurol Neurosurg Psychiatry 44:**216, 1981.
138. Mattox KL, Maningas PA, Moore EE, et al: Prehospital hypertonic saline/dextran infusion for post-traumatic hypotension: the USA multicenter trial, **Ann Surg 213:** 482, 1991.
139. McIntosh TK: Novel pharmacologic therapies in the treatment of experimental traumatic brain injury: a review, **J Neurotrauma 10:**215, 1993.
140. Memon ZI, Altura BT, Benjamin JL, et al: Predictive value of serum ionized but not total magnesium levels in head injuries, **Scand J Clin Lab Invest 55:**671, 1995.
141. Messert B, Orrison WW, Hawkins MJ, et al: Central pontine myelinolysis: considerations of etiology, diagnosis and treatment, **Neurology 29:**147, 1979.
142. Micahud LJ, Rivara FP, Longstreth WT, et al: Elevated initial blood glucose levels and poor outcome following severe brain injuries in children, **J Trauma 31:**1355, 1991.
143. Miller JD, Butterworth JF, Gudeman SK: Further experience in the management of severe head injury, **J Neurosurg 54:**289, 1981.
144. Miller M, Dalakos T, Moses AM: Recognition of partial defects in anitidiuretic hormone secretion, **Ann Intern Med 73:**721, 1970.
145. Moses AM, Blumenthal SA, Streeten DH: Acid-base and electrolyte disorders associated with endocrine disease: Pituitary and thyroid, in Arief AI, Defronzo RA,

(eds): **Fluid electrolyte and acid-base disorders,** New York: Churchill Livingstone, pp 851-892.
146. Moses M: Clinical and laboratory observations in the adult with diabetes insipidus, **Front Horm Res 13:**156, 1985.
147. Moss GS, Lowe RJ, Tilek J, et al: Colloid or crystalloid in the resuscitation of hemorrhagic shock: a controlled clinical trial, **Surgery 89:**434, 1981.
148. Myllynen P, Kivioja A, Rokkanen P, et al: Cervical spinal cord injury: The correlations of initial clinical features and blood gas analyses with early prognosis, **Paraplegia 27:**19, 1989.
149. Nakao N, Itakura T, Yokote H et al: Effect of atrial natriuretic peptide on ischemic brain edema: changes in brain water and electroyltes, **Neurosurgery 27:**39, 1990.
150. Nakashima K, Yamashita T, Kashiwagi S, et al: The effect of sodium bicarbonate on CBF and intracellular pH in man: stable Xe-CT and ^{31}P-MRS, **Acta Neurol Scand 166:**96, 1996.
151. Narins RG, Emmett M: Simple and mixed acid-base disorders: a practical approach, **Medicine (Baltimore) 59(3):**161, 1980.
152. Nearman HS, Herman ML: Toxic effects of colloids in the intensive care unit, in Carlson RW, Geheb MA, Blumer JL, et al, (eds): **Critical care clinics,** Philadelphia: W. B. Saunders, pp 713-723.
153. Needleman P, Greenwald JE: Atriopeptin: a cardiac hormone intimately involved in fluid, electrolyte, and blood-pressure homeostasis, **N Engl J Med 314:**828, 1986.
154. Nelson PB, Seif S, Gutai J, et al: Hyponatremia and natriuresis following subarachnoid hemorrhage in a monkey model, **J Neurosurg 60:**233, 1984.
155. Nelson PB, Seif SM, Maroon JC et al: Hyponatremia in intracranial disease: perhaps not the syndrome of inappropriate secretion of antidiuretic hormone (SIADH), **J Neurosurg 55:**938, 1981.
156. Norenberg MD, Leslie KO, Robertson AS: Association between rise in serum sodium and central pontine myelinolysis, **Ann Neurol 11:**128, 1982.
157. North JB, Jennett S: Abnormal breathing patterns associated with acute brain damage, **Arch Neurol 31:**338, 1974.
158. Notman DD, Mortek MA, Moses AM: Permanent diabetes insipidus following head trauma: observations on ten patients and an approach to diagnosis, **J Trauma 20:**599, 1980.
159. O'Connor LR, Wheeler WS, Bethune JE: Effect of hypophosphatemia on myocardial performance in man, **N Engl J Med 297:**901, 1977.
160. Obrist WD, Langfitt TW, Jaggi JL, et al: Cerebral blood flow and metabolism in comatose patients with acute head injury: relationship to intracranial hypertension, **J Neurosurg 61:**241, 1984.
161. Oelkers W: Hyponatremia and inappropriate secretion of vasopressin (antidiuretic hormone) in patients with hypopituitarism, **N Engl J Med 321:**492, 1989.
162. Outwater KM, Rockoff MA: Diabetes insipidus accompanying brain death in children, **Neurology 34:**1243, 1984.
163. Padilla G, Leake JA, Castro R, et al: Vasopressin levels and pediatric head trauma, **Pediatrics 83:**700, 1989.
164. Peters JP, Welt LG, Sims EAH, et al: A salt wasting syndrome associated with cerebral disease, **Trans Assoc Am Physicians 63:**57, 1950.
165. Pomeranz S, Constantini S, Rappaport ZH: Hypokalemia in severe head trauma, **Acta Neurochir 97:** 62, 1989.
166. Poole GV, Prough DS, Johnson JC, et al: Effects of resuscitation from hemorrhagic shock on cerebral hemodynamics in the presence of an intracranial mass, **J Trauma 27:**18, 1987.
167. Proctor HJ, Cairns C, Fillipo D, et al: Brain metabolism during increased intracranial pressure as assessed by niroscopy, **Surgery 96(2):**273, 1984.
168. Prough DS, Johnson JC, Stump DS, et al: Effects of hypertonic saline versus lactated Ringer's solution on cerebral oxygen transport during resuscitation from hemorrhagic shock, **J Neurosurg 64:**627, 1986.
169. Qureshi AI, Suarez JI, Bhardwaj A, et al: Use of hypertonic (3%) saline/acetate infusion in the treatment of cerebral edema: effect on intracranial pressure and lateral displacement of the brain, **Crit Care Med 26:**440, 1998.
170. Ram Z, Sadeh M, Shacked I, et al: Magnesium sulfate reverses experimental delayed cerebral vasospasm after subarachnoid hemmorrhage in rats, **Stroke 22:**922, 1991.
171. Ramming S, Shackford SR, Zhuang J, et al: The relationship of fluid balance and sodium administration to cerebral edema formation and intracranial pressure in a porcine model of brain injury, **J Trauma 37:**705, 1994.
172. Rapoport SI. A model for brain edema, in Inaba Y, Klatzo I, Spatz M, (eds): **Brain edema,** Berlin, Springer-Verlag, 1984.
173. Raymond KH, Reineck HJ, Stein JH: Sodium metabolism and maintenance of extracellular fluid volume, in Arieff AI, DeFronzo RA, (eds): **Fluid electrolyte and acid-base disorders,** New York, Churchill Livingstone, pp 39-76.
174. Reeder RF, Harbaugh RE: Administration of intravenous urea and normal saline for the treatment of hyponatremia in neurosurgical patients, **J Neurosurg 70:** 201, 1989.
175. Rettig R, Ganten D, Lang RE, et al: Brain angiotensin II: localization and possible functions, **Adv Biochem Psychopharmacol 43:**129, 1987.
176. Rimmer JM, Gennari FJ: Metabolic alkalosis, **J Intensive Care Med 2:**137, 1987.
177. Robertson CS, Goodman JC, Narayan RK, et al: The effect of glucose administration on carbohydrate metabolism after head injury, **J Neurosurg 74:**43, 1991.
178. Robertson GL: The pathophysiology of ADH secretion, in Tolis G, Labrie F, Martin JB, et al, (eds): **Clinical neuroendocrinology: a pathophysiological approach,** New York, Raven Press, 1979, p 247.
179. Robertson GL: Thirst and vasopressin function in normal and disordered states of water balance, **J Lab Clin Med 101:**351, 1983.
180. Robinson AG, Verbalis JG: Treatment of central diabetes insipidus, **Front Horm Res 13:**292, 1985.
181. Rosenfeld JV, Barnett GH, Sila CA, et al: The effect of subarachnoid hemorrhage on blood and CSF atrial natriuretic factor, **J Neurosurg 71:**32, 1989.

182. Rosner MJ, Becker DP: Origin and evolution of plateau waves, **J Neurosurg 60:**312, 1984.
183. Rosner MJ, Coley IB: Cerebral perfusion pressure, intracranial pressure, and head elevation, **J Neurosurg 65:** 636, 1986.
184. Ross EJ, Christie SBM: Hypernatremia, **Medicine (Baltimore) 48:**441, 1969.
185. Rude RK, Singer FR: Magnesium deficiency and excess, **Ann Rev Med 32:**245, 1981.
186. Ryzen E, Wagners PW, Singer FR: Magnesium deficiency in a medical ICU population, **Crit Care Med 13:** 19, 1985.
187. Salem M, Munoz R, Chernow B: Hypomagnesemia in critical illness: a common and clinically important problem, **Critical Care Clinics 7(1):**191, 1991.
188. Samson WK: Atrial natriuretic factor and the central nervous system, **Endocrinol Metab Clin North Am 16:** 145, 1987.
189. Schatzmann C, Heissler HE, Konig K, et al: Treatment of elevated intracranial pressure by infusions of 10% saline in severely head injured patients, **Acta Neurochir Suppl (Wien) 71:**31, 1998.
190. Schierhout G, Roberts I: Fluid resuscitation with colloid or crystalloid solutions in critically ill patients: a systematic review of randomised trials, **Br Med J 316:**961, 1998.
191. Schmoker JD, Zhuang J, Shackford SR: Hypertonic fluid resuscitation improves cerebral oxygen delivery and reduces intracranial pressure after hemorrhagic shock, **J Trauma 31:**1607, 1991.
192. Schrier RW, Anderson RJ: Renal sodium excretion, edematous disorders, and diuretic use, in Schrier RW (ed): **Renal and electrolyte disorders,** 2nd ed, Boston: Little, Brown, pp 65-114.
193. Schrier RW, Berl T, Anderson RH: Osmotic and nonosmotic control of vasopressin release, **Am J Physiol 236(4):**F321, 1979.
194. Schwartz WB, Bennett W, Curelop S: A syndrome of renal sodium loss and hyponatremia probably resulting from inappropriate secretion of antidiuretic hormone, **Am J Med 23:**529, 1957.
195. Serradeil-LeGal C, Lacour C, Valette G, et al: Characterization of SR 121463A, a highly potent and selective, orally active vasopressin V_2 receptor antagonist, **J Clin Invest 98:**2729, 1996.
196. Severinghaus JW, Lassen N: Step hypocapnia to separate arterial from tissue PCO_2 in the regulation of cerebral blood flow, **Circ Res 20:**272, 1967.
197. Shackford SR, Bourguignon PR, Wald SL, et al: Hypertonic saline resuscitation of patients with head injury: a prospective randomized clinical trial, **J Trauma 44:**50, 1998.
198. Sharkey PC, Perry JH, Ehni G: Diabetes insipidus following section of hypophyseal stalk, **J Neurosurg 18:** 445, 1961.
199. Sheikh AA, Matsuoka T, Wisner DH: Cerebral effect of resuscitation with hypertonic saline and a new low-sodium hypertonic fluid in hemorrhagic shock and head injury, **Crit Care Med 24:**1226, 1996.
200. Shibata S, Mori K, Teramoto S: Diabetes insipidus after surgery of intracranial arterial aneurysms, **No Shinkei Geka 6:**795, 1978.
201. Shils ME: Experimental human magnesium depletion, **Medicine (Baltimore) 48:**61, 1969.
202. Shimoda M, Yamada S, Yamamoto I, et al: Atrial natriuretic polypeptide in patients with subarachnoid haemorrhage due to aneurysmal rupture. Correlation to hyponatremia, **Acta Neurochir 97:**53, 1989.
203. Shoemaker WC, Schluchter M, Hopkins JA, et al: Comparison of the relative effectiveness of colloids and crystalloids in emergency resuscitation, **Am J Surg 142:** 73, 1981.
204. Shoemaker WC: Fluids and electrolytes in the acutelly ill adult, in Shoemaker WC, Ayres S, Grenvik A, et al, (eds): **Textbook of critical care,** 2nd ed, Philadelphia: W.B. Saunders 1989, pp 1128-1152.
205. Shucart WA, Jackson I: Management of diabetes insipidus in neurosurgical patients, **J Neurosurg 44:**65, 1976.
206. Sica D, Zawada E, Midha M, et al: Hyponatremia in the cord injured patient—a neglected phenomena, **Kidney Int 24:**137, 1984.
207. Sica DA, Culpepper RM: Case report: severe hyponatremia in spinal cord injury, **Am J Med Sci 298(5):**331, 1989.
208. Silvis SE, Paragas PD: Paresthesias, weakness, seizures, and hypophosphatemia in patients receiving hyperalimentation, **Gastroenterology 62:**513, 1972.
209. Simma B, Burger R, Falk M, et al: A prospective, randomized, and controlled study of fluid management in children with severe head injury: lactated Ringer's solution versus hypertonic saline, **Crit Care Med 26:**1265, 1998.
210. Sivakumar V, Rajshekhar V, Chandy MJ: Management of neurosurgical patients with hyponatremia and natriuresis, **Neurosurgery 34:**269, 1994.
211. Sladen A, Laver MB, Pontoppidan H: Pulmonary complications and water retention in prolonged mechanical ventilation, **N Engl J Med 279:**448, 1968.
212. Solis JM, Herranz AS, Herreras O, et al: Does taurine act as an osmoregulatory substance in the rat brain? **Neurosci Lett 91:**53, 1988.
213. Solomon RA, Post KD, McMurty JG: Depression of circulating blood volume in patients after subarachnoid hemorrhage: implications for the management of symptomatic vasospasm, **Neurosurgery 15:**354, 1984.
214. Solomon SM, Kirby DF: The refeeding syndrome: a review, **J Parenteral Enteral Nutrit 14:**90, 1990.
215. Sorensen PS, Gjerris F, Hammer M: Cerebrospinal fluid and plasma vasopressin during short-term induced intracranial hypertension, **Acta Neurochir 77:**46, 1985.
216. Sorensen PS: Studies of vasopressin in the human cerebrospinal fluid, **Acta Neurol Scand 74:**81, 1986.
217. Steardo L, Nathanson JA: Brain barrier tissues: end organs for atriopeptins, **Science 235:**470, 1987.
218. Steinbok P, Thompson GB: Metabolic disturbances after head injury: abnormalities of sodium and water balance with special reference to the effects of alcohol intoxication, **Neurosurgery 3(1):**9, 1978.
219. Sterns R, Cox M, Feig P: Internal potassium balance and the control of the plasma potassium concentration, **Medicine (Baltimore) 60:**339, 1981.
220. Sterns RH, Darbbie JD, Herndon RM: Brain dehydration and neurologic deterioration after rapid correction of hyponatremia, **Kidney Int 35:**69, 1989.

221. Sterns RH, Riggs JE, Schochet SS: Osmotic demyelineation syndrome following correction of hyponatremia, **N Engl J Med 314:**1535, 1986.
222. Sterns RH: The management of hyponatremic emergencies, in Carlson RW, Geheb MA, Zaloga GP, (eds): **Crit Care Clin 7(1):**127-142, 1991.
223. Sterrett PR, Thompson AM, Chapman AL, et al: The effects of hyperosmolarity on the blood-brain-barrier: a morphological and physiological correlation, **Brain Res 77:**281, 1974.
224. Stuart FP, Torres E, Fletcher R, et al: Effects of single, repeated and massive mannitol infusion in the dog: structural and functional changes in kidney and brain, **Ann Surg 172:**190, 1970.
225. Suarez JI, Qureshi AI, Bhardwaj A, et al: Treatment of refractory intracranial hypertension with 23.4% saline, **Crit Care Med 26:**1118, 1998.
226. Sugar O: Central neurological complications of hypoparathyroidism, **Arch Neurol Psychiatry 70:**86, 1953.
227. Symington BE: Hetastarch and bleeding complications, **Ann Intern Med 105:**627, 1986.
228. Szczepanska-Sadowska EWA: Mechanisms subserving brain water electrolyte homeostasis, **Acta Physiol Pol 40:** 301, 1989.
229. Takaku A, Shindo K, Tanaka S, et al: Fluid and electrolyte disturbances in patients with intracranial aneurysms, **Surg Neurol 11:**349, 1979.
230. Tator CH, Fehlings MG: Review of the secondary injury theory of acute spinal cord trauma with emphasis on vascular mechanisms, **J Neurosurg 75:**15, 1991.
231. Thel MC, Armstrong AL, McNulty SE, et al: Randomised trial of magnesium in in-hospital cardiac arrest, Duke Internal Medicine Housestaff, **Lancet 350:**1272, 1997.
232. Thurston HG, Sherman WR, Hauhart RE, et al: Myoinositol: a newly identified nonnitrogenous osmoregulatory molecule in mammalian brain, **Pediatr Res 26:** 482, 1989.
233. Thurston JH, Hauhart RE: Brain amino acids decrease in chronic hyponatremia and rapid correction causes brain dehydration: possible clinical significance, **Life Sci 40:**2539, 1987.
234. Todd M, Zornow MH: Effects of crystalloid and colloid infusions on intracranial pressure, **Neurosurgery 26:** 546, 1990.
235. Todd MM, Tommasino C, Moore S: Cerebral effects of isovolemic hemodilution with a hypertonic saline solution, **J Neurosurg 63:**944, 1985.
236. Tommasino C, Moore S, Todd MM: Cerebral effects of isovolemic hemodilution with crystalloid or colloid solutions, **Crit Care Med 16:**862, 1988.
237. Tranmer BI, Iacobacci RI, Kindt GW: Effects of crystalloid and colloid infusions on intracranial pressure and computerized electroencephalographic data in dogs with vasogenic brain edema, **Neurosurgery 25:**173, 1989.
238. Trost HA, Gaab MR: Plasma osmolality, osmoregulation and prognosis after head injury, **Acta Neurochir (Wien) 116:**33, 1992.
239. Tu YK, Kuo MF, Liu HM: Cerebral oxygen transport and metabolism during graded isovolemic hemodilution in experimental global ischemia, **J Neurol Sci 150:** 115, 1997.
240. Tuchschmidt J, Sharma OP: Impact of hemodynamic monitoring in a medical intensive care unit, **Crit Care Med 15:**840, 1987.
241. Turner JWA: Concentrated serum in head injuries, **Lancet 2:**557, 1941.
242. Unger T, Gohlke P, Kotrba M, et al: Angiotensin II and atrial natriuretic peptide in the brain: effects on volume and Na^+ balance, **Resuscitation 18:**309, 1989.
243. Vassar MJ, Holcroft JW: Use of hypertonic-hyperoncotic fluids for resuscitation of trauma patients, **J Intensive Care Med 7:**189, 1992.
244. Vassar MJ, Perry CA, Gannaway WL, et al: 7.5% sodium chloride/dextran for resuscitation of trauma patients undergoing helicopter transport, **Arch Surg 126:** 1065, 1991.
245. Velanovich V: Crystalloid versus colloid fluid resuscitation: a meta-analysis of mortality, **Surgery 105:**65, 1989.
246. Vianna MJ: Severe hypophosphatemia due to hypokalemia, **JAMA 215:**1497, 1971.
247. Vingerhoets F, De Tribolet N: Hyponatremia hypoosmolarity in neurosurgical patients. "Appropriate secretion of ADH" and "cerebral salt wasting syndrome," **Acta Neurochir 91:**50, 1988.
248. Virgilio RW, Rice CL, Smith DE, et al: Crystalloid vs. colloid resuscitation: is one better? **Surgery 85:**129, 1979.
249. Wade JV, Olson JP, Samson FE, et al: A possible role for taurine in osmoregulation within the brain, **J Neurochem 51:**740, 1988.
250. Wass CT, Lanier WL: Glucose modulation of ischemic brain injury: review and clinical recommendations, **Mayo Clin Proc 71:**801, 1996.
251. Weil MH: Patient evaluation, "vital signs," and initial care. Critical care: state of the art, **Fullerton Soc Crit Care Med, 1(A):**1, 1980.
252. Whang R, Oei TO, Aikawa JK, et al: Predictors of clinical hypomagnesia: hypokalemia, hypophosphatemia, hyponatremia and hypocalcemia, **Arch Intern Med 144:** 1794, 1984.
253. Wijdicks EFM, Ropper AH, Hunnicutt EJ, et al: A trial natriuretic factor and salt wasting after aneurysmal subarachnoid hemorrhage, **Stroke 22:**1519, 1991.
254. Wijdicks EFM, Van Dongen KJ, Vangijn J, et al: Enlargement of the third ventricle and hyponatraemia in aneurysmal subarachnoid haemorrhage, **J Neurol Neurosurg Psychiatry 51:**516, 1988.
255. Wijdicks EFM, Vermeulen M, Hijdra A, et al: Hyponatremia and cerebral infarction in patients with ruptured intracranial aneurysms: is fluid restriction harmful? **Ann Neurol 17:**137, 1985.
256. Wijdicks EFM, Vermeulen M, Ten Haff JA,: Volume depletion and natriuresis in patients with a ruptured intracranial aneurysm, **Ann Neurol 18:**211, 1985.
257. Wildenthal K, Mierzwiak DS, Myers RW: Effects of acute lactic acidosis of left ventricular performance, **Am J Physiol 214:**1352, 1968.
258. Williams HH, Wall BM, Horan JM, et al: Nonosmotic stimuli alter osmoregulation in patients with spinal cord injury, **J Clin Endocrinol Metab 71:**1536, 1990.

259. Wilson RF, Gibson D, Percinel AK: Severe alkalosis in critically ill surgical patients, **Arch Surg 105:**197, 1972.
260. Worthley LIG, Cooper DJ, Jones N: Treatment of resistant intracranial hypertension with hypertonic saline, **J Neurosurg 68:**478, 1988.
261. Wright D, Bond D, Hughes J: Reduction of cerebrospinal fluid pressure by concentrated lyophile serum. Further observations, **Arch Neurol Psychiatry 39:**1288, 1938.
262. Young B, Ott L, Dempsy R, et al: Relationship between admission hyperglycemia and neurologic outcome of severely brain-injured patients, **Ann Surg 210:**466, 1989.
263. Young GB, Amacher AL, Paulseth JE,: Hypophosphatemia versus brain death, **Lancet 1(1):**617, 1982.
264. Young WF, Rosenwasser RH, Vasthare US, et al: Preservation of post-compression spinal cord function by infusion of hypertonic saline, **J Neurol Anesthesiol 6:**122, 1994.
265. Zaloga GP, Chernow B, Cook D, et al: Assessment of calcium homeostasis in the critically ill surgical patient, **Crit Care Med 12:**236, 1984.
266. Zaloga GP, Chernow B, Cook D: Assessment of calcium homeostasis in the critically ill patient: the diagnostic pitfalls of the Mclean Hastings nomogram, **Ann Surg 202:**587, 1985.
267. Zaloga GP, Chernow B: Hypocalcemia in critical illness, **JAMA 256(14):**1924, 1986.
268. Zaloga GP, Wilkens R, Tourville J,: A simple method for determining physiologically active calcium and magnesium concentrations in critically ill patients, **Crit Care Med 15(9):**813, 1987.
269. Zaloga GP: Hypocalcemic crisis, **Crit Care Clin 7:** 191, 1991.
270. Zollinger RM, Skillman JJ, Moore FD: Alterations in water, colloid, and electrolyte distribution after hemorrhage, in Fox CL, Nahas GG, (eds): **Body fluid replacement in the surgical patient,** New York: Grune and Stratton, 1970, pp 2-9.
271. Zornow MH, Scheller MS, Shackford SR: Effect of hypertonic lactated Ringer's solution on intracranial pressure and cerebral water content in a model of traumatic brain injury, **J Trauma 29:**484, 1989.
272. Zornow MH, Scheller MS, Todd MM, et al: Acute cerebral effects of isotonic crystalloid and colloid solutions following cryogenic brain injury in the rabbit, **Anesthesiology 69:**185, 1988.
273. Zornow MH, Todd MM, Moore SS: The acute cerebral effects of changes in plasma osmolality and oncotic pressure, **Anesthesiology 67:**936, 1987.

CHAPTER 7

Metabolic, Nutritional, and Endocrine Aspects of Neurosurgical Intensive Care

DAVID MCKALIP

INTRODUCTION

Optimal nutritional support of the postoperative, critically ill, or injured neurosurgical patient is essential to ensure recovery from these altered metabolic states. Lengthy intracranial operations, severe head injury, and critical illness in the neurosurgical patient can be accompanied by elevations of metabolic rate, disturbances in processing of metabolic components, and potential for inadequate wound healing or recovery from central nervous system (CNS) injury. Severe head injury serves as a model for the most extreme form of metabolic disturbance associated with neurosurgical critical care and will be used for consideration of these topics in this chapter. The basic principles of metabolic and nutritional management of this population can be applied to other situations in the critically ill neurosurgical patient with variations made as needed for specific diseases.

Disturbances in endocrine physiology can also impact on the critically ill neurosurgical patient. Thyroid, adrenal, or neurohypophyseal dysfunction can lead to critical disturbances in patient homeostasis. Hormonal pathophysiology will be discussed as it relates to the management of the metabolic state in the critically ill neurosurgical patient.

METABOLISM AND NUTRITION

Normal metabolic physiology is characterized by optimal utilization of energy intake to maintain the energy needs of the individual in normal and altered homeostatic states. Calories taken in the form of carbohydrates, protein, and fats are absorbed by the gastrointestinal (GI) tract, broken down to their basic constituents, and converted to glucose for short-term energy, glycogen for less immediate needs, and fat for long-term storage of reserve calories. When the body faces a new homeostatic state requiring more energy—as may be seen in critical illness, injury, or elective surgery—metabolic processes are altered to meet these needs. In these states, end-organ energy demand may outstrip the ability of the body to supply this energy, and mobilization of protein and fat stores may occur. Failure to keep up with the body's metabolic needs as it faces this hypermetabolic state can result in loss of muscle mass, immunosuppression, and malnutrition states characterized by increased infections, poor wound healing, and weight loss. Failure to meet metabolic needs has been associated with increased mortality and morbidity in head-injured patients.[40]

Fifty years ago Cuthbertson[12] characterized the metabolic response to injury as containing ebb and flow phases.[2] The ebb phase is accompanied by depressed cardiac output due to hypovolemia and extracellular fluid sequestration and is characterized by decreased oxygen consumption, body temperature, and insulin levels. During this phase, occurring in the first 24 to 48 hours after injury, blood glucose, lactate, and free fatty acids are elevated along with circulating levels of catecholamines, glucagons, and cortisol. The body becomes insulin resistant, resulting in increased glucose levels. By the end of the first week, the flow phase begins, characterized by increased oxygen consumption, cardiac output, and body temperature. Nitrogen loss occurs, and the body experiences elevated glucose, free fatty acids, and cytokine production. The mediators of hypermetabolic states are not completely defined; however, elevated serum catecholamines[53] and cytokines such as interleukin-1, interleukin-6, and other mediators of the acute phase response are thought to contribute.[35,37,57]

Metabolic changes occurring in the neurosurgical patients have been most thoroughly studied following head injury,[29] but many of these processes are present in other neurologic diseases, such as acute ischemic events.[51] Head-injured patients have been shown to

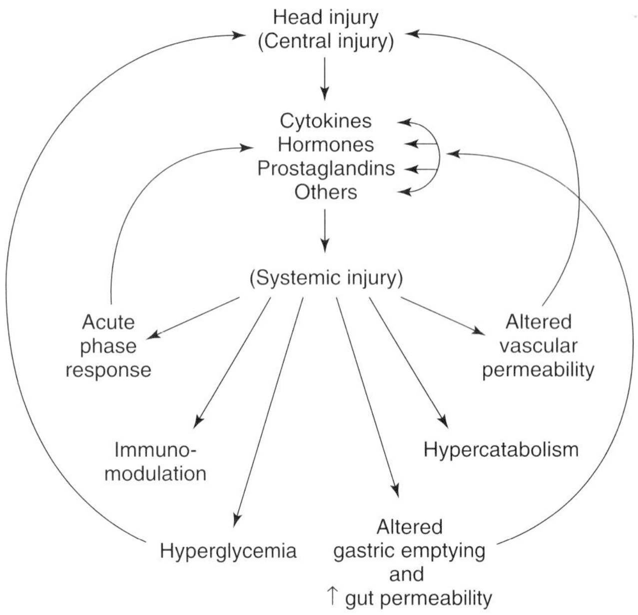

FIG. 7-1 ■ Metabolic consequences of head injury. (From Young and Ott[58] with permission.)

experience a degree of hypermetabolism not present in patients with noncranial injury.[6] Severe head injury (Glasgow Coma Scale score ≤ 8) is characterized by negative nitrogen balance, weight loss, immune depression, and depressed plasma protein levels, even in the face of adequate caloric and protein administration (Fig. 7-1).[10,35,62] Through an unclear mechanism, basal metabolic expenditure (BME) is increased an average of 40% for 3 weeks after severe head injury[35] and may be the common cause of these observed effects. Others have noted an increased metabolic rate up to a year following severe head injury.[18,62]

The spinal cord–injured patient appears to have a basal energy expenditure that is 10% to 55% lower than predicted.[27,45] It is likely that decreased oxygen consumption occurs in the denervated muscle mass, resulting in an overall lowered metabolic requirement. Basal energy expenditure measured in five quadriplegic patients revealed a requirement of only 80% of that determined using predictive formulas.[25] A higher level of spinal cord injury correlates with a lower caloric requirement.[11,27] The stroke patient appears to have an average 20% increase in energy demand, which correlates with increased serum catecholamines.[50] Metabolic response to subarachnoid hemorrhage is less well studied, but an increased metabolic rate has been noted in these patients as well.[23]

Evaluation of Nutritional Requirements and Status

To optimally nourish a patient recovering in the critical care unit, an assessment of the patient's premorbid nutritional status, current metabolic needs, and special requirements should be made. Premorbid status can be evaluated by careful history and physical examination, attending to signs or symptoms of malnourishment (e.g., alcoholism and cachexia) or obesity. Laboratory patients of the premorbidly malnourished patient may show low albumin, potassium, and magnesium levels. Current needs can be evaluated based on the underlying disease state and a determination of the patient's energy expenditure and nutrient requirements. Weight and anthropometric measurements are not reliable in the acute phase given their slow rate of change and the effect of the rapid fluid shifts associated with injury and critical illness. Skin testing may also be an unreliable technique in the acute phase.[35]

Energy Requirements

The ideal method of measuring a patient's caloric needs (in kilocalories per day) has yet to be established. It can be estimated (1) objectively with indirect calorimetry, (2) through the use predictive formulas, or (3) empirically. The goal in calculating a caloric requirement is to avoid complications associated with overfeeding (Table 7-1) or underfeeding. Although the most accurate method of measuring the patient's metabolic energy expenditure (MEE) is indirect calorimetry,[31,47] the technique requires special equipment and a person skilled in interpreting the data obtained. During indirect calorimetry, oxygen and carbon dioxide content are determined in inspired and expired gas from the patient. Oxygen consumption and carbon dioxide production is then determined using formulas with known constants. The respiratory quotient (RQ) is calculated as the ratio of VCO_2 to VO_2 and used with the 24-hour urine urea nitrogen (UUN) to calculate the source of energy predominantly used by the patient, if desired. An RQ of 0.70 indicates predominate fat usage, 0.8 protein usage, and 1.0 carbohydrate usage. The UUN is used to calculate energy derived from protein use. An RQ greater than 1 may indicate overfeeding of the patient. The energy expenditure is calculated using the

TABLE 7-1 ■ Complications of Overfeeding[46]

- Excessive CO_2 production
- Increased minute ventilation
- Respiratory failure
- Respiratory acidosis in COPD due to CO_2 retention
- Pulmonary edema
- Worsening of congestive heart failure
- Hyperglycemia
- Lipogenesis
- Gain of fluid/fat rather than lean body mass
- Fatty liver
- Uremia
- Electrolyte depletion

- $VO_2 = (Vi \times FiO_2) - (Ve \times FeO_2)$
- $VCO_2 = (Vi \times FiCO_2) - (Ve \times Fe\ CO_2)$
- $RQ = VCO_2/VO_2$
- $EE = (3.586 \times VO_2) + (1.433 \times VC02) - 1.180\ NM$

NM, Metabolized nitrogen (grams of protein intake/6.25); *VO_2,* Oxygen consumption; *VCO_2,* carbon dioxide production; *RQ,* respiratory quotient; *Fi,* fraction of inspired gas; *Fe,* fraction of expired gas; *Vi,* inspired volume; *Ve,* expired volume.

FIG. 7-2 ■ Formulas used to calculate energy requirements using data derived from indirect calorimetry.

formula in Fig. 7-2 and reflects the amount of energy expended by the patient during the metabolic study. To obtain an estimate of the energy requirement, it may be necessary for the patient to fast for 12 hours prior to the study. The test is most accurate when the patient is resting and needs no interventions that may elevate energy expenditure such as suctioning or ventilator changes.[31] The RQ can also be estimated using the Fick method with a pulmonary artery catheter, although this is less accurate.[31]

Formulas used to calculate a patient's needs have been shown to be poorly correlated with estimates of MEE determined by indirect calorimetry.[47] Formulas calculate the kilocalories required per day based on age, anthropometric data (weight, height, sex), clinical data (heart rate, days since injury, Glasgow Coma Scale [GCS] score), or known stress factors (Fig. 7-3). Of three methods compared with indirect calorimetry (%RME, Harris-Benedict, and Stress Stratification Estimate), the estimation of %RME described by Clifton correlated best, but still miscalculated the nutritional requirements in more than 40% of patients.[47]

Although the Harris-Benedict equation provides an estimate of the basal energy expenditure (BEE), the energy estimation must be modified to account for the stress of illness. In the past, the actual energy expenditure—the resting energy expenditure (REE)—has traditionally been calculated by multiplying the BEE by 30%, 60%, or 100% for patients with injury, sepsis, and burns, respectively; however, this may overestimate the amount of calories supplied, resulting in metabolic complications of overfeeding such as CO_2 overproduction, increased ventilatory de-

%RME (Clifton, 1986)[8]	• $GCS \leq 7$: %RME = 152 − 14(GCS) + 0.4(HR) + 7(DSI) • $GCS > 7$: %RME = 90 − 3(GCS) + 0.9(HR)
Harris-Benedict Equation	**Men:** kcal/24 hr = **Women:** kcal/24 hr = 66.5 + (13.8×W) + (5.0×H) − (6.8×A) 655 + (9.6×W) + (1.8×H) − (4.7×A)

W, Weight (kg); *H,* height (cm); *A,* age (yr)

FIG. 7-3 ■ Formulas for prediction of energy requirements in head injury.

mands, and hyperglycemia (see Table 7-1).[3,7,16] If indirect calorimetry is unavailable or impractical, the needs can be estimated using the REE as calculated by multiplying the BEE by 1.1 to 1.4. The patient's current body weight is used when calculating the BEE by Harris-Benedict. In the very obese patient, 120 kg can be used as the weight factor, because the nomograms used in this paradigm are less accurate over this weight.[22]

The third method of estimating caloric needs empirically uses a replacement regimen of a set number of kilocalories per kilograms of ideal body weight per day depending on the patient's clinical state. This has been estimated at 26 kcal/kg/day after craniotomy, 40 to 50 for patients with a GCS of 4 to 5, 30 to 40 for GCS 6 to 7, and 30 to 35 kcal/kg/day in patients with GCS of 8 to 12. In paraplegic patients, fewer kcal day are given (27 kcal/kg/day), and quadriplegic patients are given even less (23 kcal/kg/day).[11,27] Others have first estimated protein needs and achieved a kilocalorie to nitrogen ratio of 100 to 1 to provide the nonprotein calories.[4]

The guidelines for management of patients with severe head injuries recommend providing calories to supply 140% of the patient's BEE.[33] This is based on empiric observations of BEE in head injury patients elevated by 40% on average. In those patients in whom pharmacologic paralysis is applied, the guidelines recommend replacing at 100% of BEE; however, the metabolic needs of head injury patients can vary between 120% to 250% in the nonparalyzed state. Thus indirect calorimetry provides the most accurate method of determining metabolic needs.[47] Studies have also shown no difference in energy requirements between steroid- and nonsteroid-treated head injury patients.[35,43]

Protein Requirements

Whole body catabolism and loss of muscular protein stores are the norm during severe illness and injury. The normal protein requirements for stable healthy adults is approximately 0.6 g/kg/day; however, this is increased following injury or illness to prevent loss of lean body mass. It is estimated that initial protein replacement following injury should be in the range of 1.5 to 2.5 g/kg of ideal body weight/day.[13] In the head injury guidelines, the consensus appears to be that 15% of calories should be given as protein.[33]

Once the initial protein dose is determined, the adequacy of protein replacement can be estimated using determinations of nitrogen balance or through the monitoring of plasma proteins. Nitrogen balance should be determined weekly beginning 5 days after the level of protein support is stabilized. The patient's urine is collected for 24 hours and the total urine urea nitrogen is determined in that specimen using the formulas in Fig. 7-4.

- N (in) – protein intake/6.25 (g/day)
- N (out) – urine urea N/0.8 (g/day) + GI loss (2-4 g/day) + cutaneous loss (0-4 g/day)
- Nitrogen (N) Balance = N (in) – N (out)
- Optimal = +2 – 4 g/day

FIG. 7-4 ■ Determination of nitrogen balance.

Ideally, nitrogen balance is maintained "positive" at 2 to 4 g/day—meaning that the body has the excess protein necessary to meet its needs and avoid loss of lean body mass. Efforts to place patients into a positive nitrogen balance by providing high-protein diets have been largely unsuccessful[9] because of the nitrogen wasting state that is present for 2 to 3 weeks[35] in patients with head injury; however, Twyman and colleagues reported success in achieving a positive nitrogen balance in the first 10 days using 1 g protein per 90 calories.[51] This difficulty in placing patients in positive nitrogen balance is a consistent observation in trauma victims.[35] A recent pilot investigation of insulin-like growth factor (IGF) demonstrated that patients with severe head injury receiving IGF were able to achieve positive nitrogen balance and had improved favorable outcomes.[20]

Measurement of nitrogen balance suffers from errors that may result from unmeasured losses (resulting in artificially elevated nitrogen balance during periods of high nitrogen intake). An estimate of the body's protein state may be more accurately made by measuring serum proteins. Plasma levels of albumin, prealbumin, transferrin, and retinol-binding proteins (RBP) provide an estimate of the adequacy of protein stores available in the body[4] (Table 7-2). Proteins with shorter half lives may be more sensitive to changes in nutritional stress (transferrin, RBP, prealbumin), although albumin is the most reliable prognostic marker.[4]

Lipid Requirements

Typically 30% to 40% of calories are supplied through lipids with a starting carbohydrate/lipid ratio of 4:1 g. It is best to avoid providing more than 50% to 60% of calories as lipids because this can lead to a fat overload syndrome, which is characterized by fatty deposition in capillary beds of major organs, resulting in organ failure, thrombocytopenia, and hemolytic anemia.[21] Essential fatty acids—those containing a double bond at the ninth and terminal carbon—must be provided because they cannot be synthesized by humans. Failure to provide these omega-6 (linoleic) and omega-3 (linolenic) fatty aids in adults and children, respectively, can lead to an essential fatty acid deficiency (EFAD) in 2 to 3 weeks. Essential fatty acids are used for synthesis of arachidonic acids and the resultant prostaglandins. EFAD is characterized by diffuse dermatitis, hemolytic anemia, increased platelet aggregation, decreased wound healing, and hepatic dysfunction. Essential fatty acids are found in vegetable seed oils such as soy, safflower, and canola, staples of most commercial enteral formulas. Investigators have focused on the role of exogenous fatty acids in attenuating the inflammatory response following head injury, but outcome studies are still pending.[1,21,55]

TABLE 7-2 ■ Visceral Protein Markers[4]

Protein Marker	Normal Values	Half Life (days)
Albumin	>3.5 gm/dl	20
Transferrin	>200 mg/dl	8.5
Prealbumin	20–30 mg/dl	1.3
Retinol-binding protein	4–5 mg/dl	0.4

Electrolyte and Micronutrient Requirements

The electrolyte status of the critically ill or injured neurosurgical patient is of considerable importance and is addressed separately in this book (see Chapter 6). Malnutrition and refeeding are associated with changes in electrolyte balance, which must be carefully monitored during the critical care phase. Intracellular potassium, magnesium, and phosphorous are lost in the malnourished state. These ions may drop further when refeeding the patient with an energy deficit. In patients with premorbid malnourishment, potassium and magnesium deficiencies may already exist.

Trace elements such as zinc, copper, iron, iodine, cobalt, and selenium are required for proper functioning of enzyme complexes regulating the use of carbohydrates, fats, and proteins. In the seriously ill patient, zinc and selenium are required at higher levels.[13,30] Young and colleagues[61] demonstrated an improved outcome in head-injured patients receiving zinc supplementation, although the study may have suffered from bias in selection of patients. The administration of zinc in this study was associated with an increase in the visceral proteins prealbumin and retinol-binding protein.

Although the optimal dosing of vitamins in critically ill patients remains unclear, they must be included in enteral and parenteral formulas. Most commercially available tube feeds meet the requirement for trace micronutrients, but custom orders for total parenteral nutrition (TPN) are required to supply these. Consultation with a hospital nutrition service is the optimal way to ensure these requirements are met.

Method of Feeding

Nutrition can be maintained orally, enterally, or parenterally, and should be instituted as early as possible to prevent complications of malnourishment in the critically ill patient. When available, the gut should be used for delivering nutrition to the critically ill and injured neurosurgical patient. Complications and complexity of TPN make it a second choice in this population. In the patient without altered consciousness, oral intake with caloric and protein supplementation as needed is an available option.

Enteral Feeding

In the patient with altered mental status, oral intake may be impossible or dangerous because of inability to swallow or protect the airway from aspiration. Placement of either a gastric or small bowel feeding tube can facilitate early feeding and allow for the caloric and protein requirements to be provided. Small-bore duodenal tubes can be placed at the bedside to a premeasured length. If a "high KUB" film fails to show cannulation of the small bowel, another attempt can be made and a gastric relaxant such as metoclopromide can be used while the patient is placed with his or her right side down. If after 2 to 3 days the tube is not properly placed, fluoroscopy or endoscopy can assist with placement.

In the head-injured patient, gastric emptying is often impaired and jejunal feeding is better tolerated than feeding to the stomach.[15,26,36] A threefold increase in the rate of aspiration pneumonia was seen in head-injured patients fed into the stomach versus those fed with TPN.[62] A sixfold increase in the rate of aspiration was seen in an autopsy study of tube-fed neurologic patients.[34] In a randomized study, Graham and colleagues[15] demonstrated that patients receiving gastric feedings were less likely to reach nutritional goals compared with those receiving feedings in the small bowel. In this study, those undergoing fluoroscopically guided placement of jejunal tubes reached nutritional goals by day 3. Only half those who were gastric-fed reached nutritional goals by day 7. Gastric-fed patients were delayed until bowel sounds returned, whereas jejunally fed patients were fed even in the absence of bowel sounds. Those who achieved early jejunal feeds had shorter ICU stays and lower incidence of positive sputum cultures (defined as "bronchitis" in the study). Roberts[42] attempts a trial of gastric feedings within the first day, stating that about 75% of severely head-injured patients can tolerate this, although this is based on the personal experience of that author (personal communication). The head of the bed is kept elevated 30 to 45 degrees, and if gastric residuals are high, a small bowel tube is placed. In a recent study examining ultra-early enteral feedings (first 24 hours) in severely head-injured patients,[49] 66% of the study group (n = 27) were fed through a gastric route and had no higher incidence of aspiration pneumonia; however, this was not a primary endpoint of the study and may have suffered from a type II statistical error given the relatively low number in this analysis. Ott and colleagues[36] recently demonstrated a similar aspiration rate between tubes placed in the small bowel versus those placed in the stomach, but acknowledge that the study was inconclusive in answering this question because of a high number of variables. Because of delayed gastric emptying, poor airway protection, and serious consequences of aspiration pneumonia, the author favors feeding in the small bowel below the pyloric sphincter when possible, but acknowledges that gastric feedings can be performed if residuals are low and the head of the bed is kept elevated.

Tube feedings are usually begun at a rate of approximately 30 ml/hr and advanced every 4 hours by 10 ml/hr based on the measurements of gastric residuals according to the protocol given by Roberts.[42] If gastric residuals (measured from a nasogastric [NG] tube in a patient with a small bowel tube) are more than 150 ml, feeds are held for 2 hours and resumed when residuals are under 150 ml. Taylor and colleagues demonstrated that gastrically fed patients can have feeds advanced to a full rate within 24 hours if gastric residuals are under 200 ml.[49] Abdominal distension or poor or absent bowel sound may also prompt holding or decreasing tube feeding. A KUB may be required to diagnose an ileus, and if one is found or is prolonged, TPN may be required during bowel rest.

Diarrhea may develop secondary to the high osmolality of many tube feeds. This may be solved by diluting the feeds temporarily with water, switching to another formula, or cutting the rate of the feeds. Adding fiber to tube feeds may also help to solidify the stool contents (psyllium 30 ml up to three times a day). Additionally, it is important to rule out other causes of diarrhea such as pseudomembranous colitis or medications.

It is also important to ensure that the patient's fluid needs are being met, because enteral formulas may not contain enough free water to prevent dehydration by themselves, especially in the hypermetabolic patient. Therefore free water needs should be calculated and supplied either intravenously or as additional fluid in the feeding tube. Caution should be used when blousing the small intestine, because this may not be tolerated.

Parenteral Feedings

Patients with severe head injuries receiving TPN have improved outcomes compared with those receiving inadequate nutrition enterally.[40,63] Rapp and colleagues[40] randomized patients to receive either parenteral nutrition within 48 hours of admission or standard enteral nutrition through an NG tube when patients could tolerate feeds with low gastric residuals. Those in the enteral group failed to achieve caloric goals during the study and had far worse outcomes clinically. Young and colleagues[63] randomized 51 patients to receive either TPN or enteral nutrition and determined that there was no difference in ICP, cerebral edema, or hyperglycemia between groups. Patients receiving TPN had higher early caloric intake and positive nitrogen balance and outcomes that were more favorable at 3 months, but this did not persist at 6 or 12 months. Although these studies demonstrate that TPN is an important adjunct in providing nutrition to head-injured patients, the main conclusion from these studies should demonstrate that providing early nutrition improves outcome.

TPN should be begun when the intestinal tract is fully dysfunctional or enteral feedings are failing to provide adequate nutritional support[4] and should be delivered through a fresh, dedicated central line. Formulation of the TPN solution is usually best done together with a nutrition service; refer to a standard textbook on nutrition for complete details.[22] Formulas typically start with either 25% dextrose and 4.25% amino acids or 21% dextrose and 7% amino acids. The amino acid solution should contain 25% essential amino acids. Although some formulations contain up to 50% with high-branched chain amino acids, these have yet to be shown to improve outcome. Patients on TPN typically should receive 10% to 20% lipid emulsions at least 2 times per week. Usually, 70% of energy needs should be supplied with carbohydrates and amino acids and 30% by lipids, with at least 3% as essential fatty acids.[4,13] Feeding a patient parenterally costs nearly twice as much during a hospitalization for severe head injury.[36]

When possible, a low rate of enteral feedings should be given concomitantly to prevent mucosal atrophy and help prevent bacterial translocation across the intestinal wall. Patients with hypertriglyceridemia (>300 mg%) or pancreatitis caused by hyperlipidemia should not receive lipid infusions. Patients receiving TPN can suffer from complications associated with central lines and should have daily monitoring of electrolytes, triglycerides, and glucose levels.

Oral Feeding

When the patient regains consciousness or the faculty to swallow, efforts should be directed toward oral feeding. Evaluation by a speech pathologist may assist with this determination. A clinical evaluation of swallowing may indicate "wet" swallowing, the inability to handle liquids or solid boluses. If the clinical evaluation is equivocal or not able to be performed, evaluation with an objective study such as a barium or Gastrografin swallow may be warranted.

After a patient has begun an oral regimen, it is important to ensure adequate caloric and protein intake, which may best be accomplished by using calorie counts. If a patient deteriorates or is unable to meet his or her nutritional needs, enteral or parenteral nutrition may again be required. Supplementing a patient's diet with high-calorie and high-protein shakes may be a valuable adjunct to meeting nutritional needs (1 to 2 cans three times a day).

Timing of Feeding

Zaloga[65] recently reviewed 19 studies examining timing of nutrition and concluded that early enteral feeding was supported by a preponderance of class I evidence. In the head-injured population, it is clear that delay in meeting nutritional needs results in poor outcomes.[40] Other studies comparing TPN with enteral nutrition[17,60] similarly demonstrated that a delay in providing adequate calories and protein negatively impacted outcomes. Studies evaluating enteral nutrition techniques found that patients fed early through jejunal[15] or gastric[49] routes had faster recoveries, shorter ICU stays, and fewer infections. In a recent randomized, prospective study of severely head-injured patients, Taylor and colleagues fed study patients at a goal rate enterally from day 1 and compared outcomes with patients fed using a progressive increase in tube feed rates.[49] The patients receiving "enhanced enteral nutrition" (study group) were fed predominantly in the stomach (66%) starting at a rate of 50 to 80 ml/hr from day 1; feeds were reduced to half rate if gastric residuals were more than 200 ml over 4 hours. Study patients achieved 70% of nitrogen and energy goals within 1 week compared with control patients, who only met 50% of their requirement by day 7. The intervention patients had fewer infective complications, shorter hospital stays, and a more rapid improvement in neurologic outcome, although the final outcome was the same, neurologically.

Advances in Nutrition

Recent investigations have focused on the use of enhanced nutritional formulas or treatments to improve outcomes from neurological injury beyond what is normally achieved by simply providing for caloric and protein needs. These efforts focus on preventing hyperglycemia in the head-injured patient, modulating injury-induced hypermetabolism, or preventing infections using "immunonutrition."

Following injury, metabolic changes render the patient insulin resistant, resulting in a "diabetes of injury."[58] In animal models, hyperglycemia has been shown to exacerbate neuronal injury, presumably by increasing local lactic acid production in the brain. Hyperglycemia has been correlated with poor outcomes in head-injured patients,[59] although it is unclear if this is a direct cause of poor outcome or merely reflects a worsened metabolic state after injury.[5,14,39,54,56] Although it remains to be seen if hyperglycemia adversely affects clinical outcome in patients, several groups have focused on ensuring that hyperglycemia occurring after injury is not exacerbated.[41,48] Robertson and colleagues[44] randomly provided nutrition with or without glucose to head-injured patients and determined that cerebrospinal fluid (CSF) lactate levels were lower and the brain was more able to utilize ketone bodies in those not receiving glucose. Further studies are required to determine if managing patients without glucose in feeds[41] or intravenous solutions[48] will improve outcomes. In the meantime, it seems prudent to manage hyperglycemia in the brain-injured patient with frequent monitoring of glucose levels and insulin as needed to keep serum glucose as close to normal as possible (<200 mg%).

Excitatory amino acids also may exacerbate brain injury, although a randomized controlled study of agents that block their receptors have not show benefit.[32] Nevertheless, there are concerns over the use of glutamate in "enhanced" enteral formulas designed to prevent bacterial translocation by supplying the amino acid to the small bowel mucosa (which uses it directly for energy production). The use of glutamine-containing formulas may merit further investigation prior to routine use in the head-injured patient. Others have investigated the use of additional branched chain amino acids to improve nitrogen balance.[38] These studies have shown a deceleration in protein loss but have not yet been associated with improved outcome.[21]

Recently, investigators have studied the benefits of "immunonutrition" in preventing infections in critically ill patients, and a recent review of 12 prospective studies of immunonutrition demonstrate with class I evidence that immune-enhancing formulas improve outcomes and reduce length of hospitalization.[64] These formulas typically contain substances thought to enhance the immune system, such as dietary peptides (e.g., casein, soy), arginine, glutamine, nucleic acids, and vitamins C, E, and A, as well as omega-3 and omega-6 fatty acids. Although these results are encouraging, these formulas have not yet been fully evaluated in the head injury population.

ENDOCRINE ISSUES

The remainder of this chapter deals with the critical care of patients with primary endocrine derangements directly attributable to neurosurgical disease, and care of patients with neurosurgical disease who have underlying endocrinopathies. Sudden endocrine disturbances may occur following pituitary surgery, CNS injury, or in patients with preexisting endocrine disease who are subject to the stress of illness, injury, or elective surgery. In most cases, consultation with a specialist experienced in managing endocrinopathies in a critical care setting is valuable.

The endocrine system is driven by the hypothalamus, pituitary stalk, anterior and posterior pituitary, and endocrine glands (thyroid, adrenal, parathyroid, gonads). Complex regulation of release of hormones along various axes (e.g., adrenal, thyroid) occurs in this system as hormones are released to affect cell receptors throughout the body. For instance, the release of thyrotropin-releasing hormone (TRH) from the hypothalamus causes release of thyroid-stimulating hormone (TSH) from the anterior pituitary, which induces production of thyroxine from the thyroid. This is used by individual cells throughout the body to regulate protein production and other intracellular metabolic processes and also feeds back to the hypothalamic-pituitary axis to inhibit its own release. Derangement of this delicate balance may not cause a sudden critical illness in a healthy individual, but it may impact the ability of the patient to tolerate a systemic insult from illness, injury, or elective surgery. Conversely, acute insults of the neurohypophysis may result in sudden alteration in body homeostasis. The most profound example of this is diabetes insipidus due to arginine vasopressin (AVP) deficiency or syndrome of inappropriate antidiuretic hormone secretion (SIADH). These are discussed separately in the chapter on fluid and electrolytes (Chapter 6).

Patients with pituitary tumors usually present to the ICU after elective surgical resection. Many have severe metabolic and hormonal derangements caused by their tumors: acromegaly, Cushing's disease, and hypopituitarism, for example.[24] Removal of these tumors per se will not necessarily cause direct endocrinopathies from sudden normalization of hormonal levels, but patients may suffer acute derangements from parasellar surgery itself. For instance, injury to adrenocorticotropic hormone (ACTH) secreting cells may cause acute hypoadrenalism manifested by hyponatremia, hyperkalemia, and obtundation. Therefore, many centers routinely administer glucocorticoids because of the presumed loss of ACTH secretion, which may occur with parasellar surgery.[24] Although patients with known adrenal insufficiency would require this, Hout and colleagues[24] have advocated only administering exogenous glucocorticoids to patients with known preoperative adrenal insufficiency. They carefully monitor postoperative cortisol levels (2 to 3 times per day) and administer hydrocortisone to patients with low cortisol levels or who manifest symptoms of ACTH deficiency.

Patients with adrenal insufficiency (Addisonian crisis) secondary to pituitary tumors or other causes may manifest this when stressed. Sudden obtundation accompanied by hyponatremia and hyperkalemia may follow infection, injury, or surgery, and a diagnosis can be confirmed by cortisol levels below 20 μg/dl.[19] Other causes related to primary adrenal disease should also be considered as a source, including autoimmune adrenalitis and destruction by tuberculosis. Patients who are withdrawn from steroid therapy too quickly or who are adrenally suppressed from chronic steroid therapy may also be affected. Therapy is directed toward rapid fluid resuscitation, immediate administration of steroids, and correction of any accompanying hypoglycemia. If the diagnosis is well established, a patient can be administered a 100-mg intravenous bolus of hydrocortisone hemisuccinate followed by a 75 to 100 mg dose every 6 hours. After resuscitation, patients are tapered to 30 mg orally every 6 hours. If the diagnosis is in doubt, a cosyntropin (Cortrosyn) stimulation test may be required to determine if serum cortisol levels can rise in response to administration of the ACTH analog cosyntropin. In this case, dexamethasone (Decadron) is used for initial therapy (4 mg intravenously every 4 hours) and tapered to hydrocortisone after the test. Dexamethasone will not interact with the cortisol, which is detected 30 to 60 minutes after administration of 250 μg. Failure of cortisol to rise above 20 μg/dl indicates adrenal insufficiency. Other critically ill patients requiring acute steroid administration can include those suffering from hypopituitarism, pituitary apoplexy, or those receiving prior steroid therapy for other reasons.

Patients with known thyroid disease may have exacerbation of their underlying dysfunctional hormonal state when faced with injury, illness, or elective surgery. Thyroid hormones primarily increase metabolic activity in a patient leading to increased heart rate, temperature, and oxygen consumption. Patients with hypothyroidism may be unable to mount such a response in the face of stress, whereas hyperthyroid patients may have a hyperactive response with attendant complications.

Patients with a preexisting hypothyroid state are subject to decreased cardiac output, stroke volume, and hyponatremia when critically ill. Profoundly hypothyroid patients may lack a fever or leukocytosis when faced with an infection. More profound compromise than expected for the underlying disease or state should prompt an investigation of signs and symptoms of hypothyroidism (Table 7-3) and an inquiry to the family regarding past thyroid disease. Patients with hypothyroidism may suffer myxedema coma manifested as obtundation, nonpitting edema, hypothermia, hypoventilation, hypotension, and hypoglycemia. Management of these patients includes administration of thyroid hormones but also careful cardiovascular and pulmonary support. In the case of myxedema coma intravenous thyroxine is usually given at 500 μg initially followed by 50 μg every day and hydrocortisone may be given (100 mg q8h) in the event of coexisting adrenal insufficiency; however, this must be accompanied by aggressive hemodynamic fluid, and pulmonary management and passive warming of the cold patient. Hypothyroid patients without actual myxedema coma may still benefit from treatment with thyroid hormones orally or intravenously. Surgery may be carried out in these patients when stabilized as needed with a slight increase in complications.[28,52]

TABLE 7-3 ■ Common Signs and Symptoms of Hypothyroidism

Symptoms	Signs
• Cold intolerance	• Bradycardia
• Constipation	• Bradykinesia
• Dry skin	• Coarse hair
• Hoarseness	• Dry and coarse skin
• Lethargy	• Periorbital edema
• Parasthesias	• Delayed relaxation phase of deep tendon reflexes
• Peripheral edema	
• Weakness	
• Weight gain	

In patients with hyperthyroidism, illness, injury, or elective surgery may precipitate a thyroid storm or thyrotoxic crisis. Patients with previously unrecognized hyperthyroidism may have preexisting signs and symptoms of thyrotoxicosis (Table 7-4). A thyrotoxic crisis may manifest as hyperdynamic cardiac function (tachycardia, increased cardiac output and ejection fraction, decreased vascular resistance), arrhythmias (atrial fibrillation, supraventricular tachycardia), altered mental status, pulmonary compromise, and fever. When the diagnosis is suspected, therapy must begin immediately—prior to receiving results of confirmatory laboratory testing (elevated

TABLE 7-4 ■ Signs and Symptoms of Thyrotoxicosis

Symptoms	Signs
• Dyspnea	• Dermopathy
• Heat intolerance	• Goiter
• Hyperdefecation	• Gynecomastia
• Increased appetite	• Hyperkinesis
• Nervousness	• Hyperreflexia
• Palpitations	• Fine hair
• Scant or absent menses	• Lid retraction/lag
• Sweating	• Onycholysis
• Weakness	• Opthalmopathy
• Weight loss	• Proximal muscle weakness
	• Smooth skin
	• Thyroid bruit
	• Tremor
	• Warm, moist palms

T3 and T4 levels). Therapy usually consists of close monitoring, cardiovascular, pulmonary and fluid support, and rapid administration of antithyroid drugs, and beta-blockers. In life-threatening situations, treatment begins with propylthiouracil to inhibit thyroid hormone synthesis (800–1200 mg PO, then 200–300 q6h PO) and is accompanied by agents to inhibit thyroid hormone release (such as Lugol's solution, dexamethasone, or sodium iodide). As with other life-threatening endocrine disorders, consultation with a physician experienced in managing these diseases is prudent.

CONCLUSION

Adequate nutritional support of the critically ill neurosurgical patient requires an understanding of the patient's new metabolic state and nutritional requirements. When possible, objective measures of energy expenditure (such as indirect calorimetry) should be made and predictive formulas and empiric methods used as a secondary means of assessment. The patient should be monitored for signs of underfeeding or overfeeding. Enteral nutrition should be used as the first choice, because it is less expensive and less complicated than parenteral methods. Care should be taken when delivering enteral feeds directly to the stomach because of the risk of aspiration of gastric contents. Reaching nutrition goals as early as possible will improve patient outcomes. A nutritionist can provide indispensable service to assist in meeting a patient's nutritional needs and monitoring success of nutrition.

A patient with an underlying endocrinopathy may suffer an acute crisis in homeostasis when facing a stress such as illness, injury, or elective surgery. Attention to preexisting signs and symptoms of endocrine disease may assist in diagnosing the source of such a decompensation. Alternatively, parasellar surgery or head injury may produce a new disturbance in endocrine function. Rapid and aggressive systemic support together with administration of specific agents to replace or counteract missing or excessive hormonal levels may be required. Working together with a specialist experienced in managing critically ill patients with endocrine disease is optimal.

REFERENCES

1. Beale RJ, Bryg DJ, Bihari DJ: Immunonutrition in the critically ill: a systematic review of clinical outcome, **Crit Care Med 27:**2799–2805, 1999.
2. Bessey PQ, Downey RS, Monafo WM: Metabolic response to injury and critical illness, in Civetta JM, Taylor RW, Kirby RB, (eds): **Critical care,** ed 3, Philadelphia, 1997, Lippincott-Raven, pp 325–334.
3. Bjerke HS, Shabot MM: Glucose intolerance in critically ill surgical patients: relationship to total parenteral nutrition and severity of illness, **Am Surg 58:**728–731, 1992.
4. Byers P, Jeejeebhoy KN: Enteral and parenteral nutrition, in Civetta JM, Taylor RW, Kirby RB, (eds): **Critical care,** ed 3, Philadelphia, 1997, Lippincott-Raven, pp 457–473.
5. Chiaretti A, De Benedictis R, Langer A, et al: Prognostic implications of hyperglycaemia in paediatric head injury, **Childs Nerv Syst 14:**455–459, 1998.
6. Chiolaero R, Schutz Y, Lemarchand T, et al: Hormonal and metabolic changes following severe head injury or noncranial injury, **JPEN J Parenter Enteral Nutr 13:**5–12, 1989.
7. Christman JW, McCain RW: A sensible approach to the nutritional support of mechanically ventilated critically ill patients, **Intensive Care Med 19:**129–136, 1993.
8. Clifton GL, Robertson CS, Choi SC: Assessment of nutritional requirements of head-injured patients, **J Neurosurg 64:**895–901, 1986.
9. Clifton GL, Robertson CS, Contant CF: Enteral hyperalimentation in head injury, **J Neurosurg 62:**186–193, 1985.
10. Clifton GL, Robertson CS, Grossman RG, et al: The metabolic response to severe head injury, **J Neurosurg 60:**687–696, 1984.
11. Cox SA, Weiss SM, Posuniak EA, et al: Energy expenditure after spinal cord injury: an evaluation of stable rehabilitating patients, **J Trauma 25:**419–423, 1985.
12. Cuthbertson DP: Post-shock metabolic response, **Lancet 1:**433, 1942.
13. DeBiasse MA, Wilmore DW: What is optimal nutritional support? **New Horiz 2:**122–130, 1994.
14. Flakoll PJ, Wentzel LS, Hyman SA: Protein and glucose metabolism during isolated closed-head injury, **Am J Physiol 269:**E636–E641, 1995.
15. Grahm TW, Zadrozny DB, Harrington T: The benefits of early jejunal hyperalimentation in the head-injured patient, **Neurosurgery 25:**729–735, 1989.
16. Guenst JM, Nelson LD: Predictors of total parenteral nutrition-induced lipogenesis, **Chest 105:**553–559, 1994.
17. Hadley MN, Grahm TW, Harrington T, et al: Nutritional support and neurotrauma: a critical review of early nutrition in forty-five acute head injury patients, **Neurosurgery 19:**367–373, 1986.
18. Haider W, Lackner F, Schlick W, et al: Metabolic changes in the course of severe acute brain damage, **Eur J Intensive Care Med 1:**91, 1975.
19. Harris ME, Barrow DL: **Neuroendocrine physiology and management, neurosurgical critical care,** AANS pp 179–199, 1993.
20. Hatton J, Rapp RP, Kudsk KA, et al: Intravenous insulin-like growth factor-I (IGF-I) in moderate-to-severe head injury: a phase II safety and efficacy trial, **J Neurosurg 86:**779–786, 1997.
21. Hatton J, Ziegler TR: Nutritional support of the neurosurgical patient, in Tindall G, Cooper PR, Barrow DL, (eds): **The practice of neurosurgery,** Baltimore, 1996, Williams and Wilkins, pp 381–396.

22. Heimburger DC, Weinsier RL: **Handbook of clinical nutrition,** 3rd ed. St. Louis, 1997, Mosby.
23. Hersio K, Vapalahti M, Kari A, et al: Impaired utilization of exogenous amino acids after surgery for subarachnoid haemorrhage, **Acta Neurochir (Wien) 106:**13–17, 1990.
24. Hout WM, Arafah BM, Salazar R, et al: Evaluation of the hypothalamic-pituitary-adrenal axis immediately after pituitary adenomectomy: is perioperative steroid therapy necessary? **J Clin Endocrinol Metab 66:**1208–1212, 1988.
25. Kearns PJ, Thompson JD, Werner PC, et al: Nutritional and metabolic response to acute spinal-cord injury, **JPEN J Parenter Enteral Nutr 16:**11–15, 1992.
26. Kirby DF, Clifton GL, Turner H, et al: Early enteral nutrition after brain injury by percutaneous endoscopic gastrojejunostomy, **JPEN J Parenter Enteral Nutr 15:**298–302, 1991.
27. Kolpek JH, Ott LG, Record KE, et al: Comparison of urinary urea nitrogen excretion and measured energy expenditure in spinal cord injury and nonsteroid-treated severe head trauma patients, **JPEN J Parenter Enteral Nutr 13:**277–280, 1989.
28. Ladenson PW, Levin AA, Ridgway EC, et al: Complications of surgery in hypothyroid patients, **Am J Med 77:**261–266, 1984.
29. Loan T: Metabolic/nutritional alterations of traumatic brain injury, **Nutrition 15:**809–812, 1999.
30. Mainous MR, Deitch EA: Nutrition and infection, **Surg Clin North Am 74:**659–676, 1994.
31. Molina P, Burzstein S, Abumrad NN: Theories and assumptions on energy expenditure. Determinations in the clinical setting, **Crit Care Clin 11:**587–601, 1995.
32. Morris GF, Bullock R, Marshall SB, et al: Failure of the competitive N-methyl-D-aspartate antagonist Selfotel (CGS 19755) in the treatment of severe head injury: results of two phase III clinical trials. The Selfotel investigators. **J Neurosurg 91:**737–743, 1999.
33. **Nutritional support of brain-injured patients: Guidelines for the management of severe head injury.** New York, Brain Trauma Foundation, 1995.
34. Olivares L, Segovia A, Revuelta R: Tube feeding and lethal aspiration in neurological patients: a review of 720 autopsy cases, **Stroke 5:**654–657, 1974.
35. Ott L, Young B: Metabolic and nutritional management, in Andrews B, (ed): Neurosurgical intensive care, pp 163–177, New York, 1993, McGraw-Hill.
36. Ott L, Annis K, Hatton J, et al: Postpyloric enteral feeding costs for patients with severe head injury: blind placement, endoscopy, and PEG/J versus TPN, **J Neurotrauma 16:**233–242, 1999.
37. Ott L, McClain CJ, Gillespie M, et al: Cytokines and metabolic dysfunction after severe head injury, **J Neurotrauma 11:**447–472, 1994.
38. Ott LG, Schmidt JJ, Young AB, et al: Comparison of administration of two standard intravenous amino acid formulas to severely brain-injured patients, **Drug Intell Clin Pharm 22:**763–768, 1988.
39. Paret G, Tirosh R, Lotan D, et al: Early prediction of neurological outcome after falls in children: metabolic and clinical markers, **J Accid Emerg Med 16:**186–188, 1999.
40. Rapp RP, Young B, Twyman D, et al: The favorable effect of early parenteral feeding on survival in head-injured patients, **J Neurosurg 58:**906–912, 1983.
41. Ritter AM, Robertson CS, Goodman JC, et al: Evaluation of a carbohydrate-free diet for patients with severe head injury, **J Neurotrauma 13:**473–485, 1996.
42. Roberts PR: Nutrition in the head-injured patient, **New Horiz 3:**506–517, 1995.
43. Robertson CS, Clifton GL, Goodman JC: Steroid administration and nitrogen excretion in the head-injured patient, **J Neurosurg 63:**714–718, 1985.
44. Robertson CS, Goodman JC, Narayan RK, et al: The effect of glucose administration on carbohydrate metabolism after head injury, **J Neurosurg 74:**43–50, 1991.
45. Rodriguez DJ, Clevenger FW, Osler TM, et al: Obligatory negative nitrogen balance following spinal cord injury, **JPEN J Parenter Enteral Nutr 15:**319–322, 1991.
46. Skipper A: **Nutrition support policies, procedures, forms, and formulas,** Gaithersburg, Md, 1995, Aspen Publishers.
47. Sunderland PM, Heilbrun MP: Estimating energy expenditure in traumatic brain injury: comparison of indirect calorimetry with predictive formulas, **Neurosurgery 31:**246–252, 1992.
48. Talmor D, Shapira Y, Artru AA, et al: 0.45% saline and 5% dextrose in water, but not 0.9% saline or 5% dextrose in 0.9% saline, worsen brain edema two hours after closed head trauma in rats, **Anesth Analg 86:**1225–1229, 1998.
49. Taylor SJ, Fettes SB, Jewkes C, et al: Prospective, randomized, controlled trial to determine the effect of early enhanced enteral nutrition on clinical outcome in mechanically ventilated patients suffering head injury [see comments], **Crit Care Med 27:**2525–2531, 1999.
50. Touho H, Karasawa J, Sawada T: Metabolism in acute cerebrovascular disease, **Crit Care Med 14:**1023–1025, 1986.
51. Twyman D: Nutritional management of the critically ill neurologic patient, **Crit Care Clin 13:**39–49, 1997.
52. Weinberg AD, Brennan MD, Gorman CA, et al: Outcome of anesthesia and surgery in hypothyroid patients, **Arch Intern Med 143:**893–897, 1983.
53. Wilmore DW, Long JM, Mason AJ, et al: Catecholamines: mediator of the hypermetabolic response to thermal injury, **Ann Surg 180:**653–669, 1974.
54. Wilson RF, Tyburski JG: Metabolic responses and nutritional therapy in patients with severe head injuries, **J Head Trauma Rehabil 13:**11–27, 1998.
55. Wolfram G: The use of lipid infusions in postoperative nutrition [editorial], **Nutrition 14:**407–409, 1998.
56. Yang SY, Zhang S, Wang ML: Clinical significance of admission hyperglycemia and factors related to it in patients with acute severe head injury, **Surg Neurol 44:**373–377, 1995.
57. Young AB, Ott LG, Beard D, et al: The acute-phase response of the brain-injured patient, **J Neurosurg 69:**375–380, 1988.
58. Young B, Ott L: Nutritional and metabolic management of the head-injured patient, in Narayan RK, Wilberger JW, Povlishock JT, (eds): **Neurotrauma,** New York, 1996, McGraw-Hill, 345–363.

59. Young B, Ott L, Dempsey R, et al: Relationship between admission hyperglycemia and neurologic outcome of severely brain-injured patients, **Ann Surg 210:**466–472, 1989.
60. Young B, Ott L, Haack D, et al: Effect of total parenteral nutrition upon intracranial pressure in severe head injury, **J Neurosurg 67:**76–80, 1987.
61. Young B, Ott L, Kasarskis E, et al: Zinc supplementation is associated with improved neurologic recovery rate and visceral protein levels of patients with severe closed head injury, **J Neurotrauma 13:**25–34, 1996.
62. Young B, Ott L, Norton J, et al: Metabolic and nutritional sequelae in the non-steroid treated head injury patient, **Neurosurgery 17:**784–791, 1985.
63. Young B, Ott L, Twyman D, et al: The effect of nutritional support on outcome from severe head injury, **J Neurosurg 67:**668–676, 1987.
64. Zaloga GP: Immune-enhancing enteral diets: where's the beef? [editorial comment], **Crit Care Med 26:**1143–1146, 1998.
65. Zaloga GP: Early enteral nutritional support improves outcome: hypothesis or fact? [editorial comment], **Crit Care Med 27:**259–261, 1999.

CHAPTER 8

Infectious Disease

L.J.S. YANG
J.T. HOFF

Infectious disease in neurosurgical patients occurs when invading microorganisms overcome complex host defense mechanisms. This imbalance can occur spontaneously, resulting in the need for neurosurgical intensive care, or may result from violation of host defense mechanisms by neurosurgical procedures. Better control of infectious diseases in neurosurgical intensive care units (ICUs) depends not only on understanding the normal host-microorganism interactions but also on rapid advancements concerning its modifications in neurosurgery.

THE HOST DEFENSE SYSTEM AND ESTABLISHMENT OF INFECTIOUS DISEASE

Host-microorganism interaction refers to the complex host defense mechanisms and their reaction to invading microorganisms. Host defense mechanisms include physical barriers, chemical milieu, resident flora, inflammation, and the immunologic response. Physical surfaces such as skin, mucous membranes, and urologic and intestinal epithelial membranes are effective barriers to microbial invasion; some of these surfaces purge contaminants through reflex coughing or peristalsis. Chemical milieu inhibits microbial adherence and invasion. For example, the acidity maintained by sebaceous glands or stomach epithelium and the thick, watery environment containing immunoglobulins supplied by specialized cells in the respiratory and alimentary tract hamper invading microorganisms. Resident flora colonizing healthy physical surfaces provides yet a further impediment. Although the above defenses are usually successful in protecting the healthy host, microbial entry occurs when virulent organisms develop methods of adhering to human epithelial surface molecules and of breaching this barrier. Some organisms secrete toxins that damage barrier integrity. Others express molecules, encouraging endocytosis of the organism by the epithelium. The compromised physical and chemical defenses in the neurosurgical patient (debilitated by his condition and reliant on mechanical instrumentation and indwelling catheters, receiving a variety of antibiotics, or suffering malnutrition) facilitate microbial penetration of epithelial barriers.

Once a microorganism has entered through the epithelium, it encounters subepithelial host defenses such as the inflammatory response, the phagocytic cells, and the lymphatic system. The inflammatory response occurs with the vigorous dilation and increased permeability of the microcirculation in infected tissues. Immunoglobulins and complement proteins bind to microbes (opsonization) and stimulate the release of immune modulators (cytokines). These molecules induce further vasodilation, stimulate leukocyte chemotaxis, and promote phagocytosis by polymorphonuclear leukocytes (neutrophils, eosinophils, and basophils) and monocytes (precursors of macrophage and brain microglia). Some of these immune cells nonspecifically phagocytose foreign particles and secrete enzymes, reactive oxygen species, lipid-derived mediators, and cytokines. These agents not only kill target microbes but also injure normal tissues in the immediate vicinity. As the area and intensity of inflammation increase, the acute phase response occurs. Increased levels of corticosteroid hormones, acute phase proteins (produced by the liver), and various cytokines (see the following) result in a general rise in metabolism and sedimentation rate.

The subepithelial host defenses are remarkably successful; however, some microbes have evolved mechanisms to evade the inflammatory response. Exotoxins produced by *Streptococcus pyogenes*, *Staphylococcus aureus*, and *Clostridium* species kill neutrophils. Viruses

TABLE 8-1 ■ Partial List of Cytokine Families

Family	Members	Major Characteristics
Interleukins	IL-1α, IL-1β, IL-1ra, IL-2–IL-15	Immunoregulation in multiple tissues
Chemokines	IL-8/NAP-1, NAP-2, MIP1 α and β, MCAF/MCP-1, MGSA and RANTES	Leukocyte chemotaxis and cellular activation
Tumor necrosis factors	TNF-α and β	Tumor cytotoxicity and immunoregulation in multiple tissues
Interferons	IFN-α, β, and γ	Modulation of cell growth and intracellular viral replication
Colony-stimulating factors	G-CSF, M-CSF, GM-CSF, IL-3	Regulation of colony cell formation in bone marrow and activation of mature leukocytes
Growth factors	EGF, FGF, PDGF, ECGF, TGF-α and β	Regulation of cell growth and differentiation
Neurotrophins	BDNF, NGF, NT-3–NT-6, GDNF	Regulation of neuronal growth and differentiation
Neuropoietins	LIF, CNTF, OM, IL-6	Modulation of nervous system activity

BDNF, Brain-derived neurotrophic factor; *CNTF,* ciliary neurotrophic factor; *EGF,* epidermal growth factor; *ECGF,* endothelial cell growth factor; *FGF,* fibroblast growth factor; *GDNF,* glial-derived neurotrophic factor; *G, M,* and *GM-CSF,* ganulocyte, macrophage, and granulocyte/macrophage colony stimulating factor(s); *IFN,* interferon; *IL,* interleukin; *IL-1ra,* interleukin-1 receptor antagonist; *MCAF,* monocyte chemotactic and activating factor; *MCP,* monocyte chemotactic protein; *MGSA,* melanoma growth stimulatory activity; *MIP,* macrophage inflammatory protein; *NGF,* nerve growth factor; *NT,* neurotrophin; *NAP,* neutrophil activating protein; *OM,* oncostatin M; *PDGF,* platelet-derived growth factor; *RANTES,* regulated on activation normal expressed and secreted; *TGF,* transforming growth factor; *TNF,* tumor necrosis factor.

and *Mycobacterium* species produce lysosomal inhibition proteins that allow survival in the macrophage after phagocytosis. The capsules of *Streptococcus pneumoniae* and *Hemophilus influenzae* inhibit phagocytosis. Likewise, because the inflammatory response is unable to be optimally generated in the acutely ill neurosurgical patient, opportunistic infections by resident bacteria, fungi, and/or nosocomial agents become significant problems.

The inflammatory response is also accompanied by dilation of lymphatic capillaries. Microbes can enter into the lymphatic circulation and subsequently travel to the lymph nodes. Here, phagocytosis and filtration occur, and the immune response is triggered. The immune response comprises both the antibody- and cell-mediated components. The former is transferred by serum and the latter by lymphocytes. The antibody-mediated response targets invading microbes and depends on plasma cells (antibody-forming cells) to secrete microbe-specific antibodies in the context of appropriate cytokines: Antigens are brought and presented to the plasma cells residing in lymph nodes by circulating macrophages and other antigen-presenting cells (APCs). The resultant antibodies then circulate throughout the host and interact with the microbes, resulting in complement activation and further stimulation of the inflammatory response described previously. Deficiencies in the antibody-mediated response may occur in neurosurgical patients undergoing chemotherapy, and such patients are at particular risk for infections moderated by opsonization (e.g., infections by *S. pneumoniae* and *H. influenzae*).

In contrast, the cell-mediated response targets infected host cells. Subsets of lymphocytes perform different functions in this division of the immune response. The helper T-lymphocytes, displaying the CD4 surface receptor, coordinate the cell-mediated response. Signaled by APCs through cytokines and surface presentation of microbial antigens, the $CD4^+$ T-cells secrete additional cytokines that activate macrophages and cytolytic T-lymphocytes to selectively kill infected host cells. Compromise of cell-mediated immunity can occur in the neurosurgical patient undergoing steroid therapy[62] and in patients with acquired immunodeficiency syndrome (AIDS), causing difficulty in coping with intracellular pathogens like *Listeria monocytogenes, Cryptococcus, Toxoplasma, Aspergillus, Nocardia,* and *Mycobacterium* species.

As indicated above, the immune response relies intimately on cytokines to coordinate the potent host defenses for overcoming pathogens with minimal destruction of non-infected host tissues. Table 8-1 represents a partial list of cytokines and their major functions.[129,166] Neurosurgical procedures and neurologic disease states modify cytokine production and behavior, and these modifications may be responsible for a majority of the infectious pathology encountered in neurosurgical intensive care (Table 8-2).* Further discoveries concerning the effect of the nervous system disease on host defense mechanisms may yet improve the outcomes of neurosurgical patients afflicted with infectious disease.

SYSTEMIC INFECTIONS IN NEUROINTENSIVE CARE

Pathogenesis and Prevention of Systemic Infection in Critically Ill Patients

Nosocomial infections in ICU patients account for more than 20% of hospital infections, although these patients occupy fewer than 10% of hospital beds.[37] According to the National Nosocomial Infections Surveil-

*References 11,84,87,99,109,122,129,163,172,181,182,184,185,190,202,248,255,256,259,271,295,296,297

TABLE 8-2 ■ Cytokine Synthesis in Brain

Stimulus	Cytokines Produced	Cell Source
Peripheral infection, endotoxin	IL-1β, IL-6	Neurons, microglia
CNS infectious disease	IL-1β, IL-6, TNF-α, TGF-β, IFN-γ, MIP-1, MIP-2	Microglia, astrocytes
Brain tumors*	IL-1α and β, IL-1ra	Glioblastoma, possibly gliomas and meningiomas
	IL-6	Astrocytoma, glioblastoma, possibly macrophages
	IL-8	Astrocytoma, glioblastoma
	IL-10	50% of primary brain tumors
	G-CSF, GM-CSF	Astrocytoma, glioblastoma
	M-CSF	Glioblastoma
	TGF-β	Glioblastoma
Brain injury	IL-1β, IL-2, IL-6, TNF-α, IL-8, LIF, NGF, FGF, PDGF, EGF, TGF-β	Microglia, possibly neurons
Convulsants	IL-1β, IL-6, TNF-α, LIF	Possibly neurons
Ischemia	IL-1β, IL-6, FGF, TGF-β, possibly, TNF	Neurons, perivascular cells, possibly microglia
Multiple sclerosis	IL-1β, IL-2, IL-6, TNF-α and β, IFN-γ	Glia, lymphocytes
Down syndrome	IL-1β	Microglia
Alzheimer's disease	IL-1b, IL-2, IL-6, possibly FGF	Microglia, possibly macrophages

*Data acquired from primary tumor cells, cell lines, and stimulated tumor cells.

EGF, epidermal growth factor; *FGF,* fibroblast growth factor; *IFN,* interferon; *IL,* interleukin; *IL-1ra,* interleukin-1 receptor antagonist; *G, M, GM-CSF,* ganulocyte, monocyte colony stimulating factor; *LIF,* leukemia inhibitory factor; *MIP,* macrophage inflammatory protein; *NGF,* nerve growth factor; *PDGF,* platelet-derived growth factor; *TGF,* transforming growth factor; *TNF,* tumor necrosis factor.

lance (NNIS) data, urinary tract infections, pneumonia, surgical-site infections, and primary bloodstream infection are most common.[78] These infections may be acquired by patients in ICUs or may necessitate ICU care. Many risk factors contribute to this statistic, some characteristic of the setting, others of the patients involved. Understanding the risk factors contributing to the significant infectious rates in ICUs aids in the development of effective prevention strategies. General infection control practices are discussed here; those involving specific devices or systems are discussed in the sections to follow.

The ICU concentrates high-risk patients in small areas. It houses a large number of varied health care workers, many of whom rotate among several ICUs. Major risk factors for cross infection in the ICU setting are the physicians, nurses, and other staff who carry out frequent interventions or invasive procedures on ICU patients. Nosocomial bacterial spread, sometimes epidemic, can result from the variable commitment to hand washing, allowing bacteria and other pathogens to be carried from patient to patient. Although many reports have revealed hand washing discipline to be poor,[107,154,175] hand washing continues to be "the single most important procedure for preventing nosocomial infection."[95,153] The Centers for Disease Control and Prevention (CDC) recommends hand antisepsis by surgical scrub or alcohol-based emulsions before placement of invasive devices, in addition to routine hand washing with antiseptic soaps.[72,76,213] CDC "Standard Precautions" recommend routine glove use when touching body fluids, including blood, secretions, excretions, and body fluid–contaminated items, and removal of gloves and hand washing before working with another patient.[95] The efficacy of routine gown use in control of infectious transmission remains uncertain except in situations in which splashing of body fluids is likely.[30,241] Other risk factors inherent to the ICU setting include the level of crowding, the degree of asepsis of maintenance and monitoring devices, as well as the proper sterilization of irrigation solution, sinks, ventilators, and other environmental surfaces. Frequent antibiotic use in the ICU predisposes this setting to microbes that acquire antibiotic resistance because of selective pressure. Effective surveillance of infection control habits and the appropriate review of antimicrobial utilization have significantly decreased the rate of infection in compliant hospital systems.[68]

Factors inherent to the ICU patient also increase the incidence of infectious disease. As mentioned above, the underlying neurological or neurosurgical illness can alter cytokine activity, leading to attenuation of the patient's host defenses. Underlying systemic illnesses such as diabetes and renal insufficiency, malnutrition, or immunosuppression impair the immune response. Medications used to treat the underlying diseases also affect the immune response. Even those used for ulcer prophylaxis may sufficiently alter normal flora and result in superinfection. Normal physical and chemical barriers to infection are compromised in ICU patients, the skin by trauma or surgical procedures and the mucosa by endotracheal tubes, nasogastric tubes, and urethral catheters. Percutaneous indwelling vascular catheters, drains, or monitoring devices invade normally sterile sites and provide inlets for infectious pathogens. Attempts to reestablish the patient's normal physiological status as well as attention to the aseptic placement and subsequent maintenance of the above devices may prevent infections in ICU patients.

Patients who undergo extensive surgical procedures occupy a significant number of ICU beds. Many neurosurgical procedures have prolonged operative/anesthesia times or involve the insertion of foreign bodies. Both are risks for postoperative infections including wound infections, respiratory tract infections, urinary tract infections, and bacteremia. According to reports from the NNIS system, patients undergoing craniotomies have the third highest rate of nosocomial infections.[257] Foreign bodies such as intracranial pressure monitors expose neurosurgical ICU patients to an increased infection risk.[205,293] Draining systems have more infectious complications compared with non-draining systems.[13] The association between infection and duration of use remains controversial.[205,293] Therefore, standard protocols have not been definitively established regarding the duration of use or the routine changing of these monitors. Likewise, efficacy of prophylactic antibiotics has yet to be demonstrated.[13,121] Further research and increasing awareness of the factors contributing to infection in the neurosurgical ICU patient will facilitate the development of effective prevention strategies.

Pneumonia

Pneumonia is the most common nosocomial infection in intensive care units,[74] and it is associated with the greatest morbidity and mortality.[110] The escalating need for endotracheal intubation and mechanical ventilation to support critically ill neurosurgical patients increases the incidence of nosocomial pneumonia as well as the length of hospital stays and cost.

Pneumonia occurs when virulent organisms overcome normal lung protective mechanisms to access distal airways. An inflammatory response is generated, and immune cells accumulate in the peripheral bronchi and alveoli. The subsequent production of purulent sputum and consolidation is detectable by radiography. Fever and leukocytosis are common. In ICU patients, aspiration and endotracheal intubation are the most common risk factors for developing pneumonia. Patients with decreased level of consciousness or loss of epiglottic and cough reflexes because of their neurosurgical illness or neurotrauma aspirate oropharyngeal or gastrointestinal bacteria. Endotracheal intubation inhibits the effective clearance of oral secretions and damages airway mucosa. Even with the use of low-pressure, high-volume cuffs, leakage of oropharyngeal secretions around the cuff is common and exposes the distal lung to potential pathogens.[228]

Pathogens that cause pneumonia in ICU patients dependent on mechanical ventilation include *Pseudomonas aeruginosa*, *S. aureus*, *Acinetobacter* species, and *Enterobacteriaceae*.[97] However, in patients reliant on mechanical ventilation after head trauma or after undergoing neurosurgery, *S. aureus* is most common.[214,217] Anaerobes are also common pathogens in neurosurgical patients with decreasing mental status who are predisposed to aspiration.

The diagnosis of pneumonia by lung histology remains the gold standard.[16] However, obtaining adequate lung tissue is often impractical and costly. Therefore, pneumonia is most commonly detected by noninvasive modalities such as endotracheal aspiration or radiographic examination. Routine bacterial cultures of endotracheal aspirates suctioned through an endotracheal tube or tracheostomy are commonly used but often unreliable.[180] Quantitative cultures with a diagnostic threshold of at least 10^6 CFU/ml coupled with microscopic analysis of the aspirate increases the specificity of detection.[180]

Therapeutic strategies for treatment of suspected nosocomial pneumonia are based on the knowledge of concurrent illnesses, prior antibiotic treatment, and length of ICU stay. The American Thoracic Society recommends that empiric management of pneumonia in ICU patients on mechanical ventilation include an aminoglycoside or ciprofloxacin, an antipseudomonal agent, and an agent effective against methicillin-resistant *S. aureus* (MRSA).[3] When or if the pathogens causing pneumonia are known, optimal treatment is selected to cover the antibiotic susceptibilities of these organisms.

Potential prevention of nosocomial ventilator-associated pneumonia has been extensively investigated. Although many nonantibiotic measures such as drainage of subglottic secretions, use of the semirecumbent position, prevention of gastric microbial overgrowth by stress-ulcer prophylaxis, early enteral feeding, and early tracheostomy have been studied, none have yet proven effective.[179,254]

Sinusitis

Sinusitis is problematic in ICU patients requiring mechanical ventilation (with endotracheal or nasotracheal tubes) and nasogastric drainage. These patients may have multiple organ system disease with impairment of host defenses, and they usually undergo multiple invasive interventions. Bacterial strains found in lower airways are also found in upper airways, predisposing patients requiring nasal cannulation to sinus infection. Head injuries and facial fractures predispose patients to sinusitis by directly introducing foreign material or potentially pathogenic organisms into the exposed sinuses. Common organisms causing sinusitis in the ICU are *S. aureus*, *P. aeruginosa*, enteric gram-negative bacteria, and *Streptococcus* species.[282] Patients with sinusitis present with unexplained fever and purulent nasal drainage. Diagnosis depends on microbiological analysis and culture, although techniques to collect uncontaminated specimens are yet to be standardized.[282] Direct antroscopy of the paranasal sinuses is currently considered the most reliable means of diagnosis.[152] Sinus computed tomography (CT) and/or ultrasound are more practical.[134,139] Treatment relies on knowledge of the organisms involved and their antibiotic susceptibilities. Removal of foreign objects from the nasal cavity when possible reduces the risk of developing sinusitis. Prompt therapy is necessary to prevent spread of infection, leading to osteomyelitis, subdural empyema, meningitis, and brain abscess.[50]

Urinary Tract Infection

Urinary tract infection is the second most common nosocomial infection in the ICU, responsible for approximately 40% of all infections.[204,281] Urinary catheters in neurosurgical patients with decreased mental status or those who have undergone major neurosurgical procedures predispose these patients to infection by compromising the mucosa and normal protective mechanisms. Risk factors for the development of urinary tract infection include a long duration of catheterization, systemic antibiotics, female sex, diabetes mellitus, and open-drainage systems. Aerobic gram-negative bacilli, yeast, and *P. aeruginosa* are the most common pathogens.[204] *Bacteriuria* refers to the colonization of the urinary tract and bacterial invasion (occurring in 10% to 20% of catheterized patients), whereas *urinary tract infection* refers specifically to the presence of more than 10^5 colony-forming units (CFU) of bacteria per milliliter of urine associated with fever, dysuria, urgency, frequency, pyuria, hematuria, and/or suprapubic tenderness (occurring in 2% to 6% of catheterized patients).[94] Diagnosis of urinary tract infection is achieved through microbiological examination and quantitative cultures. Treatment depends on the susceptibilities of the responsible organism(s). Early treatment is necessary to prevent complications such as systemic urosepsis.

Bloodstream Infection

Primary bloodstream infections (BSIs) are responsible for 13% of nosocomial ICU infections.[78] The most frequent source of BSI are intravascular devices, with 90% of these infections related to central venous catheters.[167] Central venous catheters are often used in the neurosurgical ICU for treatment of patients with subarachnoid hemorrhage and vasospasm. The use of these catheters, especially multiluminal catheters, increases the risk of developing BSI two- to thirtyfold.[116,136] Presence of the catheter in the femoral vein results in the highest rates of colonization and infection, followed by presence in the internal jugular vein and the subclavian vein.[21] In certain circumstances, an alternative to the central venous catheter, the peripherally inserted central catheter (PICC), can be used with fewer complications and lower incidence of infection.[212]

Although aseptic insertion of the catheter decreases the incidence of catheter-related BSIs, delaying colonization of the skin at the entry site is crucial. Topical application of antimicrobial agents at the insertion site significantly decreases the incidence of infection.[57] Diligent attention to the aseptic care of hub-related manipulations also reduces infection. The use of central venous catheters for total parenteral nutrition (TPN) increases the incidence of infection because TPN fluids support the growth of gram-negative aerobic bacilli and fungi.[231] Lastly, the use of transparent dressings allows for easy inspection of the catheter site but seemingly provides no advantage because catheter-related BSIs rarely show localized signs of infection.[57]

Diagnosis is accomplished by culturing blood (from a peripheral site as well as through the catheter itself) and the catheter tip; however, in the clinical setting of possible BSI, most clinicians remove the suspicious catheter and begin empiric antibiotic therapy. The most likely pathogens are coagulase-negative staphylococci, *S. aureus*, *Enterobacter*, and *P. aeruginosa*.[57] Appropriate combinations for therapy include vancomycin and an antibiotic providing anaerobic gram-negative coverage (gentamicin, levofloxacin, Zosyn, second- or third-generation cephalosporins). The usual duration of therapy after removal of the catheter varies from 7 to 14 days. If BSI is complicated by endocarditis, antibiotic therapy is instituted for 4 to 8 weeks.[9]

BACTERIAL INFECTIONS OF THE CENTRAL NERVOUS SYSTEM

The central nervous system expresses infection differently than other organs because of several anatomic and physiologic features unique to it. These features may help or hinder the host, depending on the mode of insult. For example, the skull protects the brain against trauma but does not allow for swelling, so that raised intracranial pressure results in herniation. Cerebrospinal fluid (CSF) cushions the brain but is responsible for hydrocephalus and is a potent medium for the multiplication and dissemination of pathogens throughout the entire CNS. The blood-brain barrier (BBB), formed by tightly apposed endothelium, provides a stable intraparenchymal milieu but leaves the brain an immunologically privileged site (except at the choroid plexus, where fenestrated endothelium allows more indiscriminate passage of plasma proteins or pathogens). Finally, the absence of lymphatic drainage provides immunologic insulation but allows the CNS to suffer from accumulated edema.

CNS infections are commonly thought of in two general categories. (1) Infection of the structures surrounding the parenchyma, including the meninges, meningeal spaces, and overlying bone, results in generalized involvement of the CNS and significant global deficits in CNS function. (2) Infection of the parenchyma of the brain and spinal cord leads to focal neurological deficits and/or evidence of increased intracranial pressure. Although these categories are usually separable, the progression of infection to multiple compartments with both global and focal symptoms can occur. For example, a meningoencephalitis results if unchecked meningitis extends into the brain.

Subgaleal Abscess

Subgaleal abscess forms from infection of the space between the galea of the scalp and the pericranium. Infection is usually initiated by contamination of a scalp wound by staphylococci, streptococci, and anaerobic organisms as a result of traumatic injury or at a surgical site. Abscess formation is signaled by localized scalp tenderness and swelling. Dissemination of the infection results in fever, lymphadenopathy, and/or facial swelling. In the absence of penetrating injury to the skull, intracranial extension is rare, although secondary osteomyelitis is known to occur. Treatment includes surgical drainage and debridement coupled with antibiotics.

Osteomyelitis

Osteomyelitis of the skull develops from extension of an established local infection (e.g., external otitis, mastoiditis, or sinusitis), from direct contamination of the skull at operation or after trauma, or rarely from a distant source such as the respiratory or urinary tract by hematogenous spread. An established skull infection may extend inward to produce an epidural abscess or outward into the subgaleal space.[262] Osteomyelitis of the skull base can result from malignant external otitis, leading to cranial nerve palsies, sigmoid sinus thrombosis, meningitis, and death. Diabetes and immune suppression increase the incidence of osteomyelitis and the likelihood of associated complications. Diagnosis relies on clinical presentation, culture of purulent drainage, and measurement of the erythrocyte sedimentation rate (ESR). CT, magnetic resonance imaging (MRI), or radionuclide scans confirm the diagnosis by showing bony involvement and are helpful in following the progression of the disease. Common pathogens include staphylococci, anaerobic streptococci, and, increasingly, pseudomonads. Treatment consists of drainage, debridement of infected bone, and appropriate antibiotics for at least 6 weeks.

Osteomyelitis of the spine contributes to approximately 1% of all cases of osteomyelitis[6] and results from insidious systemic infection, direct trauma, or surgery. The incidence of postoperative osteomyelitis after lumbar discectomy is 0.7% to 0.8%, and the addition of instrumentation increases the incidence to 6% to 8%.[203] The disease presents most often with pain as the initial symptom, usually associated with localized muscle spasm. Neurological signs (e.g., myelopathy and radiculopathy) usually occur late in the progression of the disease. Signs of systemic illness, such as fever, increased ESR, and leukocytosis, may be present. Diagnostic delays often occur. Clinical suspicion is most important in establishing the diagnosis, and obtaining the previous history of bacteremia from phlebitis or urinary infection may be helpful. Radiological studies are useful for both aiding in the diagnosis and for following the progression of the disease. Plain radiographic films and CT scans show focal destruction, including irregular endplates and disc space narrowing, or collapse of the vertebral bodies within 3 to 6 weeks after the onset of infection. Radionuclide scans show abnormal foci of nuclide uptake before any changes are obvious on plain radiographs. MRI remains the most accurate radiological technique showing both abnormalities in the bone as well as surrounding soft tissues. Confirmation of the diagnosis requires percutaneous aspiration and culture of the offending agent. *S. aureus* is the usual pathogen, although *Escherichia coli*, *Pseudomonas*, and *Proteus* are also common.[203] Most cases are successfully treated with immobilization and appropriate antibiotics for at least 4 to 6 weeks, with the goals being prevention or reversal of neurological deficit, pain relief, spinal stability, and prevention of relapse.[6,58] Open surgery is indicated in the 10% to 20% of patients in whom significant neurological deficits or deformities potentially leading to deficits are present.[41,77] An anterior approach is usually indicated for direct access to the infected tissues; involvement of the posterior elements is much less common.[6,203] Severe kyphotic deformities may require additional spinal fusion with instrumentation. Serial sedimentation rates and radiological studies are valuable for following response to therapy.

Epidural Abscess

Intracranial epidural abscess, a focal collection of purulent material between the cranium and the dura mater, is a rare complication of traumatic or operative contamination of epidural tissue. More commonly, it results from extension of adjacent osteomyelitis. Intact dura inhibits transdural extension. Common organisms responsible for this infection include anaerobes, aerobic streptococci, staphylococci, *S. pneumoniae*, *H. influenzae*, and gram-negative bacilli.[264] Treatment consists of drainage, debridement, and systemic antibiotics.

Spinal epidural abscesses represent approximately 67% of all spinal infections[6] and constitutes a neurosurgical emergency in the context of progressive neurological compromise. This disease presents as purulent collections on the dorsal or ventral surfaces of the dural sac. Systemic infection and hematogenous spread are the primary mode of pathogenesis, although epidural abscesses may also result from local osteomyelitis. Postoperative epidural abscesses represent about 16% of all epidural abscesses.[14] Symptoms include localized pain, radiculopathy, and myelopathy resulting from compression by the purulent mass or associated vascular changes. Diagnosis relies on clinical judgment in the setting of fever, elevated ESR, and leukocytosis. Radiological studies, especially MRI, can confirm the diagnosis and evaluate the extent of the epidural mass. The most common pathogen remains *S. aureus*, followed by anaerobic bacteria and gram-negative bacilli.[6,111] Treatment consists of urgent surgical decompression and abscess drainage followed by specific antibiotic therapy for at least 4 to 6 weeks.[6] Suggested antibiotics for empiric therapy before the antibiotic sensitivities are known are shown in Table 8-3.[99,173,264] Recovery of neurological function is directly related to the duration and severity of impairment prior to surgery.[141,275]

Meningitis

Bacterial meningitis is a purulent infection of the subarachnoid space. It generally presents as an acute, fulminating illness characterized by fever, headache, nausea, vomiting, and nuchal rigidity. Coma occurs in about 5% to 10% of cases, and its development carries a poor prognosis. Seizures occur in approximately 20% of patients, and cranial nerve palsies occur in 5%. Untreated bacterial meningitis is essentially fatal. CSF examination shows polymorphonuclear leukocytosis, elevated protein, and depressed glucose. CSF Gram stain demonstrates the causative organism in 75% of cases, and rapid latex agglutination tests are available for several common pathogens. Tests, incorporating polymerase chain reaction (PCR) for amplification of bacterial DNA, are especially useful for those patients who have received antibiotics and are being developed for routine laboratory use.[264] The current gold standard continues to be CSF culture, which provides a diagnosis in 90% of cases and is indispensable in characterizing the antibiotic sensitivity of the pathogen. Depressed level of consciousness, especially when associated with papilledema or focal neurological deficits, should lead

TABLE 8-3 ■ Intracranial Abscess and Empyema: Causative Organisms and Empiric Therapy by Source of Infection

Source	Common Organisms	Empiric Therapy
Otitis media/mastoiditis	Streptococci (anaerobic and aerobic), *Bacteroides fragilis*, Enterobacteriaceae, *P. aeruginosa*	Third-generation cephalosporin + metronidazole +- penicillin
Paranasal sinusitis	Streptococci (aerobic and anaerobic), *Bacteroides* spp., Enterobacteriaceae, *Haemophilus* spp. *Staphylococcus aureus*, *Fusobacterium*	Third-generation cephalosporin + metronidazole
Dental infection/ manipulation	Streptococci, *Fusobacterium, Bacteroides* spp.	Penicillin + - metronidazole
Trauma/ neurosurgery	*S. aureus, S. epidermidis,* Enterobacteriaceae, streptococci, *Pseudomonas aeruginosa*, *Clostridium* spp.	Antistaphylococcal penicillin + third-generation cephalosporin or vancomycin + third-generation cephalosporin
Meningitis	*Listeria monocytogenes, Citrobacter diversus*	Ampicillin + third-generation cephalosporin
Cyanotic heart disease	Streptococci, *Haemophilus* spp.	Ampicillin
Pyogenic lung disease	Streptococci, *Nocardia asteroides*, *Actinomyces, Fusobacterium, Bacteroides*	Penicillin or third-generation cephalosporin + metronidazole
Bacterial endocarditis	Viridans streptococci, *S. aureus*, enterococci, *Haemophilus* spp.	Antistaphylococcal penicillin, ampicillin, or vancomycin +- aminoglycoside
Gastrointestinal source	Enterobacteriaceae	Third-generation cephalosporin
T-cell deficiency	*Toxoplasma Gondii, Nocardia, L. monocytogenes*	Variable (pyrimethamine + sulfadiazine in AIDS)
Neutropenia	Enterobacteriaceae, *P. aeruginosa*	Third-generation cephalosporin, meropenem

the investigator to CT evaluation prior to lumbar puncture to rule out a mass lesion or hydrocephalus. Diffuse intracranial hypertension, in the absence of a mass lesion, is not a contraindication to lumbar puncture. Physical evaluation should include careful examination for contiguous sites of inflammation such as otitis and sinusitis and for causes of bacteremia like endocarditis. Blood cultures may be positive.

The primary cause of bacterial meningitis is leptomeningeal invasion by bloodborne bacteria that colonize the nasopharyngeal mucosa of the host. The common meningeal pathogens are all encapsulated bacteria. After colonizing the nasopharynx, the encapsulated bacteria traverse the epithelium and gain access to the bloodstream. Encapsulation inhibits phagocytosis by neutrophils; thus common meningeal pathogens demonstrate the ability to maintain a transient bacteremia. The subsequent mechanism, by which bacteria in the bloodstream gain access to the leptomeninges and subarachnoid space, is largely unknown. Another source of bacterial meningitis is direct extension from otorhinologic infections, although its incidence has declined markedly with the advent of effective early antibiotic therapy of otitis and sinusitis. Infrequently, meningitis is caused by direct inoculation during penetrating trauma.

The widespread used of vaccines within the last decade has changed the microbiology of the illness in children.[265] During the 1970s to 1980s, *H. influenza* was the pathogen in nearly 50% of cases. Since the introduction of the Hib polysaccharide polyribosylribitol phosphate vaccine, a decrease of approximately 85% in the incidence of *H. influenza* meningitis has been reported.[1,34] In fact, several surveys report that *S. pneumoniae* and *Neisseria menigitidis* have surpassed *H. influenza* as the more common causes of childhood bacterial meningitis.[35,235] Likewise, in adults, the microbiology continues to change. Nosocomial infection and neurosurgical procedures or implants are becoming more prominent sources, and gram-negative bacilli have overtaken *S. pneumoniae* as a cause of adult meningitis.[265]

The treatment for acute bacterial meningitis, outlined in Table 8-4, depends on the primary source of the infection, the age of the patient, the causative organism, and its antibiotic sensitivity.* Treatment should be directed to both the CSF infection and the primary source. Meningitis that occurs secondary to bacteremia and direct otorhinal extension tends to be

*References 59,99,173,178,211,235,264,268

TABLE 8-4 ■ **Meningitis: Empiric Therapy by Age and Common Organisms**

Source	Common Organisms	Empiric Therapy
SPONTANEOUS		
Neonate	*E. coli*, group B streptococci, *L. monocytogenes, S. agalactiae, K. pneumoniae*	Ampicillin + third-generation cephalosporin or ampicillin + aminoglycoside
1-3 months	*E.coli*, group B streptococci, *L. monocytogenes, H. influenzae, S. pneumoniae, S. agalactiae, N. meningitidis*	Ampicillin + third-generation cephalosporin or Trimethoprim/sulfamethoxazole + chloramphenicol or vancomycin + third-generation cephalosporin
3 mo−18 yr	*H. influenzae, N. meningitidis, S. pneumoniae**	Third-generation cephalosporin or vancomycin or ampicillin + chloramphenicol
18−50 yr	*S. pneumoniae,** *N meningitidis*	Third-generation cephlosporin or vancomycin or ampicillin + chloramphenicol
Over 50 yr	*S. pneumoniae,** *N. meningitidis, L. monocytogenes*, gram-negative bacilli	Ampicillin + third-generation cephalosporin or vancomycin
INJURY		
Closed skull (+/-CSF leak)	*S. pneumoniae,** other streptococcus, *H. influenzae*	Ampicillin + third-generation cephalosporin
Penetrating	*S. aureus, S. epidermidis, Streptococcus* spp.*, gram-negative bacilli	Vancomycin + third-generation cephalosporin
POSTOPERATIVE		
	S. aureus, S. epidermidis, gram-negative bacilli	Vancomycin + third-generation cephalosporin

* For penicillin resistant *S. pneumoniae* (MIC ≥2 g/ml), vancomycin + third-generation cephalosporin or rifampin + vancomycin or third-generation cephalosporin +/− rifampin is recommended.

caused by organisms frequently seeding the nasopharynx. Meningitis occurring after a traumatic brain injury and skull fracture, with or without CSF otorhinorrhea, is most often caused by *S. pneumoniae*. Meningitis that develops following a penetrating wound is usually caused by staphylococcal, streptococcal, or gram-negative organisms.

Empiric therapy is subsequently modified when the causative organism is identified (Table 8-5). Penicillin G and ampicillin have been found to be equally efficacious in the majority of *S. pneumoniae* and *N. meningitidis* infections, except in the case of penicillin-resistant *S. pneumoniae*, for which treatment includes vancomycin and a third-generation cephalosporin. The increasing prevalence of beta-lactamase–producing *H. influenzae*, currently around 25%, led to the adoption of the ampicillin and chloramphenicol regimen for empiric therapy. Ceftriaxone and cefotaxime have been shown to be as efficacious and are endorsed as the treatments of choice in neonates and children.[268,298] Although cefuroxime, a second-generationcephalosporin, had been commonly used for *H. influenzae*, it is no longer recommended for CNS infections because of delayed CSF sterilization and a report of *H. influenzae* meningitis developing during systemic therapy.[8,61,155] *L. monocytogenes* is not sensitive to cephalosporins, and the recommended treatment is ampicillin or penicillin G. An alternative is trimethoprim -sulfamethoxazole. Patients with *S. aureus* meningitis should be treated with nafcillin or oxacillin, with vancomycin being reserved for methicillin-resistant strains and for *S. epidermidis*. Gram-negative bacillary meningitis is best treated with third-generation cephalosporins. Duration of therapy for meningitis is generally empiric and based on tradition, usually 7 to 14 days for the major meningeal pathogens and 21 days for gram-negative bacillary infections.[269]

Prevention of meningitis has become an increasingly prevalent practice. Housemates of patients with meningitis are at high risk for secondary disease. Rifampin is the recommended prophylaxis for *H. influenza* and *N. meningitidis*.[112] Single doses of ceftriaxone and ciprofloxacin are also effective.[56]

TABLE 8-5 ■ Specific CNS Bacterial Pathogens and Antimicrobial Therapy

Organism	Drug of Choice	Alternatives
Streptococcus pneumoniae—penicillin susceptible	Penicillin G (or ampicillin)	Third-generation cephalosporin, chloramphenicol
Streptococcus pneumoniae—penicillin resistant	Vancomycin	Third/fourth-generation cephalosporin, imipenem, meropenem
S. pyogenes	Penicillin G, V +/− gentamicin	Third-generation cephalosporin, chloramphenicol, erythromycin
S. group B	Penicillin G +/− gentamicin	Third-generation cephalosporin, chloramphenicol, erythromycin
S. faecalis	Penicillin G +/− gentamicin	Vancomycin + gentamicin
Staphylococcus aureus		
Methicillin-sensitive	Nafcillin	Oxacillin, vancomycin, clindamycin, erythromycin, fluoroquinolones
Methicillin-resistant	Vancomycin	Teicoplanin, Trimethoprim-sulfamethoxazole, ciprofloxacin
Staphylococcus epidermidis	Vancomycin +/− rifampin	Teicoplanin
Listeria monocytogenes	Ampicillin +/− aminoglycoside	Trimethoprim-sulfamethoxazole
Clostridium difficile	Vancomycin	Metronidazole, Bacitracin
N. meningitidis	Penicillin G	Chloramphenicol, third-generation cephalosporin
H. influenza		
Beta-lactamase-negative	Ampicillin	Third-generation cephalosporin
Beta-lactamase-positive	Ceftriaxone, ampicillin + chloramphenicol	Chloramphenicol
Enterobacteriaceae (Escherichia, Klebsiella, Proteus, Serratia)	Anti-pseudomonal penicillin + antipseudomonal aminoglycoside or imipenem or meropenem	Ticarcillin/clavulanate, or piperacillin/tazobactam or Ciprofloxacin
P. aeruginosa	Third generation cephalosporin +/− aminoglycoside, antipseudonal penicillin	Piperacillin + aminoglycoside, imipenem
Bacteroides	Metronidazole	Clindamycin, vancomycin

Routine adjunctive therapy of bacterial meningitis with corticosteroids remains controversial despite numerous studies[96,208,265,304]; however, many clinicians feel that it is reasonable to use dexamethasone in infants and children with *H. influenzae* meningitis and in adult patients with positive CSF Gram stains and symptoms of raised intracranial pressure.[268] The suggested dose is 0.15 mg/kg IV every 6 hours for 2 to 4 days.

Subdural Empyema

Subdural empyema refers to the collection of purulent material between the dura mater and the arachnoid mater. This disease contributes to 15% to 20% of all focal intracranial infections[264] and has a 10% to 20% mortality rate.[123,240] Subdural empyema commonly occurs as a complication of direct trauma, neurosurgical procedures, and sinusitis, otitis, and mastoiditis. Infection spreads rapidly across the brain in the subdural space, limited only by dural adhesions. The enlarging purulent material acts as a mass lesion, resulting in increased intracranial pressure and compression of underlying parenchyma. Ultimately, hydrocephalus and cerebral edema ensue, and thrombosis of venous cavities leads to parenchymal infarction.

Patients suffering the sequelae of subdural empyema present initially with fever and headache, and progress to focal neurological deficits and seizures. Cranial nerve palsies, especially those nerves vulnerable because of their location, are common. Raised intracranial pressure is reflected by the presence of nausea and vomiting and mental status changes. Diagnosis relies on radiological examination. CT and MRI reveal abnormal signal of the expanded subdural space, often with displacement of underlying brain. Lumbar puncture is forbidden in patients with suspected or known subdural empyema. Common pathogens include anaerobes, streptococci, staphylococci, *H. influenzae* and gram-negative bacilli, singly or in combination.[264] Management of subdural empyema in the context of neurological compromise depends on surgical evacuation. Primary craniotomy with wide exposure, aggressive subdural exploration, and careful debridement of purulent material from the brain surface yields better clinical results than a minimal bur hole drainage.[82,174] Cultures obtained during surgery dictate long-term antibiotic treatment. Table 8-3 provides recommendations for empiric therapy before antibiotic sensitivities are available. For small, asymptomatic subdural fluid collections, empiric antibiotic therapy may be sufficient.[199]

Subdural empyema of the cervical spine is a rare entity presenting with neck pain, leukocytosis, and radiculopathy/myelopathy. Established recommendations for treatment of this disorder have been delayed by the paucity of reported cases; however, cervical laminectomy with durotomy and drainage followed by intravenous antimicrobial administration seems reasonable.[157]

Brain Abscess

Brain abscess refers to the focal intraparenchymal collection of purulent material that accounts for approximately 1% to 2% of all intracranial space-occupying lesions.[201] Although the incidence declined with the advent of antibiotics, it may again be rising because of the recent rapid increase in immunocompromised hosts. Brain abscess results from inoculation by direct trauma, neurosurgical procedure, hematogenous spread, or infection in adjacent anatomy. In fact, the common sources include infections in the paranasal sinuses, middle ear, and mastoid. These lesions are typically solitary and located in the frontal or temporal lobes. Multiple brain abscesses suggest hematogenous seeding from distant sources including bacterial endocarditis, lung disease, and gastrointestinal (GI) infections. Penetrating trauma can cause brain abscess formation relatively soon after trauma, although progression may be delayed for years.[219] The progression of infection has been described in four stages.[33] Infection begins with the *early cerebritis stage*, reflected by a focal area of parenchymal inflammation and edema. The *late cerebritis stage* is characterized by the development of a necrotic center. The *early capsule stage* ensues with the formation of a ring-enhancing capsule accompanied by peripheral gliosis. Finally, the *late capsule stage* refers to the presence of a well-established circumscribed abscess. Uninterrupted progression through the four stages usually takes place within 2 to 3 weeks.

The classic presentation of patients with brain abscess is similar to that of other intracerebral space-occupying lesions; however, the time course tends to be more acute, with 75% of patients presenting within 2 weeks.[227] Constant refractory headache is apparent in 70% to 97% of patients.[189,195,227,299] Fever is present in approximately 50% of patients.[189,227,299] As intracranial pressure rises, nausea and vomiting become prominent, as does altered mental status. Papilledema is seen. The location of the abscess dictates the focal neurologic deficit. Cerebellar abscess can present with ataxia and nystagmus. Seizures occur in 30% to 50% of patients.[169,189,227]

Diagnosis of brain abscess relies primarily on radiologic study; lumbar puncture is contraindicated because of mass effect and the risk of herniation, and it is of little clinical value because the sensitivity is less than 10%.[264] In fact, CT imaging is touted to be responsible for the decline in mortality rate of this disease to less than 15% over the last few decades.[169,222] The appearance of brain abscess on CT parallels the stages described above[173,288]; however, CT findings may mimic those seen with neoplasms or other granulomatous diseases. MRI appears to be not only more specific, but also more sensitive, especially in the posterior fossa because of the absence of bone artifact. The distinction of abscess fluid from CSF on MRI may be important if intraventricular rupture is suspected.

The pathogen responsible depends on the site of the initiating infection, the patient's medical condition, and the patient's locale. Overall, the most common organisms remain streptococci, *Enterobacter*, anaerobes, *S. aureus*, and fungi, with 30% to 60% of cases harboring multiple organisms. In immunocompromised patients undergoing bone marrow or solid organ transplants, *Aspergillus* species is prominent.[113] Patients with AIDS or other diseases of T-cell immunity are especially susceptible to infections with intracellular organisms, including *Toxoplasma* species, *Nocardia* species, *Mycobacterium* species, and *Cryptococcus neoformans*.

The goals of therapy include the early identification of the pathogen and its antibiotic sensitivity, sterilization of the CNS and the primary site, rapid correction of mass effect, and resolution of brain edema. Absolute indications for surgery and the adjuvant use of steroids remain controversial. During cerebritis and the early stage of encapsulization, or in high surgical risk patients with small abscesses and a known causative organism, medical therapy with the appropriate parenteral antibiotic may be sufficient (see Table 8-3).[99,173,223,264] Otherwise, the preferred treatment is surgical drainage of the purulent material by either aspiration or excision and a minimum of 4 weeks of antibiotics.[251] Surgery may reduce the mass effect and thereby reduce the most critical and dangerous aspect of this infection. Surgery also allows identification of the causative organism in 60% to 80% of cases, provided that cultures are processed carefully for both aerobic and anaerobic organisms. Preoperative antibiotics should not be given when an operation will be performed without delay because of the likelihood of sterile cultures. Although surgical excision has been shown to have a lower recurrence rate, most authorities recommend image-guided stereotactic aspiration of brain abscesses, reserving excision for solitary, superficial lesions, those that contain a foreign body, or those for which aspiration fails.[115,169,215,250]

Postoperative Infections

All the pyogenic infections described in this section may develop after neurosurgical procedures. Although drainage of an infected wound is a time-honored surgical principle, that method must be modified when applied to infections of the CNS. Because the dura is a critical barrier between the CSF and the external environment, drainage of an infected neurosurgical wound cannot be instituted unless the dura is sealed.

Subdural empyema can be a serious postoperative complication after bur hole exploration, craniotomy, or halo pin placements.[92] The infection is usually confined to the operative site and is commonly caused by *S. aureus* and *S. epidermidis*. It is rarely fulminant and is often detected by its subgaleal extension. Treatment includes debridement, drainage, and antibiotics. If a bone plate exists, it should be removed.

Meningitis complicates approximately 0.34% of cases following craniotomy and is usually caused by *S. aureus, S. epidermidis,* and gram-negative bacilli.[38] Postcraniotomy nosocomial gram-negative bacillary meningitis is a serious infection usually caused by highly resistant organisms such as *Pseudomonas*, *Enterobacter*, and *Klebsiella* species. Mortality approaches 70% and requires prompt institution of antibiotic therapy. Vancomycin combined with a third-generation cephalosporin provide a broad spectrum of activity while awaiting specific pathogen identification. Intraventricular aminoglycosides are justified in critically ill patients.[187]

Eradication of infection becomes more difficult when prosthetic materials or CSF shunt implants are involved. Shunt infections occur in 5% to 15% of the shunt procedures performed and occur in 15% to 25% of hydrocephalic patients with shunts.[4,216,279,303] *S. epidermidis* and *S. aureus* are the most frequently identified organisms; however, in infants, *Enterobacteriaceae* species are also encountered.

In general, a foreign body should be removed when infection is discovered. Sometimes, however, infections can be cleared in the presence of a shunt, provided the infection is indolent and the shunt essential.[86,104] Combined systemic and intrathecal antibiotics are usually necessary to cure the infection and salvage the shunt or prosthetic material. Pending a sensitivity profile, current therapy for shunt infections caused *by S. epidermidis* is vancomycin, for *S. aureus* (methicillin sensitive) it is intravenous nafcillin, and for gram-negative enteric bacilli it is a third-generation cephalosporin such as cefotaxime. When the patient fails to respond to antibiotic therapy, removal of all hardware and external CSF drainage is often required to eradicate the infection.

Antibiotic Prophylaxis

Antibiotics have been used in neurosurgery for many years to prevent infection, although unbiased data for the efficacy of prophylaxis was scarce. Historically, few fair attempts were made to acquire the data for the following reasons.[36] First, the incidence of infection in neurosurgery is relatively low, reportedly 3% to 4%; therefore, an appropriate study would require very large numbers of patients to detect a significant difference between regimens. Second, ethical concerns dictate that many surgeons use antimicrobial prophylaxis because they feel that any potential for infection could be devastating. Third, some infections present as a delayed complication, and therefore the true incidence is difficult to ascertain. Lastly, some studies were ruled invalid because of the lack of stringency in the study protocol; however, more recently, several better executed studies (including prospective, double-blinded, controlled trials) suggest that the postoperative infection rate in patients undergoing elective craniotomies who receive antibiotic prophylaxis is significantly less than that of the placebo group.[27,40,71,272,302] Controversy continues, however, because even these studies do not meet the sample size required to reach a conclusive opinion.[36] Likewise, the optimal antimicrobial regimen is yet to be established. Many different agents have been used intravenously, still others applied directly to the wound.[230] Although many reports suggest these strategies are effective, direct comparative studies have yet to be done.

Therefore, for clean, nonimplant neurosurgery, the most reasonable approach to antibiotic prophylaxis accounts for the nature and susceptibilities of the likely bacterial pathogens. *S. aureus* is associated with 52% of infections, gram-negative bacilli with 16%, coagulase-negative staphylococci with 15%, streptococci with 9%, and numerous other species for the remaining 8%.[36] Vancomycin combined with an aminoglycoside would provide effective coverage[98,114,236] except that the widespread use of vancomycin would not be endorsed by most infectious disease experts because of the potential for development of resistance against an agent that has been uniformly effective for gram-positive bacteria. Additionally, multiresistant strains of *S. aureus* and gram-negative bacilli are uncommon in neurosurgery. Therefore, the general practice of using intravenous first- or second-generation cephalosporins perioperatively is broadly supported.[125,218,229,261] An established regimen of antibiotic dosing is likewise elusive. General conclusions, gathered from the reports in neurosurgery and those made in comparison with other types of surgery, suggest that a single preoperative dose with at most one or two postoperative doses is adequate.[36]

In implant neurosurgery, particularly in the case of CSF shunt surgery, rates of infection are higher, averaging 10% to 15%. Established use of prophylactic antibiotics would be an obvious strategy except that the number of studies showing prophylaxis to be effective parallel those showing it to be ineffective.[36] Again, the most rational approach would be to consider the pathogens most responsible and direct antibiosis appropriately. Nearly 90% of shunt infections are associated with coagulase-negative staphylococci (60% of these multiresistant), followed by *S. aureus*, aerobic gram-negative bacilli, streptococci, *Propionobacterium acnes*, and *Corynebacterium* species.

In the case of CSF leak associated with trauma, 11% to 25% of patients become infected.[156,161] CSF rhinorrhea is frequently associated with infection. The reported time course of infection varies widely, from 1 week to 1 year.[36] The primary pathogen is *S. pneumoniae*. As above, the data surrounding the use of antibiotic prophylaxis are conflicting,[165] as are several recommendations published.[60,145,247] The use of antibiotic prophylaxis in the case of CSF fistulae remains at the discretion of the individual neurosurgeon.

Antibiotics for Infections in Neurosurgical Patients

The need to provide broad-spectrum antimicrobial activity usually leads to combination empiric therapy, which is changed to more specific therapy based on culture and sensitivity results. In the critically ill patient with CNS infection, the need for CNS penetration is crucial in some situations. Table 8-5 summarizes well-tested therapy options following organism identification prior to confirmation of sensitivity.* The parenteral dose of antibiotics is summarized in Table 8-6.

Ampicillin and penicillin G achieve good CSF levels in the face of inflammation and are most commonly used in neurosurgical settings for treating uncomplicated meningitis. The penicillinase-resistant penicillins such as methicillin, nafcillin, and oxacillin are cen-

*References 59,99,173,178,221,237,264,269.

TABLE 8-6 ■ Antibiotic Doses for CNS Infection in Adults

Antibiotic	Daily Dose	Dosing Interval (h)
Penicillin G	20–40 million units	4
Ampicillin	12 g	4
Nafcillin, oxacillin	9–12 g	4
Vancomycin	2–4 g	12
Piperacillin	300 mg/kg body weight	4
Ceftriaxone	50 mg/kg body weight or 4 g	12
Cefotaxime	8–12 g	4–6
Ceftizoxime	6–9 g	8
Ceftazidime	6–12 g	8
Gentamicin, tobramycin	5 mg/kg body weight	8
Amikacin	14 mg/kg body weight	12
Trimethoprim/ sulfamethoxazole	10 mg (Tmp)/ kg body weight	12
Chloramphenicol	4–6 g	6
Rifampin	0.6–1.2 g	12–24
Metronidazole	30 mg/kg body weight	6

tral to the treatment of suspected or proven *S. aureus* infection. These compounds have no activity against gram-negative bacilli or *Streptococcus faecalis* but do inhibit *S. pyogenes* and *S. pneumoniae* at achievable concentrations.

Methicillin-resistant *S. aureus* strains appear to have altered penicillin-binding proteins, making them resistant to all penicillins and cephalosporins. Vancomycin, a glycopeptide antibiotic, is the only antibiotic that consistently shows sensitivity to this strain and to coagulase-negative *S. epidermidis*. Another glycopeptide, teicoplanin, is eliminated more slowly, is better tolerated, and is more potent than vancomycin.

The antipseudomonal penicillins play a role in therapy of ICU infections because of the frequency of *P. aeruginosa* in various clinical circumstances. Piperacillin is active against *P. aeruginosa* and also provides activity for other gram-negative pathogens such as *Klebsiella* and *Enterobacteraceae*. The expanded spectrum of piperacillin has made it a popular agent in ICU settings, most commonly in combination with an aminoglycoside.

The third-generation cephalosporins continue to be important in the therapy of patients with complicated neurosurgical conditions. Cefotaxime and cetriaxone have good CSF penetration, allowing treatment of many episodes of gram-negative meningitis previously requiring intrathecal therapy. *Klebsiella*, *Proteus*, *Serratia*, and *Enterobacter* species are usually sensitive to these extended spectrum cephalosporins; however, the concentrations achieved are not sufficient to be predictably active for staphylococci.

Metronidazole provides excellent activity for anaerobic bacteria including *Bacillus fragilis* and penetrates the CNS well. Neurotoxicity including ataxia has been noted and can be confusing when this agent is used in a regimen for CNS infection, but fortunately side effects are rare. In addition to excellent *B. fragilis* activity, clindamycin is a good antistaphylococcal agent. Other unproven but promising antibiotics in the treatment of resistant gram-negative CNS infections include fluoroquinolones, imipenem, and aztreonam.

VIRAL INFECTIONS OF THE CENTRAL NERVOUS SYSTEM

Viruses are obligate intracellular parasites that are classified by their nucleic acid type and are subdivided by the size and shape of their protein coat. There are 10 groups of RNA viruses and 5 groups of DNA viruses. RNA viruses replicate in the cell cytoplasm, whereas DNA viruses, except poxviruses, replicate in the cell nucleus. Viral infection is established when susceptible cells displaying particular receptors bind to the complementary viral glycoprotein ligands.

Viruses usually enter the body through the mucous membranes of the respiratory, gastrointestinal, or urinary tracts. Breach of the epidermis is necessary for transmission through this barrier. Some viruses remain confined to mucosal surfaces, whereas others disseminate widely throughout the lymphatic and circulatory systems. Viral entry into the CNS occurs along peripheral nerves and via the bloodstream. The peripheral neural route is important for the migration and dissemination of rabies, herpes simplex, and varicella zoster viruses. In the presence of viremia, viruses reach brain parenchyma despite the BBB created by endothelial cells. Once the particles enter the CNS, they must reach susceptible cells that they can successfully infect. Not all cell types in the CNS are vulnerable to attack by a given virus, and progression of the disease depends on intimate viral contact with host cells expressing the appropriate receptor.

Clinical neurological disease depends on viral effects on the infected cells. Herpes simplex virus (HSV) causes profound changes in cellular protein metabolism, resulting in early cell death. Other viruses produce little change in basal cellular metabolism but cause alterations in functional metabolism, such as the production of enzymes and neurotransmitters leading to abnormalities of specialized neural physiologic functions. Yet other viruses may persist for long periods in the CNS before producing any evidence of disease. This long latency is most commonly seen with DNA viruses and is associated with chronic infections, such as subacute sclerosing panencephalitis caused by the measles virus and progressive multifocal leukoencephalopathy caused by papovavirus.

The variety of symptoms in viral diseases is due to the differing vulnerability of CNS cell populations to the various viruses. The high degree of specialization and complexity of CNS cell membranes can explain the unique vulnerability of certain groups of neurons and glia to specific viruses. For example, the rabies virus involves the limbic system neurons but not neocortical neurons; papovaviruses selectively attack oligodendrocytes; and HSV localizes to the temporal lobes but can successfully infect a wide variety of cell types. Most viral infections of the CNS are caused by viruses common in the general population and are usually associated with a benign and self-limited course. Breakdown of usual host defense mechanisms during viral infection of the CNS is implied by the presence of virus-specific within the CNS. A major therapeutic advance has been the development of killed and attenuated viral strains for immunization against polio, mumps, and measles.

Viral meningitis, the most common sequelae of CNS viral infection, presents as aseptic meningitis. Enteroviral meningitis can begin abruptly with no prodrome, occasionally with symptoms resembling a mild subarachnoid hemorrhage, which may lead to an initial neurosurgical referral. As with meningitis, viral encephalitis is usually mild and self-limited; occasionally, patients present with depressed levels of consciousness, seizures, focal weakness, paralysis, ataxia, or nystagmus. Serious consequences, even death, can occur from HSV encephalitis, the equine encephalitides, and polio.

Viral diseases and viral-associated diseases that may be encountered in neurosurgical practice include HSV encephalitis, Reye's syndrome, and human immunodeficiency virus (HIV) infection. These will be considered in greater detail. Specific drugs for the treatment of viral diseases are under development, and a number of newer agents that have shown promise in early clinical investigation will be discussed with respect to these diseases.

Herpes Simplex Encephalitis

Herpes simplex virus (HSV) is a DNA virus with two antigenically distinct subtypes, HSV type 1 and HSV type 2. Respiratory droplets and saliva spread HSV-1; it is the agent of the ubiquitous and benign recurrent cold sore of the oral mucosa. Approximately 90% of adults have circulating antibodies to HSV-1 and about 25% have recurrent cold sores; however, this seemingly benign virus can demonstrate enhanced CNS virulence and cause necrotizing encephalitis. HSV-2 is spread by sexual contact; it is the cause of genital mucosal lesions and can result in systemic infection in the newborn, including diffuse encephalitis. Neonatal herpes is probably transferred from the infected mother during birth. In adults, HSV-2 is also associated with a recurrent aseptic meningitis (Mollaret's meningitis).

HSV-1 can remain in a dormant state in the cell bodies of trigeminal ganglion sensory neurons, reactivating intermittently to cause mucocutaneous lesions around the mouth. The virus reaches the trigeminal ganglion by retrograde axoplasmic transport up the axons supplying the area of the oral lesion. Fever, injury, exposure to ultraviolet light, and trauma to the trigeminal nerve can reactivate the dormant virus. While in the dormant state, viral particles are unable to be isolated, although the viral DNA is preserved within the host cells. However, viral replication occurs rapidly on reactivation.

HSV-1 encephalitis is the primary cause of fatal sporadic encephalitis in the United States. The mortality rate is approximately 70% if untreated, much higher than most encephalitides.[290] The relationship of HSV-1 encephalitis to oral herpes infection is unclear. Rarely, patients have an active oral lesion at the time of onset of encephalitis. A past history of herpetic lesions is present in 25% of patients, similar to the general population. The mechanism of CNS infection involves HSV-1 invasion of the nasal epithelium and migration along axons of the olfactory tract to the frontal and temporal lobes.[188] Subsequent invasion and lysis of both glial and neuronal cells indicate disease progression.

Approximately 90% of patients show early neurological signs indicating frontotemporal localization—hallucinations, behavioral abnormalities, and personality change. Fever and headache are almost universal in the early presentation, as are seizures. Memory impairment, implying bilateral basal temporal involvement, is present in many patients. Focal motor deficits, usually in the face and arm, may occur, and aphasia is common if the dominant frontotemporal region is involved. As the disease progresses, the frontotemporal region becomes edematous and the swollen brain resembles an intracranial mass, leading to increased intracranial pressure and uncal herniation. Coma, an age greater than 30 years, and delay in antiviral therapy contribute to a poor prognosis.[188]

An electroencephalogram (EEG) may help confirm a focal process by demonstrating periodic paroxysmal discharges or slow wave complexes in one or both temporal lobes. CT scans may show decreased attenuation in one or both temporal lobes as early as the third day of the disease. This decreased attenuation represents edema and necrosis found in the areas of encephalitis. The use of contrast agents can show areas of abnormal enhancement surrounding the low-density areas. MRI is more sensitive for documenting early edematous changes and hastens the recognition of nonhemorrhagic HSV encephalitis.[194]

Definitive diagnosis of HSV encephalitis had depended on histologic or culture results from brain biopsy. However, despite great sensitivity and specificity, the invasive surgical procedure is controversial and rarely used. CSF examination is now used to establish the diagnosis of HSV encephalitis. CSF pleocytosis is reflected by the presence of a mixture of neutrophils and mononuclear cells, predominantly the latter. Red blood cells, very rare in other encephalitides, are frequently present. Protein is moderately elevated, and glucose is normal. HSV cultures are rarely positive from CSF and take too long to be of early diagnostic value; however, PCR amplification of HSV DNA in CSF specimens is now the recognized gold standard for diagnosing HSV CNS infections.[258]

The treatment of choice for HSV encephalitis remains acyclovir. Acyclovir is an acyclic analog of guanosine that inhibits viral DNA synthesis by binding to the viral DNA polymerase following phosphorylation in infected cells. Therapy (30 mg/kg/day q8h for at least 10 days) should begin as soon as the diagnosis is suspected, because delay in the start of therapy may drastically affect patient morbidity.[289] An equally important factor in the treatment of this disease is the control of increased ICP associated with frontotemporal edema. Intravenous fluids must be carefully monitored, and the judicious use of hyperventilation, steroids, osmotic diuretics, and intracranial pressure monitoring remain essential in the treatment regimen.

Acquired Immunodeficiency Syndrome

Worldwide, 20 million adults and 2 million children are infected with HIV, and one third to one half of these individuals will develop CNS involvement before death.[159,192] In fact, neurological disease is the AIDS defining illness in 10% to 20% of cases.[25,32] These statistics underestimate the actual frequency of CNS involvement; in postmortem examinations of AIDS patients, 75% of cases show pathologic signs of nervous system involvement.[108,191,198]

The common neurological manifestations of HIV infection can be divided into those that result directly from HIV infection and those that result indirectly from immunosuppression. Discussed below are the neurological sequelae of AIDS that are of potential neurosurgical interest.

Primary Neurological Sequelae of HIV Infection

The primary neurological sequelae of HIV infection include meningitis, encephalopathy/dementia, and myelopathy. Two types of meningitis have been described: (1) an acute febrile syndrome similar to mononucleosis that presents within days to weeks of initial HIV exposure, and (2) a subacute aseptic meningitis around the time of seroconversion. Symptoms of the acute form of meningitis or meningoencephalitis include headache, meningismus, photophobia, seizures, and depressed mental status. CSF pleocytosis is mononuclear, and culture is positive in about 50% of the cases.[176] Symptoms of the subacute form include chronic headaches, usually without meningeal signs. CSF characteristics are similar to that of the acute form except that anti-HIV antibodies can usually be detected.[124] However, abnormal CSF finding are common in asymptomatic HIV-infected individuals and may not predict the subsequent development of neurological disease.[159,171]

HIV-1 encephalopathy is now the leading cause of dementia in those younger than 60 years of age,[135,177] and afflicted patients usually die within 6 months after onset.[120] HIV encephalopathy presents with a progressive global dementia associated with headaches, increasing social isolation, and loss of sexual drive. In addition to cognitive decline, painful peripheral dysesthesias and motor impairment can occur. Overall, adult HIV encephalopathy is a subcortical dementia with global cognitive decline, psychomotor impairment, and motor and behavioral abnormalities. In children affected with this disorder, developmental delay and/or loss of motor and intellectual milestones are seen. Motor weakness, ataxia, myoclonus, and seizures accompany HIV encephalopathy in children. Gross pathology shows diffuse brain atrophy with enlargement of CSF spaces and occasional meningeal fibrosis. Microscopically, white matter pallor results from perivascular demyelination accompanied by astrocytic reaction. Multinucleate giant cells appear to be a hallmark of the disease. Radiological studies of the brain reflect the pathologic abnormalities. Sulcal and ventricular enlargement are seen on CT imaging, and demyelination in the periventricular white matter and centrum semiovale are seen on MRI. CSF studies can show increased protein and mononuclear pleocytosis. HIV-specific antibody and HIV antigen may be present in the CSF. Azidothymidine and zidovudine can result in improvement of HIV encephalopathy.[79]

HIV myelopathy often presents with extremity weakness, gait difficulties, and incontinence of bowel and bladder. These sequelae of HIV infection are clinically underrecognized and often not detected until late in the course of HIV infection. Pathologic examination shows demyelination and spongy degeneration affecting the lateral and posterior columns more than the anterior columns. Associated microvacuolization of the white matter results from intramyelin swelling. Central chromatolysis of the anterior horn cells may also occur. MRI of the spinal cord is used to exclude other structural causes of myelopathy, and the diagnosis of HIV myelopathy is often a diagnosis of exclusion in the context of known or presumed HIV infection. Specific treatment of HIV myelopathy outside the realm of systemic treatment of HIV infection has not been established.

Opportunistic Neoplasms of the CNS in AIDS

CNS lymphoma is the second most frequent intracerebral mass lesion in AIDS patients.[79,158] The incidence of primary CNS lymphoma has risen rapidly over the past 20 years because of the increasing numbers of AIDS patients. CNS lymphoma was reported to be the AIDS defining illness in 16% of cases.[17] Affected patients present with mental status changes, memory loss, lethargy, dysphasia, seizures, and cranial nerve palsies. Pathological examination reveals high-grade immunoblastic lymphomas. The primary treatment remains radiation therapy.

Opportunistic Infections of the CNS in AIDS

Bacteria that cause opportunistic CNS infection in AIDS include *Mycobacterium* species and *Treponema*. *Mycobacterium tuberculosis* has been reported to cause CNS tuberculosis in up to 2.4% of HIV-infected patients with CNS disease.[25] CNS tuberculosis manifests clinically as meningismus with fever, altered mental status, and seizures. Pathologic examination reveals tuberculomas, cerebral abscesses, and meningitis. Patients with CNS disease caused by *Mycobacterium avium-intracellulare* mass lesions occur more commonly than meningitis.[159] CT and MRI show ring-enhancing lesions and diffuse signal abnormalities. CSF studies may show no abnormalities. Spinal cord abscesses resulting from mycobacteria have also been reported in AIDS.[73] Treatment of mycobacterial infection with a multiple drug regimen for a minimum of 9 months has generally resulted in improvement.[48]

Positive *Treponema pallidum* serologies in AIDS patients approximate 50% frequency in some institutions.[159] Treponeme CNS infection in the context of HIV infection presents as acute neurosyphilis, in which the usually delayed secondary and tertiary symptoms occur after a much shortened period. Meningovascular syphilis and general paresis have been reported to occur within 4 months of the primary infection, even when the patients were treated with penicillin prior to the onset of neurological symptoms.[137] Other unusual neurological sequelae of *Treponema* infection include syphilitic meningomyelitis, polyradiculopathy, and cerebral gliomas.[22,151] Diagnosis and subsequent evaluation of high-dose penicillin G treatment efficacy relies on both serum and CSF VDRL titers.

Common viral opportunistic infection in AIDS patients include JC virus and cytomegalovirus (CMV), both of which have been associated for years with immunosuppressed or immunodeficient patients with impaired cell-mediated immunity. JC virus is a papovavirus that causes progressive multifocal leukoencephalopathy (PML), characterized by demyelination, pleomorphic giant astrocytes, and abnormal oligodendrocytes. In HIV-infected patients, the reported incidence of PML ranges from 0.5% to 4.2%.[23,149,160,244] Patients afflicted with PML present most often with mental status changes and dysphasia, although a variety of other symptoms, including visual disturbances, ataxia, vertigo, and headache, are not uncommon. Radiological examination reveals white matter abnormalities predominantly in the parietooccipital region. CSF studies rarely reveal abnormalities. Diagnosis is usually obtained by brain biopsy. Definitive therapy of PML has yet to be established, although many antiviral agents have been tried.[24,149,183,224]

Cytomegalovirus is associated with subacute encephalopathy in HIV-infected patients. The pathology of this entity is characterized by microglial nodules in the subcortical gray matter and viral inclusions in capillary endothelia, astrocytes, and neurons. Gancyclovir remains the mainstay of treatment.[159,224]

The most common fungal opportunist of HIV-infected patients is *Cryptococcus neoformans* with an incidence approximating 10%.[244] As in non-AIDS patients (see section on fungal infections), meningitis is the primary sequela.[148] Infection generally occurs by inhalation, resulting in a primary pulmonary site of infection. Meningitis results from reactivation and spread of primary disease. AIDS patients present with typical symptoms of meningitis, with rare focal findings. Pathology is characterized by a basilar meningitis with opacifications of meninges and diffuse brain edema. Cystic lesions representing budding yeast may be seen in the superficial layers of the cortex with little surrounding inflammation. CSF is characterized by increased protein and decreased glucose. Diagnosis relies on specific stains of the CSF with India ink with a sensitivity of greater than 90%.[306] Treatment relies on amphotericin B, flucytosine, and fluconazole.[224]

Parasitic infection with *Toxoplasma gondii* occurs in up to 40% of neurologically ill AIDS patients.[23] Toxoplasmosis is the most common cause of intracerebral mass lesions in HIV-infected patients.[280] The lack of cell-mediated immunity allows for the release and circulation of invasive trophozoites and establishment of encephalitis. Neurological symptoms present as focal deficits within the context of diffuse encephalopathy. Hemiparesis associated with headache, confusion, and lethargy is common. Radiological imaging reveals multiple ring-enhancing lesions with surrounding edema and mass effect. Most lesions occur in the cerebral hemispheres and basal ganglia.[193] CSF examination reveals mononuclear pleocytosis and decreased glucose. Serologic studies are usually indicative of toxoplasmosis. Definitive diagnosis is reached by brain biopsy. Therapy includes pyrimethamine and sulfadiazine.[224]

Reye's Syndrome

Although it is not a viral infection of the CNS, Reye's syndrome is a viral-associated illness in which neurosurgical intervention is often lifesaving. Reye's syndrome is a rare, noninflammatory encephalopathy associated with hepatic microvesicular fatty infiltration and severe hyperammonemia that occurs almost exclusively in children. First described in 1963, the syndrome is characterized by an unremarkable prodromal viral illness followed by abrupt onset of encephalopathy, usually after only 3 days.[101] Hepatomegaly is usually present, and laboratory examination reveals elevated serum ammonia, elevated AST and ALT, lactic acidemia, and prolonged prothrombin time. CSF examination is unremarkable. Decerebrate posturing and hyperventilation become prominent as the disease progresses. EEG shows widespread neuronal dysfunction, reflecting the severity of the process, and is useful in staging the disease when combined with clinical criteria.[164]

The agent of the disease and the cause of the biochemical abnormalities are not clearly understood but are thought to be multifactorial. In almost all cases the encephalopathic phase is preceded by a respiratory illness or chickenpox. Epidemics of influenza B or A and varicella are associated with outbreaks of Reye's syndrome.[143] Six epidemiological studies have documented a close relationship between aspirin usage for the prodromal viral symptoms and the subsequent development of Reye's syndrome.* The annual number of reported cases has decreased sharply since 1980: the total number of reported cases was only 25 in 1989, despite a substantial influenza B epidemic.[47] This decline is coincident with increased public awareness of aspirin's association with Reye's syndrome and a decrease in the use of aspirin-containing medication in children.[47]

The most important factor in the pathogenesis of the encephalopathy in Reye's syndrome appears to be hyperammonemia. Liver clearance of ammonia is decreased by destruction of the urea cycle enzymes. The arterial ammonia level may be as high as 1000 μg/100ml and is directly related to the depth of coma, the severity of EEG abnormality, and the mortality rate.[54] Examination of the brain shows cytotoxic cerebral edema with swelling of astrocyte foot processes and no signs of interstitial edema, inflammation, or demyelination.[26]

Cerebral edema is almost universal in fatal cases, and the high mortality in Reye's syndrome patients is closely associated with increasing intracranial pressure (ICP). Reversal of coma and reduction in mortality has been documented when ICP monitoring and vigorous attempts to lower ICP are added to the protocols of supportive treatments.[145,275] Mannitol has been shown to be effective in ICP management, whereas corticosteroids appear to be ineffective.

PRION INFECTIONS OF THE CENTRAL NERVOUS SYSTEM

Prion infections comprise a group of diseases affecting the central nervous system in which the "infectious agent" is the abnormal conformation (associated with mutations or insertions in the prion gene) of a prion protein found normally on cell surfaces.[210,211] These diseases, often referred to as the spongiform encephalopathies, ultimately progress to severe neurodegeneration with uniformly fatal outcomes. The incidence of Creutzfeldt-Jakob disease (CJD), the most common human prion disease, has been reported as one per million population.[127,147,292] The variable clinical phenomena of the different prion diseases is presented in the following. Diagnosis of these diseases continues to rely on pathologic examination of biopsied brain.

CJD presents as a rapidly progressive global dementia with characteristic triphasic EEG complexes associated with behavioral changes, movement disorders, or focal neurological deficits. The mean age of onset is 65 years of age with a mean duration of illness before death of 5 months.[215] Pathologic studies show CJD to be a neuronal disease primarily affecting gray matter of the cerebral hemispheres, although thalamic involvement has been reported.[147]

Variant CJD presents with initial psychiatric symptomatology including anxiety and depression leading to a rapidly progressing cerebellar syndrome.[67,292] The mean age of onset is 27 years, with a mean duration of illness before death of 16 months.[133] Spongiform changes occur primarily in the basal ganglia with florid amyloid plaques containing the abnormal prion protein. Additionally, the abnormal prion protein can be found in lymphoid tissues such as lymph nodes, tonsils, and spleen.

Fatal familial insomnia presents as severe insomnia associated with symptoms of autonomic dysregulation, including hyperthermia, tachycardia, hypertension, and hyperhydrosis.[91] Destruction of the thalami with astrogliosis is common. Spongiform changes and amyloid deposits are rare.

Gerstmann-Straussler-Scheinker syndrome presents with cerebellar ataxia, slowly progressive dementia, and movement disorder. An abundance of amyloid plaques are found in the brain, especially in the cerebellum.[133]

Kuru presents as profound cerebellar ataxia associated with emotional lability, with rare dementia[89] thought to be associated with ritualistic cannibalism in Papua New Guinea. The cessation of these practices has resulted in dramatically decreased incidence of this prion disease.

Diagnosis of the prion diseases has relied primarily on pathological examination of brain tissues using strict diagnostic criteria.[39] The most sensitive method is Western blot detection of the abnormal prion protein. Early detection relies on immunostaining of the abnormal protein in biopsied brain tissues with microscopic confirmation. For prion diseases in which the abnormal protein is found in lymphoid tissues, lymph nodes or tonsils can be used as tissue sources. Examination of cerebrospinal fluid by radioimmunoassay for prion protein markers is promising,[119,130] although the clinical reliability and specificity have yet to be demonstrated. EEG shows slow waves progressing to triphasic waves, periodic sharp wave complexes, and ultimately isoelectric waves. CT or MRI may assist in diagnosis by demonstrating severe atrophic changes, which occur over several months. Other sporadic changes on MRI, including contrast enhancement and hyperintense signals in the basal ganglia, have been described.[238] Positron emission tomography is reported to demonstrate decreased cortical metabolism that precedes the atrophic changes seen on MRI.[200]

Transmission of prion disease in the United States has primarily occurred via iatrogenic procedures.[53,127] All reported cases of human-to-human transmission of CJD resulted from allogeneic dura mater grafts, corneal grafts, pituitary derivative injections, and intracranial surgical procedures using instruments subjected to inappropriate disinfection protocols.[146] Recommendations for the disinfection of neurosurgical instruments

*References 85,117,118,131,249,277.

involving high-temperature moist-heat sterilization have been published.[270] Transmissibility of prion diseases by blood or from other species is yet to be definitively characterized.

The treatment of prion disease remains theoretical. Several compounds have been reported to inhibit abnormal prion protein accumulation after experimental infection in vitro.[45,46] Compounds that interfere with the conversion of the normal prion into the abnormal conformation is also promising.[51] Successful treatment will ultimately rely on further knowledge about these confounding diseases.

FUNGAL INFECTIONS OF THE CENTRAL NERVOUS SYSTEM

Fungi are ubiquitous organisms in the environment with low virulence that become pathogenic during particular circumstances, including suppression of cell-mediated immunity, neutropenia, and prolonged systemic antibiotic therapy. The reported incidence of fungal infections in the United States is increasing due to more awareness of such infections, better diagnostic techniques, increased travel to and from regions of endemic infection, the increasing numbers of ICU patients using prolonged systemic antibiotics, and especially the increasing numbers of immunosuppressed patients.[301]

Fungal infections may be divided into those caused by pathogenic fungi (e.g., *Histoplasma*, *Blastomyces*, and *Coccidiodes*) or by opportunistic fungi (e.g., *Candida, Torulopsis, Aspergillus, Mucoraceae, Cryptococcus,* and *Phycomycetes*).[63] Involvement of the CNS may be disseminated, causing meningitis or meningoencephalitis, or it may be focal, causing granulomatous abscesses. Fungal infections of the CNS remain relatively rare, and discussed in the following are those encountered more commonly in the United States.

Cryptococcosis

C. neoformans, a common soil organism, is the most common cause of fungal meningitis in the United States, primarily because of the AIDS epidemic.[242] Cryptococcal infection has been reported in all age groups, but two thirds of cases occur between the ages of 30 and 50 years.[228] The respiratory tract is the primary site of infection, and hematogenous dissemination is the most common source of CNS infection. CNS infection occurs most commonly as meningitis, but brain abscesses and granulomas have also been reported.[233] Cryptococcal meningitis presents differently in AIDS patients versus non-AIDS patients.[49,207,226] AIDS patients present with the minimal nonfocal findings of headache, fever, and lethargy. Non-AIDS patients present with severe headache, nausea, vomiting, meningeal signs, and depressed mental status in addition to focal abnormalities including papilledema, cranial nerve palsies, and reduced visual acuity resulting from raised intracranial pressure.[138]

In non-AIDS patients, CSF pleocytosis is lymphocytic, CSF protein is elevated, and CSF glucose is reduced. In AIDS patients, CSF white blood cell counts remain low and often CSF glucose is normal. Culture for *C. neoformans* from CSF is productive for both AIDS and non-AIDS patients. CSF india ink smears are positive in 50% to 75% of non-AIDS patients with cryptococcal meningitis and in up to 88% in AIDS patients.[242] Serologic testing by latex agglutination of the cryptococcal polysaccharide antigen has an overall sensitivity and specificity of nearly 100%.[28] CT or MRI helps to detect signs of basilar inflammation, intracranial mass lesions, or hydrocephalus.

Treatment of cryptococcal meningitis in non-AIDS patients relies on combination therapy with amphotericin B (0.3 mg/kg/day) with flucytosine (150 mg/kg/day) for 6 weeks.[69] The poor response of AIDS patients to amphotericin B has led to the practice of reducing the course of amphotericin B with or without flucytosine for 2 weeks followed by fluconazole (440 mg/day) to complete a 10-week course.[242] Fluconazole (200 mg/day) is the agent of choice used to prevent relapse of cryptococcal meningitis in patients with AIDS.

Coccidiomycosis

Coccidiodies immitis is found in the semiarid soils of the southwestern United States, Mexico, and Central and South America. Infection occurs almost invariably by the respiratory tract; person-to-person transmission has not been reported. Systemic dissemination occurs in approximately 0.5% of patients within 6 months after the initial infection.[5] Of these patients, 30% to 50% have meningitis.[186,242] Disseminated coccidiomycosis is associated with extremes of age, non-Caucasian race, and immunosuppression.[266] Systemic coccidiomycosis, in a person with evidence of HIV, has been classified as an AIDS-defining illness.

Coccidiodal meningitis presents commonly as headache associated with fever, confusion, seizures, personality changes, and focal cranial nerve palsies. Meningeal signs have been reported in only 30% of cases.[242] CNS coccidiomycosis is often not recognized until the disease is well established, with a thick proteinaceous basal cistern exudate resulting in subsequent cranial nerve palsies and hydrocephalus.

Examination of CSF shows a predominant mononuclear and/or eosinophilic pleocytosis.[232,253] CSF protein is elevated, and CSF glucose is decreased. Culture of CSF for the fungus is positive in only 20% to 50% of patients. Diagnosis of systemic coccidiomycosis relies on the complement fixation test for CSF antibody to the fungus. At least 70% of patients with early disease and almost all patients with disease progression show significant antibody titers.[5,29] In patients with coccidiodal meningitis, CSF antibody titers parallel the course of meningeal disease. In AIDS patients, appropriate antibodies may not develop in either serum or CSF.

Treatment of coccidiodal meningitis relies on both intravenous and intrathecal amphotericin B.[29,242] The usual intrathecal dose is 0.5 mg three times per week for 15 weeks. When combined with intrathecal corticosteroids, doses of 1 to 1.5 mg can be used. Therapy is discontinued when CSF is normal for 1 year. Because of the toxicities associated with amphotericin B, studies regarding the use of fluconazole and itraconazole continue.[90,267]

Candidiasis

Candida albicans rarely causes disease in healthy individuals, although it is a common constituent of oropharyngeal flora. There are more than 150 species of this organism, but only 10 have been reported as human pathogens; of these, *C. albicans* is most commonly associated with CNS disease. CNS infection usually results from spread of intestinal, urinary, or vascular catheter infection[162] in patients with immunodeficiencies or altered host defenses. CNS involvement in patients with systemic candidiasis has been reported to be approximately 50%.[242]

CNS *Candida* infection usually presents as multiple cerebral microabscesses. *Candida* meningitis is less common, occurring in less than 15% of patients with CNS candidiasis[18,162,278] and presents with fever and signs of meningeal irritation. *Candida* has also been reported to cause a higher rate of meningitis in AIDS patients and in patients with shunts.[75,107,301]

CSF pleocytosis is predominantly neutrophilic. Cultures and smears are often positive. Serologic testing of serum or CSF is not currently reliable.

Treatment of choice for CNS *Candida* infection remains amphotericin B (0.6 mg/kg/day) with or without flucytosine.[18,162] Surgical resections of granulomas or abscesses following institution of medical therapy have also shown favorable outcomes.[132]

Histoplasmosis

Histoplasma capsulatum is endemic to the river valleys of the Ohio, Mississippi, and St. Lawrence rivers and along the Appalachian Mountains in North Carolina and Virginia. Histoplasmosis is diagnosed more commonly in those younger than 3 years and those older than 40 years, and in males more than females. The source of infection is the respiratory tract. Only a small number of non-AIDS patients develop systemic infection; however, more than 90% of AIDS patients have disseminated infection.[287] CNS histoplasmosis occurs in up to 24% of patients with disseminated histoplasmosis in the form of meningitis, solitary or multiple granulomas.[226]

CNS histoplasmosis presents as generalized headache, confusion, decreased level of consciousness, ataxia, and seizures. Focal neurological deficits including cranial nerve palsies are also seen. Meningeal signs occur in fewer than 10% of cases.

CSF examination shows a mild neutrophilic or lymphocytic pleocytosis.[266,283] CSF protein is elevated, and CSF glucose is reduced. CSF smears and cultures are of low yield. Tests detecting antibodies to *Histoplasma* by both complement fixation and radioimmunoassay have excellent sensitivity but low specificity. Tests detecting the *Histoplasma* polysaccharide antigen (HPA) in blood, CSF, and urine are being developed and standardized.[284–286]

Treatment of systemic and CNS histoplasmosis relies on intravenous amphotericin B (0.7–1.0 mg/kg/day for >5 weeks).[207,266,287] Intrathecal administration does not improve the efficacy of treatment. In AIDS patients, intravenous amphotericin B is given at doses of 1 to 1.5 g over 6 to 8 weeks, followed by maintenance azole antifungal therapy.

Blastomycosis

Blastomyces dermatitidis is endemic to the Ohio, Mississippi, and St. Lawrence River valleys. The organism enters the body through the respiratory tract. The incidence of blastomycosis is highest in middle-aged men.[242] CNS blastomycosis presents in 3% to 10% of patients with disseminated blastomycosis as a late and fulminant complication, resulting in meningitis or abscess formation.

CSF evaluation for blastomycosis is usually nondiagnostic. A reliable serologic test is yet to be developed, and other tests (e.g., complement fixation, immunodiffusion) have been useful for epidemiological assessments but not for clinical diagnosis.[31] Diagnosis of CNS blastomycosis is essentially derived from clinical judgment in the setting of disseminated blastomycosis.

Again, amphotericin B is the mainstay of treatment for this fungal infection. For patients with CNS involvement, doses of 0.3 to 0.6 mg/kg/day for 6 to 8 weeks are recommended.[103,266] The use of intrathecal amphotericin B and azoles remains a last resort.

Aspergillosis

Aspergillus species are the most common fungi in the environment. In immunocompromised patients, aspergillosis is becoming increasingly prevalent, with a mortality of greater than 90%.[52] CNS aspergillosis has become the second most common fungal infection of the CNS in AIDS patients. The usual source of disseminated disease is the respiratory tract via hematogenous spread. CNS disease has been reported in the forms of mycotic aneurysms, brain abscesses, osteomyelitis, discitis, and meningitis.[10,12,52,147,150]

Amphotericin B is the suggested medical therapy. Standard regimens are yet to be established. In case of discrete intracranial masses, craniotomy for resection combined with medical therapy has been described with favorable outcomes.[52,104] In general, the prognosis for patients with widely disseminated aspergillosis with CNS involvement is poor.

Phycomycetes

Although hematologic spread is the usual route for most fungal CNS infections, CNS infections by *Zygomyces*, particularly mucormycosis, can result from direct contamination of the brain by adjacent infected tissues (e.g., orbits and paranasal sinuses). Mucormycosis presents as diffuse fungal encephalitis, especially in patients with diabetes mellitus and AIDS. This disease preferentially involves the cerebral vasculature, resulting in ischemia, thrombosis, and infarction as well as inflammation. Treatment includes debridement of the infected and devitalized tissues and systemic amphotericin B. Prognosis remains poor despite aggressive therapy.

Actinomycosis

Actinomyces israelii is a gram-positive anaerobic bacterium found in normal oral flora. It is discussed in this section because of its historical categorization as a fungal infection. CNS actinomycosis is rare, with only 70 reported cases between 1937 and 1987.[243] CNS actinomycosis presents as brain abscesses, meningitis or meningoencephalitis, actinomycoma, subdural empyema, and epidural abscesses.[88,243] Treatment includes surgical drainage when appropriate and intravenous penicillin for 3 to 4 months.

Nocardiosis

Nocardia is a gram-positive aerobe found in soil and decaying vegetables, also historically categorized as a fungus-like bacteria. With the emergence of the AIDS epidemic, the number of reported cases is increasing.[168] Nocardiosis is primarily contracted by inhalation, and CNS nocardiosis is acquired by hematogenous spread.[83] Of patients with disseminated nocardial infections, 15% to 44% have cerebral abscesses.[19,129,142,239] Purulent meningitis also occurs. Recommended treatment includes surgical drainage combined with sulfonamide antibiotic therapy.[169]

PARASITIC INFECTIONS OF THE CENTRAL NERVOUS SYSTEM

Although parasitic infection of the CNS is relatively uncommon in North America and Western Europe, it is a major cause of disease worldwide. Once CNS infestation occurs, treatment options are limited and remain mostly palliative. Often, the CNS becomes infected as a complication of primary infection in another organ system. The infections described in the following are limited to those of particular concern in neurosurgery.

Neurocysticercosis

Neurocysticercosis (NC) is the most common parasitic infection of the CNS.[65] The tapeworm *Taenia solium* is the parasitic agent. Both the adult *T. solium* pork tapeworm (taeniasis) and its larval stages (cysticercosis) are found in humans. Taeniasis causes intestinal infection; however, cysticercosis is a highly neurotropic infection, acquired by ingesting tapeworm eggs shed in human feces, not by ingesting pork.

Four principal forms of NC have been described: parenchymal, ventricular, meningeal, and racemose.[80] Parenchymal cysts are found more commonly in the gray matter than the spinal cord, more commonly in the cerebrum than the cerebellum, and are 3 to 15 mm in diameter.[2,43,70] Ventricular cysts, singly or in clusters, adhere to the ventricular wall or float freely in the cerebrospinal fluid (most commonly found in the fourth ventricle).[43,252] Subarachnoid cysts have been described as present not only in the subarachnoid spaces, but adherent to the pia or within the cortical parenchyma.[197] Racemose cysts are found in clusters in the basal cisterns, often obstructing the flow of CSF.

The clinical manifestations of NC range from asymptomatic infection to severe disabling disorders and vary with the location of the cysts. Parenchymal NC presents as seizures, focal deficits, and cognitive decline. Motor weakness is common, along with brainstem dysfunction, cerebellar ataxia, and sensory deficits. Cranial nerve palsies, involuntary movements, cavernous sinus syndrome, and hydrocephalus have also been described.[246] Cysticercotic encephalitis, in which hundreds to thousands of cysts cause intense inflammation, is a particularly severe form of parenchymal NC and presents with a clinical syndrome identical to viral encephalitis. Ventricular cysts adherent to the ventricular wall can result in ependymitis, and clusters of cysts filling the fourth ventricle cause hydrocephalus. Subarachnoid cysts trigger the inflammatory response within the subarachnoid spaces and are associated with occlusive endarteritis of thamostriate, middle cerebral, and internal carotid arteries.[64,220]

Racemose cysts lead to arachnoiditis, endarteritis, cranial neuropathies, and hydrocephalus.[55,70,197,263]

The diagnosis of neurocysticercosis is based on clinical, immunodiagnostic, and radiographic findings. CSF studies show high opening pressures, pleocytosis with lymphocytic or eosinophilic predominance, or decreased glucose. Enzyme-linked immunosorbent assay (ELISA) and enzyme-linked immunoelectrotransfer blot (EITB) of both serum and CSF are helpful, but their low sensitivity and specificity is limiting.[15] CT and MRI have significantly improved the detection of NC lesions. Lesions on CT appear singly or multiply, calcified or low density, or ring-enhancing with contrast, depending on the variable pathologic forms. MRI is superior for detecting cisternal and intraventricular cysts.[260,305]

Treatment of NC centers on controlling the clinical symptoms of seizures with antiseizure medications, the reduction of cerebral edema with steroids, and the relief of hydrocephalus or mass lesions with surgery. Supplementation of symptomatic therapy with praziquantel and albendazole has significantly improved the outcome of patients suffering from NC.[93,273] Adjunctive steroids to prevent the potent inflammatory reaction triggered by the acute destruction of the parasites is critical.[245]

Echinococcosis (Hydatid Cysts)

Echinococcus granulosus and *E. multilocularis* infect the CNS, leading to hydatid cyst disease. Echinococcus is a ubiquitous parasite that infects man as the intermediate host and the dog as the primary host. The eggs pass from the gastrointestinal tract to the liver, where embryos develop into hydatid cysts. These cysts then disseminate to other organ systems. In the CNS, solitary parenchymal cysts are generally seen. Intraventricular and meningeal cysts are rare.[7] Involvement of the spinal cord is also rare.[44]

Common clinical signs and symptoms of hydatid disease include hemiparesis, motor deficits, decreased mental status, and seizures.[140] When *Echinococcus* invades the spine, radicular pain, motor and sensory deficits, and decreasing bladder function can be seen.

Diagnosis of CNS hydatid cyst disease is based on the epidemiologic context, serologic testing, and neuroimaging. On radiologic studies, *E. granulosus* hydatid cysts appear as spherical cystic lesions with clearly defined borders, with little ring enhancement.[66] *E. multilocularis* infection is described radiologically as an indistinct, semisolid mass with central necrosis and calcification.[106] MRI allows for the detection of the pericystium and the multiplicity of cysts with surrounding edema.[198]

Treatment of hydatid cyst disease includes surgical removal of the offending parasite. Superficial cysts are removed by flushing the pericystic space with normal saline. Deeper cysts are removed with the germinal membrane. Spillage of cyst contents should be avoided because liberated protoscoleces lead to active secondary infection. Surgical treatment of spinal disease is complicated by the need to remove large sections of infected vertebral bone.[81] Although medical treatment with mebendazole and albendazole has been reported effective against extracerebral disease, their successful use in cerebral disease remains uncertain.[20,140]

Amebic Brain Abscess and Meningoencephalitis

Amebic infections of the central nervous system are rare but are associated with high morbidity and mortality. Most amebic CNS infections are caused by *Naegleria* or *Acanthamoeba* protozoans.

Naegleria amebas cause a primary amebic meningoencephalitis (PAM). The organisms live in soil and fresh water, but have been found in swimming pools, domestic water supplies, septic systems, and home humidifiers.[170] *Naegleria* amebas attach to the olfactory neuroepithelium, migrate along the unmyelinated olfactory nerves to enter the subarachnoid space, and then spread to other parts of the CNS. Hemorrhagic necrosis of the olfactory bulbs, purulent leptomeningitis, and encephalitis result. Symptoms include severe headaches, fever, seizures, and coma. CT shows enhancement of affected regions with intravenous contrast medium. Diagnosis is established by examination of CSF showing low glucose, leukocytosis, and detection of the amoebae. Treatment relies on amphotericin B, often dosed through intraventricular reservoirs.[275]

Acanthamoebae cause encephalitis with abscess formation, usually in immunocompromised patients, referred to as granulomatous amebic encephalitis (GAE). These pathogens are ubiquitous. The likely source of infection is the repiratory tract and the route hematogenous. Patients with GAE present with symptoms of a mass lesion and signs of encephalitis. Brain biopsy remains the crux of diagnosis. Treatment of multiple mass lesions is surgical, because no effective chemotherapy protocols have been definitively established.[42]

REFERENCES

1. Adams WG, Deaver KA, Cochi SL, et al: Decline of childhood Haemophilus influenzae type b (Hib) disease in the Hib vaccine era, **JAMA 269:**221, 1993.
2. Akiguchi I, Fujiwara T, Matsuyama H, et al: Intramedullary spinal cysticercosis, **Neurology 29:**1531, 1979.
3. American Thoracic Society: Hospital-acquired pneumonia in adults: diagnosis, assessment of severity, ini-

tial antimicrobial therapy, and preventive strategies. A consensus statement, **Am J Respir Crit Care Med 153:**1711, 1996.
4. Ammirati M, Raimondi AJ: Cerebrospinal fluid shunt infections in children. A study on the relationship between the etiology of hydrocephalus, age at the time of shunt placement, and infection rate, **Childs Nerv Syst 3:**106, 1987.
5. Ampel NM, Wieden MA, Galgiani JN: Coccidioidomycosis: clinical update, **Rev Infect Dis 11:**897, 1989.
6. Antunes JL: Infections of the spine, **Acta Neurochir 116:**179, 1992.
7. Arana-Iniguez R: Echinococcus, in Vinken P, Bruyn G, (eds): **Infections of the nervous system. Part III: Handbook of clinical neurology,** vol. 35, Amsterdam: North Holland Publishing, 1978, p 175.
8. Arditi M, Herold BC, Yogev R: Cefuroxime treatment failure and Haemophilus influenzae meningitis: case report and review of literature, **Pediatrics 84:**132, 1989.
9. Arnow PM, Quimosing EM, Beach M: Consequences of intravascular catheter sepsis, **Clin Infect Dis 16:**778, 1993.
10. Artico M, Pastore FS, Polosa M, et al: Intracerebral Aspergillus abscess: case report and review of the literature, **Neurosurg Rev 20:**135, 1997.
11. Asadullah K, Woiciechowsky C, Docke WD, et al: Immunodepression following neurosurgical procedures, **Crit Care Med 23:**1976, 1995.
12. Assaad W, Nuchikat PS, Cohen L, et al: Aspergillus discitis with acute disc abscess, **Spine 19:**2226, 1994.
13. Bader MK, Littlejohns L, Palmer S: Ventriculostomy and intracranial pressure monitoring: in search of a 0% infection rate, **Heart Lung 24:**166, 1995.
14. Baker AS, Ojemann RG, Swartz MN, et al: Spinal epidural abscess, **N Engl J Med 293:**463, 1975.
15. Barry M, Kaldjian LC: Neurocysticercosis, **Semin Neurol 13:**131, 1993.
16. Baselski VS, el-Torky M, Coalson JJ, et al: The standardization of criteria for processing and interpreting laboratory specimens in patients with suspected ventilator-associated pneumonia, **Chest 102:**571S, 1992.
17. Baumgartner JE, Rachlin JR, Beckstead JH, et al: Primary central nervous system lymphomas: natural history and response to radiation therapy in 55 patients with acquired immunodeficiency syndrome, **J Neurosurg 73:**206, 1990.
18. Bayer AS, Edwards JE Jr., Seidel JS, et al: Candida meningitis. Report of seven cases and review of the english literature, **Medicine 55:**477, 1976.
19. Beaman BL, Burnside J, Edwards B, et al: Nocardial infections in the United States, 1972–1974, **J Infect Dis 134:**286, 1976.
20. Behari S, Banerji D, Phadke RV, et al: Multiple infected extradural parasellar hydatid cysts, **Surg Neurol 48:**53, 1997.
21. Bergen GA, Toney JF: Infection versus colonization in the critical care unit, **Crit Care Clin 14:**71, 1998.
22. Berger, JR: Spinal cord syphilis associated with human immunodeficiency virus infection: a treatable myelopathy, **Am J Med 92:**101, 1992.
23. Berger JR, Kaszovitz B, Post MJ, et al: Progressive multifocal leukoencephalopathy associated with human immunodeficiency virus infection. A review of the literature with a report of sixteen cases, **Ann Intern Med 107:**78, 1987.
24. Berger JR, Levy R, Dix R: AIDS and immunocompromised states, in Schlossberg D, (ed): **Infections of the central and peripheral nervous system,** Berlin: Springer-Verlag, 1990, p 268.
25. Berger JR, Moskowitz L, Fischl M, et al: Neurologic disease as the presenting manifestation of acquired immunodeficiency syndrome, **South Med J 80:**683, 1987.
26. Blisard KS, Davis LE: Neuropathologic findings in Reye syndrome, **J Child Neurol 6:**41, 1991.
27. Blomstedt GC, Kytta J: Results of a randomized trial of vancomycin prophylaxis in craniotomy, **J Neurosurg 69:**216, 1988.
28. Boom WH, Piper DJ, Ruoff KL, et al: New cause for false-positive results with the cryptococcal antigen test by latex agglutination, **J Clin Microbiol 22:**856, 1985.
29. Bouza E, Dreyer JS, Hewitt WL, et al: Coccidioidal meningitis. An analysis of thirty-one cases and review of the literature, **Medicine 60:**139, 1981.
30. Boyce JM, Jackson MM, Pugliese G, et al: Methicillin-resistant Staphylococcus aureus (MRSA): a briefing for acute care hospitals and nursing facilities. The AHA Technical Panel on Infections within Hospitals, **Infect Control Hosp Epidemiol 15:**105, 1994.
31. Bradsher RW: Blastomycosis, **Clin Infect Dis 14(Suppl 1):**S82, 1992.
32. Bredesen DE, Levy RM, Rosenblum ML: The neurology of human immunodeficiency virus infection, **Q J Med 68:**665, 1988.
33. Britt RH, Enzmann DR, Yeager AS: Neuropathological and computerized tomographic findings in experimental brain abscess, **J Neurosurg 55:**590, 1981.
34. Broadhurst LE, Erickson RL, Kelley PW: Decreases in invasive Haemophilus influenzae diseases in US Army children, 1984 through 1991, **JAMA 269:**227, 1993.
35. Broome C, Wenger J, Schuchat A, et al: Changing epidemiology of bacterial meningitis in the United States, in **Thirty-sixth Interscience Conference on Antimicrobial Agents and Chemotherapy,** American Society for Microbiology, New Orleans, 1996.
36. Brown EM: Antimicrobial prophylaxis in neurosurgery, **J Antimicrob Chemother 31(Suppl B):**49, 1993.
37. Brown R, Colodny S, Drapkin M, et al: One-day prevalence study of nosocomial infections, antibiotic usage, and selected infection control practices in adult medical/surgical intensive care units in the United States, in Fifth annual meeting of the Society for Healthcare Epidemiology: abstracts, **Infect Control Hosp Epidemiol April (suppl),** 1995.
38. Buckwold FJ, Hand R, Hansebout RR: Hospital-acquired bacterial meningitis in neurosurgical patients, **J Neurosurg 46:**494, 1977.
39. Budka H, Aguzzi A, Brown P, et al: Neuropathological diagnostic criteria for Creutzfeldt-Jakob disease (CJD) and other human spongiform encephalopathies (prion diseases), **Brain Pathol 5:**459, 1995.

40. Bullock R, Van Dellen JR, Ketelbey W, et al: A double-blind placebo-controlled trial of perioperative prophylactic antibiotics for elective neurosurgery, **J Neurosurg 69:**687, 1988.
41. Cahill DW, Love LC, Rechtine GR: Pyogenic osteomyelitis of the spine in the elderly, **J Neurosurg 74:**878, 1991.
42. Campbel S: Amebic brain abscess and meningoencephalis, **Semin Neurol 13:**153, 1993.
43. Cardenas J: Pathologic and radiologic findings, **J Neurosurgery 19:**635, 1962.
44. Carrea R, Murphy G: Primary hydatid cyst of the spinal cord, **Acta Neurol Latinoam 10:**308, 1964.
45. Caughey B: Scrapie associated PrP accumulation and its prevention: insights from cell culture, **Br Med Bull 49:**860, 1993.
46. Caughey B, Ernst D, Race RE: Congo red inhibition of scrapie agent replication, **J Virol 67:**6270, 1993.
47. Centers for Disease Control and Prevention: Reye syndrome surveillance—United States, 1989, **JAMA 265:**960, 1991.
48. Chaisson RE, Schecter GF, Theuer CP, et al: Tuberculosis in patients with the acquired immunodeficiency syndrome. Clinical features, response to therapy, and survival, **Am Rev Respir Dis 136:**570, 1987.
49. Clark RA, Greer D, Atkinson W, et al: Spectrum of cryptococcus neoformans infection in 68 patients infected with human immunodeficiency virus, **Rev Infect Dis 12:**768, 1990.
50. Clayman GL, Adams GL, Paugh DR, et al: Intracranial complications of paranasal sinusitis: a combined institutional review, **Laryngoscope 101:**234, 1991.
51. Cohen FE, Pan KM, Huang Z, et al: Structural clues to prion replication, **Science 264:**530, 1994.
52. Coleman JM, Hogg GG, Rosenfeld JV, et al: Invasive central nervous system aspergillosis: cure with liposomal amphotericin B, itraconazole, and radical surgery—case report and review of the literature, **Neurosurgery 36:**858, 1995.
53. Collins SJ, Masters CL: Transmissibility of Creutzfeldt-Jakob disease and related disorders, **Sci Prog 78:**217, 1995.
54. Corey L, Rubin RJ, Hattwick MA: Reye's syndrome: clinical progression and evaluation of therapy, **Pediatrics 60:**708, 1977.
55. Couldwell WT, Zee CS, Apuzzo ML: Definition of the role of contemporary surgical management in cisternal and parenchymatous cysticercosis cerebri, **Neurosurgery 28:**231, 1991.
56. Cuevas LE, Hart CA: Chemoprophylaxis of bacterial meningitis, **J Antimicrob Chemother 31(Suppl B):**79, 1993.
57. Cunha BA: Intravenous line infections, **Crit Care Clin 14:**339, 1998.
58. Currier B, Eismont F: Infections of the spine, in Rothman R, Simeone F, (eds): **The spine,** Philadelphia: W.B. Saunders, 1992, p 1319.
59. Dagbjartsson A, Ludvigsson P: Bacterial meningitis: diagnosis and initial antibiotic therapy, **Pediatr Clin North Am 34:**219, 1987.
60. Dagi T, George E: The management of cerebrospinal fluid leaks, in Schmidek H, Sweet W, (eds): **Operative neurosurgical techniques,** vol. 1, Philadelphia: W.B. Saunders, 1988, p 57.
61. Dajani AS, Pokowski LH: Delayed cerebrospinal fluid sterilization, in vitro bactericidal activities, and side effects of selected beta-lactams, **Scand J Infect Dis (Suppl)73:**31, 1990.
62. Dauch WA, Krex D, Heymanns J, et al: Peri-operative changes of cellular and humoral components of immunity with brain tumour surgery, **Acta Neurochir 126:**93, 1994.
63. Dean DA, Burchard KW: Fungal infection in surgical patients, **Am J Surg 171:**374, 1996.
64. Del Brutto OH: Cysticercosis and cerebrovascular disease: a review, **J Neurol Neurosurg Psychiatry 55:**252, 1992.
65. Del Brutto OH, Sotelo J: Neurocysticercosis: an update, **Rev Infect Dis 10:**1075, 1988.
66. Demir K, Karsli AF, Kaya T, et al: Cerebral hydatid cysts: CT findings, **Neuroradiology 33:**22, 1991.
67. Deslys JP, Lasmezas CI, Streichenberger N, et al: New variant Creutzfeldt-Jakob disease in France, **Lancet 349:**30, 1997.
68. Dieckhaus KD, Cooper BW: Infection control concepts in critical care, **Crit Care Clin 14:**55, 1998.
69. Dismukes WE, Cloud G, Gallis HA, et al: Treatment of cryptococcal meningitis with combination amphotericin B and flucytosine for four as compared with six weeks, **N Engl J Med 317:**334, 1987.
70. Dixon H, Lipscomb F: Cysticercosis: an analysis and follow-up of 450 cases, **Med Res Counc Spec Rep Ser 299:**1, 1961.
71. Djindjian M, Lepresle E, Homs JB: Antibiotic prophylaxis during prolonged clean neurosurgery. Results of a randomized double-blind study using oxacillin [see comments], **J Neurosurg 73:**383, 1990.
72. Doebbeling BN, Stanley GL, Sheetz CT, et al: Comparative efficacy of alternative hand-washing agents in reducing nosocomial infections in intensive care units, **N Engl J Med 327:**88, 1992.
73. Doll DC, Yarbro JW, Phillips K, et al: Mycobacterial spinal cord abscess with an ascending polyneuropathy, **Ann Intern Med 106:**333, 1987.
74. Edwards J, Jarvis W: The distribution of nosocomial infections by site and pathogen in adult and pediatric intensive care units in the United States 1986–1990, in **Third Decennial International Conference on Nosocomial Infections, Centers for Disease Control and the National Foundation for Infectious Diseases,** Atlanta, abstract B19, 1990.
75. Ehni WF, Ellison RTD: Spontaneous Candida albicans meningitis in a patient with the acquired immune deficiency syndrome, **Am J Med 83:**806, 1987.
76. Ehrenkranz NJ: Bland soap handwash or hand antisepsis? The pressing need for clarity, **Infect Control Hosp Epidemiol 13:**299, 1992.
77. Emery SE, Chan DP, Woodward HR: Treatment of hematogenous pyogenic vertebral osteomyelitis with anterior debridement and primary bone grafting, **Spine 14:**284, 1989.

78. Emori TG, Gaynes RP: An overview of nosocomial infections, including the role of the microbiology laboratory, **Clin Microbiol Rev 6:**428, 1993.
79. Epstein MF, Leviton A, Kuban KC, et al: Bilirubin, intraventricular hemorrhage, and phenobarbital in very low birth weight babies, **Pediatrics 82:**350, 1988.
80. Escobar A: The pathology of neurocysticercosis, in Palacios E, Rodriguez-Carbajal J, Taveras J, (eds): Cysticercosis of the central nervous system, Springfield, Ill: Charles C. Thomas, 1983, p 27.
81. Ferris BD, Scott JE, Uttley D: Hydatid disease of the vervical spine, **Clin Orthop 207:**174, 1986.
82. Feuerman T, Wackym PA, Gade GF, et al: Craniotomy improves outcome in subdural empyema, **Surg Neurol 32:**105, 1989.
83. Filice G, Simpson G: Management of nocardia infections, in Remington J, Swartz M, (eds): **Current clinical topics in infectious diseases,** vol. 5, New York: McGraw-Hill, 1984, p 49.
84. Finklestein SP, Caday CG, Kano M, et al: Growth factor expression after stroke, **Stroke 21:**(III)122, 1990.
85. Forsyth BW, Horwitz RI, Acampora D, et al: New epidemiologic evidence confirming that bias does not explain the aspirin/Reye's syndrome association, **JAMA 261:**2517, 1989.
86. Frame PT, McLaurin RL: Treatment of CSF shunt infections with intrashunt plus oral antibiotic therapy, **J Neurosurg 60:**354, 1984.
87. Frei K, Nadal D, Fontana A: Intracerebral synthesis of tumor necrosis factor-alpha and interleukin- 6 in infectious meningitis, **Ann N Y Acad Sci 594:**326, 1990.
88. Funaki B, Rosenblum JD: MR of central nervous system actinomycosis, **AJNR Am J Neuroradiol 16:**1179, 1995.
89. Gajdusek D: **N Engl J Med 974:** 1957.
90. Galgiani JN, Catanzaro A, Cloud GA, et al: Fluconazole therapy for coccidioidal meningitis. The NIAID-Mycoses Study Group, **Ann Intern Med 119:**28, 1993.
91. Gambetti P: Fatal familial insomnia and familial Creutzfeldt-Jakob disease: a tale of two diseases with the same genetic mutation, **Curr Top Microbiol Immunol 207:**19, 1996.
92. Garfin SR, Botte MJ, Triggs KJ, et al: Subdural abscess associated with halo-pin traction, **J Bone Joint Surg [Am] 70:**1338, 1988.
93. Garg RK, Nag D: Intramedullary spinal cysticercosis: response to albendazole: case reports and review of literature, **Spinal Cord 36:**67, 1998.
94. Garibaldi RA, Mooney BR, Epstein BJ, et al: An evaluation of daily bacteriologic monitoring to identify preventable episodes of catheter-associated urinary tract infection, **Infect Control 3:**466, 1982.
95. Garner JS: Guideline for isolation precautions in hospitals. The Hospital Infection Control Practices Advisory Committee, **Infect Control Hosp Epidemiol 17:**5, 1996.
96. Geiman BJ, Smith AL: Dexamethasone and bacterial meningitis. A meta-analysis of randomized controlled trials, **West J Med 157:**27, 1992.
97. George DL: Epidemiology of nosocomial pneumonia in intensive care unit patients, **Clin Chest Med 16:**29, 1995.
98. Geraghty J, Feely M: Antibiotic prophylaxis in neurosurgery. A randomized controlled trial, **J Neurosurg 60:**724, 1984.
99. Gilbert D, Moellering R, Sande M: **The Sanford guide to antimicrobial therapy,** Vienna, Va: Antimicrobial Therapy, 1999.
100. Giulian D, Tapscott, MJ: Immunoregulation of cells within the central nervous system, **Brain Behav Immun 2:**352, 1988.
101. Glasgow JF, Jenkins JG, Hicks EM, et al: The prognosis of Reye's syndrome in Ireland. Can it be improved? **Ir J Med Sci 155:**111, 1986.
102. Gombert ME, Landesman SH, Corrado ML, et al: Vancomycin and rifampin therapy for Staphylococcus epidermidis meningitis associated with CSF shunts: report of three cases, **J Neurosurg 55:**633, 1981.
103. Gonyea EF: The spectrum of primary blastomycotic meningitis: a review of central nervous system blastomycosis, **Ann Neurol 3:**26, 1978.
104. Goodman ML, Coffey RJ: Stereotactic drainage of Aspergillus brain abscess with long-term survival: case report and review, **Neurosurgery 24:**96, 1989.
105. Gower DJ, Crone K, Alexander E Jr., et al: Candida albicans shunt infection: report of two cases, **Neurosurgery 19:**111, 1986.
106. Grabbe E, Kerb P, Heller M: Human echinococcosis: diagnostic value of computed tomography, **Tropenmed Parasitol 32:**35, 1981.
107. Graham M: Frequency and duration of handwashing in an intensive care unit, **Am J Infect Control 18:**77, 1990.
108. Gray F, Gherardi R, Scaravilli F: The neuropathology of the acquired immune deficiency syndrome (AIDS). A review, **Brain 111:**245, 1988.
109. Griffin WS, Stanley LC, Ling C, et al: Brain interleukin 1 and S-100 immunoreactivity are elevated in Down syndrome and Alzheimer disease, **Proc Natl Acad Sci U S A 86:**7611, 1989.
110. Gross PA, Neu HC, Aswapokee P, et al: Deaths from nosocomial infections: experience in a university hospital and a community hospital, **Am J Med 68:**219, 1980.
111. Guerrero IC, Slap GB, MacGregor RR, et al: Anaerobic spinal epidural abscess. Case report, **J Neurosurg 48:**465, 1978.
112. Haemophilus influenza infections, in Peter G, (ed): **1994 Red Book: Report of the Committee on Infectious Diseases,** Elk Grove Village, Ill: American Academy of Pediatrics, 1994, p 203.
113. Hagensee ME, Bauwens JE, Kjos B, et al: Brain abscess following marrow transplantation: experience at the Fred Hutchinson Cancer Research Center, 1984–1992, **Clin Infect Dis 19:**402, 1994.
114. Haines SJ, Goodman ML: Antibiotic prophylaxis of postoperative neurosurgical wound infection, **J Neurosurg 56:**103, 1982.
115. Haines SJ, Mampalam T, Rosenblum M, et al: Cranial and intracranial bacterial infections, in Youmans J, (ed): **Neurological surgery,** Philadelphia: W.B. Saunders, 1990.
116. Haley RW, Schaberg DR, Von Allmen SD, et al: Estimating the extra charges and prolongation of hospitaliza-

tion due to nosocomial infections: a comparison of methods, **J Infect Dis 141:**248, 1980.
117. Hall SM: Reye's syndrome and aspirin: a review, **Br J Clin Pract Suppl 70,** 1990.
118. Halpin TJ, Holtzhauer FJ, Campbell RJ, et al: Reye's syndrome and medication use, **JAMA 248:**687, 1982.
119. Harrington MG, Merril CR, Asher DM, et al: Abnormal proteins in the cerebrospinal fluid of patients with Creutzfeldt-Jakob disease, **N Engl J Med 315:**279, 1986.
120. Harrison M, McArthur J: HIV-associated dementia complex, in Harrison M, McArthur J, (eds): **AIDS and neurology,** New York: Churchill Livingstone, 1995.
121. Hickman KM, Mayer BL, Muwaswes M: Intracranial pressure monitoring: review of risk factors associated with infection, **Heart Lung 19:**84, 1990.
122. Hillhouse EW, Mosley K: Peripheral endotoxin induces hypothalamic immunoreactive interleukin-1 beta in the rat, **Br J Pharmacol 109:**289, 1993.
123. Hlavin ML, Kaminski HJ, Fenstermaker RA, et al: Intracranial suppuration: a modern decade of postoperative subdural empyema and epidural abscess, **Neurosurgery 34:**974, 1994.
124. Hollander H, Stringari S: Human immunodeficiency virus-associated meningitis. Clinical course and correlations, **Am J Med 83:**813, 1987.
125. Holloway KL, Smith KW, Wilberger JE Jr., et al: Antibiotic prophylaxis during clean neurosurgery: a large, multicenter study using cefuroxime, **Clin Ther 18:**84, 1996.
126. Holman RC, Khan AS, Kent J, et al: Epidemiology of Creutzfeldt-Jakob disease in the United States, 1979–1990: analysis of national mortality data, **Neuroepidemiology 14:**174, 1995.
127. Holmes SJ, Ironside JW, Shalet SM: Neurosurgery in a patient with Creutzfeldt-Jakob disease after pituitary derived growth hormone therapy in childhood, **J Neurol Neurosurg Psychiatry 60:**333, 1996.
128. Hooper DC, Pruitt AA, Rubin RH: Central nervous system infection in the chronically immunosuppressed, **Medicine 61:**166, 1982.
129. Hopkins, SJ, Rothwell N J: Cytokines and the nervous system. I: Expression and recognition, **Trends Neurosci 18:**83, 1995.
130. Hsieh G, Kenney K, Gibbs CJ, et al: The 14-3-3 brain protein in cerebrospinal fluid as a marker for transmissible spongiform encephalopathies, **N Engl J Med 335:**924, 1996.
131. Hurwitz ES, Barrett MJ, Bregman D, et al: Public Health Service study of Reye's syndrome and medications. Report of the main study, **JAMA 257:**1905, 1987.
132. Ilgren EB, Westmorland D, Adams CB, et al: Cerebellar mass caused by candida species. Case report, **J Neurosurg 60:**428, 1984.
133. Ironside JW: Prion diseases in man, **J Pathol 186:**227, 1998.
134. Jannert M, Andreasson L, Holmer NG, et al: Ultrasonic examination of the paranasal sinuses, **Acta Otolaryngol Suppl 389:**1, 1982.
135. Janssen RS, Nwanyanwu OC, Selik RM, et al: Epidemiology of human immunodeficiency virus encephalopathy in the United States, **Neurology 42:**1472, 1992.
136. Jarvis WR, Edwards JR, Culver DH, et al: Nosocomial infection rates in adult and pediatric intensive care units in the United States. National Nosocomial Infections Surveillance System, **Am J Med 91:**185S, 1991.
137. Johns DR, Tierney M, Felsenstein D: Alteration in the natural history of neurosyphilis by concurrent infection with the human immunodeficiency virus, **N Engl J Med 316:**1569, 1987.
138. Johnston SR, Corbett EL, Foster O, et al: Raised intracranial pressure and visual complications in AIDS patients with cryptococcal meningitis, **J Infect 24:**185, 1992.
139. Jorissen M: Recent trends in the diagnosis and treatment of sinusitis, **Eur Radiol 6:**170, 1996.
140. Kammerer WS: Echinococcosis affecting the central nervous system, **Semin Neurol 13:**144, 1993.
141. Kaufman DM, Kaplan JG, Litman N: Infectious agents in spinal epidural abscesses, **Neurology 30:**844, 1980.
142. Khalili AH: Nocardial brain abscess: a case report, **J Neurol 227:**115, 1982.
143. Kilpatrick-Smith L, Hale DE, Douglas SD: Progress in Reye syndrome: epidemiology, biochemical mechanisms and animal models, **Dig Dis 7:**135, 1989.
144. Kindt GW, Waldman J, Kohl S, et al: Intracranial pressure in Reye syndrome. Monitoring and control, **JAMA 231:**822, 1975.
145. Klastersky J, Sadeghi M, Brihaye J: Antimicrobial prophylaxis in patients with rhinorrhea or otorrhea: a double-blind study, **Surg Neurol 6:**111, 1976.
146. Korczyn AD: Prion diseases, **Curr Opin Neurol 10:**273, 1997.
147. Kountakis SE, Kemper JV Jr., Chang CY, et al: Osteomyelitis of the base of the skull secondary to Aspergillus, **Am J Otolaryngol 18:**19, 1997.
148. Kovacs JA, Kovacs AA, Polis M, et al: Cryptococcosis in the acquired immunodeficiency syndrome, **Ann Intern Med 103:**533, 1985.
149. Krupp LB, Lipton RB, Swerdlow ML, et al: Progressive multifocal leukoencephalopathy: clinical and radiographic features, **Ann Neurol 17:**344, 1985.
150. Kurino M, Kuratsu J, Yamaguchi T, et al: Mycotic aneurysm accompanied by aspergillotic granuloma: a case report, **Surg Neurol 42:**160, 1994.
151. Lanska MJ, Lanska DJ, Schmidley JW: Syphilitic polyradiculopathy in an HIV-positive man, **Neurology 38:**1297, 1988.
152. Laranne JE, Penttila MA, Paakkala TA, et al: Diagnostic value of plain radiographs in chronic maxillary sinusitis: a comparison between radiological and endoscopic findings in 75 patients, **Rhinology 30:**205, 1992.
153. Larson EL: APIC guideline for handwashing and hand antisepsis in health care settings, **Am J Infect Control 23:**251, 1995.
154. Larson EL, McGeer A, Quraishi ZA, et al: Effect of an automated sink on handwashing practices and attitudes in high-risk units, **Infect Control Hosp Epidemiol 12:**422, 1991.
155. Lebel MH, Hoyt MJ, McCracken GH Jr.: Comparative efficacy of ceftriaxone and cefuroxime for treatment of bacterial meningitis, **J Pediatr 114:**1049, 1989.

156. Leech PJ, Paterson A: Conservative and operative management for cerebrospinal-fluid leakage after closed head injury, **Lancet 1:**1013, 1973.
157. Levy ML, Wieder BH, Schneider J, et al: Subdural empyema of the cervical spine: clinicopathological correlates and magnetic resonance imaging. Report of three cases, **J Neurosurg 79:**929, 1993.
158. Levy R, Janssen R, Bush T: Neuroepidemiology of AIDS, in Rosenblum M, Levy R, Bredesen D, (eds): **AIDS and the nervous system,** New York: Raven Press, 1988, p 13.
159. Levy RM, Berger JR: Neurosurgical aspects of human immunodeficiency virus infection, **Neurosurg Clin N Am 3:**443, 1992.
160. Levy RM, Bredesen DE, Rosenblum ML: Neurological manifestations of the acquired immunodeficiency syndrome (AIDS): experience at UCSF and review of the literature, **J Neurosurg 62:**475, 1985.
161. Lewin, W: **Br J Surg 42:**1, 1954.
162. Lipton SA, Hickey WF, Morris JH, et al: Candidal infection in the central nervous system, **Am J Med 76:**101, 1984.
163. Logan A, Berry M: Transforming growth factor-beta 1 and basic fibroblast growth factor in the injured CNS, **Trends Pharmacol Sci 14:**337, 1993.
164. Lovejoy FH Jr., Smith AL, Bresnan MJ, et al: Clinical staging in Reye syndrome, **Am J Dis Child 128:**36, 1974.
165. MacGee EE, Cauthen JC, Brackett CE: Meningitis following acute traumatic cerebrospinal fluid fistula, **J Neurosurg 33:**312, 1970.
166. Maher JJ: Cytokines: overview, **Semin Liver Dis 19:**109, 1999.
167. Maki, D: in Bennett J, Brachman P, (eds): Hospital infections, Boston: Little, Brown, 1992, p 849.
168. Mamelak AN, Obana WG, Flaherty JF, et al: Nocardial brain abscess: treatment strategies and factors influencing outcome, **Neurosurgery 35:**622, 1994.
169. Mampalam TJ, Rosenblum ML: Trends in the management of bacterial brain abscesses: a review of 102 cases over 17 years, **Neurosurgery 23:**451, 1988.
170. Marciano-Cabral F: Biology of naegleria spp, **Microbiol Rev 52:**114, 1988.
171. Marshall DW, Brey RL, Cahill WT, et al: Spectrum of cerebrospinal fluid findings in various stages of human immunodeficiency virus infection, **Arch Neurol 45:**954, 1988.
172. Mathiesen T, Grane P, Lindgren L, et al: Third ventricle colloid cysts: a consecutive 12-year series, **J Neurosurg 86:**5, 1997.
173. Mathisen GE, Johnson JP: Brain abscess, **Clin Infect Dis 25:**763, 1997.
174. Mauser HW, Van Houwelingen HC, Tulleken CA: Factors affecting the outcome in subdural empyema, **J Neurol Neurosurg Psychiatry 50:**1136, 1987.
175. Mayer JA, Dubbert PM, Miller M, et al: Increasing handwashing in an intensive care unit, **Infect Control 7:**259, 1986.
176. McArthur JC: Neurologic manifestations of AIDS, **Medicine 66:**407, 1987.
177. McArthur JC, Hoover DR, Bacellar H, et al: Dementia in AIDS patients: incidence and risk factors. Multicenter AIDS Cohort Study, **Neurology 43:**2245, 1993.
178. McCracken GH Jr.: Current management of bacterial meningitis, **Pediatr Infect Dis J 8:**919, 1989.
179. McRitchie DI, Matthews JG, Fink, MP: Pneumonia in patients with multiple trauma, **Clin Chest Med 16:**135, 1995.
180. Meduri GU: Diagnosis and differential diagnosis of ventilator-associated pneumonia, **Clin Chest Med 16:**61, 1995.
181. Merrill JE, Chen IS: HIV-1, macrophages, glial cells, and cytokines in AIDS nervous system disease, **Faseb J 5:**2391, 1991.
182. Merrill JE, Kono DH, Clayton J, et al: Inflammatory leukocytes and cytokines in the peptide-induced disease of experimental allergic encephalomyelitis in SJL and B10.PL mice, **Proc Natl Acad Sci U S A 89:**574, 1992.
183. Miller JR, Barrett RE, Britton CB, et al: Progressive multifocal leukoencephalopathy in a male homosexual with T-cell immune deficiency, **N Engl J Med 307:**1436, 1982.
184. Minami M, Kuraishi Y, Yabuuchi K, et al: Induction of interleukin-1 beta mRNA in rat brain after transient forebrain ischemia, **J Neurochem 58:**390, 1992.
185. Minami M, Kuraishi Y, Yamaguchi T, et al: Immobilization stress induces interleukin-1 beta mRNA in the rat hypothalamus, **Neurosci Lett 123:**254, 1991.
186. Mischel PS, Vinters HV: Coccidioidomycosis of the central nervous system: neuropathological and vasculopathic manifestations and clinical correlates, **Clin Infect Dis 20:**400, 1995.
187. Mombelli G, Klastersky J, Coppens L, et al: Gram-negative bacillary meningitis in neurosurgical patients, **J Neurosurg 59:**634, 1983.
188. Morawetz RB, Whitley RJ, Murphy DM: Experience with brain biopsy for suspected herpes encephalitis: a review of forty consecutive cases, **Neurosurgery 12:**654, 1983.
189. Morgan H, Wood MW, Murphey F: Experience with 88 consecutive cases of brain abscess, **J Neurosurg 38:**698, 1973.
190. Morganti-Kossmann MC, Kossmann T, Wahl SM: Cytokines and neuropathology,**Trends Pharmacol Sci 13:**286, 1992.
191. Moskowitz LB, Hensley GT, Chan JC, et al: The neuropathology of acquired immune deficiency syndrome, **Arch Pathol Lab Med 108:**867, 1984.
192. Nath A, Geiger J: Neurobiological aspects of human immunodeficiency virus infection: neurotoxic mechanisms, **Prog Neurobiol 54:**19, 1998.
193. Navia BA, Petito CK, Gold JW, et al: Cerebral toxoplasmosis complicating the acquired immune deficiency syndrome: clinical and neuropathological findings in 27 patients, **Ann Neurol 19:**224, 1986.
194. Neils EW, Lukin R, Tomsick TA, et al: Magnetic resonance imaging and computerized tomography scanning of herpes simplex encephalitis. Report of two cases, **J Neurosurg 67:**592, 1987.

195. Nielsen H, Gyldensted C, Harmsen A: Cerebral abscess. Aetiology and pathogenesis, symptoms, diagnosis and treatment. A review of 200 cases from 1935–1976, **Acta Neurol Scand 65:**609, 1982.
196. Nielsen SL, Petito CK, Urmacher CD, et al: Subacute encephalitis in acquired immune deficiency syndrome: a postmortem study, **Am J Clin Pathol 82:**678, 1984.
197. Nieto D: Cysticercosis of the nervous system. Diagnosis by means of the spinal fluid complement fixation test, **Neurology 6:**725, 1956.
198. Nurchi G, Floris F, Montaldo C, et al: Multiple cerebral hydatid disease: case report with magnetic resonance imaging study, **Neurosurgery 30:**436, 1992.
199. Obana WG, Rosenblum ML: Nonoperative treatment of neurosurgical infections, **Neurosurg Clin N Am 3:**359, 1992.
200. Ogawa T, Inugami A, Fujita H, et al: Serial positron emission tomography with fludeoxyglucose F 18 in Creutzfeldt-Jakob disease, **AJNR Am J Neuroradiol 16:**978, 1995.
201. Osenbach RK, Loftus CM: Diagnosis and management of brain abscess, **Neurosurg Clin N Am 3:**403, 1992.
202. Osuka K, Suzuki Y, Saito K, et al: Changes in serum cytokine concentrations after neurosurgical procedures, **Acta Neurochir 138:**970, 1996.
203. Ozuna RM, Delamarter RB: Pyogenic vertebral osteomyelitis and postsurgical disc space infections, **Orthop Clin North Am 27:**87, 1996.
204. Paradisi F, Corti G, Mangani V: Urosepsis in the critical care unit, **Crit Care Clin 14:**165, 1998.
205. Paramore CG, Turner DA: Relative risks of ventriculostomy infection and morbidity, **Acta Neurochir 127:**79, 1994.
206. Patterson TF, Andriole VT: Current concepts in cryptococcosis, **Eur J Clin Microbiol Infect Dis 8:**457, 1989.
207. Perfect J: Diagnosis and treatment of fungal meningitis, in Scheld W, Whitley R, Durack D, (eds): **Infections of the central nervous system,** New York: Raven Press, 1991, p 729.
208. Prasad K, Haines T: Dexamethasone treatment for acute bacterial meningitis: how strong is the evidence for routine use? **J Neurol Neurosurg Psychiatry 59:**31, 1995.
209. Prusiner SB: Biology and genetics of prion diseases, **Annu Rev Microbiol 48:**655, 1994.
210. Prusiner SB: Transgenetics of prion diseases, **Curr Top Microbiol Immunol 206:**275, 1996.
211. Quagliarello VJ, Scheld WM: Treatment of bacterial meningitis, **N Engl J Med 336:**708, 1997.
212. Raad I, Davis S, Becker M, et al: Low infection rate and long durability of nontunneled silastic catheters. A safe and cost-effective alternative for long-term venous access [see comments], **Arch Intern Med 153:**1791, 1993.
213. Recommendations for preventing the spread of vancomycin resistance. Hospital Infection Control Practices Advisory Committee (HICPAC), **Infect Control Hosp Epidemiol 16:**105, 1995.
214. Rello J, Ausina V, Castella J, et al: Nosocomial respiratory tract infections in multiple trauma patients. Influence of level of consciousness with implications for therapy, **Chest 102:**525, 1992.
215. Renier D, Flandin C, Hirsch E, et al: Brain abscesses in neonates. A study of 30 cases, **J Neurosurg, 69:**877, 1988.
216. Renier D, Lacombe J, Pierre-Kahn A, et al: Factors causing acute shunt infection. Computer analysis of 1174 operations, **J Neurosurg 61:**1072, 1984.
217. Reusser P, Zimmerli W, Scheidegger D, et al: Role of gastric colonization in nosocomial infections and endotoxemia: a prospective study in neurosurgical patients on mechanical ventilation, **J Infect Dis 160:**414, 1989.
218. Rimoldi RL, Haye W: The use of antibiotics for wound prophylaxis in spinal surgery, **Orthop Clin North Am 27:**47, 1996.
219. Rish BL, Caveness WF, Dillon JD, et al: Analysis of brain abscess after penetrating craniocerebral injuries in Vietnam, **Neurosurgery 9:**535, 1981.
220. Rodriguez-Carbajal J, Del Brutto OH, Penagos P, et al: Occlusion of the middle cerebral artery due to cysticercotic angiitis, **Stroke 20:**1095, 1989.
221. Roos K: Meningitis as it presents in the elderly: Diagnosis and care, **Geriatrics 45:**63, 1990.
222. Rosenblum ML, Hoff JT, Norman D, et al: Decreased mortality from brain abscesses since advent of computerized tomography, **J Neurosurg 49:**658, 1978.
223. Rosenblum ML, Hoff JT, Norman D, et al: Nonoperative treatment of brain abscesses in selected high-risk patients, **J Neurosurg 52:**217, 1980.
224. Roullet E: Opportunistic infections of the central nervous system during HIV-1 infection (emphasis on cytomegalovirus disease), **J Neurol 246:**237, 1999.
225. Sabetta JR, Andriole VT: Cryptococcal infection of the central nervous system, **Med Clin North Am 69:**333, 1985.
226. Salaki JS, Louria DB, Chmel H: Fungal and yeast infections of the central nervous system. A clinical review, **Medicine 63:**108, 1984.
227. Samson DS, Clark K: A current review of brain abscess, **Am J Med 54:**201, 1973.
228. Sanderson PJ: The sources of pneumonia in ITU patients, **Infect Control 7:**104, 1986.
229. Savitz MH, Katz SS: Rationale for prophylactic antibiotics and neurosurgery, **Neurosurgery 9:**142, 1981.
230. Savitz SI, Savitz MH, Goldstein HB, et al: Topical irrigation with polymyxin and bacitracin for spinal surgery, **Surg Neurol 50:**208, 1998.
231. Scheckelhoff DJ, Mirtallo JM, Ayers LW, et al: Growth of bacteria and fungi in total nutrient admixtures, **Am J Hosp Pharm 43:**73, 1986.
232. Schermoly MJ, Hinthorn DR: Eosinophilia in coccidioidomycosis, **Arch Intern Med 148:**895, 1988.
233. Schmidt S, Reiter-Owona I, Hotz M, et al: An unusual case of central nervous system cryptococcosis, **Clin Neurol Neurosurg 97:**23, 1995.
234. Schoendorf KC, Adams WG, Kiely JL, et al: National trends in Haemophilus influenzae meningitis mortality and hospitalization among children, 1980 through 1991, **Pediatrics 93:**663, 1994.
235. Segreti J, Harris AA: Acute bacterial meningitis, **Infect Dis Clin North Am 10:**797, 1996.

236. Shapiro M, Wald U, Simchen E, et al: Randomized clinical trial of intra-operative antimicrobial prophylaxis of infection after neurosurgical procedures, **J Hosp Infect 8:**283, 1986.
237. Shelton M, Marks W: Bacterial meningitis: an update, **Neurol Clin 8:**605, 1990.
238. Shyu WC, Lee CC, Hsu YD, et al: Panencephalitic Creutzfeldt-Jakob disease. Unusual presentation of magnetic resonance imaging and proton magnetic resonance spectroscopy, **J Neurol Sci 138:**157, 1996.
239. Simpson GL, Stinson EB, Egger MJ, et al: Nocardial infections in the immunocompromised host: A detailed study in a defined population, **Rev Infect Dis 3:**492, 1981.
240. Singh B, Van Dellen J, Ramjettan S, et al: Sinogenic intracranial complications, **J Laryngol Otol 109:**945, 1995.
241. Slaughter S, Hayden MK, Nathan C, et al: A comparison of the effect of universal use of gloves and gowns with that of glove use alone on acquisition of vancomycin-resistant enterococci in a medical intensive care unit, **Ann Intern Med 125:**448, 1996.
242. Slavoski LA, Tunkel AR: Therapy of fungal meningitis, **Clin Neuropharmacol 18:**95, 1995.
243. Smego RA Jr.: Actinomycosis of the central nervous system, **Rev Infect Dis 9:**855, 1987.
244. Snider WD, Simpson DM, Nielsen S, et al: Neurological complications of acquired immune deficiency syndrome: analysis of 50 patients, **Ann Neurol 14:**403, 1983.
245. Sotelo J: Treatment of brain cysticercosis, **Surg Neurol 48:**110, 1997.
246. Sotelo J, Guerrero V, Rubio F: Neurocysticercosis: a new classification based on active and inactive forms. A study of 753 cases, **Arch Intern Med 145:**442, 1985.
247. Spetzler R, Zabramski J: Cerebrospinal fluid fistulae:their management and repair, in Youmans J, (ed): **Youmans neurological surgery,** vol. 4, Philadelphia: W.B. Saunders, 1990, p 2269.
248. Stahel PF, Kossmann T, Joller H, et al: Increased interleukin-12 levels in human cerebrospinal fluid following severe head trauma, **Neurosci Lett 249:**123, 1998.
249. Starko KM, Ray CG, Dominguez LB, et al: Reye's syndrome and salicylate use, **Pediatrics 66:**859, 1980.
250. Stephanov, S: Surgical treatment of brain abscess, **Neurosurgery 22:**724, 1988.
251. Stephanov S, Joubert MJ: Large brain abscesses treated by aspiration alone, **Surg Neurol 17:**338, 1982.
252. Stern WE: Neurosurgical considerations of cysticercosis of the central nervous system, **J Neurosurg 55:**382, 1981.
253. Stevens D: Coccidiodes immitis, in Mandell G, Bennett J, Dolin R, (eds): Principles and practice of infectious diseases, New York: Churchill Livingstone, 1994, p 2365.
254. Stoutenbeek CP, Van Saene HK: Nonantibiotic measures in the prevention of ventilator-associated pneumonia, **Semin Respir Infect 12:**294, 1997.
255. Strauss S, Bauer J, Ganter U, et al: Detection of interleukin-6 and alpha 2-macroglobulin immunoreactivity in cortex and hippocampus of Alzheimer's disease patients, **Lab Invest 66:**223, 1992.
256. Suzuki M, Endo S, Inada K, et al: Inflammatory cytokines locally elevated in chronic subdural haematoma, **Acta Neurochir 140:**51, 1998.
257. Swartz MN: Hospital-acquired infections: diseases with increasingly limited therapies, **Proc Natl Acad Sci U S A 91:**2420, 1994.
258. Tang YW, Mitchell PS, Espy MJ, et al: Molecular diagnosis of herpes simplex virus infections in the central nervous system, **J Clin Microbiol 37:**2127, 1999.
259. Taupin V, Toulmond S, Serrano A, et al: Increase in IL-6, IL-1 and TNF levels in rat brain following traumatic lesion. Influence of pre- and post-traumatic treatment with Ro5 4864, a peripheral-type (p site) benzodiazepine ligand, **J Neuroimmunol 42:**177, 1993.
260. Teitelbaum GP, Otto RJ, Lin M, et al: MR imaging of neurocysticercosis, **AJR Am J Roentgenol 153:**857, 1989.
261. Tenney JH, Vlahov D, Salcman M, et al: Wide variation in risk of wound infection following clean neurosurgery. Implications for perioperative antibiotic prophylaxis, **J Neurosurg 62:**243, 1985.
262. Thomas JN, Nel JR: Acute spreading osteomyelitis of the skull complicating frontal sinusitis, **J Laryngol Otol 91:**55, 1977.
263. Torrealba G, Del Villar S, Tagle P, et al: Cysticercosis of the central nervous system: clinical and therapeutic considerations, **J Neurol Neurosurg Psychiatry 47:**784, 1984.
264. Townsend GC, Scheld WM: Infections of the central nervous system, **Adv Intern Med 43:**403, 1998.
265. Townsend GC, Scheld WM: The use of corticosteroids in the management of bacterial meningitis in adults, **J Antimicrob Chemother 37:**1051, 1996.
266. Treseler CB, Sugar AM: Fungal meningitis, **Infect Dis Clin North Am 4:**789, 1990.
267. Tucker RM, Denning DW, Dupont B, et al: Itraconazole therapy for chronic coccidioidal meningitis, **Ann Intern Med 112:**108, 1990.
268. Tunkel AR, Scheld WM: Acute bacterial meningitis, **Lancet 346:**1675, 1995.
269. Tunkel AR, Wispelwey B, Scheld W: Bacterial meningitis: Recent advances in pathophysiology and treatment, **Ann Intern Med 112:**610, 1990.
270. Van Asten JA, Geertsma RE, Dorpema JW: Prions and hospital infections, **Lancet 347:**966, 1996.
271. van Dam AM, Brouns M, Louisse S, et al: Appearance of interleukin-1 in macrophages and in ramified microglia in the brain of endotoxin-treated rats: a pathway for the induction of non-specific symptoms of sickness? **Brain Res 588:** 291, 1992.
272. Van Ek B, Dijkmans BA, Van Dulken H, et al: Antibiotic prophylaxis in craniotomy: a prospective double-blind placebo-controlled study, **Scand J Infect Dis 20:**633, 1988.
273. Vazquez V, Sotelo J: The course of seizures after treatment for verebral cysticercosis, **N Engl J Med 327:**696, 1992.
274. Venes JL, Shaywitz BA, Spencer DD: Management of severe cerebral edema in the metabolic encephalopathy of Reye-Johnson syndrome, **J Neurosurg 48:**903, 1978.
275. Verner EF, Musher DM: Spinal epidural abscess, **Med Clin North Am 69:**375, 1985.

276. Visvesvara GS, Stehr-Green JK: Epidemiology of free-living ameba infections, **J Protozool 37:**25S, 1990.
277. Waldman RJ, Hall WN, McGee H, et al: Aspirin as a risk factor in Reye's syndrome, **JAMA 247:**3089, 1982.
278. Walsh TJ, Hier DB, Caplan LR: Fungal infections of the central nervous system: comparative analysis of risk factors and clinical signs in 57 patients, **Neurology 35:**1654, 1985.
279. Walters BC, Hoffman HJ, Hendrick EB, et al: Cerebrospinal fluid shunt infection. Influences on initial management and subsequent outcome, **J Neurosurg 60:**1014, 1984.
280. Wanke C, Tuazon CU, Kovacs A, et al: Toxoplasma encephalitis in patients with acquired immune deficiency syndrome: diagnosis and response to therapy, **Am J Trop Med Hyg 36:**509, 1987.
281. Weinstein RA: Epidemiology and control of nosocomial infections in adult intensive care units, **Am J Med 91:**179S, 1991.
282. Westergren V, Lundblad L, Hellquist HB, et al: Ventilator-associated sinusitis: a review, **Clin Infect Dis 27:**851, 1998.
283. Wheat LJ, Batteiger BE, Sathapatayavongs B: Histoplasma capsulatum infections of the central nervous system. A clinical review, **Medicine 69:**244, 1990.
284. Wheat LJ, Connolly-Stringfield P, Kohler RB, et al: Histoplasma capsulatum polysaccharide antigen detection in diagnosis and management of disseminated histoplasmosis in patients with acquired immunodeficiency syndrome, **Am J Med 87:**396, 1989.
285. Wheat LJ, Kohler RB, Tewari RP: Diagnosis of disseminated histoplasmosis by detection of Histoplasma capsulatum antigen in serum and urine specimens, **N Engl J Med 314:**83, 1986.
286. Wheat LJ, Kohler RB, Tewari RP, et al: Significance of Histoplasma antigen in the cerebrospinal fluid of patients with meningitis, **Arch Intern Med 149:**302, 1989.
287. Wheat LJ, Slama TG, Zeckel ML: Histoplasmosis in the acquired immune deficiency syndrome, **Am J Med 78:**203, 1985.
288. Whelan MA, Hilal SK: Computed tomography as a guide in the diagnosis and follow-up of brain abscesses, **Radiology 135:**663, 1980.
289. Whitley RJ, Alford CA, Hirsch MS, et al: Vidarabine versus acyclovir therapy in herpes simplex encephalitis, **N Engl J Med 314:**144, 1986.
290. Whitley RJ, Cobbs CG, Alford CA Jr., et al: Diseases that mimic herpes simplex encephalitis. Diagnosis, presentation, and outcome. NIAD Collaborative Antiviral Study Group, **JAMA 262:**234, 1989.
291. Will RG, Alperovitch A, Poser S, et al: Descriptive epidemiology of Creutzfeldt-Jakob disease in six European countries, 1993–1995. EU Collaborative Study Group for CJD, **Ann Neurol 43:**763, 1998.
292. Will RG, Ironside JW, Zeidler M, et al: A new variant of Creutzfeldt-Jakob disease in the UK, **Lancet 347:**921, 1996.
293. Winfield JA, Rosenthal P, Kanter, RK, et al: Duration of intracranial pressure monitoring does not predict daily risk of infectious complications, **Neurosurgery 33:**424, 1993.
294. Wispelwey B, Scheld WM: Brain abscess, **Semin Neurol 12:**273, 1992.
295. Woiciechowsky C, Asadullah K, Nestler D, et al: Different release of cytokines into the cerebrospinal fluid following surgery for intra- and extra-axial brain tumours, **Acta Neurochir 139:**619, 1997.
296. Woiciechowsky C, Schoning B, Daberkow N, et al: Brain-IL-1beta induces local inflammation but systemic anti-inflammatory response through stimulation of both hypothalamic- pituitary-adrenal axis and sympathetic nervous system, **Brain Res 816:**563, 1999.
297. Woodroofe MN, Sarna GS, Wadhwa M, et al: Detection of interleukin-1 and interleukin-6 in adult rat brain, following mechanical injury, by in vivo microdialysis: evidence of a role for microglia in cytokine production, **J Neuroimmunol 33:**227, 1991.
298. Word BM, Klein JO: Therapy of bacterial sepsis and meningitis in infants and children: 1989 poll of directors of programs in pediatric infectious diseases, **Pediatr Infect Dis J 8:**635, 1989.
299. Yang SY: Brain abscess: a review of 400 cases, **J Neurosurg 55:**794, 1981.
300. Yogev R, Davis AT: Neurosurgical shunt infections. A review, **Childs Brain 6:**74, 1980.
301. Young RF, Gade G, Grinnell V: Surgical treatment for fungal infections in the central nervous system, **J Neurosurg 63:**371, 1985.
302. Young RF, Lawner PM: Perioperative antibiotic prophylaxis for prevention of postoperative neurosurgical infections. A randomized clinical trial, **J Neurosurg 66:**701, 1987.
303. Younger JJ, Simmons JC, Barrett FF: Operative related infection rates for ventriculoperitoneal shunt procedures in a children's hospital, **Infect Control 8:**67, 1987.
304. Yurkowski PJ, Plaisance KI: Prevention of auditory sequelae in pediatric bacterial meningitis: a meta-analysis, **Pharmacotherapy 13:**494, 1993.
305. Zee CS, Segall HD, Miller C, et al: Unusual neuroradiological features of intracranial cysticercosis, **Radiology 137:**397, 1980.
306. Zuger A, Louie E, Holzman RS, et al: Cryptococcal disease in patients with the acquired immunodeficiency syndrome. Diagnostic features and outcome of treatment, **Ann Intern Med 104:**234, 1986.

CHAPTER 9

Head Injury Management

Brian T. Andrews

INTRODUCTION

Head injury is a major public health problem in the United States, accounting for more than a third of all deaths caused by trauma and an estimated 70,00 to 90,000 patients per year with long-term disability.[22] The recent era of head injury management has seen a remarkable decrease in the mortality rate from severe head injuries, to as low as 20% to 30% in modern series.* This is probably not because of advances in surgical technology, but rather improved pre-hospital care, diagnosis, use of computed tomography (CT),[56] and, of particular importance, advances in the intensive care of such patients. Monitoring of intracranial pressure,[56,57,60,62] perfusion pressure,[67,69,70] and reversal or prevention of the detrimental effects of hypoxia, hypotension, and hypoperfusion of the brain have been essential to the improvements seen over time. In addition, recent novel treatment methods, such as therapeutic hypothermia,[11,47,48,75,76] and resurgence of older techniques, such as early decompressive craniectomy[23,87] may be adding to the improvement in mortality and quality of outcome in those many patients that do survive a serious head injury.

MILD, MODERATE AND SEVERE HEAD INJURY

Head injuries are most commonly categorized by the level of consciousness as determined with the Glasgow Coma Scale (GCS)[80] (see Chapter 3). It is useful to categorize head injuries as mild, moderate, and severe, because this generally defines the level of treatment applied to the patient.[1] Patients with mild head injury, constituting the vast majority of the head injured population, have a relatively normal level of consciousness following the insult (GCS of 13–15); at worst they are slightly lethargic and confused, but able to communicate and follow commands.

A moderate head injury is present when patients have a more severely altered level of consciousness, but are not in coma (GCS of 9–12). Such patients are usually quite lethargic or obtunded but arousable to vocal and noxious stimulation. Such patients must be carefully evaluated not only for head injury but also for complications such as drug intoxication, hypoxia or hypercarbia, and metabolic abnormalities. These patients have a more severe structural brain injury (defined in the following text), and are at greater risk for delayed deterioration caused by complications such as the development of an intracranial hematoma or cerebral swelling and for secondary insults such as hypoxia, hypercarbia, hypotension, and acidosis.

Severe head injury is defined as having occurred in patients rendered comatose by the trauma (GCS of 8 or less). Such patients do not open their eyes, have no intelligible speech, and do not follow commands. They may be able to localize painful stimuli, but with decreasing GCS they may have only complex flexion, flexor posturing, extensor posturing, or complete flaccidity to noxious stimulation. Not infrequently with severe brain injury there may be a life-threatening structural brain injury, as well as important secondary injury mechanisms such as hypoxia, hypercarbia, and acidosis that must be reversed with ICU care.[1] Injury to other organ systems must also be quickly recognized and treated.

BRAIN INJURY MECHANISMS

Trauma to the head may initiate a variety of injury mechanisms. An abrupt change in angular momentum often causes an immediate diffuse brain injury as the outer cortex rotates, injuring neurons and shearing ax-

*References 11, 47, 48, 70, 75-77

ons as they enter the underlying white matter.[24,28] Such diffuse axonal injury may also occur between the white matter and deeper subcortical structures, such as the basal ganglia and thalamus, and within the upper brainstem as the entire cerebrum rotates on this axis. If extremely mild, this shearing force may result in nothing more than transient loss of consciousness; if more severe, it may cause more extensive cellular and axonal injury and more profound and persistent neurological deficits.

Recently, additional damage to axons has been identified, termed *delayed axotomy,* that may continue for up to 24 hours after the time of injury.[24] The precise mechanism for this delayed axonal damage is not clear; it has been postulated that calcium-activated proteases, termed *calpains,* may play a crucial role.[37] Axonal damage may also have important effects on altering the brain's responsiveness to subsequent secondary ischemic damage.[79] Future treatment will be directed at ways to limit secondary axotomy.

Direct impact against the adjacent irregular calvaria may result in cerebral contusions, particularly at the frontal, temporal, and occipital lobes; occasionally there is injury at the impact site (coup) and at the opposite pole of the brain (contrecoup).[28] Depressed skull fractures or penetrating injury is also associated with cerebral lacerations. Mechanical impact leads to neuronal depolarization, and cellular energy failure followed by ion flux, including a marked rise in extracellular calcium, and the abnormal release of neurotransmitters, including the excitatory amino acids glutamate and aspartate.[51,79] A variety of additional biochemical and neurochemical changes then occur, resulting in lipolysis, proteolysis, the breakdown of cellular membranes, cytoskeletal disruption and phosphorylation.[51,79]

The initial impact of the injury is largely on neurons and their functional interconnections, but there are also important influences on glia and the cerebral vasculature.[79] It has become clear that such primary brain trauma is intrinsically linked to additional delayed events, such as cellular apoptosis, secondary axotomy, and wallerian degeneration, as well as vascular events, such as global and regional cellular ischemia.[29,36,79] The interaction between traumatic and ischemic mechanisms occurs very early in the process of damage.

Hypoxia and cerebral ischemia commonly occur in association with severe head injury, but may occur with moderate or mild injury accompanied by additional systemic insults, such as cardiopulmonary dysfunction or multiple injury.[29] Recent investigations have shown that there may be global cerebral ischemia, generally occurring very early after injury,[5] particularly before the evacuation of a significant mass lesion. Transient diffuse ischemia may be documented when brain oxygenation is measured continuously, and has been shown to occur in almost every severely head-injured patient regardless of the quality of intensive care.[79]

Sustained focal ischemia may occur underlying a subdural hematoma both prior to and following evacuation,[73] and in zones that surround cerebral contusions and intracerebral hematomas.[72,73] Conventional CT may not show this zone, which may represent cytotoxic edema and devitalized brain, for many hours following injury.

After head injury there is an enhanced sensitivity to further injury as a result of cerebral ischemia, even in the mildly traumatized brain. A period of ischemia that produces no permanent damage in the uninjured brain can result in permanent structural damage in a brain previously injured, even mildly.[36] Systemic hypoxia has also been shown to be much more damaging to the injured brain than the uninjured one by aggravating the ischemic insult.[34,35]

These recent data emphasize the fact that cerebral ischemia is a critical component of secondary injury following a closed head trauma and that episodes of systemic hypoxia may be damaging. Intensive care management must focus all effort on the maintenance of blood pressure, oxygen tension, normalization of hypercarbia, and acidosis, to minimize these effects. They justify the use of the ICU for the initial management of patients with mild or moderate injury if there is any chance of cardiopulmonary dysfunction that may add an hypoxic-ischemic insult to the brain injury.

WHOM TO ADMIT TO THE ICU

There is general agreement that all patients with severe closed head injury (CHI) and open calvarial or penetrating injuries to the skull (that are deemed salvageable), and post-craniotomy patients should be admitted to the intensive care unit for observation and initial care.[1] Most patients with moderate injury are also placed initially in the ICU[1]; however, there are regional and interhospital differences regarding the use of the ICU for monitoring patients with mild CHI.[17,27,42]

Whereas some patients with mild CHI are discharged for observation in the home setting, and others are placed on the general hospital ward for observation, there are several good reasons for admitting at least selected patients with mild injury to the ICU. Patients with mild head injury and significant systemic trauma, particularly to the chest, with a risk of hypoxia or cardiopulmonary instability, should be admitted to the ICU until they are stable to maintain optimal oxygenation and perfusion of the brain.[36]

Patients harboring linear or depressed skull fractures have a much higher risk of developing a surgically significant intracranial hematoma. Dacey and colleagues[17] have noted that in the presence of a defined skull fracture, nearly 20% of patients required an operative intervention, compared with only 1% of those without fracture.

A hemorrhagic intracranial lesion identified on an initial CT scan after mild CHI also places the patient at definite risk for subsequent neurological deterioration because of progression of these pathological areas,[27] particularly in children.[4,42] Thus one can reasonably argue that patients with a non–basilar-type skull fracture or any hemorrhagic lesion on an initial CT scan should be admitted to the ICU for initial observation for at least 24 hours.

Children, particularly infants and younger children, in whom the clinical examination may be hampered by lack of language skills or difficulty with interpretation of clinical symptoms, should always be placed into a specialized pediatric ICU where the physician and nursing staff are familiar with the differences in caring for patients of this age group.[33]

NEUROLOGICAL MONITORING

A detailed discussion of neurological monitoring can be found in Chapter 3. During the course of ICU care, neurological status is assessed at least hourly to identify any signs of deterioration. A uniform method of examination and record keeping with a standardized form should be used to avoid errors of omission. Delayed complications of head injury, such as the development of intracranial hematomas, enlargement of contusions, or cerebral edema, increases in intracranial pressure, or the occurrence of hypoxia or ischemia may all be reflected by a decrease in the level of consciousness or the onset of new or worsened localizing deficits, such as a hemiparesis or pupillary anisocoria.[1] Generally a decrease of two or more points in the Glasgow Coma Score and/or the presence of new localizing deficits are considered significant and should prompt an immediate assessment of the potential causes for deterioration. Hypoxia, hypotension, acidosis, electrolyte imbalance (particularly hyponatremia), and seizures must all be corrected; a CT of the brain should also be considered to evaluate for the presence of new intracranial mass lesions.

Accurate neurological monitoring may prove to be difficult in some patients because of extreme agitation, requiring the use of sedatives or pharmacologic paralysis to prevent them from injuring themselves or causing elevations in intracranial pressure (ICP). I have found that for sedation, an intravenous infusion of propofol has proven very useful because it is safe for patients with brain injury and has an extremely short half-life, allowing it to be stopped and an accurate examination performed within a brief period.[38] The benzodiazepines should be avoided if possible, because of their longer half-life. For the severely agitated patient who is intubated and undergoing controlled ventilation, for purposes of controlling ICP temporary therapeutic paralysis may be used rather than propofol; an intravenous infusion of short-acting paralytics such as vecuronium can be used. The paralytic can be stopped at routine intervals, such as every 3 to 4 hours, to allow neurological assessment. For patients in therapeutic barbiturate coma, propofol sedation, or paralysis with vecuronium, ICP monitoring should be used to allow identification of intracranial complications.[1,63]

CARDIOPULMONARY MONITORING AND MANAGEMENT

The goal of cardiopulmonary monitoring is to ensure adequacy of oxygenation, cardiac output, and tissue perfusion. Oxygenation is monitored in several ways, including the examination of respiratory function, pulse oxymetry, and arterial blood gas analysis. The six breathing patterns that may be associated with severe head injury are reviewed in Chapter 3. In the neonatal ICU (NICU), breathing patterns should be monitored hourly, whether or not the patient is intubated or being mechanically ventilated. Bedside pulse oximetry should also be used hourly or as needed to maintain optimal arterial oxygenation. Assessment of arterial blood gases for measurement of PaO_2, $PaCO_2$, pH, and bicarbonate concentration may be obtained from arterial puncture or indwelling arterial catheters. In mechanically ventilated patients, the end-tidal CO_2 tension in expired gas may be measured to approximate the $PaCO_2$. This may be particularly useful in settings of increased ICP, in which hyperventilation is being used temporarily.

Systemic Arterial Pressure Monitoring

Patients with severe head injury, who have undergone a craniotomy, or those with multisystem trauma or cardiopulmonary failure should initially have indwelling arterial catheters.[44,85] This allows continuous monitoring of blood pressure and heart rate and calculation of cerebral perfusion pressure (CPP) if concurrent ICP monitoring is being used (CPP = mean arterial pressure − ICP).[1,67,69,70]

Central Venous Pressure Monitoring

Central venous pressure (CVP) monitoring is important to assess volume status and avoid dehydration. Placement of a catheter into the superior vena cava and measurement of right ventricular end-diastolic pressure provide an estimate of volume status if ventricular compliance is normal.[85,86] A CVP of less than 5 usually suggests dehydration. It is my practice to use CVP catheters in younger severely head-injured patients, in whom precise control of cerebral perfusion is necessary.[1,67,69,70]

Pulmonary Artery Pressure Monitoring

In older patients or those with ventricular disease, it is preferable to use a pulmonary artery (PA) catheter to estimate volume status.[45,85] This is more extensively discussed in Chapter 1. An optimal PA wedge pressure is approximately 12 to 14 mm Hg. Patients with a spinal cord injury resulting in neurogenic hypotension may also benefit by the use of a PA catheter to assist in volume management, as may severely head-injured patients with multisystem injury or acute respiratory distress syndrome (ARDS), in whom cardiopulmonary failure is likely.

MANAGEMENT OF RESPIRATORY FAILURE

Systemic complications such as hypoxia, hypercarbia, and acidosis must be prevented or rapidly identified and corrected. In patients with head injury, respiratory failure may be a result of upper airway obstruction or pulmonary problems such as atelectasis, pneumonia, or chest wall trauma.

Therapy to Improve Arterial Oxygenation

Obtunded or comatose patients often develop atelectasis. Among the simplest measures to prevent this is manual repositioning of the patient on an hourly basis, to improve atelectasis and lung perfusion.[46] Oxygen delivery systems may be used to increase FiO_2. Nasal cannulas provide less supplemental oxygen than open face masks; fitting face masks with a nonrebreathing device can provide even higher concentrations of O_2 if needed. Endotracheal intubation provides maximal O_2 concentration.

Indications for Endotracheal Intubation

An FiO_2 greater than 0.50 is best delivered through endotracheal intubation and use of mechanical ventilation.[46] Intubation also protects the patient from aspiration of gastric contents and secretions, as well as upper airway obstruction. Both these indications are usually present in patients that are deeply obtunded or comatose. Intubation is recommended in all patients with severe head injury.[1,2] In addition, patients are often initially intubated after craniotomy for traumatic mass lesions. Those with severe underlying pulmonary diseases may also require endotracheal intubation.[45,46] A detailed discussion of the types of intubation, the various modes of ventilation, and the weaning of mechanical ventilation may be found in Chapter 1.

HYPERVENTILATION

In patients with severe head injury with documented clinical deterioration, immediate endotracheal intubation is indicated. Moderate hyperventilation may be initiated, under the assumption that there is an intracranial mass lesion present, and should be used if clinical signs of transtentorial herniation exist.[1,7] Hyperventilation is usually continued until imaging studies, such as CT, are completed or ICP monitoring is established. Initial arterial PCO_2 is maintained in the range of 25 to 30 mm Hg to provide cerebral vasoconstriction and decrease elevated ICP. Extreme hyperventilation should be avoided because it may not result in further vasoconstriction[40,53,66] and may produce regions of cerebral ischemia,[15,16] as well as metabolic complications from excessive serum alkalosis.

After initial identification and treatment of surgical mass lesions or elevated ICP, using ventricular drainage, osmolar therapy, intravenous mannitol, perfusion pressure management, or other measures, gradual normalization of arterial PCO_2 is optimal. Continuous hyperventilation loses its effect after 20 to 24 hours, as arterial and cerebrospinal fluid (CSF) pH, as well as arteriolar caliber and cerebral blood volume, return to normal.[10,40,53] Return to a more normal $PaCO_2$ then results in overdilation of arterioles and aggravation of ICP elevation.[53] Thus continuous hyperventilation should always be avoided because it becomes ineffective.

In severely head-injured patients without clinical deterioration, the use of prophylactic hyperventilation should be avoided.[7] Normal $PaCO_2$ levels (35-40 mm Hg) should be maintained during the initial evaluation period and hyperventilation reserved for any subsequent decline. This avoids potential aggravation of any secondary ischemic injury during the early phase of management.[5,29,73,74]

MANAGEMENT OF CIRCULATORY DYSFUNCTION

As important as maintaining normal pulmonary physiology is the maintenance of an adequate blood pressure, circulation, and tissue perfusion. Cerebral ischemia caused by compressive mass lesions or elevated ICP is exacerbated by systemic hypotension, which decreases cerebral perfusion pressure.*

Types of Circulatory Failure in Neurotrauma

Hypovolemic shock is most common in the setting of multisystem injury or intraoperative blood loss with inadequate replacement. Clinical findings include low blood pressure, tachycardia, and signs of peripheral

*References 1, 2, 68, 69, 73, 74.

vasoconstriction such as skin pallor and poor capillary refill.[86] The treatment is rapid fluid resuscitation employing isotonic crystalloid volume expanders such as lactated Ringer's solution.

Even in the presence of severe head injury, adequate volume resuscitation is far more important than the fear of excessive fluid overload. CVP measurement may be utilized to guide volume resuscitation. After initial volume resuscitation, an assessment of anemia is necessary to begin adequate replacement of blood volume. A hematocrit of approximately 30% to 33% is optimal.[1]

Cardiogenic shock caused by primary loss of cardiac function may occur as a result of blunt chest trauma with a cardiac contusion or concurrent myocardial ischemia.[45,86] Such patients usually require the use of a PA catheter to optimize volume status and cardiac output and often require use of pharmacological agents that reduce arrhythmias, improve cardiac perfusion, such as nitroglycerin, or reduce afterload on the heart, such as dopamine.[45]

Obstructive shock, caused by obstruction to blood flow such as large pulmonary emboli, and distributive shock, as a result of systemic causes of decreased systemic vascular resistance such as sepsis, are more rare but must be considered in patients with systemic hypotension. Refer to reviews of these topics for further details.[45]

Treatment of Systemic Hypertension

The treatment of hypertension is controversial. In settings in which cerebral ischemia and elevated ICP are not issues, the blood pressure should generally be kept at the patient's usual baseline, even if previously hypertensive. Post-injury or postoperative hypertension is often a result of pain, which should be treated with appropriate analgesics; persistent severe hypertension should lead to reassessment for possible cerebral ischemia or ICP elevation. If these have been ruled out, blood pressure is generally maintained at less than 180 mm Hg using short-acting intravenous β-blockers, such as esmolol or labetalol, or sodium nitroprusside.[1] When compared with nitroprusside, β-blockers achieve similar control of hypertension with improved control of ICP and CPP.[61]

In settings in which cerebral ischemia or elevated ICP are potential problems, hypertension should not be treated unless it is extreme, such as a systolic pressure over 220 mm Hg. Treatment of hypertension in this setting may lower CPP, aggravating ischemia. β-Blockers such as esmolol or labetalol are optimal[61]; nitroprusside should be avoided in the setting of elevated ICP because it may aggravate increased ICP as a result of cerebral vasodilation and increased cerebral blood volume.[14,18]

Intracranial Pressure Monitoring and Management

The pathophysiology and management of elevated ICP have been reviewed in detail in Chapter 4. We monitor ICP in all patients with a severe head injury (GCS of 8 or less) and in all those who undergo a craniotomy for evacuation of an acute traumatic mass lesion.* At times patients with a moderate or even mild head injury may be considered for ICP monitoring, such as if they have highly worrisome abnormalities predictive of elevated ICP on CT scanning,[55,82] if they have episodes of hypotension or hypoxia as a result of severe systemic trauma, or if they are at risk for a secondary ischemic insult to the injured brain.[1]

Monitoring of ICP has several major advantages. It immediately identifies elevations in ICP, which can result in a decrease in CPP, defined as mean arterial pressure − ICP.[67,69,70] Treatment of ICP above 20 mm Hg has been widely recommended[1,57,63,67,70] to maintain a CPP of 70 mm Hg or greater.[67,69,70]

Monitoring ICP also provides an early warning of complications that may elevate ICP, such as delayed intracerebral hemorrhage, cerebral edema, or hydrocephalus. ICP monitoring is of particular use in deeply comatose patients, in whom the neurological examination may not reflect such complications.

Methods of ICP Monitoring

Detailed methodologies of ICP monitoring are reviewed elsewhere.† Bedside monitoring can be achieved using a percutaneous catheter placed into the frontal horn of the lateral ventricle through a twist drill or burr hole.[60] A ventricular catheter remains the optimal monitor for ICP both because of its accuracy and because it allows for drainage of CSF as a means to control ICP.[1,60,70] A fiberoptic catheter (Camino catheter) can also be placed, using a twist-drill technique, into the brain tissue or ventricle.[62]

Patients having undergone a craniotomy may have catheters placed either into the lateral ventricle or into the subdural space.[1,2,60] Those within the ventricle are probably the most accurate and allow CSF drainage as a method of ICP control. Monitors are usually left in place until the ICP has been normalized for at least 24 hours after treatment of elevated ICP has ceased.

Treatment of Elevated ICP

Elevated ICP is treated first by ruling out treatable intracranial mass lesions, such as hematomas, using appropriate imaging studies. The initial use of hyperventilation was outlined earlier; it is continued only until other measures have been introduced. Medical treat-

*References 1, 2, 57, 62, 69, 71.
†References 1, 2, 57, 60, 62, 63.

ment of elevated ICP includes the use of CSF drainage, therapeutic sedation,[25,63] intravenous mannitol,[1,54,63] hyperosmolar therapy, and perfusion pressure management.[67,69,70] In selected patients, barbiturates[1,2,21,83] or controlled hypothermia[11,47,48,75,76] may also be of use.

Therapeutic sedation, and at times neuromuscular paralysis, are a standard treatment for patients with elevated ICP, particularly if they are agitated or coughing excessively in a fashion that elevates ICP. The most commonly used drug for sedation is morphine; in general the benzodiazepines are avoided because they mask neurological function. Recent Class 1[7] evidence shows propofol to be more effective than morphine in maintaining lower ICP in severely head-injured patients, with less need for other measures to lower ICP; at delayed follow-up examinations, a trend toward more favorable outcomes was also observed.[38]

Mannitol is administered as an intermittent intravenous bolus (0.25-1.0 gm/kg body weight) as often as every 4 to 6 hours. Where the blood-brain barrier is intact, mannitol remains in the intravascular and extracellular spaces[1,63]; it has a number of effects, including an immediate increase in circulating blood volume and blood pressure, reduced blood viscosity, improved blood flow, and arteriolar vasoconstriction, in regions of the brain where autoregulation is intact.[54] Patients with a low initial CPP respond better to mannitol than those with a higher CPP, suggesting that the increase in systolic blood pressure and CPP allow direct cerebral vasoconstriction.[68]

Hyperosmolar therapy involves decreasing the extracellular volume within the brain, by initial use of mannitol, to provide an osmotic diuresis in addition to its effects noted above. Free-water intake is also limited, and at times other diuretics are used, such as furosemide.[1,63] The goal is not clinical dehydration, which may decrease CPP, but rather a euvolemic state with increased serum sodium, osmolality, and serum tonicity. A serum sodium level of 145 to 155 mEq/L and serum osmolality of 300 to 330 mOsm/L are optimal. To avoid excessive dehydration, central venous pressure should be monitored and isotonic fluids such as normal saline or salt-poor albumin administered to keep the CVP at 2 to 5 mm Hg.

Perfusion pressure management, as described by Rosner,[67,69,70] involves the active elevation of blood pressure, using volume expansion and vasopressors such as norepinephrine, to increase CPP, improving cerebral blood flow and allowing vasoconstriction in regions where autoregulation remains intact. This may directly lower ICP. Even in vascular regions where autoregulation is no longer intact, elevating CPP may prevent additional ischemic brain injury. The absolute blood pressure needed to improve perfusion varies; in some patients a CPP of 80 to 90 mm Hg is necessary before an ICP decrease is noted. Clinical results to date in patients with severe head injury suggest that perfusion pressure management not only improves control of ICP elevation, but may also improve functional survival and outcome.[67,69] However, because a prospective, randomized, and controlled study of this modality has never been accomplished, the results remain controversial and this method is considered only as a second-tier therapeutic option in the *Guidelines for the Management of Severe Head Injury*.[7]

Barbiturate coma has been used to successfully treat elevated ICP when other methods have failed.[21,59,83] Barbiturates reduce ICP by decreasing cerebral metabolism, oxygen use, and blood flow.[21,59,83] The usual dosage of pentobarbital is initially a bolus of 10 mg/kg body weight, followed by an infusion of 1.5 mg/kg/hr. Serum pentobarbital levels should be monitored and the dose adjusted to maintain a serum level of approximately 3 mg/dl. Systemic hypotension caused by myocardiac suppression can be expected, requiring the additional use of intravenous vasopressors and intravascular monitoring using a Swan-Ganz catheter.[21,59,63,83] Such patients are routinely intubated, on controlled ventilation, and must have ICP monitoring in place, because the possibility of neurological examination is lost as a result of the pharmacological effects of the drug. Barbiturates have been shown to effectively reduce elevated ICP when virtually all other measures have failed.[21,59] The *Guidelines for the Management of Severe Head Injury*[7] indicate that barbiturate therapy may be considered in hemodynamically stable patients with refractory elevations in ICP. However, Ward and colleagues[83] have reported that in a prospective, controlled trial of barbiturate coma for severe head injury, there was no difference in the incidence or duration of elevated ICP compared with other measures and no improvement in survival with its use.

Therapeutic hypothermia, when used to moderate levels (32-35° C), has been shown to lower intracranial pressure[48,75,76] and appears to improve outcome in patients with severe head injury.[11,47] Like barbiturates, hypothermia decreases cerebral metabolism, oxygen utilization, and blood flow. A thermistor is needed within the brain, as well as in the pulmonary artery, to adequately monitor cerebral and core body temperatures. The maintenance of hypothermia may be difficult, requiring external cooling blankets and gastric ice water lavage in some cases. Shiozaki and colleagues[76] have shown that after failure of all conventional measures, mild hypothermia was effective in preventing progressive ICP elevation in patients with intracerebral mass lesions and a maximal ICP of less than 40 mm Hg; hypothermia was not effective at all for patients with diffuse cerebral swelling or a maximal ICP of 40 mm Hg or greater. More recent results reported by Clifton[11] also indicate that there are significant toxicities of hypothermia, as well as a lack of effectiveness in certain patient groups. Currently the use of mild to moderate hypothermia remains a second-tier therapeutic option in the *Guidelines for the Management of Severe Head Injury*.[7]

Hyperventilation with Jugular Venous Oxygen Monitoring

When all the above measures have failed, return to the use of hyperventilation (Pa_{CO_2} below 25 mm Hg) can be considered. Optimally this is done using jugular venous oxygen saturation monitoring[13,15,16,25,72] or other measures of cerebral blood flow[49] to allow identification of the development of cerebral ischemia as a result of induced vasoconstriction.

Decompressive craniectomy, either unilateral[31,65,87] or bilateral,[26,64] has been performed for many years, usually as a last resort for intractable elevated ICP; when used in this way, it is not surprising that the results have often been poor, with a perception that functional survival is not improved.[12] More recently Gaab and colleagues[23] and others have shown that patients with refractory ICP elevation and swelling without major areas of infarction or contusion have responded well to decompressive craniectomy, both in effectively lowering ICP[64,87] and in improved morbidity and mortality.[31,64] I have found that earlier use of these techniques, before extreme elevations in ICP have occurred, seem to be the most effective. The removed bone flap can be stored in a freezer (−70° C) or placed in the patient in a subcutaneous abdominal pouch for storage and later replacement.

Additional Neurological Monitors Used in the Intensive Care Unit

In addition to ICP monitoring, a number of other methods have been developed to monitor the state of cerebral blood flow and perfusion at the bedside. Cerebral blood flow (CBF) measurement can be performed directly at the bedside in the ICU using the xenon-133 clearance technique[49] and provides accurate assessment of regional cerebral blood flow at a single time. CBF measurement may be useful for patients with head injury; Martin and colleagues[49] have documented the variety of states that may be identified, from frank hyperemia to ischemia, after severe head injury. The measurement of CBF directly allows specific management for each individual patient's exact needs.

The state of cerebral perfusion can be assessed in another way, using arteriojugular venous difference in oxygen content (j-$AVDO_2$).[13,15,16,25,72] In states of relatively inadequate perfusion, the j-$AVDO_2$ increases as more oxygen is extracted from the circulation; in states of excessive perfusion for demand (so-called luxury perfusion), the j-$AVDO_2$ decreases as less oxygen is extracted. Cruz[16] has shown that such measurements in patients with severe head injury allow rapid identification of complications that result in secondary brain ischemia, such as elevated ICP or systemic hypoxia. The degree of therapeutic hyperventilation can also be optimized with j-$AVDO_2$ measurement so as to counteract posttraumatic cerebral hemodynamic changes, such as luxury perfusion syndrome, and avoid inducing cerebral ischemia.[33] One limitation of this technique is that it assesses global cerebral perfusion and may not identify areas of regional ischemia.[13,15,16,25,72]

Recently Cormio and colleagues[13] have shown that severely head-injured patients with a low j-$AVDO_2$, suggesting hyperemia, had a significantly higher CBF and lower cerebral metabolic rate than other groups, as well as a worse prognosis than those with a normal j-$AVDO_2$.

Several other methods of bedside blood flow and oxygenation analysis have been developed for patients with head injury, including transcranial Doppler,[58,84] cortical-surface blood flow measure using thermal diffusion methods,[8,25] optical spectroscopy,[50] and near-infrared spectroscopy.[39] Recently the clinical feasibility of direct measurement of brain tissue partial pressure of oxygen (PO_2) and pH has been reported.[52] All these methods have certain advantages and limitations but have not yet become widely utilized for bedside monitoring. Transcranial Doppler is useful because it can identify the presence of arterial vasospasm associated with traumatic subarachnoid hemorrhage and is useful to confirm the presence of brain death by verification of the absence of intracranial blood flow.[58] Direct measurement of brain tissue PO_2 may become more widespread as a result of the recent availability of commercially produced monitors that are easily placed into brain parenchyma.

Recently Menzel and colleagues monitored brain tissue PO_2 and pH and measured brain tissue lactate levels using microdialysis.[52] They showed that markedly elevated lactate levels are common in brain tissue after severe head injury, suggesting the occurrence of anaerobic metabolism. Increasing PaO_2 by raising inspired FIO_2 to 100% increased brain tissue PO_2 and lowered mean tissue lactate levels by 40%, implying a shift to aerobic metabolism.

Optimally measurement of ICP, CPP, cerebral blood flow, and brain tissue PO_2 provides the practitioner the data needed at the bedside to correct intracranial physiology by adjustment of blood pressure, Pa_{CO_2}, PaO_2, and pH and normalizing of ICP.

METABOLIC MANAGEMENT

Problems of metabolism are common after severe head injury. Serum electrolytes and osmolality are routinely monitored every 6 to 12 hours for the first 36 to 48 hours of ICU management. Fluid requirements include three basic components: maintenance needs, initial deficits, and ongoing losses. The choice of maintenance fluids is influenced by neurosurgical patients' unique predisposition to impaired water excretion and resulting hyponatremia. In patients with injury confined to the central nervous system (CNS), intravenous fluids are initiated using isotonic solutions, such as 0.9% normal saline or Ringer's lactate, at a rate lower than would be used for patients with systemic trauma. Careful monitoring of electrolytes, body weight, hemodynamics, urine output, and renal function are then needed to titrate appropriate maintenance fluids to maintain a euvolemic state. Glucose-containing solutions should be avoided because clinical studies in patients with head injury have suggested that hyperglycemia is associated with a poorer outcome.[1,3]

The most common problem encountered is electrolyte imbalance, most often hyponatremia or hypernatremia.[3,17] Hypernatremia and a hyperosmolar state may result from the frequent use of mannitol or other diuretics, combined with restriction of free-water intake to prevent cerebral edema. Excessive hypernatremia may result in neuronal dysfunction in addition to cardiopulmonary and renal complications. The serum sodium should generally be kept below 150 mEq/L and the hyperosmolar state below 330 mOsm/L. Excessive hypernatremia is managed with free-water replacement using a hypotonic crystalloid solution, such as 0.21% or 0.45% normal saline.

Hyponatremia is extremely common as a result of inappropriately elevated secretion of antidiuretic hormone (ADH) in patients after head injury and other major brain insults (so-called syndrome of inappropriate ADH [SIADH]).[17,41] Such patients receiving an infusion of hypotonic fluids at routine maintenance levels will retain excessive free water and develop hyponatremia. Hyponatremia may aggravate cerebral edema and ICP elevation and, if severe, induce seizures.[17] Serum sodium must be monitored and hyponatremia treated with fluid restriction or, if extreme, 3% saline infusion and furosemide to remove excessive free water.[17,41]

More rarely, patients may develop hyponatremia without an excess of free water and may in fact become clinically dehydrated. Such cerebral salt wasting results from urinary losses of both sodium and free water, probably as a result of excessive release of atrial natriuretic factor.[3,41] Cerebral salt wasting has been described in patients with head injury and after pituitary surgery.[3] Treatment requires volume reexpansion using isotonic or hypertonic solutions with correction of the dehydrated state. Thus, when evaluating a patient with hyponatremia, volume status must be carefully assessed for evidence of free water excess (SIADH) or dehydration (cerebral salt wasting).

Other complications encountered after head injury include diabetes insipidus, most often as a result of trauma to the pituitary stalk or clinical brain death with loss of hypothalamic function. Defined as excessive output (>200 ml/hr) of diluted urine (specific gravity of <1.005), combined with rising serum sodium (to >145 mEq/L), diabetes insipidus should be treated with exogenous replacement of ADH using aqueous pitressin or DDAVP.[17]

Hyperglycemia, a component of acute-phase and stress response, is also encountered frequently in the neurosurgical ICU and may be exacerbated by enteral or parenteral feeding. Hyperglycemia is associated with a poorer outcome after head injury as a result of elevating intracellular lactate caused by anaerobic metabolism.[1,17] Glucose is not routinely added to maintenance fluids, and serum glucose is monitored daily at first; hyperglycemia greater than 200 mg/100 ml is treated with a sliding-scale insulin regimen.

NUTRITIONAL MANAGEMENT

After head injury, institution of early nutrition is beneficial. In patients with severe head injury a negative nitrogen balance rapidly develops as a result of hypermetabolism and hypercatabolism.[30,32] Intake of both calories and protein is required to avoid significant weight loss and muscle atrophy. Inadequate nutrition also results in impaired immune function, poor wound healing, anemia, and increased incidence of infection.[32]

Initially after an injury, enteral feeding may not be tolerated because of paralytic ileus or anesthesia; CNS complications such as elevated ICP may further delay return of normal gut function. Some have recommended that total parenteral nutrition (TPN) be initiated early in the management of patients who do not tolerate enteral feedings to meet nutritional requirements and replace catabolic losses.[32] Among head-injured patients, comparison of TPN with enteral feedings have shown improved nitrogen balance but no change in survival when TPN was utilized.[32]

The expense and complications of TPN use have led some to initiate enteral hyperalimentation as early as 24 to 36 hours after injury, by placing a nasojejunal tube under fluoroscopic guidance.[30] In this fashion, improved caloric intake and nitrogen balance can be achieved, even in the absence of bowel sounds. It remains my practice to attempt to initiate enteral feedings by way of a nasogastric tube as soon as possible; if after 24 hours bowel sounds have not returned, the tube is advanced under fluoroscopic guidance into the jejunum to begin nasojejunal feeding. TPN is reserved for patients with multisystem injury or severe cachexia or those that cannot tolerate any form of enteral feeding for the first 3 or 4 days after insult.

ANTICONVULSANTS

For patients with severe head injuries, the initial use of prophylactic or therapeutic anticonvulsants has been routine because of the high potential for seizures and the potential for complications should a seizure occur.[1] The drug most often used in this setting has been phenytoin (Dilantin), given in an initial loading dosage of 15 to 18 mg/kg body weight, followed by 5 mg/kg daily thereafter. Phenytoin has the advantages of a rapid parenteral route of administration, low incidence of severe side effects, and efficacy against the types of seizures that occur in these settings.

Temkin and colleagues[81] have shown that prophylactic treatment with phenytoin for a full year after head injury was no more effective in preventing seizures than treatment for only the first 7 days. Treatment for the first week prevented early posttraumatic epilepsy, which is most common after penetrating injuries such as gunshot wounds, depressed skull fractures and in those with focal posttraumatic hematomas. Thereafter a patient can be monitored without treatment for delayed posttraumatic epilepsy and only treated should seizures occur. It has become my practice to treat patients with severe head injury only for the first 7 days and not to treat patients with mild or moderate head injury, nontraumatic hemorrhages, or cerebral infarction at all unless seizures occur.

Although phenytoin is generally safe, some side effects are common, particularly mild cognitive impairment. This is usually not a problem in the ICU setting but may be a limitation during the rehabilitative period of care. Other side effects include rash, fever, blood dyscrasias, and Stevens-Johnson syndrome.[1] Anticonvulsants used as an alternative to phenytoin include carbamazepine (Tegretol), which cannot be given parenterally, and phenobarbital, which causes severe sedation. Recently available is gabapentin (Neurontin), an oral anticonvulsant structurally related to γ-aminobutyric acid (GABA).[6] The role of gabapentin in the acute care of the neurosurgical patient has not yet been established.

OTHER CONSIDERATIONS

Pulmonary and urinary tract infections are the most common problems encountered in the ICU after severe head injury; these problems are addressed in other chapters of this book. Patients intubated for more than 5 days commonly get pneumonia. Urinary tract infections usually result from bladder catheterization. Both sources of infection should be assessed periodically by performing appropriate diagnostic studies, including stains and cultures.

Infections related to the CNS insult itself or craniotomy are much more rare but include meningitis, brain abscess, and epidural and subdural empyemas. The decision to use perioperative prophylactic antibiotics is both controversial and beyond the scope of this chapter. In the ICU setting, patients with externalized intracranial catheters have often been treated with broad-spectrum antibiotics such as the cephalosporins; however, scientific evidence that this is useful is lacking. With the emerging problems of bacterial resistance to antibiotics, suppressive or prophylactic antibiotic use in the ICU should generally be avoided and infections treated as specifically as possible.

Patients with CNS insults resulting in paralysis form a particularly high-risk group for the development of deep venous thrombosis and subsequent potential pulmonary embolism.[78] It is my practice to place both compressive hose and pneumatic stockings on all patients before craniotomy and continuously in the neurosurgical ICU thereafter, so as to minimize the risk until the patient is mobile and ambulatory. The use of prophylactic anticoagulants is generally avoided unless the patient is at extreme risk, such as having a known hypercoagulable state or quadriplegia. In these settings the therapies discussed earlier, combined with minidose heparin (5000 U SQ bid) and use of an oscillating bed provide maximal prophylaxis.[20] The platelet count should be monitored because thrombocytopenia may complicate the use of heparin. For patients that develop documented thrombosis or pulmonary emboli, complete heparinization may be dangerous because of the potential for precipitating intracranial or intraspinal hemorrhage, and vena caval interruption by way of a caval filter may be necessary.

Disseminated intravascular coagulation (DIC) is also a potentially life-threatening complication of severe head injury. DIC may occur as a result of the widespread activation of coagulation caused by massive intravascular release of cell membrane phospholipids, cytokines, and tissue factor, which results in systemic generation of thrombin.[43] The pathogenesis and treatment of this disorder is reviewed by Levi and Cate.[43]

Gastrointestinal hemorrhage is also a risk after coma-inducing head-injury. Chan and colleagues[9] have defined five high-risk categories for stress ulceration in postoperative neurosurgical patients. These include preoperative coma, age over 60 years, CNS infection, the presence of SIADH, and reoperation. They performed a prospective, controlled, double-blinded study of the use of the histamine-2 blocker parenteral ranitidine in such high-risk patients and showed a significantly decreased incidence of gastrointestinal hemorrhage. It is my practice to initiate such medications (ranitidine, famotidine, or cimetidine) upon the institution of steroid treatment, after severe head or spinal cord injury, after routine craniotomy, and in the high-risk groups defined above.

REFERENCES

1. Andrews BT: The intensive care management of patients with head injury, in Andrews, BT (eds): **Neurosurgical Intensive Care.** New York: McGraw-Hill, 1993, pp 227-242.
2. Andrews BT, Pitts LH: **Traumatic Transtentorial Herniation.** New York: Futura Press, 1991.
3. Andrews BT, Tyrell JB, Fitzgerald P, et al: Cerebral salt wasting after pituitary exploration: report of a case, **Neurosurgery 18:**469-471, 1986.
4. Bonadio WA, Smith DS, Hillman S: Clinical indicators of intracranial lesions on computed tomographic scans in children with parietal skull fracture, **Am J Dis Child 143:**194-196, 1989.
5. Bouma GJ, Muixelaar JP, Stringer WA, et al: Ultra-early evaluation of regional cerebral blood flow in severely head-injured patients using xenon-enhanced computed tomography, **J Neurosurg 77:**360-368, 1992.
6. Browne TR: Efficacy and safety of gabapentin, in Chadwick D (ed): **New Trends in Epilepsy Management: The role of Gabapentin.** Royal Society of Medicine Services International Congress and Symposium Number 198, 1993.
7. Bullock R, Chesnut RM, Clifton G, et al: **Guidelines for the Management of Severe Head Injury.** New York: Brain Trauma Foundation Publishers, 1995.
8. Carter LP, Grahm T, Bailes JE, et al: Continuous postoperative monitoring of cortical blood flow and intracranial pressure, **Surg Neurol 36:**36-38, 1991.
9. Chan KH, Lai EC, Tuen H, et al: Prospective double-blind placebo controlled randomized trial on the use of ranitidine in preventing postoperative gastroduodenal complications in high-risk neurosurgical patients, **J Neurosurg 82:**413-417, 1995.
10. Christensen MS: Acid-base changes in cerebrospinal fluid and blood, and blood volume changes following prolonged hyperventilation in man, **Br J Anaesth 46:**348-351, 1974.
11. Clifton GL, Allen S, Barrodale P, et al: A phase II study of moderate hypothermia in severe brain injury, **J Neurotrauma 10:**263-273, 1993.
12. Cooper PR, Rovit RL, Ransohoff J: Hemicraniectomy in the treatment of acute subdural hematoma: a reappraisal, **Surg Neurol 5:**25-28, 1976.
13. Cormio M, Valadka AB, Robertson C: Elevated jugular venous oxygen saturation after severe head injury, **J Neurosurg 90:**9-15, 1999.
14. Cottrell JE, Patel K, Turndorf H, et al: Intracranial pressure changes induced by sodium nitroprusside in patients with intracranial mass lesions, **J Neurosurg 48:**329-334, 1978.
15. Cruz J: Combined continuous monitoring of systemic and cerebral oxygenation in acute brain injury: preliminary observations, **Crit Care Med 21:**1225-1232, 1993.
16. Cruz J: On-line monitoring of global cerebral hypoxia in acute brain injury. Relationship to intracranial hypertension, **J Neurosurg 79:**228-233,1993.
17. Dacey R, Alves WM, Rimel RW, et al: Neurosurgical complications after apparently minor head injury: assessment of risk in a series of 610 patients, **J Neurosurg 65:**203-210, 1986.
18. Darby JM, Nelson PB: Fluid, electrolyte and acid-base balance in neurosurgical intensive care, in Andrews BT (ed): **Neurosurgical Intensive Care.** New York: McGraw-Hill, 1993, pp 133-162.
19. Davis RF, Douglas ME, Heenen TJ, et al: Brain tissue pressure measurement during sodium nitroprusside infusion, **Crit Care Med 9:**17-19, 1981.
20. Dickman CA, Sonntag VKH: The intensive care management of spinal cord injury, in Andrews BT (ed): **Neurosurgical Intensive Care.** New York: McGraw-Hill, 1993, pp 243-249.
21. Eisenberg HM, Frankowski RF, Conant CF et al: High-dose barbiturate control of elevated intracranial pressure in patients with severe head injury, **J Neurosurg 69:**15-19, 1988.
22. **Federal Interagency Head Injury Task Force Report.** Washington DC: US Department of Health and Human Services, 1989.
23. Gaab MR, Rittierodt M, Lorenz M, et al: Traumatic brain swelling and operative decompression: implications for the management of severe head injuries, **Acta Neurochir (Wein) 51:**394-396, 1990.
24. Gentleman SM, Roberts GW, Gennarelli TA, et al: Axonal injury: a universal consequence of fatal closed head injury, **Acta Neuropath (Berl) 89:**537-543, 1995.
25. Gopinath S, Valadka A, Contant CF, et al: Relationship between global and cortical cerebral bloodflow in patients with head injuries, **Neurosurgery 44:**1273-1279, 1999.
26. Gower DJ, Lee KS, McWhorter JM: Role of subtemporal decompression in severe closed head injury, **Neurosurgery 23:**417-422, 1988.
27. Graham DI: Neuropathology of head injury, in Narayan R, Wilberger J, Povlishock JT: **Neurotrauma.** New York: McGraw-Hill, 1996, pp 43-69.
28. Graham DI, Adams JH, Nicoll JAR, et al: The nature, distribution and causes of traumatic brain injury, **Brain Pathol 5:**397-406, 1995.
29. Graham DI, Ford I, Adams JH, et al: Ischemic brain damage is still common in fatal non-missile head injury, **J Neurol Neurosurg Psychiatry 52:**346-350, 1989.
30. Grahm TW, Zadrozny DB, Harrington T: The benefits of early jejunal hyperalimentation in the head-injured patient, **Neurosurgery 25:**729-732, 1989.
31. Guerra WKW, Gaab MR, Dietz H, et al: Surgical decompression for traumatic brain swelling. indications and results, **J Neurosurg 90:**1187-1196, 1999.
32. Hadley MN, Grahm TW, Harrington T, et al: Nutritional support and neurotrauma. A critical review of early nutritional support in forty-five acute head injury patients, **Neurosurgery 19:**367-371, 1986.
33. Hammer G, Lindsey JN: The neurosurgical pediatric patient, in Andrews BT (ed): **Neurosurgical Intensive Care.** New York: McGraw-Hill, 1993, pp 391-413.

34. Ishige N, Pitts LH, Berry I, et al: Effect of hypoxia on traumatic brain injury in rats: alterations in neurological function, brain edema, and cerebral bloodflow, **J Cereb Bloodflow Metab 7:**759-767, 1987.
35. Ishige N, Pitts LH, Hashimoto T, et al: Effect of hypoxia on traumatic brain injury in rats. Part 1: Changes in neurological function, electroencephalograms and histopathology, **Neurosurgery 20:**848-853, 1987.
36. Jenkins LW, Moszynski K, Lyeth BG, et al: Increased vulnerability of the mildly traumatized rat brain to cerebral ischemia: the use of controlled secondary ischemia to identify common or different mechanisms contributing to mechanical and ischemic brain injury, **Brain Res 477:**211-224, 1989.
37. Kampfl A, Posmantur RM, Zhao X, et al: Mechanisms of calpain proteolysis following traumatic brain injury: implications for pathology and therapy. A review and update, **J Neurotrauma 14:**121-134, 1997.
38. Kelly DF, Goodale DB, Williams J, et al: Propofol in the treatment of moderate and severe head injury: a randomized, prospective double-blinded pilot trial, **J Neurosurg 90:**1042-1052, 1999.
39. Kirkpatrick PJ, Smielewski P, Czosnyka M, et al: Near-infrared spectroscopy use in patients with head injury, **J Neurosurg 83:**963-970, 1995.
40. Lassen NA: Brain extracellular pH: the main factor controlling cerebral blood flow, **Scand J Clin Lab Invest 22:**247-250, 1968.
41. Lester MC, Nelson PB: Neurological aspects of vasopressin release and the syndrome of inappropriate secretion of antidiuretic hormone, **Neurosurgery 8:**735-739, 1981.
42. Levi L, Guilburd JN, Linn S, et al: The association between skull fracture, intracranial pathology and outcome in pediatric head injury, **Br J Neurosurg 5:**617-625, 1991.
43. Levi M, Cate H: Disseminated intravascular coagulation, **N Engl J Med 341:**586-592, 1999.
44. Luce J: Cardiopulmonary physiology and management in neurosurgical intensive care, in Andrews BT (ed): **Neurosurgical Intensive Care.** New York: McGraw-Hill, 1993, pp 1-30.
45. Luce JM, Hopewell PC: Critical care medicine, in Wyngaarden JB, Smith LH, Bennett JC, et al (eds): **Cecil's Textbook of Medicine,** 19th ed. Philadelphia: WB Saunders, 1992, pp 459-476.
46. Luce JM, Tyler LM, Pierson DJ: **Intensive Respiratory Care.** Philadelphia: WB Saunders, 1984.
47. Marion DW, Obrist WD, Carlier PM, et al: The use of therapeutic moderate hypothermia for patients with severe head injuries: a preliminary report, **J Neurosurg 79:**354-362, 1993.
48. Marion DW, Penrod LE, Kelsey SF et al: Treatment of traumatic brain injury with moderate hypothermia, **N Engl J Med 336:**540-546, 1997.
49. Martin NA, Doberstein C, Zane C: Posttraumatic cerebral arterial spasm: transcranial Doppler ultrasound, cerebral blood flow and angiographic findings, **J Neurosurg 77:**575-583, 1992.
50. McCormick P, Stewart M, Goetting MG, et al: Regional cerebrovascular oxygen saturation measured by optical spectroscopy in humans, **Stroke 22:**569-602, 1991.
51. McIntosh TK, Smith DH, Meany DF et al: Neuropathological sequelae of traumatic brain injury: relationship to neurochemical and biochemical mechanisms, **Lab Invest 74:**315-342, 1996.
52. Menzel M, Doppenberg EMR, Zauner A, et al: Increased inspired oxygen concentration as a factor in improved brain tissue oxygenation and tissue lactate levels after severe head injury, **J Neurosurg 91:**1-10, 1999.
53. Muizelaar JP, van der Poel HG, Li Z, et al: Pial arteriolar vessel diameter and CO_2 reactivity during prolonged hyperventilation in the rabbit, **J Neurosurg 69:**923-927, 1988.
54. Muizelaar JP, Wei EP, Kontos HA, et al: Mannitol causes compensatory cerebral vasoconstriction and vasodilation in response to blood viscosity changes, **J Neurosurg 59:**822-825, 1983
55. Murphy A, Teasdale E, Matheson M, et al: Relationship between CT indices of brain swelling and intracranial pressure after head injury, in Ishii S, Nagai H, Brock M (eds): **Intracranial Pressure.** Berlin: Springer-Verlag, 1983, pp 562-565.
56. Narayan RK, Greenberg RP, Miller JD, et al: Improved confidence of outcome prediction in severe head injury: a comparative analysis of the clinical examination, multi-modality evoked potentials, CT scanning, and intracranial pressure, **J Neurosurg 54:**751-762, 1981.
57. Narayan RK, Kishore PR, Becker DP, et al: Intracranial pressure: to monitor or not to monitor? A review of our experience with severe head injury, **J Neurosurg 56:**560-566, 1982.
58. Newell DW, Grady S, Sirotta P, et al: Evaluation of brain death using transcranial Doppler, **Neurosurgery 24:**509-513, 1989.
59. Nordstrom CH, Messeter K, Sunbarg G, et al: Cerebral blood flow, vasoreactivity, and oxygen consumption during barbiturate therapy in severe traumatic brain lesions, **J Neurosurg 68:**424-427, 1988.
60. North B, Reilly P: Comparison among three methods of intracranial pressure recording, **Neurosurgery 18:**730-734, 1986.
61. Orlowski JP, Shiesley D, Vidt DG, et al: Labetalol to control blood pressure after cerebrovascular surgery, **Crit Care Med 16:**765-768, 1988.
62. Ostrup RC, Luerssen TG, Marshall LF, et al: Continuous monitoring of intracranial pressure with a miniaturized fiberoptic device, **J Neurosurg 67:**206-207, 1987.
63. Pitts LH, Andrews BT: Intracranial pressure monitoring and treatment of intracranial hypertension, in Wood L (ed): **Principles of Critical Care Medicine.** New York: McGraw-Hill, 1992, pp 2985-3011.
64. Polin RS, Shaffrey ME, Bogaev CA, et al: Decompressive bifrontal craniectomy in the treatment of severe refractory posttraumatic cerebral edema, **Neurosurgery 41:**84-92, 1999.
65. Ransohoff J, Benjamin MV, Gage EL, et al: Hemicraniectomy in the management of acute subdural hematoma, **J Neurosurg 34:**70-76, 1971.

66. Reivich M: Arterial P_{CO_2} and cerebral hemodynamics, **Am J Physiol 25:**206-210, 1964.
67. Rosner MJ: Pathophysiology and management of increased intracranial pressure, in Andrews BT (ed): **Neurosurgical Intensive Care.** New York: McGraw-Hill, 1993, pp 57-112.
68. Rosner MJ, Coley I: Cerebral perfusion pressure: a hemodynamic mechanism of mannitol and the postmannitol hemogram, **Neurosurgery 21:**147-149, 1987.
69. Rosner MJ, Daughton S: Cerebral perfusion pressure management in head injury, **J Trauma 30:**933-937, 1990.
70. Rosner MJ, Rosner SD, Johnson AH: Cerebral perfusion pressure: management protocol and clinical results, **J Neurosurg 83:**949-962, 1995.
71. Saul TG, Ducker TB: Effect of intracranial pressure monitoring and aggressive treatment on mortality in severe head injury, **J Neurosurg 56:**498-503, 1982.
72. Schroder ML, Muizelaar JP, Bullock MR, et al: Focal ischemia due to traumatic contusion documented by stable xenon CT and ultrastructural studies, **J Neurosurg 82:**966-971, 1995.
73. Schroder ML, Muizelaar JP, Kuta AJ: Documented reversal of global ischemia immediately after removal of an acute subdural hematoma: report of 2 cases, **J Neurosurg 80:**324-327, 1994.
74. Sheinberg M, Kanter MJ, Robertson CS, et al: Continuous monitoring of jugular venous oxygen saturation in head injured patients, **J Neurosurg 76:**212-218, 1992.
75. Shiozaki T, Sugimoto H, Taneda M, et al: Effect of mild hypothermia on uncontrolled intracranial hypertension after severe head injury, **J Neurosurg 79:**363-368, 1993.
76. Shiozaki T, Sugimoto H, Taneda M, et al: Selection of severely head injured patients for mild hypothermia, **J Neurosurg 89:**206-211, 1998.
77. Sosin DM, Sneizek JE, Waxweiler RJ: Trends in death associated with traumatic brain injury, 1979 through 1992, **JAMA 273:**1778-1780, 1995.
78. Swann KW, Black PM: Deep vein thrombosis and pulmonary emboli in neurosurgical patients: a review, **J Neurosurg 61:**1055-1062, 1984.
79. Teasdale GM, Graham DI: Craniocerebral trauma: protection and retrieval of the neuronal population after injury, **Neurosurgery 43:**723-738, 1998.
80. Teasdale GM, Jennet B: Assessment of coma and impairment of consciousness: A practical scale, **Lancet 2:**81-84, 1974.
81. Temkin NR, Dikmen SS, Wilensky AJ, et al: A randomized, double-blind study of phenytoin for the prevention of post-traumatic seizures, **N Engl J Med 323:**497-500, 1990.
82. Toutant SM, Klauber MR, Marshall LF, et al: Absent or compressed basal cisterns on first CT scan: ominous predictors of outcome in severe head injury, **J Neurosurg 61:**691-694, 1984.
83. Ward JD, Becker DP, Miller JD, et al: Failure of prophylactic barbiturate coma in the treatment of severe head injury, **J Neurosurg 62:**203-206, 1985.
84. Weber M, Grolimund P, Seiler RW: Evaluation of posttraumatic cerebral blood flow velocities by transcranial Doppler ultrasonography, **Neurosurgery 27:**106-112, 1990.
85. Williams FC, Spetzler RF: Hemodynamic monitoring in the neurosurgical intensive care unit, **Clin Neurosurg 35:**101-107, 1987.
86. Wisner DH: The intensive care management of multisystem injury, in Andrews BT (ed): **Neurosurgical Intensive Care.** New York: McGraw-Hill, 1993, pp 251-290.
87. Yoo DS, Kim DS, Cho KS, et al: Ventricular pressure monitoring during bilateral decompression with dural expansion, **J Neurosurg 91:**953-959, 1999.

CHAPTER 10

Spinal Cord Injury Management

ASH SINGHAL
ANDREW BAKER
MICHAEL G. FEHLINGS

Spinal cord injury (SCI) is a devastating event that has dramatic impact on the functional and psychosocial well-being of the survivor. Historically, tracing back to the times of the ancient Egyptians and the Edwin Smith papyrus, physicians held to the belief that SCI and quadriplegia were "ailments not to be treated."[83] However, the modern era of care and management of the SCI patient began in World War II in England, leading to the development of specialized treatment centers for such injuries.[32,38]

The impact of this condition is enormous, with great worldwide variation in published incidence rates, from 6 per million[43] to 57.8 per million.[54] In the United States there are 40 new cases per million per year, with an average of 10,000 new cases diagnosed per year.[5,16,39] There is a strong male preponderance, between 71% and 80%, and youth preponderance, with an average age of 31.5 years.[5,16,39] Approximately 62% of cases have incomplete or complete paraplegia, and 38% of cases have incomplete or complete tetraplegia.

After the initial resuscitation (including commencement of methylprednisolone protocol) and radiographical investigation of the spinal cord–injured patient (and in selected cases, surgical decompression or stabilization), the management shifts to the intensive care unit (ICU). This chapter focuses on this post-trauma phase of management. The ICU medical and nursing staff must anticipate acute complications of SCI and in certain cases play an active role in the prevention of intermediate and long-term complications. A systems approach must be taken, with consideration of complications in the respiratory, cardiovascular, gastrointestinal, genitourinary, and integumentary systems. In addition, the ICU medical and nursing staff must be vigilant regarding delayed neurological worsening, which in most instances requires prompt assessment and treatment by the neurosurgeon. Psychiatric sequelae are also common, with suicide rates 10 times higher in SCI survivors than in age-matched peers.[64] However, these are not discussed in detail in this chapter.

RESPIRATORY MANAGEMENT

Respiratory management consists of airway and ventilator management and diagnosis and treatment of respiratory complications.

Airway

In many instances the patient arrives in the ICU already intubated. However, if this is not the case, the adequacy of the airway must frequently be assessed. Patients who are conversant, without hoarseness or stridor, typically have unobstructed airways. However, many patients with acute SCI also have closed head injuries and associated depressed level of consciousness. If this is the case, the threshold for intubation should be quite low. These patients have an increased risk of regurgitation of stomach contents and aspiration pneumonitis, compounded by gastrointestinal paresis, which develops soon after injury.[33] A variety of techniques for intubation may be used; the goals of these techniques are prevention of neck manipulation and prevention of gastric content aspiration. One acceptable choice is topical local anesthesia followed by blind or fiberoptic-assisted nasotracheal intubation (although prolonged nasotracheal intubation is inadvisable because of higher risks of sinus infections).

Alternatively, rapid-sequence intubation can be attempted, using a short-acting induction agent such as a barbiturate and a neuromuscular blocking agent with cricoid pressure application, with or without fiberoptic assistance. Neither method is conclusively associated with more or less manipulation of the neck or risk of neurological morbidity.[57,72] One special note must be made regarding succinylcholine. This depolarizing muscle relaxant has been shown to cause a massive release of skeletal muscle potassium after SCI.[14,68,70] Such a potassium release has caused cardiac arrest in some SCI patients. This response is believed to be caused by denervation as a result of the proliferation of extrajunctional acetylcholine receptors at the motor endplate.[14,68,70] This response may last at least 3 to 6 months and might be present as early as 48 hours after injury. As such, except in the initial 48 hour period after SCI, nondepolarizing neuromuscular blockers are not recommended.

Ventilation

After intubation or ensuring that the patient's airway is protected, the adequacy of ventilation must be assessed. Tachypnea, cyanosis, and use of accessory muscles are all signs of respiratory failure. Continuous pulse oximetry should be employed and arterial blood gases determined to rule out hypercarbia and hypoxemia.

Patients with high cervical lesions have significant mechanical respiratory dysfunction. Lesions at C4 and above cause rapid respiratory failure unless immediate resuscitation is started. After such an SCI, only the muscles innervated by the spinal accessory cranial nerves can function (sternocleidomastoid and trapezius), with dysfunction of the abdominal and intercostal muscles and diaphragm. Paradoxical abdominal movement with inspiratory inward displacement of the abdomen signals the presence of diaphragmatic dysfunction.[56] In addition to insufficient vital capacities, respiratory muscle dysfunction results in inadequate cough and therefore inadequate ability to clear respiratory secretions. Lung volumes are further diminished in the recumbent position as a result of the cephalad displacement of the diaphragm by the weight of the abdominal contents. As a result of these factors, patients with high cervical SCI typically require prolonged mechanical ventilation to prevent hypoxia, hypercarbia, and atelectasis. There is general agreement that positive pressure ventilation is required when Po_2 is less than 55 mm Hg on 50% oxygen, if Pco_2 is greater than 45, or if respiratory rate is greater that 35.[3,65] One assessment tool that can be used to monitor the awake, cooperative patient is serial measurement of vital capacity. Vital capacity is the amount of gas that can be expired after maximal inspiration and includes tidal volume and inspiratory and expiratory reserve volumes. In a patient who is previously ventilating well without mechanical assistance, a drop in vital capacity to less than 10 to 15 ml/kg should raise a red flag that the patient is beginning to tire and might require mechanical ventilation.[65]

The type of mechanical ventilation varies depending on each patient and his or her level of consciousness. Assist control or intermittent mandatory ventilation is required in the patient with minimal respiratory effort. These ventilator settings can be programmed to deliver full-minute ventilation. Other patients with adequate respiratory effort who fatigue easily (as manifested by increasing respiratory rate and decreasing tidal volume) might tolerate support ventilation such as intermittent mandatory ventilation at a low rate or pressure support.[3] In any event, patients with high cervical SCI should be considered for early tracheostomy.

Patients with cervical cord lesions below C4 with maintained diaphragmatic activity can still suffer significant respiratory compromise. Intercostal muscles, supplied by T1-T12, and abdominal muscles, supplied by T7-L1, are paralyzed, resulting in inspiratory and expiratory muscle weakness. Total lung capacities are reduced up to 25% and vital capacity is reduced up to 55%, with expiratory reserve volume reduced up to 80% during the acute phase of the injury.[3] The patient's position might affect ventilation as well. Patients who are well ventilated while supine might desaturate and become tachypneic when sitting. When upright, in contrast to the accessory respiratory muscles, the hemidiaphragms are at a disadvantageous position.[10]

Vital capacity begins to improve as early as 3 to 5 days after SCI, with rapid improvement in the initial month and then gradual improvement over the subsequent 6 months.[37] This is likely a result of the transition from chest wall flaccidity to spasticity, which decreases paradoxical chest wall movement.[10]

Patients with lower cervical cord injuries or thoracic or lumbar cord injuries do not typically require mechanical ventilation, unless for associated chest trauma, pulmonary edema, pneumonia, or acute respiratory distress syndrome (ARDS). However, patients with lower cervical or upper or lower thoracic SCI still are at increased risk of pneumonia because of impaired cough and clearance of respiratory secretions.[52]

Weaning patients off the ventilator is a complex problem that merits a chapter of its own. In general, in SCI patients the following criteria assist the intensive care physician in deciding if a patient is ready to wean[47]: vital capacity greater than 10 ml/kg, tidal volume greater than 5 ml/kg, peak inspiratory pressure greater than 20 cm H_2O, and respiratory rate less than 30 breaths/min. Weaning the SCI patient can be accomplished by leaving the patient off the ventilator for increasing periods of time, for example, of a T-piece, or by decreasing the rate of intermittent mandatory ventilation.[65]

Respiratory Complications

Pulmonary complications are the most common cause of morbidity and mortality after acute SCI.[7,65] The most frequent complications include neurogenic pulmonary edema, deep vein thrombosis/pulmonary embolism, and pneumonia.

Neurogenic Pulmonary Edema

Neurogenic pulmonary edema is seen in up to 44% of SCI patients after resuscitation of spinal shock.[58] It is characterized by a rapidly developing pulmonary edema, with protein levels in the air spaces approaching that found in the plasma. The mechanism might involve increased pulmonary capillary leak, resulting from increased sympathetic activity.[58,75]

Patients with this condition present with hypoxia and large amounts of foamy endotracheal secretions. The goal of management is to treat the underlying pulmonary edema without permitting hypotension while maintaining adequate oxygenation and ventilation. Treatment usually includes urgent endotracheal intubation, pulmonary toilet (with or without bronchoscopy), positive end–expiratory pressure to open collapsed airways, and diuresis, guided by central venous pressure monitoring or pulmonary capillary wedge pressure monitoring by Swan-Ganz catheterization.

Deep Vein Thrombosis/Pulmonary Embolism

Pulmonary embolism is one of the most common causes of death after spinal cord injury.[17,30,76,81] In a large multicenter review of more than 1400 SCI patients, a 15% incidence of clinically recognized deep vein thrombosis (DVT) and 5% rate of clinically recognized pulmonary embolus (PE) was found.[81] The rate of non–clinically recognized DVT may be more than 67%.[30] Although the risk is clearly greater during the acute phase, the risk continues through the rehabilitation phase up to at least 3 months after injury.[11,41,46] Because of these dramatically high incidences, The American College of Chest Physicians has recommended that all patients with acute SCI be treated with low-molecular-weight heparin prophylaxis.[28] Intermittent pneumatic compression of the calf has not been shown to be as effective in prevention of DVT,[35] and low-molecular-weight heparin is more effective than unfractionated heparin.[31,34] After the acute phase, the patients may be converted from low-molecular-weight heparin to oral anticoagulation with warfarin (Coumadin), although this has not been studied in detail.[28]

Because of the lack of sensation below the level of injury, the ICU medical and nursing staff must be particularly vigilant for the onset of the signs of DVT, including unexplained fever, leg edema and increase in leg circumference, redness, and increase in skin temperature. A low index of suspicion should be maintained and Doppler ultrasonography obtained rapidly when the condition is suspected. Treatment of proximal DVT, with full anticoagulation and placement of an inferior vena cava filter, must be instituted promptly to minimize the risk of embolization and PE.

Because of the SCI, the patient with PE may not present with typical chest pain. Tachycardia, tachypnea, desaturation, abrupt changes in arterial blood gases, and typical electrocardiogram changes should all raise the suspicion of PE. Other possible signs include hemoptysis, cyanosis, hypotension, loud S2 or S3, or S4 gallop. After a high-probability ventilation-perfusion scan or positive pulmonary angiography, full anticoagulation should be commenced to prevent extension of the thrombus/embolus.

Pneumonia

As discussed previously, patients with acute cervical SCI are at significantly increased risk for developing pneumonia as a result of loss of lung volumes (atelectasis), inability to cough and clear secretions, prolonged intubation, and immobility. Pneumonia is a frequent complication and cause of death, affecting 5% to 20% of all cervical SCI patients during the initial hospital admission.[18,29] Like DVT/PE, early measures to prevent the condition are indicated, with positive end–expiratory pressure to minimize atelectasis, aggressive chest physiotherapy, and sterile endotracheal suctioning. In the early phase, insertion of a nasogastric tube and suction of stomach contents are indicated because of gastric atony.[33] It should be mentioned that endotracheal suctioning may, in rare cases, cause significant bradycardia, a side effect that can be attenuated by adequate preoxygenation.[3,55] In addition, ventilatory muscle training and frequent sighs have been advocated as measures to prevent pneumonia.[25,26]

Pneumonia in SCI patients shows a preponderance to the left lower lobe,[72] likely as a result of the more acute angle of the left mainstem bronchus. Fever, leukocytosis, and purulent sputum are the common findings in SCI patients with pneumonia, with few developing any symptoms, such as cough, because of the paralysis of respiratory muscles.[59]

CARDIOVASCULAR MANAGEMENT

After initial resuscitation and management of any ongoing causes of hemorrhagic shock, many SCI patients continue to have hypotension. Up to 68% of cervical SCI patients are hypotensive (two consecutive systolic blood pressure measurements of less than 90 mm Hg) in the acute phase.[48] This ongoing hypotension has variously been described as spinal shock or neurogenic shock. The pathophysiology can be attributed to loss of supraspinal regulatory control, reduced sympathetic activity, and peripheral α-adrenoceptor hyperresponsiveness.[74]

There are many experimental laboratory studies suggesting that blood pressure elevation improves spinal cord blood flow,[19-21,36] but so far no human studies have demonstrated an outcome benefit from aggressive management of blood pressure in the acute phase, including in the ICU. However, it is generally accepted that systolic pressures lower than 90 mm Hg should be treated aggressively, with crystalloid fluid resuscitation and, if necessary, with inotropic support. One group advocates aggressive management of blood pressure, with routine Swan-Ganz catheterization and fluid loading and inotropic support based on systemic vascular resistance indices and cardiac index.[50]

In addition to neurogenic shock, many patients, up to 71%, suffer from bradycardia, with 20% requiring inotropic support to maintain systolic pressures.[63,84]

GASTROINTESTINAL MANAGEMENT

Patients with spinal cord injuries frequently encounter sequelae pertaining to the gastrointestinal (GI) system, the two most frequent being alteration in gastrointestinal motility and stress ulcer/gastrointestinal hemorrhage. Preventative measures can be taken in the ICU to address these potentially life-threatening complications.

Decreased motility is seen in all trauma patients, and SCI patients in particular. Nasogastric tube insertion and suction of stomach contents and secretions should be undertaken as soon as possible. Once suctioned amounts begin to fall, indicating returning motility, enteral nutrition can be slowly introduced.

It is estimated that the incidence of GI ulceration or hemorrhage in the spinal cord injury population is between 2% and 20%.[1] Harvey Cushing, in 1932,[15] reported 11 cases of GI ulceration or perforation, or hemorrhage, associated with neurological disease, and these ulcers have subsequently borne his name, Cushing's ulcers. Many have proposed a neurogenic basis for this significant complication, with persistent vagal activity unopposed by sympathetic outflow.[2] Patients with cervical spine injures, as opposed to thoracolumbar injuries, are more prone to ulceration/hemorrhage.[2,42,69,80] The most common time course for bleeding is within the first month after injury, and within this time it appears that the first 10 days are the most susceptible period.[33,49,80]

The optimal management for the prevention of GI ulceration/hemorrhage is under debate. It is not known which agent is best or what dosing schedule for the existing agents provides maximal benefit. Antacids have long been the mainstay of preventative therapy. Several older studies have shown that hypersecretion of gastric acid is associated with ulceration in the neurosurgical patient.[4,15,40,60,82] Raising the pH to 4 recently has been shown to decrease the incidence of GI hemorrhage.[8] Agents such as magnesium hydroxide, aluminum, or aluminum-magnesium mixtures are options in raising gastric pH by direct neutralization of acid. Given in the high doses and frequency (e.g., q4-6h) necessary to elevate pH in the critically ill patients, some side effects may be seen, including diarrhea, constipation, hypophosphatemia (these agents bind phosphate), and metabolic alkalosis.

Numerous studies have been performed on antacids for ulcer/hemorrhage prophylaxis, and large metaanalyses, specifically in critical care patients, have demonstrated that antacid therapy is safe and efficacious.[13,79]

Histamine receptor antagonists (cimetidine, ranitidine, and famotidine) have also been studied extensively as prophylactic agents in critical care patients. The reversible inhibition of parietal cell histamine receptors (type 2) is the mechanism of reduced acid secretion. Numerous studies have demonstrated that these histamine antagonists decrease the rate of GI hemorrhage in critical care patients compared with placebo.[3] Whether or not these agents are more effective in prophylaxis remains controversial.[85]

A third type of agent to be considered is sucralfate, which is a combination of sucrose, sulfate, and aluminum hydroxide. It exerts a protective benefit by binding to gastric mucosa, increasing its hydrophobicity, as well as increasing the viscosity of the gastric mucus.[67,85] One study found that sucralfate (1g PO/NG q6h) was more effective than ranitidine (50 mg IV q6h) in preventing GI ulceration in ICU patients, including those with central nervous system (CNS) injuries.[23] Two metaanalyses showed no difference between sucralfate and antacids but a significant benefit of both over histamine blockers.[78,79]

There has been some debate concerning possible increased incidence of nosocomial pneumonia with the use of pH-altering ulcer prophylaxis. This effect is likely secondary to an increase in oropharyngeal and stomach bacterial colonizations as pH levels rise.[12,22] Several studies have demonstrated no difference among the antacids, histamine blockers, and sucralfate,[27,53,62] although two metaanalyses have shown a modestly decreased incidence of pneumonia with sucralfate.[13,79]

Enteral nutrition may play a role in prevention of stress ulceration compared with parenteral nutrition. One retrospective study showed that SCI patients who are fed enterally have a significantly lower incidence of ulceration,[44] although there is a study that showed no difference.[6] In general, if enteral nutrition is possible in the ICU, it is preferable to parenteral nutrition.

GENITOURINARY MANAGEMENT

Initially after acute SCI the bladder is hypotonic. As the acute phase passes, the type of neurogenic bladder that develops depends on the level of the injury. Lesions rostral to the sacral spinal cord typically produce a hypertonic bladder.[1,71,77] Poor coordination between the detrusor and the urinary sphincter results in incomplete emptying, which can result in progressively increasing urinary volumes.[1,71,77] This can result in autonomic dysreflexia, a life-threatening condition associated with lack of central inhibition of sympathetic outflow, in response to a stimulus such as bladder distention. Symptoms include sweating, headache, hypertension, and bradycardia. However, in the ICU, where almost all SCI patients are catheterized or undergo intermittent catheterization, this is not usually a concern.

Bacteriuria is almost universal in SCI patients. When fever is present in the ICU patient, urinary infection must be ruled out.[59]

INTEGUMENTARY MANAGEMENT

Decubitus ulcers are a major problem in SCI patients, and prevention is the mainstay of treatment. With immobility, low blood pressure, and decreased skin perfusion, SCI patients can develop ulcers on a rigid spine board in less than 6 hours.[17,74] ICUs should have a standard protocol that includes turning the patients (with the safety of the spine in mind), air flotation beds, and frequent inspection of likely afflicted areas, such as the sacrum, greater trochanter, ischial tuberosities, lateral malleoli, and heels.

CONCLUSION

Advances in critical care techniques have greatly reduced the morbidity and mortality from spinal cord injury. The ICU medical and nursing staff must take a systems approach to the management of these patients and must carefully consider prophylactic measures that can be taken, as well as be attentive for the numerous complications that might develop.

REFERENCES

1. Abdel-Azim M, Sullivan M, Yalla SV: Disorders of bladder function in spinal cord disease, **Neurol Clin 9**:727-740, 1991.
2. Albert TJ, Levine MJ, Balderston RA, et al: Gastrointestinal complications in spinal cord injury, **Spine 16**:S522-S525, 1991.
3. Borel CO, Guy J: Ventilatory management in critical neurologic illness, **Neurol Clin 13(3)**:627-644, 1995.
4. Bowen JC, Fleming WH, Thompson JC: Increased gastrin release following penetrating central nervous system injury, **Surgery 75**:720-724, 1974.
5. Bracken MB, Freeman DH, Hellenbrand K: Incidence of acute traumatic hospitalized spinal cord injury in the United States, 1970-77, **Am J Epidemiol 113**:615-622, 1981.
6. Cannon LA, Heiselman DE, Gardner WG, et al: Prophylaxis of upper gastrointestinal tract bleeding in mechanically ventilated patients: a randomized study comparing the efficacy of sucralfate, cimetidine, and antacids, **Arch Intern Med 147**:2101-6, 1987.
7. Carter RE: Respiratory aspects of spinal cord injury management, **Paraplegia 25**:262-266, 1987.
8. Chan K, Lai ECS, Tuen H, et al: Prospective double-blind placebo-controlled randomized trial on the use of ranitidine in preventing postoperative gastroduodenal complications in high-risk neurosurgical patients, **J Neurosurg 82**:413-417, 1995.
9. Chan K, Mann KS, Lai ECS, et al: Factors influencing the development of gastrointestinal complications after neurosurgery: results of multivariate analysis, **Neurosurgery 25**:378-382, 1989.
10. Chen CF, Lien IN, Wu MC: Respiratory function in patients with spinal cord injuries: effects of posture, **Paraplegia 28**:81-86, 1990.
11. Colachis SC, Clinchot DM: The association between deep venous thrombosis and heterotopic ossification in patients with acute traumatic spinal cord injury, **Paraplegia 31**:507-512, 1993.
12. Cook DJ, Laine LA, Guyatt GH, et al: Nosocomial pneumonia and the role of gastric pH: a meta-analysis, **Chest 100**:7-13, 1991.
13. Cook DJ, Witt LG, Cook RJ, et al: Stress ulcer prophylaxis in the critically ill: A meta-analysis, **Am J Med 91**:519-527, 1991.
14. Cooperman LH, Strobel GE, Kennell EM: Massive hyperkalemia after administration of succinylcholine, **Anesthesiology 32**:161-167, 1970.
15. Cushing H: Peptic ulcers and the interbrain. **Surg Gynecol Obstet 55**:1-34, 1932.
16. DeVivo MJ: Causes and cost of spinal cord injury in the United States, **Spinal Cord 35**:809-813, 1997.
17. DeVivo MJ, Black KJ, Stover SL: Causes of death during the first 12 years after spinal cord injury, **Arch Phys Med Rehabil 74**:248-254, 1993.
18. DeVivo MJ, Kartus PL, Stover SL, et al: Cause of death for patients with spinal cord injuries, **Arch Intern Med 149**:1761-1766, 1989.
19. Ducker TB, Salcman M, Daniell HB: Experimental spinal cord trauma, III: therapeutic effect of immobilization and pharmacologic agents, **Surg Neurol 10**:71-76, 1978.
20. Ducker TB, Salcman M, Lucas JT, et al: Experimental spinal cord trauma, II: blood flow, tissue oxygen, evoked potentials in both paretic and plegic monkeys, **Surg Neurol 10**:64-70, 1978.
21. Ducker TB, Salcman M, Perot PL, et al: Experimental spinal cord trauma, I: correlation of blood flow, tissue oxygen and neurologic status in the dog, **Surg Neurol 10**:60-63, 1978.
22. du Moulin GC, Paterson DG, Hedley-Whyte J, et al: Aspiration of gastric bacteria in antacid-treated patients: a

frequent cause of postoperative colonization of the airway, **Lancet 1:**242-245, 1982.
23. Eddleston JM, Vohra A, Scott P, et al: A comparison of the frequency of stress ulceration and secondary pneumonia in sucralfate or ranitidine treated intensive care unit patients, **Crit Care Med 19:**1491-1496, 1991.
24. Epstein N, Hood DC, Ransohoff J: Gastrointestinal bleeding in patients with spinal cord trauma: Effects of steroids, cimetidine, and mini-dose heparin, **J Neurosurg 54:**16-20, 1981.
25. Estenne M, De Troyer A: Cough in tetraplegic subjects: an active process, **Ann Intern Med 112:**22-28, 1990.
26. Estenne M, Knoop C, Vanaerenbergh J, et al: The effect of pectoralis muscle training in tetraplegic subjects, **Am Rev Respir Dis 139:**1218-1222, 1989.
27. Fabian TC, Boucher BA, Croce MA, et al: Pneumonia and stress ulceration in severely injured patients: a prospective evaluation of the effects of stress ulcer prophylaxis, **Arch Surg 128:**185-191, 1993.
28. Fifth ACCP Consensus Conference on Antithrombotic Therapy, **Chest 114(5):**S542-543, 1998.
29. Fishburn MJ, Marino RJ, Ditunno JF: Atelectasis and pneumonia in acute spinal cord injury, **Arch Phys Med Rehabil 71:**197-200, 1990.
30. Geerts WH, Code KI, Jay RM, et al: A prospective study of venous thromboembolism after major trauma, **N Engl J Med 331:**1601-1606, 1994.
31. Geerts WH, Jay RM, Code KI, et al: A comparison of low-dose heparin with low-molecular-weight heparin as prophylaxis against venous thromboembolism after major trauma, **N Engl J Med 335:**701-707, 1996.
32. Geisler WO, Jousse AT, Wynne-Jones M, et al: Survival in traumatic spinal cord injury, **Paraplegia 21:**364-373, 1983.
33. Gore RM, Mintzer RA, Calenoff L: Gastrointestinal complications of spinal cord injury, **Spine 6:**538-544, 1981.
34. Green D, Lee MY, Lim AC, et al: Prevention of thromboembolism after spinal cord injury using low-molecular weight heparin, **Ann Intern Med 113:**571-574, 1990.
35. Green D, Rossi EC, Yao JST, et al: Deep vein thrombosis in spinal cord injury: effect of prophylaxis with calf compression, aspirin, and dipyridamole, **Paraplegia 20:**227-233, 1982.
36. Guha A, Tator CH: Acute cardiovascular effects of experimental spinal cord injury, **J Trauma 28:**481-490, 1988.
37. Haas F, Axen K, Pineda H, et al: Temporal pulmonary function changes in cervical cord injury, **Arch Phys Med Rehabil 66:**139-144, 1985.
38. Heinemann AW, Yarkony GM, Roth EJ, et al: Functional outcome following spinal cord injury: a comparison of specialized spinal cord injury center vs general hospital short-term care, **Arch Neurol 46:**1098-1102, 1989.
39. Kalsbeek WD, McLaurin RL, Harris BSH, et al: The National Head and Spinal Cord Injury Survey: major findings, **J Neurosurg (suppl):**S19-31, 1980.
40. Kamada T, Fusamoto H, Kawano S, et al: Gastrointestinal bleeding following head injury: a clinical study of 433 cases, **J Trauma 17:**44-47, 1977.
41. Kim SW, Charallel JT, Park KW, et al: Prevalence of deep venous thrombosis in patients with chronic spinal cord injury, **Arch Phys Med Rehabil 75:**965-968, 1994.
42. Kiwerski J: Bleeding from the alimentary canal during management of spinal cord injury patients, **Paraplegia 24:**92-96, 1986.
43. Knutsdottir S: Spinal cord injuries in Iceland 1973-1989. A follow up study, **Paraplegia 31:**68-72, 1993.
44. Kuric J, Lucas CE, Ledgerwood AM, et al: Nutritional support: a prophylaxis against stress bleeding after spinal cord injury, **Paraplegia 27:**140-145, 1989.
45. LaCroix J, Infante-Rivard C, Jenicek M, et al: Prophylaxis of upper gastrointestinal bleeding in intensive care units: a meta-analysis, **Crit Care Med 17:**862-869, 1989.
46. Lamb GC, Tomski MA, Kaufman J, et al: Is chronic spinal cord injury associated with increased risk of venous thromboembolism? **J Am Paraplegia Soc 16:**153-156, 1993.
47. Lamid S, Ragalie GF, Welton K: Respirator-dependent quadriplegics: problems during the weaning period, **J Am Paraplegia Soc 8:**33-37, 1985.
48. Lehmann KG, Lane JG, Piepmeier JM, et al: Cardiovascular abnormalities accompanying acute spinal cord injuries in humans: incidence, time course and severity, **J Am Coll Cardiol 10:**46-52, 1986.
49. Leramo OB, Tator CH, Hudson AR: Massive gastroduodenal hemorrhage and perforation in acute spinal cord injury, **Surg Neurol 17:**186-190, 1982.
50. Levi L, Wolf A, Belzberg H: Hemodynamic parameters in patients with acute cervical cord trauma: description, intervention, and prediction of outcome, **Neurosurgery 33(6):**1007-1017, 1993.
51. Levine BA, Sirinek KR, McLeod CG, et al: The role of cimetidine in the prevention of stress-induced gastric mucosal injury, **Surg Gynecol Obstet 148:**399-402, 1979.
52. Luce JM: Medical management of spinal cord injury, **Crit Care Med 13:**126-131, 1985.
53. Martin LF, Booth FVM, Karlstadt RG, et al: Continuous intravenous cimetidine decreased stress-related upper gastrointestinal hemorrhage without promoting pneumonia, **Crit Care Med 21:**19-30, 1993.
54. Martins F, Freitas F, Martins L, et al: Spinal cord injuries—epidemiology in Portugal's central region, **Spinal Cord 36:**574-578, 1998.
55. Mathias CJ: Bradycardia and cardiac arrest during tracheal suction—mechanisms in tetraplegic patients, **Eur J Int Care Med 2:**147-156, 1976.
56. McMichan JC, Michel L, Westbrook PR: Pulmonary dysfunction following traumatic quadriplegia: recognition, prevention, and treatment, **JAMA 243:**528-531, 1980.
57. Meschino A, Devitt JH, Kock JP, et al: The safety of awake tracheal intubation in cervical spine injury, **Can J Anaesth 39:**114-117, 1992.
58. Meyer GA, Berman IR, Doty IB, et al: Hemodynamic responses to acute quadriplegia with or without chest trauma, **J Neurosurg 34:**168, 1971.
59. Montgomerie JZ: Infections in patients with spinal cord injuries, **Clin Inf Dis 25:**1285-1292, 1997.
60. Norton L, Greer J, Eiseman B: Gastric secretory response to head injury, **Arch Surg 101:**200-204, 1970.
61. Peura DA, Johnson LF: Cimetidine for prevention and treatment of gastroduodenal mucosal lesions in patients in an intensive care unit, **Ann Intern Med 103:**173-177, 1985.
62. Pickworth KK, Falcone RE, Hoogeboom JE, et al: Occurrence of nosocomial pneumonia in mechanically venti-

lated trauma patients; a comparison of sucralfate and ranitidine, **Crit Care Med 21:**1856-1862, 1993.
63. Piepmeier JM, Lehmann KM, Lane JG: Cardiovascular instability following acute cervical spinal cord trauma, **Cent Nerv Syst Trauma 2:**153-160, 1985.
64. Rish BL, Dilustro JF, Salazar AM, et al: Spinal cord injury: a 25-year morbidity and mortality study, **Mil Med 162:**141-148, 1997.
65. Schmitt J, Midha M, McKenzie N: Medical complications of spinal cord disease, **Neurol Clin 9:**779-795, 1991
66. Shuman RB, Schuster DP, Zuckerman GR: Prophylactic therapy for stress ulcer bleeding: a reappraisal, **Ann Intern Med 106:**562-567, 1987.
67. Slomiany BL, Piotrowski J, Okazaki K, et al: Nature of the enhancement of the protective qualities of gastric mucus by sucralfate, **Digestion 44:**222-231, 1989.
68. Smith RB, Grenvik A: Cardiac arrest following succinylcholine administration in patients with central nervous system injuries, **Anesthesiology 33:**558-560, 1970.
69. Soderstrom CA, Ducker TB: Increased susceptibility of patients with cervical cord lesions to peptic gastrointestinal complications, **J Trauma 25:**1030-1038, 1985.
70. Stone WA, Beach TP, Hamelburg W: Succinylcholine—danger in the spinal-cord-injured patient, **Anesthesiology 32:**168-169, 1970.
71. Stover SL, Lloyd LK, Waites KB, et al: Neurogenic urinary tract infection, **Neurol Clin 9:**741-755, 1991.
72. Suderman VS, Crosby ET, Lui A: Elective oral tracheal intubation in the cervical spine-injured adult, **Can J Anaesth 38:**785-789, 1991.
73. Sugarman B: Atelectasis in spinal cord injured people after initial medical stabilization, **J Am Paraplegia Soc 8:**47-50, 1985.
74. Teasell RW, Arnold JM, Krassioukov A, et al: Cardiovascular consequences of loss of supraspinal control of the sympathetic nervous system after spinal cord injury, **Arc Phys Med Rehabil 81:**506-516, 2000.
75. Theodore J, Robin ED: Speculations on neurogenic pulmonary edema (NPE), **Am Rev Respir Dis 113:**405-411, 1976.
76. Tribe CR: Causes of death in the early and late stages of paraplegia, **Paraplegia 1:**19-47, 1963.
77. Trop CS, Bennett CJ: Autonomic dysreflexia and its urological implications: a review, **J Urol 146:**1461-1469, 1991.
78. Tryba M: Prophylaxis of stress ulcer bleeding. A meta-analysis, **J Clin Gastroenterol 13(Suppl 2):**S44-S55, 1991.
79. Tryba M: Sucralfate versus antacid or H2-antagonists for stress ulcer prophylaxis: a meta-analysis on efficacy and pneumonia rate, **Crit Care Med 19:**942-949, 1991.
80. Walters K, Silver JR: Gastrointestinal bleeding in patients with acute spinal injuries, **Int Rehabil Med 8:**44-47, 1986.
81. Waring WP, Karunas RS: Acute spinal cord injuries and the incidence of clinically occurring thromboembolic disease, **Paraplegia 29:**8-16, 1991.
82. Watts CC, Clark K: Gastric acidity in the comatose patient, **J Neurosurg 30:**107-109, 1969.
83. Wilkins RH (ed): The Edwin Smith surgical papyrus, in **Neurosurgical Classics.** Park Ridge, IL: American Association of Neurological Surgeons, 1992, pp 1-5.
84. Winslow EB, Lesch M, Talano JV, et al: Spinal cord injuries associated with cardiopulmonary complications, **Spine 11:**809-812, 1986.
85. Lu WY, Rhoney DH, Boling WB, et al: A review of stress ulcer prophylaxis in the neurosurgical intensive care unit, **Neurosurgery 41:**416-425, 1997.

CHAPTER 11

Multisystem Injury Management

ROBERT MACKERSIE
ANDRE CAMPBELL
BRIAN T. ANDREWS

The intensive care management of complex, multisystem injury poses a challenge for even the most experienced clinician. For purposes of discussion in this textbook, multisystem trauma is considered in the context of concomitant traumatic brain injury (TBI) and/or spinal cord injury (SCI). The combination of neurological injury and abdominal, chest, or pelvic trauma often creates a particularly difficult situation in which the synergistic effects of shock, hypoxia, and ongoing hemorrhage may profoundly worsen the outcome from the injured brain or spinal cord. For this reason, the margin of therapeutic error in the initial management of these patients is small, and close attention to detail becomes of paramount importance.

The intensive care management of trauma patients begins in the emergency department during the initial resuscitation. The classic prioritization reflected by the mnemonic "ABC" (airway, breathing, circulation) recognizes the importance of proper treatment sequencing and the interdependence of the cardiopulmonary systems during acute critical injury. This organized approach is well described in the advanced trauma life support course sponsored by the American College of Surgeons, which has become a standard educational tool for physicians involved in the early management of major trauma. During the resuscitation phase, cardiopulmonary homeostasis is restored, the initial therapy for the injured brain or spinal cord begun, and the diagnosis of potential life- and limb-threatening injuries undertaken.

Ongoing resuscitation may extend to the operating room and/or the intensive care unit. Defining endpoints to resuscitation and establishing monitoring appropriate to these endpoints (discussed later in this chapter) typically compose the early management of the patient in the ICU. Once resuscitation is completed, the focus in the ICU typically turns to the monitoring and prevention of postinjury complications, including secondary neurological injury. The following discussion considers the intensive care management of the poly-trauma patient with associated neurological injury in the resuscitation, operative, and ICU phases of care.

RESUSCITATIVE PHASE

Airway and Breathing

Establishing a protected airway remains a priority in all forms of resuscitation to prevent cellular death resulting from inadequate oxygenation. For trauma, the additional precaution to this priority is cervical spine (c-spine) immobilization. Assessment begins by determining if there is airway obstruction. Partial obstruction is indicated by sonorous or gurgling upper airway sounds. Complete obstruction, on the other hand, is indicated by the lack of air movement. Patient attempts at breathing against this obstruction manifest with intercostal chest wall retraction and tracheal tugging. Obstruction may be due to extrinsic causes such as foreign bodies, hemorrhage, or emesis. With the loss of consciousness and the loss of muscle tone the tongue becomes a potential obstructing structure to the airway, which can be relieved with a jaw thrust lift maneuver. Edema of the oropharyngeal and laryngeal structures from neck and facial trauma or retrotracheal hemorrhage caused by cervical spinal injury may obstruct the airway.

If simple jaw thrust or oral- or nasopharyngeal airway devices do not provide relief of airway obstruction, intubation is indicated to establish a protected airway. Intubation is also indicated for respiratory failure or for airway protection in the setting of altered consciousness. Potential for airway risks in the immediate future, such as facial and laryngeal edema from thermal injury, is an indication for semi-elective intubation. This potentially avoids a difficult and possibly traumatic intubation and the need for an alternate surgical airway.

Respiratory insufficiency or failure can be classified as either a ventilatory or oxygenation problem. Ventilatory failure may be due to neurological injury or a mechanical failure within the thorax such as a hemo- or pneumothorax. Carbon dioxide retention is typically followed by hypoxemia. Hypoxemia may be corrected initially with supplemental oxygen, but the ventilatory failure cannot be corrected without mechanical ventilation. Oxygenation failure can be defined by an arterial Po_2 less than 60 mm Hg or an oxygen saturation less than or equal to 90% or by an A-a gradient. The differential diagnoses for hypoxemic failure include ventilatory insufficiency, diffusion/gas exchange abnormality (edema), ventilation-perfusion (V/Q) mismatch, increased pulmonary shunt (pulmonary contusion), and poor cardiac output (shock).

If time permits, assessment of the airway should include considerations for past medical history of difficult intubation, comorbid diseases, medications, and drug and alcohol history. Existing traumatic injuries such as c-spine fracture or facial and basal skull fractures have implications for a physically difficult airway. Poor thyromental distance, dentition, jaw opening, and a receding mandible should be noted so that the need for special equipment and personnel can be anticipated.

Endotracheal intubation is reviewed fully in Chapter 1. The preferred route of emergency intubation is orotracheal. This can be performed rapidly, safely, and reliably with in-line stabilization of the neck. Intubation should be preceded by preoxygenation, cricoid pressure, administration of anesthetic and chemical paralysis, and rapid sequence induction. The need for anesthesia is to avoid the reflex increase in intracranial pressure that occurs with the stimulus of intubation. Nasotracheal intubation, on the other hand, is not as successful or safe. Intubation in the case of c-spine and craniofacial fractures can be done by bronchoscopy if time permits. If orotracheal intubation has failed (after three experienced attempts) or is not possible because of injury, then cricothyroidotomy is the only practical choice.

Reestablishing Perfusion: The Treatment of Shock States

The definition of shock is based on poor tissue perfusion or the lack of it. Poor perfusion may be present despite normal blood pressure. Cell dysfunction and death occur when the supply of oxygen and nutrients does not meet tissue demand. Effective tissue perfusion is either the result of a reduction in cardiac output, microvascular maldistribution of blood flow, or a defect in the substrate use at the cellular level. Multiple organ dysfunction and ultimately death may be the complications without proper intervention.

There are four major categories of shock: hypovolemic, cardiogenic, extracardiac, obstructive, and distributive. Historically, hemorrhage from trauma was the first type of hypovolemic shock to be recognized and remains the common cause of death for multiple trauma patients under 45 years of age. Cardiogenic shock is more commonly recognized in the older population as a result of myocardial ischemia but may occur as the manifestation of traumatic cardiac contusion or valve disruption. Extracardiac obstruction includes tension pneumothorax and pericardial tamponade. Spinal cord trauma results in distributive shock as a result of peripheral vasodilation.

In textbooks, clinical manifestations of hypovolemic shock are frequently graded regarding severity of intravascular volume loss but should not necessarily be used as a stringent guide to diagnosis and therapy. Minimal blood loss of less than 10% to 15% frequently demonstrates no changes in vital signs in healthy patients. A loss of 20% to 30% will manifest with an increase in heart rate, orthostatic hypotension, and mental status changes such as agitation and confusion.[3]

As blood volume decreases by 30% to 40%, hypotension accompanying tachycardia is present. The respiratory rate rises to compensate for increasing metabolic acidosis from greater tissue ischemia. Low urine output, as well as pale, cool, and clammy skin, is another manifestation of poor organ perfusion. A blood loss greater than 40% is most severe and means almost certain death.[3]

Hemodynamic responses to blood loss are different in children and the elderly. Children have the ability to maintain blood pressure for a long time. Therefore hypotension may present very late with ongoing tachycardia that may be mistakenly attributed to pain and other distress. Internal blood loss must be clinically ruled out. The elderly have compromised reserve, and hypertension is usually normal in this population. Interpretation of a relatively low blood pressure without tachycardia can also be confusing if the patient is taking a beta-blocker for underlying hypertension.

A right-sided heart catheter will suggest a fall in ventricular preload with decreased central venous pressure (CVP) and wedge pressure in hemorrhagic shock. Cardiac output is compromised with compensatory increased systemic vascular resistance (SVR). Because of decreased oxygen delivery and increased metabolic demand, mixed venous oxygen saturation is decreased. SVR depends on vasoconstriction, which in turn is regulated by sympathetic innervation and neuroendocrine hormones. The body's protective mechanism compromises perfusion to the periphery to preserve blood flow to the heart and brain. Kidney perfusion is sacrificed despite the consequence of renal damage and failure. Decreased gut perfusion has multiple complications frequently seen in the "shocky" ICU patient such as ischemic gut, erosive gastritis, and acalculous cholecystitis. Severe hypovolemic and other forms of shock are linked to myocardial depression from decreased coronary perfusion and the release of inflammatory mediators (tumor necrosis factor [TNF], interleukin-1 [IL-1]) that are cardiodepressants. Thus develops a vicious circle of further myocardial depression, decreased contractility leading to decreased ejection fraction, and lower mean arterial pressure.

Cellular injury results from ischemia and accompanying inflammatory reaction that leads to oxygen-free radical production. These free radicals damage cell membranes by inactivating proteins and DNA and upregulating the inflammatory response. Below a critical oxygen delivery level (8-10 ml O_2/min/kg), anaerobic glycolysis provides only inefficient production of adenosine triphosphate (ATP) (2 ATP versus 36 ATP with aerobic glycolysis). The ATP-dependent ion transport proteins are then unable to maintain transmembrane gradients, resulting in intracellular acidosis and lactate production, cell dysfunction or death, and, on a larger scale, organ failure. Serum lactate and base deficit have been used as a predictive marker of outcome and a guide to therapy. Lactate, however, may not be a very reliable indicator in patients with liver disease, thiamine deficiency, alkalosis, or septic conditions that do not necessarily reflect tissue ischemia.

The first priority in the management of any type of shock is maintaining an airway to ensure adequate ventilation and delivery of supplemental oxygenation. At least two large-bore intravenous (IV) lines should be in place for crystalloid administration. Preferably, there should be no injury between the IV access and the heart. Monitoring equipment such as ECG, blood pressure cuff, and oxygen saturation should be in place to gauge responses to therapy. Trendelenburg positioning has no consistent effect on venous return or SVR in any form of shock. Use of inotropic agents before restoring intravascular volume is a dangerous practice. A Swan-Ganz catheter can be a very effective tool to help guide hemodynamic therapy, but it is also important to understand the specific mechanism of effect of inotropic and vasoconstrictive drugs and what the goal effect is.[24]

Blood pressure, central venous pressure, and wedge pressure are inadequate indicators of adequate resuscitation in view of the compensatory mechanisms in young people. Better clinical indicators of end-organ perfusion include adequate urine output, normal heart rate, and normal mental status. Laboratory indicators such as normal or supranormal oxygen delivery and consumption and the correction of lactate and base deficit aid in the measurement of resuscitation endpoints.

Based on the Fick equation, the difference between the arterial and mixed venous oxygen content is a measure of global body oxygen/metabolic demand. In terms of the total body, normal mixed venous saturation is between 65% to 75% and the corresponding oxygen extraction ratio is 25% to 35%. Less than normal mixed saturation or high oxygen extraction ratio indicates supply-dependent oxygen consumption. This inference is not always true. In trauma and sepsis, although the O_2 delivery is high or normal after resuscitation, lactic acidosis (anaerobic metabolism) and organ dysfunction happen in any case A high mixed venous saturation may be a reflection of shunting or altered oxygen metabolism.

Crystalloid Solutions

Normal saline and Ringer's lactate are the mainstays in acute fluid resuscitation. They are least viscous and can be administered cheaply and quickly. These crystalloids primarily fill the interstitial space, replacing the volume lost from the interstitial space to the intravascular space during hemorrhage. These interstitial fluids can result in excessive edema, weight gain, tissue compartment syndromes, decreased chest wall compliance, and pulmonary edema.

Normal saline is isotonic and has a higher pH than Ringer's lactate solution, which has additional bicarbonate, potassium, calcium, and lactate but offers no additional advantage over normal saline. Ringer's lactate is also incompatible with certain drugs and with calcium administration.

There is a growing concern about overhydration with crystalloids, with its attendant complications. Hypertonic saline and colloids offer the advantage of rapid fluid redistribution into the intravascular space with a great deal less volume (one fourth the volume of normal saline).[13] Hemodilution and decreased blood viscosity do occur along with an overall increased venous return. Hypertonic saline (7.5%) may also have cell dehydrating effects, a negative inotropic effect, and an unclear affect on the immune function.[17,37]

Colloid Solutions

The advantage of colloid agents are that they stay in the intravascular space more readily than crystalloid and therefore can more directly increase intravascular volume and assist cardiac output. Colloids include albumin, hetastarch, pentastarch, and dextrans. Albumin has a half life of 16 hours with a plasma expansion effect but usually leaks out into the interstitium, thus having no advantage over crystalloids. Hetastarch and pentastarch are effective volume expanders but have shorter half lives than albumen and have been known to cause anaphylactic reactions, coagulopathy, and increased amylase. Dextran is a larger molecule that promotes fibrinolysis and decreased platelet aggregation. Overall there has been no difference in survival rates with the use of colloid solutions, and they remain very expensive volume expanders in comparison with crystalloids.[31]

Transfusion and Autotransfusion

Transfusion of blood-banked products is still not without significant risks, including viral infection and transfusion reactions. Transfusion reactions include fever, chills, anaphylaxis, hemolysis, and fatal hemorrhage.

Massive shed blood loss can be collected and retransfused to the trauma patient. Blood from a hemothorax is normally depleted of fibrinogen, platelets, and clotting factors and is less likely to be contaminated. The blood can be collected via chest tube into commercially available collection devices attached to a pleurovac system. The reservoir contains sodium citrate. In this situation the unwashed blood cells can be reinfused through a special filter back to the patient without any further anticoagulation.

Blood shed from the repair of spinal, abdominal, or retroperitoneal injuries often contain high levels of particulate matter and clotting factors, so the red cells need to be specially processed in a cell saver after vacuum collection and mixed with a diluted heparin solution. The red cells are centrifuged, collected, washed, and rinsed with normal saline and can be stored or returned to the patient in concentrated packed-cell form.

Hypothermia, Coagulopathy, and Metabolic Acidosis

Hypothermia is an insidious problem in hemorrhagic shock. Severe hypothermia (core temperature lower than 32° C) is associated with 100% mortality in trauma patients, and morbidity is significant with any temperature lower than 34° C. Hypothermia is made worse by resuscitation with cold fluids and the evaporative heat loss from open body cavities during surgery. Another contributing factor is the loss of the protective shivering mechanism with the use of muscle relaxants. Hypothermia has a number of effects on functions such as coagulation, hemodynamics, and nervous system.[28]

Hypothermia affects all aspects of coagulation. Sequestration significantly decreases platelet count and is particularly severe at body temperatures lower than 20° C. Platelet function and clotting factor activity are also reversibly decreased. Replacement of platelets or clotting factors by transfusion are futile endeavors unless the patient is normothermic.

Hypothermia also has a negative inotropism paralleling falling temperatures, increasing irritability, and susceptibility to ventricular tachycardia and fibrillation. Bradycardic arrhythmias decaying to asystole with severe hypothermia are also observed. The use of cardiotonic drugs has little to no effect with decreased body temperature.

There is conflicting opinion regarding the speed and method of rewarming.[28] The use of warmed fluids and external body warmers are the most common. Aggressive and costly methods include hemodialysis and cardiopulmonary bypass.[40] Bypass offers the advantage of maintaining tissue perfusion and oxygenation regardless of the cardiac rhythm.[40] The beneficial effects of rewarming with hemodialysis and bypass remain controversial.

Coagulopathy, beyond that caused by hypothermia, is frequently induced from overall consumption of factors and platelets and dilution from massive blood transfusions. Platelets, fresh frozen plasma (FFP), or cryoprecipitate should be rationally used based on the clinical situation and results of appropriate laboratory tests. It is best to follow specific indications for transfusion of any banked blood product in trauma. Platelet counts less than 50,000 in the presence of active bleeding and after a replacement of more than 1.5 times normal volume in transfused blood should receive 4 to 8 units of platelets. Fibrinogen less than 100 mg/dl should be corrected with cryoprecipitate, which has a higher fibrinogen level than fresh frozen plasma. Prothrombin time greater than 1.5 times normal values or an international normalized ratio (INR) greater than 2 should be corrected with FFP. Brain injury provokes a special situation, possibly resulting from the release of tissue thromboplastins, and may lead to disseminated intravascular coagulation (DIC).

DIC is hemostatic failure with a tendency to bleed accompanied by a paradoxical tendency for microvasculature clotting. It is characterized as diffuse oozing or non-surgically correctable bleeding. Laboratory characteristics include a elevated prothrombin time (PT) and partial thromboplastin time (PTT), fibrinogen less than 50 mg/dl, severe thrombocytopenia (<50,000), and increased fibrin degradation products. It can occur following massive bleeding and transfusion, severe head injury, and any other cause of systemic inflammatory response. Treatment is primarily supportive, focusing on precipitating factors such as brain injury and infection or controlling the source of surgical bleeding. Coagulation factors are replaced with FFP and cryoprecipitate. More controversial is the use of heparin to prevent microvascular clotting in hopes of arresting ongoing end-organ deterioration. ε-Aminocaproic acid, which inhibits plasmin activity and could stabilize clot formation, has been advocated as well.

Metabolic acidosis in the trauma setting primarily originates from the basic definition of the shock state: inadequate oxygen supply to meet metabolic demands. An arterial pH less than 7.2 lowers the threshold for life-threatening arrhythmias and has a negative effect on contractility. Its only advantage is a shift in the oxygen-hemoglobin association curve to the right. If tissue hypoxia is the major culprit, attention should also be focused on ensuring adequate oxygen delivery to meet metabolic rate.

There are both opposing and supportive arguments for the use of sodium bicarbonate for the correction of metabolic acidosis. One problem is the high sodium concentration and osmolality of sodium bicarbonate solutions and the resulting complications of hypernatremia (e.g., seizures, exacerbation of cerebral edema). Severe alkalemia can result if not used carefully, resulting in cardiac arrhythmia. The resulting increase in carbon dioxide production worsens pH with resulting respiratory acidosis, and the bicarbonate actually worsens lactate production from the enhanced conversion of amino acids to lactate. Lastly, it has been shown that there is no improved survival rate associated with bicarbonate use.

Proponents of bicarbonate therapy argue that it is safe if titrated properly; that it should be used for pH less than 7.1; and that rises in Pco_2 are often not a problem for mechanically ventilated patients, whose gas exchange is supported. Bicarbonate therapy is certainly beneficial and indicated in cases of renal tubular acidoses, in which bicarbonate loss in the urine is the primary cause of metabolic acidosis.

ICU PHASE: PREVENTING AND MANAGING COMPLICATIONS

Acute Lung Injury and Acute Respiratory Distress Syndrome

Since its first historical description as early as World War I, the mortality associated with acute respiratory distress syndrome (ARDS) has decreased from 90% to 40%,[42] but despite a growing understanding of the pathophysiology of ARDS and the inflammatory process in general, the outcome of ARDS has not greatly changed in the last decade. Mortality has remained at an average of 50%. Despite the development of new and more complicated ventilator modes and still largely experimental therapies,[25] the management of acute lung injury and ARDS has remained a largely supportive and costly endeavor. Primary causative infection and inflammatory injury must be treated at the same time. There were no preventative treatments or effective therapy to alter the outcome of this illness until recently. The practice of mechanical ventilator support and alternate therapy continue to evolve.

Acute lung injury (ALI) and ARDS are both defined by oxygenation failure but differ in terms of severity. Oxygenation can be quantified in terms of the Pao_2/Fio_2 ratio obtained by an arterial blood gas measurement. The normal ratio is 450 to 500. Oxygenation failure is worse in ARDS in which the Pao_2/Fio_2 ratio is less than or equal to 200. ALI, by consensus definition, is greater than 200 but less than 300. The pathophysiology of both begin with a direct or indirect inflammatory injury to the lung. Direct lung injuries include traumatic pulmonary contusion, pneumonia, and aspiration pneumonitis. If this inflammatory injury to the lung is severe enough, it may lead to global consequences such as multiple organ failure. Indirect lung injury can result from an overwhelming inflammatory process elsewhere in the body such as intraabdominal sepsis or pancreatitis. The release of cytokines from complement-activated neutrophils causes a seemingly uncontrolled cascade of further inflammatory injury, cell membrane damage, and microvascular coagulation. The production of nitric oxide from a variety of cells leads to the production of superoxide radicals, which further damage cell membranes by lipid peroxidation.

ARDS is frequently described in three phases: exudative, proliferative, and fibrosing. For the lungs, the exudative process initially occurs with the appearance of hemorrhagic, proteinaceous secretions containing inflammatory cells and cellular debris. This manifests in a typical radiographic appearance of diffuse bilateral pulmonary infiltrates. The flooding of alveoli results in V/Q mismatching and increased dead space, which is one of the root mechanisms of hypoxemic failure. Surfactant function is altered by mixing with exudative material. Without the effective surface tension induced by surfactant lining, alveoli have an increased tendency to collapse. With cell membrane damage, the integrity of the capillary endothelial barrier is decreased and results in pulmonary edema and decreased lung compliance. Lung compliance is further worsened in the later fibroproliferative phases. The breakdown in cellular barriers is thought to promote bacterial translocation and bacteremia. Vascular changes also occur at the pulmonary arteriolar level with vasoconstriction and microthrombotic processes; they can also cause significant increases in pulmonary artery pressures that can adversely affect heart function, particularly in those patients with preexisting right-sided cardiomyopathy. Increased shunting is another significant mechanism of hypoxemic failure. Vascular changes in the lung promote shunting and add to oxygenation impairment.

Ventilator Practices in ARDS

To accommodate the resulting oxygenation failure, there is an increased demand and work of breathing that eventually leads to respiratory failure such that intubation and mechanical ventilatory support are invariably needed. Traditionally, ventilator practices stress the priority of higher than normal tidal volumes with the goal of correcting P_{CO_2}, arterial pH, and oxygenation.[4,42] This longtime standard is at the risk of overstretching normal alveolar units, which are still present even in patients with ARDS, with the use of high ventilatory pressures and air trapping with intrinsic positive end-expiratory pressure (PEEP) and barotrauma.[10] Normal lungs respond with an inflammatory reaction to this classic overstretching. Awareness of lung injury from overstretching has logically led to newer ventilator strategies such as low tidal volume, which allow for decreased airway pressure and less air trapping.[4,7,25] Disadvantages of a low or near normal tidal volume strategy include the increased tendency of alveolar units to collapse, the repetitive opening and closing action experienced at a lower starting volume, and decreased lung compliance. This cyclical trauma is also thought to initiate the inflammatory process. PEEP becomes very important in this strategy to stent the alveoli open and work at a better functional residual capacity. Another disadvantage of low tidal volume strategy is the necessity to employ permissive hypercapnia, which is usually well tolerated except for specific instances when it is not desirable, such as the head-injured patient who has elevated intracranial pressure (ICP).

The National Institutes of Health (NIH) ARDS net study[2] enrolled 861 patients who fit the diagnosis of ARDS. These patients were randomized to either conventional mechanical ventilation with high tidal volume (12 ml/kg) or to a low tidal volume (6 ml/kg) strategy. Patients excluded were those who could not tolerate hypercapnia (head-injured patients), those with an already high mortality rate from their primary disease, and those who were unlikely to wean because of neuromuscular disorders. The two groups had no major differences in age, race, gender, hemodynamics requiring pressors, or baseline pulmonary mechanics. This study showed a significant 22% decrease in mortality in the low tidal volume group (30%) compared with the higher tidal volume group (40%). Ventilator-free days and organ failure–free days were also improved. The inflammatory process as implied by IL-6 levels seemed also to be less with the lower tidal volume. This finding indicates that less initial inflammation may be important in determining outcome.

The results of the NIH-ARDS net study implies that the standard traditional approach of higher tidal volumes is harmful. Until proven otherwise, ventilator strategies should be geared toward lower or near normal tidal volumes. Surprisingly, hypercapnia was often modest and well tolerated in the low tidal volume group. PEEP and intravascular fluid status still remain important variables and the next follow-up with the ARDS study includes a look at both these factors with the low tidal volume strategy.

Positive End–Expiratory Pressure in ARDS

The use of early PEEP to improve outcome has not been effective but remains an important tool to improve oxygenation and thus allow the lowering of F_{IO_2} and limiting of oxygen toxicity. PEEP is meant to stent the alveoli open in functional position to prevent collapse and closing at end expiration.[10] It is important to remember that PEEP does not correct pulmonary edema. High PEEP and overall high airway pressures worsen V/Q mismatch. Too high a PEEP will have a deleterious effect on cardiac output and may aggravate already elevated ICP in those with head injury. Optimal amounts of PEEP will have minimal barotrauma and not adversely affect oxygen delivery for a given F_{IO_2}. A way to judge the effective level of PEEP is to titrate it based on improved arterial oxygen saturation and the resulting effects on hemodynamics.

Fluid Restriction in ARDS

Early fluid restriction has not been proven to improve outcome and may in fact be harmful.[42] A euvolemic state has proven to improve outcomes. Also, optimal fluid status is needed to maintain organ perfusion, particularly in the kidney. Invasive hemodynamic monitoring may be required to help monitor oxygen.

Inflammatory Modification in ARDS

Drug therapies have remained experimental.[1,41,42] Steroids have been proven to have no benefit in the early stages of ARDS but may help influence the later interstitial fibroproliferative stage (7-10 days after the onset of ARDS).[26] The use of monoclonal antibodies against cytokines such as TNF and the interleukins remains experimental, and so far the results have been disappointing.[1]

Antiinflammatory and antioxidant therapy such as ibuprofen, N-acetylcysteine, and allopurinol are still being investigated.[42] Surfactant therapy has been more successful in pediatric RDS than in the adult population for reasons that may have to do with the basic difference in the pathophysiology of the conditions.[42]

Other potential directions of treatment of ARDS include the use of inhaled nitric oxide,[1] prone positioning of the patient to decrease lung consolidation, the use of extracorporeal membrane oxygenation,[18,22] and partial liquid lung ventilation techniques.[15,35] Hyperbaric oxygen therapy and the use of synthetic hemoglobin to improve oxygen-carrying capacity are also being investigated. All these methods remain experimental.

Ventilator Weaning

Intubated patients should be reevaluated daily for the need for mechanical ventilatory support. This topic is more fully discussed in Chapter 1. If the patient is clinically improving and capable of spontaneous breathing, weaning from the ventilator should begin as soon as possible. The original reason for respiratory decompensation should be resolving or resolved. There are four main criteria that should be met before weaning is contemplated.

First, gas exchange, particularly the ability to oxygenate with minimal supplemental settings should be present. This is indicated with a PaO_2/FiO_2 ratio of 200 or greater with an FiO_2 less than or equal to 0.5 and PEEP less than or equal to 5. There are five main mechanisms causing oxygenation failure: V/Q mismatching, shunting, diffusion defects in gas exchange, low FiO_2, and poor cardiac output. The original mechanism for respiratory failure should improve before weaning is contemplated.

Second, the patient must be hemodynamically stable with no need for vasopressors. Suboptimal cardiac function has adverse consequences for weaning success. Cardiogenic pulmonary edema adversely affects gas exchange, so ventilator weaning is unlikely to be successful until adequately controlled. In addition, the diaphragm is the most important muscular component in spontaneous breathing, because its contraction generates the negative intrapleural pressure needed for lung inflation during the inspiratory cycle. If perfusion and oxygen delivery are suboptimal, diaphragmatic and other accessory muscle functions are compromised.

A third weaning criteria is that the patient must have an adequate drive to breathe and protect the airway. The patient should not be overly sedated or narcotized, causing brainstem respiratory center depression.[20] Neuromuscular blockade should be reversed. Metabolic problems, including severe metabolic alkalosis and hypothyroidism, need to be corrected to provide the drive to breathe. Head-injured patients must be adequately awake to both protect their airway and breathe spontaneously.

Fourth and last, the patient must be able to sustain alveolar ventilation with minimal support. Problems may include factors such as high spinal cord injury, conduction abnormalities, neuromuscular junction problems, and decreased muscle strength. Serum abnormalities such as Ca^{++}, K^{+}, Mg^{+}, and PO_4 have a negative effect on muscle function and the ability to wean. Overfeeding can increase CO_2 production and the load to breathe. Another factor that increases the work needed to breathe is agitation. Although preserving the drive to breathe is important, sedation may still be required when agitation caused by pain or anxiety is thought to be the primary cause of weaning failure.[23] This may manifest as an increase in respiratory rate and tidal volume. An increased respiratory rate and decreased lung volume may help to distinguish problems with muscle strength. Haloperidol, a sedating drug with no respiratory depressive effects, can be used as an additional or alternate drug to benzodiazepines and narcotics.

Weaning protocols vary according to physician preference and style, but there are two main approaches.[19] One approach is to gradually decrease mechanical support. A popular method in this approach is to wean with synchronized intermittent mandatory ventilation (SIMV) in which ventilator rate is decreased gradually. Pressure support (e.g., a continuous positive airway pressure [CPAP] of 5 mm Hg) can also be added to SIMV and eventually reduced to minimal levels. The second approach to weaning is spontaneous breathing trials of increasing duration using a T-piece with flow-by oxygen, pressure support, or CPAP. A T-piece has a disadvantage, however, because patients are fully disconnected from the ventilator and its monitoring alarms. Patients may require pressure support to overcome the resistance of the endotracheal tube itself. Specific measured parameters are used to predict the success of weaning and extubation; these are reviewed in Chapter 1.

Extubation should be considered if the patient is weaned from mechanical ventilation. Patients need to be awake, able to clear secretions, and protect their own airway. Direct laryngoscopy and flexible bronchoscopy to evaluate the airway may be required before extubation is considered. Excessive oral and pharyngeal edema may force a delay of extubation until this has resolved. A leak test, performed by letting the endotracheal tube cuff down and plugging the tube itself, may offer an idea of just how obstructing are the tissues around the tube. The leak test can be quantified by measuring the airway pressure required to produce an air leak. A low leak pressure of less than 12 to 15 mm Hg suggests a potentially patent airway after extubation.

Alternate airway management with tracheostomy should be considered if the patient requires prolonged intubation. Timing of tracheostomy has remained a controversial issue but should be a consideration after the first week if intubation and mechanical support continue to be a necessity. Tracheostomy offers the advantages of less resistance and dead space and better patient comfort and oral care than an orotracheal tube. Percutaneous tracheostomy can easily be done at the bedside.

Pulmonary Artery Catheters

Pulmonary artery or Swan-Ganz catheters are reviewed more fully in Chapter 2. It remains uncertain if there is an impact on mortality rate and cost-benefit to the use of these catheters in patients after systemic traumatic injuries.[16,27] Recent advances include the capability to monitor cardiac output and mixed venous saturation continuously and to measure right ventricular ejection fraction.[9] Other modifications include Doppler capability and cardiac pacing.[24] The main function of the pulmonary artery catheter is to guide therapy for optimal hemodynamic intervention to maintain tissue perfusion and oxygenation. There are significant technical limitations to these catheters; these limitations are reviewed in Chapter 2.

The goals of a pulmonary artery catheter are not the same in every clinical situation. With the assistance of inotropic pressor agents, a mean arterial pressure (MAP) of at least 70 should be ideal for a coronary perfusion, but a higher MAP may be desirable to increase cerebral perfusion pressure in the setting of high ICP.

Complications of pulmonary catheters include those attendant to central line placement, cardiac perforation, endocardial and valvular injury, heart block, arrhythmias, pulmonary artery rupture, air embolism, and infection.[16] The presence of a right-sided heart valve prosthesis is a contraindication to insertion.

Alternative technologies to obtain hemodynamic information include thoracic impedance and transesophageal echocardiography. So far there is limited experience with these techniques in the intensive care of patients with multisystem injuries.

Abdominal Compartment Syndrome

Abdominal compartment syndrome is a complication that is increasingly recognized in the critical care setting. This phenomenon consists of elevated intraabdominal pressure and associated multiple organ system dysfunction, which is often reversible with timely operative abdominal decompression. Because of varied clinical recognition, the reported mortality rate has ranged from 10% to 68%. Normal intraabdominal pressure, which can be measured from the intraperitoneal cavity directly, ranges from subatmospheric to atmospheric and is affected by the normal respiratory cycle.

The causes of increased intraabdominal pressure are many. In trauma, intraabdominal and retroperitoneal bleeding can be causes of increased abdominal volume and pressure. In hemorrhagic shock with massive fluid resuscitation, third space fluids result in bowel edema, increasing the volume within the compartment. Forced primary closure of the abdominal wall after a laparotomy can result in increased abdominal pressure, which may worsen with further edema and bleeding. This is a common postoperative problem that clinically presents itself with increasing abdominal girth, respiratory dysfunction, and hemodynamic compromise.

Respiratory dysfunction is the first manifestation of abdominal compartment syndrome.[36] The diaphragm is elevated and excursion is compromised from increased abdominal volume. Thoracic compliance, total lung capacity, functional residual capacity, and residual volume all are decreased. The patient manifests increased difficulty breathing, leading to respiratory distress and ultimately ventilatory and hypoxic failure. In the intubated patient, increased pressure is required to deliver the same tidal volume.

This increased intrathoracic pressure has a negative effect on cardiac output.[36] Compression of the intraabdominal inferior vena cava (IVC) and thoracic superior vena cava (SVC) and IVC decreases venous return and thereby decreases stroke volume. CVP, pulmonary wedge pressure, and pulmonary vascular resistance (PVR) are increased because of the transmitted pressure. A decreased systemic blood pressure from decreased cardiac output is accompanied by compensatory tachycardia and increased systemic vascular resistance (SVR). These deleterious effects on respiratory and cardiovascular function are reversible with abdominal decompression.

Renal function is affected by decreased cardiac output and direct compression of the kidneys. Renal perfusion and glomerular filtration decrease with resulting oliguria progressing to anuria. Compression compromises venous return and affects the ureters, causing postobstructive renal failure. The ischemic effects on renal function are not always reversible with abdominal decompression.

Intraabdominal organ perfusion is also affected by increased compartment pressure greater than 15 mm Hg for the hollow viscera. This ischemic injury promotes breakdown of the gut barrier and bacterial translocation leading to bacteremia. Portal and hepatic arterial pressure are affected at pressures greater than 20 mm Hg, with a negative effect on liver perfusion and function. The abdominal wall itself is also affected with decreased perfusion of the musculature and an increase in wound infection, dehiscence, and necrotizing fasciitis.

Currently, the most accepted and least invasive way to measure abdominal pressure is the measurement of bladder pressure via an indwelling Foley catheter. Reflecting the intraabdominal compartment, bladder pressure greater than 25 mm Hg is of concern. Pressure greater than 35 mm Hg with multiple organ dysfunction is considered an emergency.

Controversy exists regarding patient management based on bladder pressure measurements. Although hemodynamic effects have been shown to occur at pressures of 25 mm Hg, not all surgeons agree to intervene if there are no signs of organ failure. The consensus for intervention seems to be a bladder pressure of greater than 35 mm Hg and evidence of clinical deterioration. Therapeutic intervention is decompression of the abdominal compartment. A midline fascial incision is made and the abdominal contents are contained and protected with temporary materials. This can be done at the bedside if bowel ischemia is not suspected.

Stress Ulcer Prophylaxis

Stress gastritis is a prevalent problem in the critically ill. An estimated 50% of critical care patients develop stress ulcers within 48 hours of admission.[14] Stress gastritis is distinguished by small superficial mucosal erosions that begin in the proximal stomach and can progress to the duodenum. These erosions have a tendency to bleed and may perforate if located in the relatively thin-walled duodenum. Typically, patients have no premorbid history of gastrointestinal problems and usually have normal acid secretion. Bleeding is usually clinically occult; overt bleeding occurs in up to 15% of patients, with only a small percentage requiring blood transfusion. The incidence of life-threatening hemorrhage has dramatically decreased with the use of prophylactic therapy.

The mechanism of stress gastritis may stem from a combination of factors, but poor splanchnic blood flow seems to be most important. Gastric mucosal turnover occurs every 2 to 3 days. When this process is interrupted by inadequate nutrient supply, denuded surfaces appear and eroded superficial vessels result in bleeding. Other erosive mechanisms include increased gastric acid production, decreased bicarbonate and mucus production, and altered prostaglandin synthesis. Patients particularly prone to stress gastritis are those on prolonged mechanical ventilation;[11] those with multiple organ dysfunction, major trauma, and central nervous system (CNS) injury (Cushing's ulcer); burn patients with injuries to more than 35% of their body surface area (Curling's ulcer); and those with a history of bleeding ulcer.

Prevention of stress gastritis has had a great impact on prevention of life-threatening bleeding. Therapeutic options are many and include medications that alter gastric pH and control acid excretion, as well as cytoprotective agents. H_2 receptor antagonists and proton pump inhibitors are most effective in altering and maintaining an alkaline gastric pH. Sucralfate, given nasogastrically (NG) or by mouth (PO), has mucosal protective properties but does not alter gastric pH or acid secretion. There is a disadvantage of increasing gastric pH in that gastric flora normally suppressed in an acidic environment may increase with a more alkaline pH. Also, aspiration pneumonia in the mechanically ventilated patient may be increased with acid suppression.[14]

Early enteral nutrition should be considered in the armamentarium of stress ulcer prophylaxis with its protective trophic effect and preservation of immunological function in the intestinal lining. The relative risk of stress gastritis has been proven to decrease with early feeding. Upper gastrointestinal bleeding is suspected with an unexplained decreasing hematocrit and confirmed with the presence of gross blood on nasogastric suctioning. Along with hemodynamic support with crystalloid and blood replacement and correction of any coagulopathy, diagnostic gastroscopy should be done to identify the source of bleeding and rule out other causes; in addition, bleeding should be controlled using thermal methods or injection of sclerosing agents. Diffuse bleeding of stress gastritis may not be amenable to endoscopic interventions. If endoscopic treatment is unsuccessful, selective visceral angiography should be performed for selective vasopressin infusion or embolization of gastric arteries. Surgery is reserved for perforation and failure to control bleeding with the treatments discussed earlier. No one operation has been proven the best, but unless an acid-reducing procedure is included, the rate of recurrent bleeding remains quite high.

Colonic Ileus

Additional abdominal complications can include motility problems such as colonic ileus (Ogilvie's syndrome) and acalculous cholecystitis. Ogilvie's syndrome consists of nonobstructive colonic distention. Neurohormonal derangement is thought to be the mechanism of this pseudo-obstruction. Parasympathetic inhibition or sympathetic excitation result in the loss of peristaltic activity. Anticholinergics, antidepressants, and narcotic analgesics are contributing factors, as are potassium and magnesium deficiencies.

Early recognition and correction of Ogilvie's syndrome is important to avoid colonic ischemia and perforation. The abdomen is typically distended, with decreased bowel sounds. Right lower quadrant tenderness and elevated white cell count may indicate impending ischemic cecal perforation. A flat plate of the abdomen will show a distended air-filled colon. The cecum is the thinnest and most likely portion of the colon to perforate when a critical diameter between 8 and 12 cm is reached. Most cases do not require surgical intervention. Fluid resuscitation, correction of metabolic abnormalities, and elimination of offending drugs is a start. Nasogastric suctioning and a rectal tube assist decompression. Prokinetic agents such as guanethidine and neostigmine may help. Colonoscopy allows additional mechanical decompression of the colon. Exploratory laparotomy is necessary in the setting of potential ischemia and perforation.

Acalculous Cholecystitis

Acute acalculous cholecystitis in the multitrauma patient is potentially lethal. Stagnant bile and gallbladder ischemia are thought to be the mechanisms of inflammation initially, but secondary bacteremia may develop. Trauma patients are particularly vulnerable, especially if enteral feeding is not established. The diagnosis is often delayed by nonspecific rises in liver enzymes, fever, and elevated white cell count, and poorly localized pain in the postlaparotomy and unconscious head-injured patients. Imaging studies of the abdomen may show pericholecystic fluid and a gallbladder wall thickening of 3 mm or greater. Hepatobiliary iminodiacetic acid (HIDA) scanning can confirm the diagnosis but has a false positive rate of greater than 50%. Definitive treatment is with open or laparoscopic cholecystectomy, at which time cholangiography may be performed to rule out bile duct stones. Percutaneous cholecystostomy for drainage is an option for patients at particularly high operative risk.

Stress Metabolism and Nutrition

Metabolism and nutritional therapy are discussed more completely in Chapter 7. Hypermetabolism of critical illness is the overamplification of stress response. Stresses such as trauma, infection, and shock bring about the release of hormones and inflammatory mediators, which results in net protein catabolism. In comparison with simple starvation, glycogen and fat stores are used first. The efferent portion of the neuroendocrine axis responds by releasing catecholamine, cortisol, and glucagon, which are important in understanding the metabolic changes in nutrient balance.

Loss of lean body mass has detrimental implications. Approximately .5 to 1 pound of muscle per day can be lost in cases of severe trauma and will manifest biochemically as an increase in nitrogen loss in the urine. Loss of more than 10% of lean body mass has severe implications in terms of immune response and mortality. Loss of 20% to 30% of lean body mass is associated with failure to wean from mechanical ventilation, decreased wound healing, and severe muscular weakness. Loss of 40% is associated with 100% mortality, with death commonly a result of infectious complications such as pneumonia. Fortunately, the majority of trauma patients are premorbidly healthy and well nourished.

Manipulation of the Metabolic Rate

Treatment of hypermetabolic response includes limiting the focus of inflammation and aggressive nutritional support.[5] Treatment includes drainage of infection and removal of devitalized and ischemic tissue. Experimental therapies include agents that manipulate metabolic rate. Beta-blockers can decrease metabolic rate by 25% and may be of benefit as long as cardiac output and oxygen delivery are monitored and not adversely compromised. Anabolic steroids allow an increase in muscle mass but drawbacks include steroid toxicity. Growth hormone has been shown to improve wound healing in burn patients and may improve ventilator weaning and maintenance of lean body mass. Although promising, growth hormone therapy is expensive and hyperglycemia can result from increased insulin resistance.

Nutritional Needs

Nutrition is reviewed more completely in Chapter 7. Nutrition should be implemented as soon as possible, particularly if there is preexisting malnutrition or expected prolonged hypermetabolism. Nutritional therapy in the critically ill trauma patient should be implemented within 48 hours if possible. Enteral feeding is preferable.[32] Postlaparotomy patients generally have an ileus and should start enteral nutrition within 6 to 7 days. Enteric nutritional delivery has been shown to decrease infectious complications and costs. Direct stimulation of the enterocytes helps maintain gut mucosa. Maintaining the mucosal barrier is a defense against bacterial translocation and the development of complications. The easiest access route is via placement of a small-caliber feeding tube in the nose or mouth. Duodenal or jejunal placement of the feeding tip allows bypass of an atonic stomach, reaching nutritional goals sooner by directly feeding the small bowel. The disadvantages of the enteral route include the risk of chemical aspiration, persistent ileus, and diarrhea. Whereas total parenteral nutrition (TPN) has been popular in the past, disadvantages include complications with central line placement, increased risk of infection, and metabolic and electrolyte imbalances. There is some data suggesting that TPN in patients with head injury may worsen increased ICP. Monitoring metabolic and nutritional needs are reviewed in Chapter 7.

Deep Venous Thromboses and Pulmonary Embolism

Deep venous thrombosis (DVT) is a common problem with the potential complication of life-threatening pulmonary embolism (PE). The incidence of pulmonary embolism can vary from 1% to 10% depending on the number of risk factors. Similarly, the rate of life-threatening PE can vary from 0.5% to 5% of cases of DVT. Outcome from PE is dependent on the burden of thrombus, size of the occluded vessel, and cardiopulmonary reserve. It is estimated that 30% of patients with PE die within 30 minutes of the event as a result of hypoxia and right-sided heart failure. Mortality from PE has significantly decreased with anticoagulation prophylaxis. This cannot be neglected in multisystem trauma.

Virchow's triad of stasis, endothelial damage, and hypercoagulation is an important concept in understanding the risk factors for DVT. Prolonged immobility as a result of systemic and extremity injuries are a major risk factor of DVT, as are spinal cord injury with paralysis and abdominal surgery of more than 30 minutes duration. Other important risk factors include age, history of previous DVT, pelvic surgery, and pelvic and lower extremity fracture. Vascular access catheters are known to be the cause of DVT in sites other than the lower extremities, such as the subclavian vein. Mechanisms for hypercoagulation in trauma patients include a decrease in antithrombin III activity. Some patients also have proteins C and S deficiencies, antiphospholipid antibodies, and Factor V, placing them at increased risk for DVT and PE.

Signs and symptoms of lower extremity DVT include fever, leg edema, palpable thrombosed venous cord, and Homan's sign (pain with dorsiflexion of the ankle). DVT may be clinically silent and require further studies to document its presence. Ultrasound with Doppler flow detection is noninvasive and reliable for diagnosis of DVT.

Signs and symptoms of pulmonary embolism can occur with or without clinical evidence of a lower extremity DVT. Dyspnea, tachypnea, tachycardia, hypotension, chest pain, and syncope are clinical signs of PE, although all are nonspecific. Arterial blood gas measurements may show respiratory alkalosis and relative hypoxemia. Chest x-ray studies may be normal or nonspecific with evidence of effusion or atelectasis. If severe enough, dilated central pulmonary vessels may be in evidence.

The customary test for the diagnosis of PE is a ventilation-perfusion scan. A negative study excludes the diagnosis of PE and a high probability scan confirms the diagnosis. Low- to moderate-probability V/Q scans pose a diagnostic problem that may prompt additional tests such as a pulmonary angiogram. Pulmonary angiogram remains the gold standard for the diagnosis of PE and arguably should be the first test performed to obtain a definitive answer as soon as possible if there are concerns about starting anticoagulant therapy or other interventions.

Other tests for the diagnosis of PE are emerging, such as helical computed tomography (CT) scanning of the chest.[29,33] This has the potential of high sensitivity and specificity for the detection of a clot in primary and secondary order pulmonary veins but requires IV contrast and interpreter experience. Magnetic resonance imaging (MRI) is another alternative; MRI does not require intravenous contrast but is more cumbersome for the critically ill patient.

The management of PE may require intubation and mechanical ventilation. Because of attendant right ventricular failure, IV fluid administration needs to be carefully controlled. Inotropic agents may be needed to support the hemodynamically unstable patient. Anticoagulation is used to decrease the risk of further clot formation and more emboli. Therapy needs to be started within the first 24 hours to be effective. Typically an infusion of heparin is begun to achieve an international normalized ratio (INR) of 2 to 3.

Contraindications to anticoagulation include an increased risk of bleeding complications and hypersensitivity to heparin. Heparin-induced thrombocytopenia from presumed antibodies to heparin can also occur. The low platelet count reverses when heparin is stopped. If further pulmonary emboli occur despite therapeutic levels of anticoagulation, then anticoagulant therapy is considered a failure and indication for placement of a vena cava filter by an interventional radiologist. Generally, the anticoagulation is then stopped. Surgical embolectomy, thromboembolytic therapy, and suction catheter embolectomy may be indicated to decrease the clot burden. Surgical embolectomy requires cardiopulmonary bypass and has high morbidity and mortality. Thrombolytic therapy has a number of contraindications for increased risk of bleeding and hypersensitivity reactions to the agents and is quite costly. Contraindications include head trauma and surgeries within the past 7 days.

There are a number of measures to prophylactically decrease the DVT risk. These include low-dose subcutaneous heparin, low-molecular-weight heparin, compression stockings, and sequential compression boots. Heparin works by enhancing the anticoagulant effect of antithrombin III and is usually safe to start within 24 hours in stable patients after major trauma in the absence of coagulopathy. Low-molecular-weight heparin may be as effective in reducing the risk of DVT compared with regular heparin but risks of bleeding are thought to increase and so are avoided with CNS trauma patients. Sequential compression boots are thought to promote fibrinolytic activity and increase venous return. They are safe to use with few complications but should not be used on a limb already suspected of harboring a DVT to avoid clot migration and embolism.

Renal Failure and Renal Replacement Therapy

Acute renal failure in the critically ill has an overall associated mortality of 50%. If renal failure is a part of multiple organ failure, the mortality rate is 100%. If patients recover from their precipitating trauma, there is a good chance of recovery of renal function. Death and failure to recover renal function are associated with older age group, preexisting medical disease, infections, and liver disease. Renal failure is defined by increasing serum creatinine and urea levels and may be accompanied by lethal increases in serum potassium and other complications. Patients can be anuric (<100 ml of urine excreted/day), oliguric (100-400 ml/day), or polyuric (1 L/day). There is no specific treatment for acute renal failure; management includes renal replacement therapy as necessary.

Causes of renal failure can be classified into three broad categories: prerenal, renal, and postrenal. Prerenal causes are most commonly seen in the trauma setting from decreased renal perfusion as a result of intravascular volume depletion, such as from hemorrhage, third space losses from sepsis/inflammation, and gastrointestinal losses with accompanying inadequate fluid resuscitation. Multiple causes of renal impairment include autoimmune diseases, vascular complications (e.g., hypertension, vasculitis, renal artery thrombosis, ischemia), drug toxicity (e.g., cephalosporins, penicillins, sulfonamides, diuretics, and nonsteroidal antiinflammatory drugs [NSAIDs]), and neurotoxins (myoglobin caused by rhabdomyolysis). Anatomical obstruction to urine flow causing postrenal failure is easily ruled out with abdominal ultrasound, CT scan, or retrograde contrast studies of the genitourinary system; this can be dealt with appropriately. Abdominal compartment syndrome is also a potential cause, although its exact mechanism may include kidney ischemia and not simply compression on the outlet tracts.

Initial Approach: Prevention

The best initial approach to managing renal failure from Acute Tubular Necrosis is to optimize renal perfusion to attenuate established acute renal injury. Conversion of an oliguric state to a nonoliguric state with the use of dopamine has long been proposed.[12,30] The rationale for its use lies in theoretically increasing renal blood flow via the DA_1 receptor, thereby limiting ischemic injury and promoting urine production. The actual diuretic effect stems from inhibition of the sodium/potassium ATPase pump channel in the proximal renal tubule and ascending loop of Henle. The diuretic effect is not due to increasing glomerular filtration rate.

Rhabdomyolysis is another common and treatable cause of renal failure in the trauma patient. Muscle destruction from crush injuries or ischemia from compartment syndrome or vascular injuries present with tea- to red-colored urine and serum creatinine kinase levels greater than 10,000 IU/ml. A urinalysis for grossly positive hemoglobin is diagnostic. Treatment is presumptive with forced alkaline diuresis with crystalloid and/or mannitol for urine output rates greater than 100 ml/hr to force the myoglobin precipitate out of the renal tubules and lessen toxic exposure to the tubular cells. Mannitol has the added advantage of being an oxygen radical scavenger.

Renal Replacement Choices

The primary indication for renal replacement therapy in the critically ill patient is supportive management of the complications of renal failure: hypervolemia, electrolyte disturbances, refractory metabolic acidosis, and uremia (neurotoxic effects and pericarditis). Today there are a confusing array of choices with equally confusing acronyms, such as IHD, CHD, IUF, and SCUF, in techniques such as dialysis and ultrafiltration for solute removal.[39]

Vascular access choices for hemodialysis and ultrafiltration require large veins to allow for higher blood flow rates via large dual-lumen catheters. Venous to venous modes usually require an external pump and anticoagulation to decrease the high tendency to clot off the filters. Arterial to venous access circuits do not necessarily require these if there is sufficient driving pressure. Newer, more biocompatible membranes (non-cellulose based) have less inflammatory effects and white blood cell adhesion and thereby less drastic effects of hemodynamics (i.e., hypotension and tachycardia) and infection. Improvements in tolerance of dialysis, survival, and renal function with these filters have been demonstrated.

A hot topic is a possible new application of ultrafiltration for controlling the inflammatory response in early sepsis, which could affect morbidity and mortality.[6,38,39] There is an excess and uncontrolled activation of inflammatory cells and mediators that lead to ARDS and multiple system organ failure. Cytokine levels have previously been related to outcome and the thought has been that the removal of cytokines by hemopurification may have an effect on outcome. Depending on the pore size of the filter medium and large molecular weight, cytokine proteins such as TNF and interleukins are filtered out of the blood. There are no controlled studies to demonstrate good data, but there have been promising small case studies showing improvement in metabolic rate, decreased shunting, and better oxygenation in the case of acute lung injury and ARDS almost immediately after continuous venovenous hemofiltration (CVVH) therapy is started; however, this outcome has not been seen in all cases.[6] The actual timing of renal replacement therapy in cases of sepsis and trauma may have an important impact on clinical result. The immunological effect of filtering out all cytokines is not known, and some of these small studies have shown diverging results. Further studies are needed.

Prophylactic Antibiotics in Trauma

Major trauma has been shown to alter immune responses. Decreased chemotaxis, phagocytosis, and cell-mediated immune function, decreased in complement and immunoglobulins levels have been demonstrated in trauma. Wounds can be classified as clean, clean contaminated, and contaminated, and have different rates of infection. Clean wounds are those less than 6 hours old with no gross soilage. These have the lowest infection rate (3%). Clean contaminated wounds are clean wounds with contaminating soilage infection rate (8%). Contaminated wounds are those more than 6 hours old, and these have the highest rate of infection (25%). Risk factors in the trauma setting for surgical infection include perioperative shock, massive blood replacement, high severity of individual injuries, at least one intraabdominal injury, left colon injury, and management with colostomy.

In multisystem trauma there is controversy about specific antibiotic therapy covering specific flora during the preoperative, long intraoperative, and postoperative periods.[34] Overuse and inappropriate choices for prophylaxis and the treatment of actual infection have resulted in the emergence of resistant organisms (methicillan-resistant *Staphylococcus aureus* [MRSA], vancomycin-resistant enterococci [VRE]) and normally opportunistic fungi that are difficult to treat. It is important to monitor sensitivities of positive cultures and to pick the most specific, effective, and least toxic antibiotic.

For abdominal trauma, prophylactic treatment of gram-negative and anaerobic organisms can be covered with a single cephalosporin as well as multiple combination antibiotics. For gross intraabdominal fecal soilage, fascial laparotomy incisions should be closed and the subcutaneous layer allowed to heal by secondary intention. Inappropriate use of surgical drains (e.g., with splenectomy beds) have been proven to lead to increased incidence of abscess. Postoperative development of intraabdominal abscess present within 7 to 10 days; it can often be primarily managed with radiologically-placed percutaneous drains. Superficial wounds should be debrided and treated in an open fashion with irrigation and packing.

Orthopedic surgery uses antibiotics in particular with open fractures, which require at least 3 days of treatment with a cephalosporin. Depending on the type of contamination, anaerobic coverage for *Clostridia* species may be added. In addition, all open fractures need to be cleaned and debrided within 6 hours of admission.

A complete discussion of infectious disease management in the intensive care unit is presented in Chapter 8.

SEDATION, PARALYTICS, AND PAIN MANAGEMENT

Sedation

Sedation is frequently needed in addition to analgesia in the intensive care unit setting. Sedative drugs have a synergistic effect with pain medications and can help by lowering narcotic requirements. Sedation has an important role in controlling agitation and anxiety. Excessive delirium and agitation have implications for increased morbidity and mortality because of potentially harmful hyperdynamic responses with increased oxygen consumption. The tendency to self-harm such as self-extubation, inadvertent removal of lines and monitors, and obstruction of proper nursing care are other important considerations. Appropriate and adequate sedation remains an important aspect of hospital care; therefore a good understanding of frequently used medications in this class is necessary.

Propofol is a relatively new anesthetic agent used in head-injured patients. It is easy to titrate to a goal level of sedation, such as a Ramsay score of 3, at which point the patient is drowsy yet responsive to commands. When a propofol drip is stopped, rapid elimination allows for arousal and an accurate neurological examination. Propofol is an amnestic and hypnotic but has absolutely no analgesic properties. It is quick-acting and does have a hypotensive effect as a result of vasodilation and cardiac depression. Because it is formulated in intralipid, it makes a great culture medium; therefore the drug bottles and delivery system should be changed every 12 to 24 hours. Prolonged propofol use also increases the serum triglyceride level. There have been reported cases of pancreatitis with high dosing and prolonged use. The current recommendation is to stop propofol when the triglyceride level is greater than 300.

Benzodiazepines are frequently used in the ICU and have different characteristics. They work by binding to a portion of the γ-aminobutyric acid (GABA) receptor and enhance GABA effects.[21] More commonly used choices in the ICU setting include midazolam (Versed), diazepam (Valium), and lorazepam (Ativan). Of these, midazolam is more expensive. Its advantage is that it has a rapid onset and short duration and can be used as an infusion. Its main disadvantage is that it has an active metabolite, and its accumulation can have an effect for several days. Diazepam IV has a rapid onset but is longer acting and can accumulate because of its lipophilic characteristic. It also has an active metabolite. Lorazepam, in contrast, is intermediate in its onset and duration and has no active metabolite or accumulation. Administration problems occur as a result of the tendency of lorazepam to precipitate in intravenous solutions.

Benzodiazepines such as midazolam and lorazepam are frequently administered as continuous drips in the ICU, as opposed to intermittent boluses. The advantage of a continuous drip lies not only in ease of nursing care but also in a less disruptive, smoother course for the patient. This practice has been criticized because of the increased duration of medications after prolonged accumulation, loss of the ability to perform neurological examinations, and increased ICU stay and costs. In a recent study the use of intermittent boluses of sedatives and narcotics in the ICU was shown to modestly decrease days on mechanical ventilation, reduce the number of radiological studies of the brain, and therefore lead to shorter ICU stays and lower costs. This has not been studied specifically in trauma patients.

Flumazenil is a pure benzodiazepine receptor antagonist that is used to reverse the effect of benzodiazepines. Caution should be used when reversing the sedating effects of benzodiazepines when there is a history of chronic benzodiazepine and antidepressant use. In addition, the seizure threshold is decreased with flumazenil use.

Haloperidol is a butyrophenone neuroleptic that can be very useful in addition to benzodiazepines in controlling a delirious, delusional, and psychotic patient. It has minimal sedating effects and causes no respiratory depression. The disadvantages of haloperidol include lowering the seizure threshold; the extrapyramidal side effects include dystonia and laryngospasm, which can occur with both oral and intravenous administration. In addition, frequent and large dosing of the drug should be monitored by its effect in prolonging the QT interval, possibly leading to *torsades de pointes* or sinusoidal rhythm.

Paralytic Agents

There are specific indications for paralytic agents in the intensive care unit. Neuromuscular blocking agents can be used as a tool to decrease oxygen consumption and carbon dioxide production and help induce hypothermia by eliminating the shivering response. They can be useful when used in some modes of ventilation such as pressure control or low tidal volume breathing and permissive hypercapnia, which may be difficult for the patient to tolerate despite sedation. The risk of mechanical ventilatory barotrauma can be decreased by eliminating the portion of voluntary effort. By eliminating muscular effort, paralytics may also help control elevated intracranial pressure.

Paralytic drugs are either depolarizing agents or nondepolarizing agents. The latter are further divided into aminosteroid and benzylisoquinolinium classes. Succinylcholine is the most frequently depolarizing agent; it has a rapid onset of 60 seconds and a short duration of 7 minutes. It is best used for short procedures that require paralysis such as intubation. The dose is 1 to 1.5 mg/kg lean body weight. The competitive agonist effect on the acetylcholine receptors pre- and postneuromuscular junctions causes initial fasciculations and a transient hyperkalemia, which can be severe enough to lead to cardiac arrest. Use in quadriplegic patients or in any condition with neuromuscular abnormalities and damage is contraindicated. Succinylcholine is safe to use in the initial 24 hours after burn injury.

Nondepolarizing agents are competitive antagonists to the nicotinic acetylcholine receptor and can be given by continuous infusion or boluses. Most of these agents have a longer duration of effect. Long-term use of these agents can lead to further prolonged paralytic effect. This persistent response varies individually and can be affected by renal and liver dysfunction and whether there are active metabolites. Interaction with other drugs such as aminoglycosides, steroids, and calcium channel blockers can also influence effective duration. Monitoring and titrating the therapeutic effect involves using the train of four peripheral nerve stimulation every 1 to 2 hours. The goal is not to obtain total paralysis but one to two twitches out of four. If paralysis is maintained at this level, it is unlikely that prolonged effect will be problematic when the drug is discontinued.

Rapacuronium, rocuronium, vecuronium, and pancuronium are aminosteroids. Rapacuronium is an analog of vecuronium and has similar characteristic effects as succinylcholine. Rocuronium also has a relatively quick onset. An intubation dose of 0.5 mg/kg has a duration of 30 to 40 minutes. Rocuronium is metabolized mainly in the liver and has no active metabolites and very little cardiovascular effect. Pancuronium has a slow onset and duration of 60 to 100 minutes and is inexpensive. It does have an active metabolite and is eliminated by the liver and the kidney. It also causes increases in heart rate and blood pressure. Vecuronium has a 2- to 3-minute onset and a 25- to 45-minute duration and is another longer acting agent used for continuous drips. Vecuronium is also one of the neuromuscular blocking agents implicated with prolonged effect after chronic use.

Cisatracurium is a benzylisoquinolone with a 2- to 3-minute onset and short 20-minute duration. Its advantage is that it does not cause histamine release and has no active metabolites. It is eliminated by ester hydrolysis and Hofman elimination in the plasma. The disadvantage of this drug is tachyphylaxis and possible seizures.

Malignant hyperthermia is a rare complication linked to succinylcholine and volatile anesthetics such as halothane. It is characterized by sudden rigidity, hyperthermia (>42° C), and hypermetabolism leading to increased CO_2 production. Treatment includes cooling and administration of dantrolene. Neuroleptic malignant syndrome occurs with phenothiazines, tricyclics, and monoamine oxidase (MAO) inhibitors. It is similar to malignant hyperthermia but with a lack of muscle rigidity. The treatment is the same as for malignant hyperthermia.

Pain Control

Analgesia can take many routes and forms and is an understandable necessity following any surgery or trauma. The intramuscular route of narcotic delivery is painful and unpredictable in its absorption. The transdermal approach is available only with fentanyl and can be a useful option to wean a patient from intravenous narcotics. Patient-controlled analgesia (PCA) intravenously delivers small doses at short intervals on command; it requires an alert, cooperative, and nondelirious patient. It has been shown to be effective in maintaining a consistent blood level of narcotics with increased patient satisfaction and decreased nursing time. Epidural analgesia can offer superior pain relief, such as with patients with chest trauma as well as after laparotomy and thoracotomy. It can also be delivered on demand by the patient using a PCA pump. The other advantage offered by this route is that less narcotics are often used. The disadvantages include the risk of bleeding, infection, catheter migration, and inadvertent systemic absorption of medication. Respiratory depression and hemodynamic instability from effective sympathectomy can occur depending on the dosage. Opioids bind to receptors in the spinal cord and brain and alter the transmission of pain.[21] Tolerance to narcotics requires increased dosing, and withdrawal symptoms are not prevented by the epidural route. Local anesthetic agents are often co-administered with epidural narcotics. Bupivacaine is a frequent example. CNS toxicity, seizures, and cardiac depression and arrhythmias can complicate the use of local anesthetics.

Fentanyl is a potent drug that has a half life of 30 to 60 minutes. One hundred micrograms has the same effect as 10 mg of morphine. It has little sedating effect and no adverse cardiovascular effect because it causes no histamine release. It is a lipophilic drug, so it has a tendency to accumulate. Remifentanyl has a rapid onset and offset because of the rapid elimination by tissue esterases and can only be given intravenously. Morphine is water soluble, has a longer duration, and has an active metabolite, unlike fentanyl. It does cause histamine release and has been known to cause myoclonus and respiratory depression. Meperidine (Demerol) is not often used in the ICU setting because of the risk of significant hypotension and tachycardia secondary to histamine release. The metabolites of meperidine can be toxic, decreasing the seizure threshold and causing hyperpyrexia. This is worse in the presence of other drugs such as MAO inhibitors and phenobarbital. Hydromorphone (Dilaudid) is a semisynthetic of morphine with five to six times the potency of morphine. Its advantage lies with fewer sedating and euphoric effects. It is, however, twice as expensive as fentanyl on an equipotent basis.

NSAIDs have a very limited role in the ICU setting. They can be useful for pain related to the inflammatory process and malignant disease involving bone. Complications with NSAID use include platelet dysfunction, gastrointestinal bleeding, and renal insufficiency. Ketorolac is the only NSAID with a parenteral route. Clonidine, an α-adrenergic agonist, is sometimes used for alcohol withdrawal and to decrease pain transmission. It inhibits the release of norepinephrine at the presynaptic adrenergic fibers and thereby bypasses the hypersympathetic effects of alcohol withdrawal. The use of low-dose alcohol drips as a preventative measure for alcohol withdrawal is underway.

REFERENCES

1. Albertson TE, Marelich GP: Pharmacologic adjuncts to mechanical ventilation in acute respiratory distress syndrome, **Crit Care Clin 14(4):**581-601, 1998.
2. Amato MBP, Barbas CSV, Medeiros DM: Effect of a protective-ventilation strategy on mortality in acute respiratory distress syndrome, **N Engl J Med 338(6):**347-354, 1998.
3. Baron BJ, Scalea TM: Acute blood loss, **Emerg Med Clin North Am 14(1):**35-55, 1996.
4. Battistella FD: Ventilation in the trauma and surgical patient, **Crit Care Clin 14(4):**731-739, 1998.
5. Beale RJ, Bryg DJ, Bihari DJ: Immunonutrition in the critically ill: A systematic review of clinical outcome, **Crit Care Med 27(12):**2799-2805, 1999.
6. Bellamo R, Tipping P, Boyce N: Continuous veno-venous hemofiltration with dialysis removes cytokines from the circulation of septic patients, **Crit Care Med 21(4):**522-526, 1993.
7. Brower RG, Matthay MA, Morris A, et al: Ventilation with lower tidal volumes as compared with traditional tidal volumes for acute lung injury and the acute respiratory distress syndrome, **N Engl J Med 325:**1371-1372, 2000.
8. Cammarano WB, Marks JD, Schlobohm RM, et al: **Analgesia and Sedation Guidelines for Adult Critical Care Patients.** San Francisco: San Francisco General Hospital, 1999.
9. Cariou A, Monchi M, Dhainaut JF: Continuous cardiac output and mixed venous oxygen saturation monitoring, **J Crit Care 13(4):**198-213, 1998.
10. Chapin JC, Downs JB, Douglas ME, et al: Lung expansion, airway pressure transmission and positive end-expiratory pressure, **Arch Surg 114:**1193-1197, 1979.
11. Cook D, Heyland D, Griffith L, et al: Risk factors for clinically important upper gastrointestinal bleeding in patients requiring mechanical ventilation, **Crit Care Med 27(12):**2812-2817, 1999.
12. Denton MD, Chertow GM, Brady HR, et al: "Renal dose" dopamine for the treatment of acute renal failure: Scientific rationale, experimental studies and clinical trials, **Kidney Int 50(1):**4-14, 1996.
13. Haljameae H: Does prehospital hypertonic therapy improve the survival in trauma patients? **Lakartidningen 96(9):**1014-1017, 1999.
14. Hanisch EW, Encke A, Naujoks F, et al: A randomized trial for stress ulcer prophylaxis shows no evidence of increased pneumonia, **Am J Surg 176(5):**453-457, 1998.
15. Hirschl RB, Parent A, Tooley R, et al: Liquid ventilation improves pulmonary function, gas exchange, and lung injury in a model of respiratory failure, **Ann Surg 221(1):**79-88, 1995.

16. Ivanov R, Allen J, Calvin JE: The incidence of major morbidity in critically ill patients managed with pulmonary artery catheters: a meta-analysis, **Crit Care Med 28(3):**615-626, 2000.
17. Junger WG, Coimbra R, Liu FC, et al: Hypertonic saline resuscitation: a tool to modulate immune function in trauma patients? **Shock 8(4):**235-241, 1997.
18. Kolla S, Awad MD, Rich PB, et al: Extracorporeal life support for 100 adult patients with severe respiratory failure, **Ann Surg 226(4):**544-566, 1997.
19. Kollef MH, Shapiro SD, Silver P, et al: A randomized, controlled trial of protocol-directed vs. physician-directed weaning from mechanical ventilation, **Crit Care Med 25(4):**567-574, 1997.
20. Kress JP, Pohlman AS, O'Connor F, et al: Daily interruption of sedative infusions in critically ill patients undergoing mechanical ventilation, **N Engl J Med 342(20):**1471-1477.
21. Levine RL: Pharmacology of intravenous sedatives and opioids in critically ill patients, **Crit Care Clin 10(4):**709-731, 1994.
22. Levy FH, O'Rourke PP, Crone RK: Extracorporeal membrane oxygenation, **Int Anesthesia Res Soc 75:**1053-1062, 1992.
23. Marcy TW, Marini JJ: Respiratory distress in the ventilated patient, **Clin Chest Med 15(1):**55-73, 1994.
24. Marik PE: Pulmonary artery catheterization and esophageal Doppler monitoring in the ICU, **Chest 116(4):**1085-1091, 1999.
25. Marini JJ: Evolving concepts in the ventilatory management of acute respiratory distress syndrome, **Clin Chest Med 17(3):**555-575, 1996.
26. Meduri GU, Headly AS, Golden E, et al: Effect of prolonged methylprednisolone therapy in unresolving acute respiratory distress syndrome, **JAMA 280(2):**159-165, 1998.
27. Mimoz O, Rauss A, Nourrendine R, et al: Pulmonary artery catheterization in critically ill patients: a prospective analysis of outcome changes associated with catheter-prompted changes in therapy, **Crit Care Med 22(4):**573-579, 1994.
28. Mizushima Y, Wang P, Cioffi WG, et al: Should normothermia be restored and maintained during resuscitation after trauma and hemorrhage? **J Trauma 48(1):**58-65, 2000.
29. Novelline RA, Rhea JT, Rao PM, et al: Helical CT in emergency radiology, **Radiology 213(2):**321-339, 1999.
30. Perdue PW, Balser JR, Lipsett PA, et al: "Renal dose" dopamine in surgical patients, **Ann Surg 227(4):**470-473, 1997.
31. Porter JM, Ivantury RR: In search of the optimal endpoints of resuscitation in trauma patients: a review, **J Trauma 44(5):**908-914, 1998.
32. Raff T, Germann G, Hartmann B: The value of early enteral nutrition in the prophylaxis of stress ulceration in the severely burned patient, **Burns 23(4):**313-318, 1997.
33. Rathbun SW, Raskob GE, Whitset TL: Sensitivity and specificity of helical computed tomography in the diagnosis of pulmonary embolism: a systematic review, **Ann Intern Med 132(3):**227-232, 2000.
34. Richards MJ, Edwards JR, Culver DH, et al: Nosocomial infections in medical intensive care units in the United States, **Crit Care Med 27(5):**887-892, 1999.
35. Richman PS, Wolfson MR, Shaffer TH: Lung lavage with oxygenated perfluorochemical liquid in acute lung injury, **Crit Care Med 21(5):**768-774, 1993.
36. Ridings PC, Bloomfield GL, Blocher CR, et al: Cardiopulmonary effects of raised intra-abdominal pressure before and after intravascular volume expansion, **J Trauma 39(6):**1071-1075, 1995.
37. Rizoli SB, Kapus A, Fan J, et al: Immuno-modulatory effect of hypertonic resuscitation on the development of inflammation following hemorrhagic shock, **J Immunol 161(11):**6288-6296, 1998.
38. Sanchez-Izquierdo JA, Perez Vela, JL, Lozano Quintana MJ, et al: Cytokine clearance during venovenous hemofiltration in the trauma patient, **Am J Kidney Dis 30(4):**483-488, 1997.
39. Swartz RD, Messana JM, Orzol S, et al: Comparing continuous hemofiltration with hemodialysis in patients with severe acute renal failure, **Am J Kidney Dis 34(3):**424-432, 1999.
40. Vretenar DF, Urschel JD, Parrott JC, et al: Cardiopulmonary bypass resuscitation for accidental hypothermia, **Ann Thorac Surg 58(3):**895-898, 1994.
41. Walmrath D, Schneider T, Schemuly R, et al: Direct comparison of inhaled nitric oxide and aerosolized prostacyclin in acute respiratory distress syndrome, **Am J Respir Crit Care Med 153:**991-996, 1996.
42. Ware L, Matthay MA: The acute respiratory distress syndrome, **N Engl J Med 342(18):**1334-1349, 2000.

CHAPTER 12

Subarachnoid Hemorrhage

KEVIN C. YAO
JOSHUA B. BEDERSON

Aneurysmal subarachnoid hemorrhage (SAH) occurs in approximately 30,000 individuals per year in the United States[79] and is a devastating event with grave consequences. Population-based studies demonstrate a 30-day mortality rate following SAH of 45% and significant morbidity in one half of survivors.[1,11] Ischemic brain injury imparted by the initial hemorrhage accounts for most of these poor outcomes. However, rehemorrhage and vasospasm contribute significant morbidity and mortality in the post-hemorrhage period. Over the past decade, outcomes after SAH have improved.[18] This is due not only to improved techniques in the obliteration of aneurysms, but also to advances in the prevention and treatment of complications associated with SAH. Surgical and endovascular techniques have recently evolved such that improved outcomes in the future will depend primarily on advances made in the intensive care of SAH.

INTRACRANIAL HEMODYNAMICS OF SAH

Aneurysmal rupture is the most common cause of spontaneous SAH.[75,93] Hemodynamic stress gives rise to aneurysm formation by inducing degenerative change in the arterial wall. Major arterial branch points suffer the most turbulent blood flow and thus are the most common locations for aneurysms. Aneurysmal rupture results in subarachnoid hemorrhage (95%), intraparenchymal or intraventricular hemorrhage (50%), or subdural hemorrhage (10% to 20%).[126] Pathophysiological alterations occur in proportion to the volume of blood released. These include an increase in intracranial pressure (ICP), a decrease in cerebral perfusion pressure (CPP), a decrease in cerebral blood flow (CBF), and loss of vascular autoregulation.

ICP rises to near arterial pressure acutely following aneurysmal SAH. This rise is followed by a return toward baseline in the majority of patients. ICP measurements correlate with clinical grade and overall outcome: good-grade patients demonstrate normalization of ICP (<15 mm Hg), whereas poor-grade patients demonstrate persistent intracranial hypertension (>30 mm Hg).[7,48,57,89,121,125] As ICP rises, CPP (mean arterial pressure—ICP) falls.[20,36,38] This decrease often is not compensated in SAH because cerebral vessels lose their ability to autoregulate blood flow in response to changes in CO_2 concentrations and CPP.[121] Acute SAH-induced vasoconstriction may also contribute to ischemia in this setting, resulting in a 60% to 70% global decrease in CBF.[83] In this state, the brain is susceptible to ischemic brain injury, which is demonstrated by decreases in cerebral oxygen demand and metabolism.[16,54,78,121,] Clinical grade correlates inversely with CBF and cerebral metabolism.[27,91] Paradoxically there is an increase in total cerebral blood volume (CBV) as vessels in ischemic areas demonstrate a compensatory dilatation.[38,123] The most important cause of death after SAH is ischemic brain injury caused by the initial hemorrhage. In a population-based study, 61% of all SAH deaths occurred within 48 hours of the initial hemorrhage, with nearly half preceding medical consultation.[11] The brains of patients dying shortly after SAH demonstrate diffuse cortical ischemic change. The initial intensive care management of SAH focuses on limiting the extent of the original injury and preventing additional damage. Subsequent management addresses the neurological and medical complications of SAH, including secondary brain insults manifested as delayed ischemic deficits (DID).

DIAGNOSIS AND INITIAL MANAGEMENT OF SAH

Prompt diagnosis and treatment is paramount in the management of SAH. Within hours of onset, the consequences of misdiagnosis can be fatal. SAH is an acute event heralded by stereotyped neurological signs and symptoms.[31,120]; however, the presentation may be atypical, leading to frequent misdiagnoses. The primary symptom is sudden, severe headache described as being "the worst of my life." Brief loss of consciousness at the time of the event commonly occurs and may be followed by prolonged obtundation in more severe cases. Meningeal irritation by subarachnoid blood may cause nausea, vomiting, neck pain, or photophobia. Focal neurological signs often are not present. Several clinical grading systems for SAH help to predict prognosis. The most widely accepted is the Hunt and Hess grading scale.[55] An alternative SAH scale was proposed by the World Federation of Neurosurgical Societies to reduce interobserver variability.[112]

Prompt medical attention is essential for the treatment of SAH. Initial management in the field and emergency room involves assurance of respiratory and hemodynamic stability. Obtundation warrants endotracheal intubation. Blood pressure treatment is directed toward achieving a normotensive state in patients who often demonstrate acute, severe systolic hypertension.

The single most important diagnostic test for SAH is noncontrast computed tomography (CT). Once the patient's vital signs have been stabilized, CT should be performed. When performed on the day of symptom onset, CT detects 95% of SAH.[2] Other CT findings include cerebral edema, intracerebral hemorrhage, intraventricular hemorrhage, and hydrocephalus. The Fisher grading system helps to correlate the amount and distribution of subarachnoid blood with the subsequent development of vasospasm, one of the most important contributors to morbidity and mortality.[30] Evidence of a discrete hematoma with resultant herniation may necessitate immediate surgical evacuation and aneurysm exploration in place of further diagnostic measures. If CT fails to reveal SAH, lumbar puncture may disclose the presence of subarachnoid blood, and is mandatory in any patient in whom SAH is suspected.

Invasive intracranial pressure monitoring should be implemented in poor-grade patients (Hunt and Hess grades 4 to 5) and those with acute hydrocephalus. A ventricular catheter serves to both monitor and allow treatment of intracranial hypertension (ICP>0 mm Hg). Care is taken not to lower ICP precipitously, which may increase the pressure gradient across the aneurysm wall and cause rerupture. If ICP remains high, hyperventilation and osmotic diuretics are applied. CT angiography (CTA), magnetic resonance angiography (MRA), and digital subtraction angiography (DSA) allow examination of individual intracranial arteries for the presence of aneurysm. CTA is a recently developed technique that employs an intravenous bolus of contrast material followed by rapid sequence CT scanning. The advantages to this technique are the rapidity with which images are obtained, its noninvasiveness, and its relatively high sensitivity and specificity.[118,141] However, small aneurysms (<3 mm) may be missed and postoperative residual aneurysmal dilation may be obscured by clip artifact.[5] The amount of contrast material needed for CTA should be considered, especially in cases in which follow-up DSA may be needed the same day. One excellent application of CTA is in emergency situations, such as imminent herniation as a result of an expanding hematoma, when image acquisition time is the most crucial factor for outcome.

MRA is another noninvasive technique that relies on blood flow for visualization of the intracranial vessels. Similar to CTA, the disadvantage of MRA is its insensitivity to small (<5 mm) aneurysms. However, a recent study emphasizes the complementary roles MRA and DSA may play in the diagnosis of intracranial aneurysms.[56]

DSA remains the gold standard diagnostic modality for intracranial aneurysm and should be performed as soon as possible after the diagnosis of spontaneous SAH. An aneurysm can be identified in 95% of cases.[32] Given the 25% incidence of multiple aneurysms, a complete four-vessel angiogram should be the initial screening procedure in stable patients.[32] Vascular anatomy is examined for the aneurysm, vascular aberrancy relevant to surgical clipping, and evidence of early vasospasm. Early vasospasm portends a worse prognosis for long-term outcome. When multiple aneurysms are found, focal spasm or aneurysmal irregularity can help pinpoint the site of rupture. Additionally, focal subarachnoid blood on CT or discrete neurological deficits can aid in this determination. Early obliteration of the ruptured aneurysm is then undertaken via either direct surgical clipping or an endovascular approach.

NEUROLOGICAL CONSEQUENCES OF SAH

Rebleeding

Following the initial hemorrhage, aneurysm rebleeding and cerebral vasospasm account for the majority of morbidity and mortality in SAH. The risk of rebleeding is greatest in the first 24 hours following SAH, with an incidence of 4%.[64] Of untreated aneurysms, 20% rerupture within 2 weeks, whereas 50% rerupture within 1 month.[63,64] By 6 months the rehemorrhage risk stabilizes at 2% to 3% per year.[133] Overall, rebleeding imparts a 70% mortality and accounts for 50% of all deaths that occur more than 48 hours after the initial SAH.[76,79] Signs of rehemorrhage include worsening of existing symptoms, a new seizure, or acute neurological deterioration. When the new deficit is accompanied by an acute rise in ICP, rebleeding is the likely cause and should be confirmed by a repeat CT scan. Historically, conservative measures such as bed rest and antihypertensive medications were used to prevent rebleeding; however, these measures have been shown to be ineffective.[49,130] Early obliteration of the aneurysm is the most definitive method of preventing rebleeding. In addition, obliteration allows for more effective management of cerebral vasospasm. Consequently, early surgical intervention (within 3 days of SAH) is, in our opinion, generally warranted in the majority of good-grade patients with no limiting medical conditions.[63] Poor-grade SAH patients or those with concomitant medical complications may benefit from delayed surgery (more than 14 days after SAH). The International Cooperative Study on the Timing of Aneurysm Surgery indicated that surgical outcome was worse when undertaken 4 to 10 days after the initial hemorrhage, presumably because the brain is most vulnerable to ischemia during this period of maximum vasospasm.[63] Endovascular occlusion via detachable coils has shown promising results for poor-grade patients and poor surgical candidates by effectively preventing acute rebleeding.[17,33,39,52,67] Late surgery is an option in patients for whom endovascular occlusion is not feasible and who do not meet the criteria for early operation. Alternative surgical procedures such as aneurysm wrapping or proximal artery ligation have not proven to be effective in preventing rebleeding.

Antifibrinolytic agents have been employed to stabilize perianeurysmal clot and thereby limit recurrent hemorrhage. Early clinical trials with intravenous aminocaproic acid demonstrated efficacy in decreasing the risk of rebleeding.[3,62,119] However, this beneficial effect was negated by an increased incidence of ischemic stroke when antifibrinolysis was continued for more than 7 days.[62,113,119,127] A more recent study demonstrated the efficacy of a short course of high-dose ϵ-aminocaproic acid (EACA) in decreasing rebleeding rates prior to early aneurysm surgery without an increased risk of stroke.[71] These authors recommended an initial intravenous loading dose of 10 g of EACA once SAH is suspected, followed by a continuous infusion of 48 g daily until aneurysm obliteration. Dosages should be adjusted based on daily serum drug levels. Combination therapy involving antifibrinolytic and neuroprotective agents can increase the utility of these agents.[9]

Vasospasm

Vasospasm is prolonged cerebral arterial constriction that occurs in response to subarachnoid blood. Because SAH is focused in the basal cisterns, the most commonly involved vessels are those that lie near the base of the brain. Fisher demonstrated a correlation between thickness of subarachnoid blood clot and likelihood of subsequent vasospasm.[30] Vasospasm afflicts 70% of SAH patients, inciting ischemic symptoms in 20% to 30%.[51,61] Arterial constriction decreases CBF, producing areas of marginal perfusion that are susceptible to ischemic injury.[80] Ultimately, vasospasm leads to stroke or death in up to 15% of SAH patients who survive the original hemorrhage.[80] Vasospasm occurs in a delayed fashion, typically appearing 3 to 4 days after the initial SAH, peaking in severity at 7 to 10 days, and eventually resolving in 2 to 4 weeks.

The diagnosis of vasospasm relies on careful clinical monitoring combined with diagnostic testing. Clinically, symptoms may fluctuate and range from a subtle decreased level of alertness to focal neurological deficits or coma. Imaging of the intracranial vessels via angiography provides the definitive diagnosis by demonstrating arterial narrowing. However, angiographic spasm is not always symptomatic: approximately one half of patients with angiographic spasm remain asymptomatic. Furthermore the invasive nature of angiography, which carries a 1% to 2% risk of stroke, limits its usefulness as a monitoring technique.[23,75] Instead it should be reserved for settings in which confirmation of a clinical diagnosis is desired or interventional therapeutic techniques are needed.

The most commonly used noninvasive technique for bedside diagnosis and monitoring of vasospasm is transcranial Doppler (TCD) ultrasonography.[1,74] TCD is a technique that measures blood flow velocity in the major intracranial arteries. The Bernoulli effect predicts an inverse relationship between vessel caliber and flow velocity. Absolute elevations of TCD velocities as well as elevations relative to extracranial vessels (cervical carotid) correlate with the degree of arterial narrowing.[1,44,105] MCA velocities are normally 30 to 80 cm/sec. Elevated TCD velocities may reflect severe (>200 cm/s) or mild to moderate (120-200 cm/s) vasospasm. Acute TCD elevations often precede the onset of clinical vasospasm by 24 to 48 hours.[80] However, only low (<120 cm/s) or very high (>200 cm/s) absolute velocities consistently correlate with arterial narrowing.[124] Because most SAH patients demonstrate intermediate velocities, invasive treatment should not generally be based on TCD velocities alone.[124] Rather, the most useful role of TCD is in determining the need for further angiographic examination and in monitoring poor-grade patients in whom clinical signs of further neurological deterioration may be difficult to identify.

More recently, techniques to directly measure CBF have been used to confirm the presence of low-flow states. These techniques include xenon-133,[136] xenon-CT,[40,137] single-photon emission computed tomography (SPECT),[73] and positron emission tomography (PET).[98] Practical diagnosis and monitoring of vasospasm usually involves routine TCD daily or every other day from the onset of SAH. Angiography is performed in the postoperative period for the evaluation of surgical clipping, for diagnostic confirmation of clinical vasospasm, and for therapeutic interventional measures in refractory vasospasm.

The management of vasospasm focuses on minimizing ischemic brain injury. Approaches include removal of the irritant subarachnoid blood, prevention or reversal of vascular smooth muscle contraction, promotion of cerebral perfusion, and administration of neuroprotective agents. Several studies have confirmed a correlation between the volume of subarachnoid blood and the severity of subsequent vasospasm. Theoretically, removal of the subarachnoid clot should prevent the onset of vascular spasm. Promising experimental models using primates demonstrated the efficacy of intracisternal tissue plasminogen activator, a fibrinolytic agent, in decreasing the severity of vasospasm.[29] Several nonrandomized clinical trials subsequently demonstrated that TPA could be safely administered following aneurysm clipping.[28,68,85,102,103] However, these trials failed to demonstrate a statistically significant lower incidence of vasospasm.[138] Intraoperative removal of the subarachnoid clot by saline lavage also failed to demonstrate a significant effect on the incidence of subsequent vasospasm. Although this evidence demonstrates the limitations of TPA, it is clear from these studies that periarterial blood and its breakdown products are necessary for the development of vasospasm.[80] Continued research in this direction may produce successful prophylactic biochemical techniques for the prevention of vasospasm.

The prophylactic use of calcium-channel blocking drugs arose from the hypothesis that prevention of vascular smooth muscle contraction would limit vasospasm. In fact, several trials of the oral agent nimodipine have demonstrated consistently improved outcomes, especially in poor-grade patients.[4,94-96] As a result, nimodipine is currently the only agent available with proven clinical efficacy in decreasing the neurological sequelae of cerebral vasospasm. The FDA recently approved its use in all grades of SAH patients. It is now postulated, however, that nimodipine functions by protecting marginally ischemic neurons from excessive harmful calcium influx rather than by actually decreasing vascular spasm.[80] The usual prescription is 60 mg every 4 hours for 10 to 21 days following SAH. Its hypotensive effects may necessitate dosage reduction to 30 mg every 2 hours, or discontinuation. Another calcium-channel blocker, nicardipine, has also undergone several trials. Despite a decreased incidence of vasospasm, its injurious effects on blood pressure and volume status negated any overall benefit.[42]

Hypertensive, hypervolemic, and hemodilutional ("triple-H") therapy for vasospasm developed from the recognition that vasospastic ischemic brain injury is potentiated by hypovolemia coupled with loss of cerebrovascular autoregulation. Studies demonstrate that circulating red blood cell volume in patients with SAH is decreased.[69,77,106,109] This relative hypovolemia predisposes SAH patients to a higher incidence of DID.[109] Previous studies demonstrated that volume expansion, independent of effects on cerebral perfusion pressure, improved CBF in patients with vasospasm.[82] More recent data, however, indicate that prevention of hypovolemia rather than the induction of a hypervolemic state is the critical factor in preventing cerebral ischemia in this setting.[72] Hemodilution alone also improves both CBF and oxygen delivery by decreasing blood viscosity.[134,135] Volume expansion alone often provides adequate hemodilution to an optimal hematocrit of 30% to 33%.[37,65,86] Because of the loss of autoregulation in cerebral blood vessels, there is a direct correlation between mean arterial pressure (MAP) and CBF.[43,66,111] Several studies have demonstrated the ability of induced hypertension to reduce DID.[7,86,6,14,15,26,92,108] The combination of hypertension, hypervolemia, and hemodilution has become well accepted[72,114] despite the presence of only one published controlled trial.[100] Practical application of triple-H therapy involves volume expansion with isotonic crystalloid at full maintenance augmented with boluses of colloid (250 ml of 5% albumin every 6 hours) as needed to maintain central venous pressure between 5 to 7 mm Hg. Hematocrit is maintained between 30% to 32%. With the onset of angiographic, TCD, or clinical evidence of vasospasm in the absence of infarction or hemorrhage, hypertension is induced in a stepwise fashion until the deficit or level of consciousness improves. Pressors are weaned when either the neurological deficit resolves or ischemic infarction develops on CT scan. Fluids are maintained prophylactically for a full 2-week course following SAH. Triple-H therapy has been associated with complications including congestive heart failure, pulmonary edema, electrolyte disorders such as hyponatremia, and brain edema. Additionally, pharmacological induction of hypertension and vasoconstriction has been associated with myocardial infarction, intracranial hemorrhage, and rupture of unsecured aneurysms.

Endovascular techniques have proven to be increasingly useful not only in the primary treatment of aneurysms, but also in the treatment of vasospasm. Transluminal balloon angioplasty involves selective microcatheterization and mechanical dilation of severely narrowed cerebral arteries with an inflatable balloon. In carefully selected patients, angiographic reversal of vasospasm refractory to medical treatment has been reported to be as high as 98% to 100%.[12,53] However, many patients have distal vasospasm that is not amenable to angioplasty. The effect of dilation is long-lasting, whereas the incidence of complications, including arterial rupture, distal embolic infarction, and rerupture of unclipped aneurysms, may be relatively low in experienced centers (<6%).[10,97] The ability of angioplasty to reverse clinical symptoms is inversely related to time between onset of symptoms and institution of therapy. More significant clinical improvement is achieved when angioplasty is performed within 24 hours of neurological deterioration.[10] When instituted within 2 hours in carefully selected patients, clinical improvement is achieved in up to 70% of patients.[99] Trials of prophylactic angioplasty are ongoing.[87]

Another endovascular technique that has been employed is intraarterial infusion of papaverine. Infusion of this powerful vasodilating agent via a microcatheter has been useful in transiently reversing vasospasm, especially in distal arteries not readily accessible to angioplasty.[19,58,59] However, papaverine's short-lived effect (less than 24 hours) limits its practical use as a routine treatment for vasospasm.[24]

Experimental approaches to the treatment of vasospasm include biochemical methods to effect neuronal protection. Studies have demonstrated lipid peroxidation as an essential step in the pathogenesis of cerebral ischemia. Laboratory experiments with animal models employing antioxidants demonstrated an improvement in vasospasm; however, these results were not duplicated in a prospective randomized clinical trial using tirilazad mesylate, an antioxidant.[41] Future research promises molecular approaches to limit ischemic brain injury caused by vasospasm.

Hydrocephalus

Hydrocephalus may present acutely, subacutely, or as a late complication of SAH.[47,51] Blockage of CSF circulation by blood within the subarachnoid space may lead to acute obstructive hydrocephalus in approximately 20% of SAH patients.[117] These are typically poor-grade patients who manifest hydrocephalus either as coma or neurological deterioration.[35,84] Such symptoms warrant placement of a ventriculostomy catheter. In addition, a large percentage of poor-grade patients (Hunt and Hess grades 4 and 5) demonstrate elevated ICP even in the absence of ventriculomegaly.[7] These patents improve clinically when treated for hydrocephalus. For this reason, we believe that placement of a ventriculostomy catheter is indicated in all poor-grade SAH patients regardless of radiographic absence of ventriculomegaly. In the acute setting, care is taken not to lower ICP below 15 mm Hg because of the theoretical risk of potentiating rerupture of an unclipped aneurysm. Two thirds of patients with acute hydrocephalus improve with ventricular drainage; however, complications of infection may limit long-term outcome.[83] Prophylactic antibiotics at the time of insertion as well as routine testing of CSF for signs of infection may limit infectious complications. Hydrocephalus occurring in the subacute or late period is typically communicating rather than obstructive. Subacute hydrocephalus occurs within 1 week of SAH and is common. Because these patients may be asymptomatic, CSF drainage via ventriculostomy or lumbar drainage can be reserved for those who demonstrate neurological deterioration. Serial CT scanning often demonstrates resolution of subacute hydrocephalus without the need for permanent shunting. Up to 20% of patients surviving SAH require permanent CSF diversion.[116] Indications for ventriculoperitoneal shunting include (1) persistent symptomatic hydrocephalus in the acute or subacute period despite the absence of gross blood in the CSF or (2) the development of late hydrocephalus, within weeks to months of SAH, typically presenting as dementia, gait ataxia, or incontinence.

Seizures

Seizures occur at the time of aneurysm rupture in up to 25% of patients.[45,110] In addition, approximately 3% of patients suffer delayed seizures.[8,140] Seizures theoretically increase the risk of rerupture in patients with unsecured aneurysms and potentiate further ischemic brain injury in patients with vasospasm. Consequently, most physicians advocate the prophylactic use of anticonvulsants following SAH. However, randomized prospective trials fail to demonstrate a significant decrease in the incidence of seizure.[34,90] Nevertheless the short-term use of prophylactic anticonvulsants in SAH patients at low risk is recommended.[8] We commonly employ the prophylactic use of phenytoin following SAH for 2 weeks in low-risk patients who fail to demonstrate seizure activity. Phenobarbital is administered in the short term to patients who display intolerance to phenytoin, such as fever, rash, or hepatotoxicity. Patients with documented seizure activity or those with risk factors including a space-occupying hematoma or sizable infarct are treated with a 3-month regimen of anticonvulsants. EEG monitoring is then performed to identify the presence of a persistent seizure focus.

MEDICAL CONSEQUENCES OF SAH

SAH patients are often critically ill. Several medical complications occur as a direct result of systemic alterations induced by SAH. In addition, systemic complications related to prolonged debilitation in the critical care setting often occur.

Hyponatremia

Systemic alterations in intravascular fluid volume often occur as a result of SAH. Up to 30% of patients demonstrate hyponatremia.[128,129] Excessive sodium excretion and subsequent hypovolemia are the most common underlying causes.[77,88,131] Hypovolemia associated with cerebral salt wasting increases the susceptibility of SAH patients to ischemic injury. Hypervolemic therapy in conjunction with sodium repletion is the mainstay of treatment. Fludrocortisone, an inhibitor of natriuresis, has been useful in the correction of volume and sodium derangements.[46,132] Paradoxically, some SAH patients display hyponatremia in the setting of normovolemia or hypervolemia. This has been attributed to the syndrome of inappropriate secretion of antidiuretic hormone (SIADH). The treatment of this condition calls for fluid restriction. Distinguishing SIADH from cerebral salt wasting often requires central venous pressure monitoring and additional electrolyte measurements. Given the contradicting treatments, and the potential dangers of further volume contraction in the setting of marginally perfused brain, it is important to accurately determine and treat the cause of hyponatremia in patients with SAH.

Cardiac Complications

Cardiac complications are common following SAH.[63] Intracranial hemorrhage results in a release of catecholamines that may decrease cardiac compliance or may be directly cardiotoxic.[21,101] EKG changes are common, even in patients with no previous history of cardiac disease, and include T-wave inversions, ST segment depressions and elevations, prolonged QT interval, and prominent U waves.[13,70,81,139] Arrythmias occur in up to 30% of patients but are usually nonsustained. Elevated creatine kinase-isoenzyme levels (CPK-MB) are common as well, although the incidence of myocardial infarction is rare. Institution of hypervolemic and hypertensive therapy may aggravate myocardial ischemia.[60] Each of these abnormalities is potentially life threatening, and thus all SAH patients require close cardiac monitoring. The periods of greatest cardiac risk are during the first 48 hours following SAH and during triple-H therapy. Studies consistently show, however, that the incidence of cardiac mortality in SAH is low. Therefore no intervention, surgical or medical, should be withheld from patients with cardiac abnormalities, except in the most severe cases of life-threatening arrhythmia.[139] No controlled trials have demonstrated efficacy of prophylactic cardioprotective drugs following SAH.

Pulmonary Complications

The most common pulmonary complications of SAH are pulmonary edema, pneumonia, and pulmonary embolism. These account for half the deaths in aneurysmal SAH attributable to medical complications.[107] Pneumonia occurs in up to 20% of SAH patients. Aspiration and prolonged mechanical ventilation are the major sources of pulmonary infection in this population. Timely intubation in the face of a deteriorating mental status, appropriate antibiotic therapy, and judicious tracheostomy placement guide the treatment of pneumonia.

Pulmonary edema may be neurogenic or cardiogenic in origin. Neurogenic pulmonary edema is due to SAH-induced abnormalities in pulmonary vascular permeability. The edema fluid that results, unlike that resulting from cardiogenic pulmonary edema, is high in protein content. Positive end-expiratory pressure ventilation is frequently required to maintain adequate oxygenation. Cardiogenic pulmonary edema may occur as a result of primary cardiac failure or excessive volume expansion associated with triple-H therapy. Patients are at risk of developing cardiogenic pulmonary edema regardless of the absence of prior cardiac or pulmonary disease.[104] Carefully monitored volume expansion, with the aid of a pulmonary artery catheter in difficult cases, is indicated in all SAH patients.

Thromboembolism

SAH patients are frequently subjected to prolonged periods of bed rest and immobilization. Significant deep venous thrombosis (DVT) and pulmonary embolism (PE) complicate at least 2% of such patients.[70] Routine prophylaxis is recommended in all patients. These measures include the use of intermittent pressure stockings, low molecular weight heparin, and early mobilization. Such prophylactic measures have been shown to decrease the incidence of thromboembolism by as much as 18%.

Prospective clinical trials demonstrating the appropriate means of treatment for an established DVT or PE in the setting of SAH are lacking. Theoretically, anticoagulation may worsen the severity of aneurysmal rerupture. For this reason, vena caval filter insertion is preferred in patients with established DVT prior to treatment of the ruptured aneurysm. If anticoagulation is required in the postoperative period, intravenous heparin is instituted within 48 hours of surgery. The goal for heparinization is a PTT between 45 and 60 seconds.

Gastrointestinal Complications

Gastrointestinal bleeding caused by stress ulceration occurs in 4% of patients following SAH.[63] Poor-grade patients are at greater risk. The prophylactic use of H2 antagonists, sulcrafate, and antacids is recommended in all patients following SAH. Treatment of established stress ulceration is nasogastric lavage, fluid replacement, and transfusion.

CONCLUSION

Aneurysmal SAH is a complex pathophysiological event that has devastating consequences. Recent advances in the treatment of aneurysms and SAH-related complications have markedly improved long-term outcome, especially in good-grade patients. As we learn more about the mechanisms behind SAH and its sequelae, more rational modalities of treatment will be discovered. The future holds great improvements in patient outcome following SAH. It is the critical care setting in which most of these advances will undoubtedly be discovered and applied.

REFERENCES

1. Aaslid R, Huber P, Nornes H: Evaluation of cerebrovascular spasm with transcranial Doppler ultrasound, **J Neurosurg 60(1):**37-41, 1984.
2. Adams HP Jr, Kassell NF, Torner JC, et al: Predicting cerebral ischemia after aneurysmal subarachnoid hemorrhage: influences of clinical condition, CT results, and antifibrinolytic therapy. A report of the Cooperative Aneurysm Study, **Neurology 37(10):**1586-1591, 1987.
3. Adams HP Jr, Nibbelink DW, Torner JC, et al: Antifibrinolytic therapy in patients with aneurysmal subarachnoid hemorrhage. A report of the cooperative aneurysm study, **Arch Neurol 38(1):**25-29, 1981.
4. Allen GS, Ahn HS, Preziosi TJ, et al: Cerebral arterial spasm—a controlled trial of nimodipine in patients with subarachnoid hemorrhage, **N Engl J Med 308(11):** 619-624, 1983.
5. Anderson GB, Findlay JM, Steinke DE, et al: Experience with computed tomographic angiography for the detection of intracranial aneurysms in the setting of acute subarachnoid hemorrhage, **Neurosurgery 41(3):**522-527, 527-528, 1997.
6. Awad IA, Carter LP, Spetzler RF, et al: Clinical vasospasm after subarachnoid hemorrhage: response to hypervolemic hemodilution and arterial hypertension, **Stroke 18(2):**365-372, 1987.
7. Bailes JE, Spetzler RF, Hadley MN, et al: Management morbidity and mortality of poor-grade aneurysm patients, **J Neurosurg 72(4):**559-566, 1990.
8. Baker CJ, Prestigiacomo CJ, Solomon RA: Short-term perioperative anticonvulsant prophylaxis for the surgical treatment of low-risk patients with intracranial aneurysms, **Neurosurgery 37(5):**863-870, 870-871, 1995.
9. Beck DW, Adams HP, Flamm ES, et al: Combination of aminocaproic acid and nicardipine in treatment of aneurysmal subarachnoid hemorrhage, **Stroke 19(1):** 63-67, 1988.
10. Bejjani GK, Bank WO, Olan WJ, et al: The efficacy and safety of angioplasty for cerebral vasospasm after subarachnoid hemorrhage, **Neurosurgery 42(5):**979-986, 986-987, 1998.
11. Broderick JP, Brott TG, Duldner JE, et al: Initial and recurrent bleeding are the major causes of death following subarachnoid hemorrhage, **Stroke 25(7):**1342-1347, 1994.
12. Brothers MF, Holgate RC: Intracranial angioplasty for treatment of vasospasm after subarachnoid hemorrhage: technique and modifications to improve branch access, **AJNR Am J Neuroradiol 11(2):**239-247, 1990.
13. Brouwers PJ, Wijdicks EF, Hasan D, et al: Serial electrocardiographic recording in aneurysmal subarachnoid hemorrhage, **Stroke 20(9):**1162-1167, 1989.
14. Brown FD, Hanlon K, Mullan S: Treatment of aneurysmal hemiplegia with dopamine and mannitol, **J Neurosurg 49(4):**525-529, 1978.
15. Buckland MR, Batjer HH, Giesecke AH: Anesthesia for cerebral aneurysm surgery: use of induced hypertension in patients with symptomatic vasospasm, **Anesthesiology 69(1):**116-119, 1988.
16. Carpenter DA, Grubb RL Jr, Tempel LW, et al: Cerebral oxygen metabolism after aneurysmal subarachnoid hemorrhage, **J Cereb Blood Flow Metab 11(5):**837-44, 1991.
17. Casasco AE, Aymard A, Gobin YP, et al: **Selective endovascular treatment of 71 intracranial aneurysms with platinum coils, J Neurosurg 79(1):**3-10, 1993.
18. Cesarini KG, Hardemark HG, Persson L: Improved survival after aneurysmal subarachnoid hemorrhage: review of case management during a 12-year period, **J Neurosurg 90(4):**664-672, 1999.
19. Clouston JE, Numaguchi Y, Zoarski GH, et al: Intraarterial papaverine infusion for cerebral vasospasm after subarachnoid hemorrhage, **AJNR Am J Neuroradiol 16(1):**27-38, 1995.
20. Crompton R: Cerebral infarction following the rupture of cerebral berry aneurysm, **Brain 87:**263, 1964.
21. Cruickshank JM, Neil-Dwyer G, Stott AW: Possible role of catecholamines, corticosteroids, and potassium in production of electrocardiographic abnormalities associated with subarachnoid haemorrhage, **Br Heart J 36(7):**697-706, 1974.
22. Dion JE, Duckwiler GR, Vinuela F, et al: Pre-operative micro-angioplasty of refractory vasospasm secondary to subarachnoid hemorrhage, **Neuroradiology 32(3):** 232-236, 1990.
23. Dion JE, Gates PC, Fox AJ, et al: Clinical events following neuroangiography: a prospective study, **Stroke 18(6):**997-1004, 1987.
24. Elliott JP, Newell DW, Lam DJ, et al: Comparison of balloon angioplasty and papaverine infusion for the treatment of vasospasm following aneurysmal subarach-

noid hemorrhage [see comments], **J Neurosurg 88(2):** 277-284, 1998.
25. Eskridge JM, Newell DW, Winn HR: Endovascular treatment of vasospasm, **Neurosurg Clin N Am 5(3):** 437-447, 1994.
26. Farhat SM, Schneider RC: Observations on the effect of systemic blood pressure on intracranial circulation in patients with cerebrovascular insufficiency, **J Neurosurg 27(5):**441-445, 1967.
27. Fazl M, Houlden DA, Weaver K: Correlation between cerebral blood flow, somatosensory evoked potentials, CT scan grade and neurological grade in patients with subarachnoid hemorrhage, **Can J Neurol Sci 18(4):** 453-457, 1991.
28. Findlay JM, Weir BK, Kassell NF, et al: Intracisternal recombinant tissue plasminogen activator after aneurysmal subarachnoid hemorrhage, **J Neurosurg 75(2):** 181-188, 1991.
29. Findlay JM, Weir BK, Steinke D, et al: Effect of intrathecal thrombolytic therapy on subarachnoid clot and chronic vasospasm in a primate model of SAH, **J Neurosurg 69(5):**723-735, 1988.
30. Fisher CM, Kistler JP, Davis JM: Relation of cerebral vasospasm to subarachnoid hemorrhage visualized by computerized tomographic scanning, **Neurosurgery 6(1):**1-9, 1980.
31. Fisher CM: Clinical syndromes in cerebral thrombosis, hypertensive hemorrhage, and ruptured saccular aneurysm, **Clin Neurosurg 22:**117-147, 1975.
32. Forster DM, Steiner L, Hakanson S, et al: The value of repeat pan-angiography in cases of unexplained subarachnoid hemorrhage, **J Neurosurg 48(5):**712-716, 1978.
33. Fox AJ, Vinuela F, Pelz DM, et al: Use of detachable balloons for proximal artery occlusion in the treatment of unclippable cerebral aneurysms, **J Neurosurg 66(1):** 40-46, 1987.
34. Foy PM, Chadwick DW, Rajgopalan N, et al: Do prophylactic anticonvulsant drugs alter the pattern of seizures after craniotomy? **J Neurol Neurosurg Psychiatry 55(9):**753-757, 1992.
35. Graff-Radford NR, Torner J, Adams HP Jr, et al: Factors associated with hydrocephalus after subarachnoid hemorrhage. A report of the Cooperative Aneurysm Study, **Arch Neurol 46(7):**744-752, 1989.
36. Graham DI, Macpherson P, Pitts LH: Correlation between angiographic vasospasm, hematoma, and ischemic brain damage following SAH, **J Neurosurg 59(2):**223-230, 1983.
37. Grotta JC: Current status of hemodilution in acute cerebral ischemia [editorial]. **Stroke 18(4):**689-690, 1987.
38. Grubb RL Jr, Raichle ME, Eichling JO, et al: Effects of subarachnoid hemorrhage on cerebral blood volume, blood flow, and oxygen utilization in humans, **J Neurosurg. 46(4):**446-453, 1977.
39. Guglielmi G, Vinuela F, Dion J, et al: Electrothrombosis of saccular aneurysms via endovascular approach. Part 2: Preliminary clinical experience [see comments], **J Neurosurg 75(1):**8-14, 1991.
40. Gur D, Wolfson SK Jr, Yonas H, et al: Progress in cerebrovascular disease: local cerebral blood flow by xenon enhanced CT, **Stroke 13(6):**750-758, 1982.
41. Haley EC Jr, Kassell NF, Apperson-Hansen C, et al: A randomized, double-blind, vehicle-controlled trial of tirilazad mesylate in patients with aneurysmal subarachnoid hemorrhage: a cooperative study in North America, **J Neurosurg 86(3):**467-474, 1997.
42. Haley EC Jr, Kassell NF, Torner JC: A randomized trial of nicardipine in subarachnoid hemorrhage: angiographic and transcranial Doppler ultrasound results. A report of the Cooperative Aneurysm Study, **J Neurosurg 78(4):**548-553, 1993.
43. Handa Y, Hayashi M, Takeuchi H, et al: Time course of the impairment of cerebral autoregulation during chronic cerebral vasospasm after subarachnoid hemorrhage in primates, **J Neurosurg 76(3):**493-501, 1992.
44. Harders AG, Gilsbach JM: Time course of blood velocity changes related to vasospasm in the circle of Willis measured by transcranial Doppler ultrasound, **J Neurosurg 66(5):**718-28, 1987.
45. Hart RG, Byer JA, Slaughter JR, et al: Occurrence and implications of seizures in subarachnoid hemorrhage due to ruptured intracranial aneurysms, **Neurosurgery 8(4):**417-421, 1981.
46. Hasan D, Lindsay KW, Wijdicks EF, et al: Effect of fludrocortisone acetate in patients with subarachnoid hemorrhage, **Stroke 20(9):**1156-1161, 1989.
47. Hasan D, Vermeulen M, Wijdicks EF, et al: Management problems in acute hydrocephalus after subarachnoid hemorrhage, **Stroke 20(6):**747-753, 1989.
48. Hayashi M, Marukawa S, Fujii H, et al: Intracranial hypertension in patients with ruptured intracranial aneurysm, **J Neurosurg 46(5):**584-590, 1977.
49. Henderson WG, Torner JC, Nibbelink DW: Intracranial aneurysms and subarachnoid hemorrhage—report on a randomized treatment study. IV-B. Regulated bed rest—statistical evaluation, **Stroke 8(5):**579-589, 1977.
50. Heros RC, Zervas NT, Varsos V:Cerebral vasospasm after subarachnoid hemorrhage: an update, **Ann Neurol 14(6):**599-608, 1983.
51. Heros RC: Acute hydrocephalus after subarachnoid hemorrhage **Stroke 20(6):**715-717, 1989.
52. Higashida RT, Halbach VV, Barnwell SL, et al: Treatment of intracranial aneurysms with preservation of the parent vessel: results of percutaneous balloon embolization in 84 patients [see comments], **AJNR Am J Neuroradiol 11(4):**633-640, 1990.
53. Higashida RT, Halbach VV, Dowd CF, et al: Intravascular balloon dilatation therapy for intracranial arterial vasospasm: patient selection, technique, and clinical results, **Neurosurg Rev 15(2):**89-95, 1992.
54. Hino A, Mizukawa N, Tenjin H, et al: Postoperative hemodynamic and metabolic changes in patients with subarachnoid hemorrhage, **Stroke 20(11):**1504-1510, 1989.
55. Hunt WE, Hess RM: Surgical risk as related to time of intervention in the repair of intracranial aneurysms, **J Neurosurg 28(1):**14-20, 1968.
56. Jager HR, Mansmann U, Hausmann O, et al: MRA versus digital subtraction angiography in acute subarachnoid haemorrhage: a blinded multireader study of prospectively recruited patients, **Neuroradiology 42(5):** 313-326, 2000.

57. Jakubowski J, Bell BA, Symon L, et al: A primate model of subarachnoid hemorrhage: change in regional cerebral blood flow, autoregulation carbon dioxide reactivity, and central conduction time, **Stroke 13(5):**601-611, 1982.
58. Kaku Y, Yonekawa Y, Tsukahara T, et al: Superselective intra-arterial infusion of papaverine for the treatment of cerebral vasospasm after subarachnoid hemorrhage [see comments], **J Neurosurg 77(6):**842-847, 1992.
59. Kassell NF, Helm G, Simmons N: Treatment of cerebral vasospastic actions of oxyhemoglobin by ascorbic acid, Neurosurgery **28:**33, 1991.
60. Kassell NF, Peerless SJ, Durward QJ, et al: Treatment of ischemic deficits from vasospasm with intravascular volume expansion and induced arterial hypertension, **Neurosurgery 11(3):**337-343, 1982.
61. Kassell NF, Sasaki T, Colohan AR, et al: Cerebral vasospasm following aneurysmal subarachnoid hemorrhage, **Stroke 16(4):**562-572, 1985.
62. Kassell NF, Torner JC, Adams HP Jr: Antifibrinolytic therapy in the acute period following aneurysmal subarachnoid hemorrhage. Preliminary observations from the Cooperative Aneurysm Study, **J Neurosurg 61(2):**225-230, 1984.
63. Kassell NF, Torner JC, Haley EC Jr, et al: The International Cooperative Study on the Timing of Aneurysm Surgery. Part 1: Overall management results, **J Neurosurg 73(1):**18-36, 1990.
64. Kassell NF, Torner JC: Aneurysmal rebleeding: a preliminary report from the Cooperative Aneurysm Study, **Neurosurgery 13(5):**479-481, 1983.
65. Kee DB, Wood JH: Influence of blood rheology on cerebral circulation, in Wood JH (ed): **Cerebral Blood Flow: Physiologic and Clinical Aspects**. New York: McGraw-Hill, 1987, p 173.
66. Kindt GW, Youmans JR, Albrand O: Factors influencing the autoregulation of the cerebral blood flow during hypotension and hypertension, **J Neurosurg 26(3):**299-305, 1967.
67. Kinugasa K, Mandai S, Terai Y, et al: Direct thrombosis of aneurysms with cellulose acetate polymer. Part II: Preliminary clinical experience [see comments], **J Neurosurg 77(4):**501-507, 1992.
68. Kodama N, Sasaki T, Kawakami M: Prevention of vasospasm: cistern irrigation therapy with urokinase and ascorbic acid, in Sano K, et al (eds): **Cerebral Vasospasm**. Tokyo: University of Tokyo Press, 1990, p 292-296.
69. Kudo T, Suzuki S, Iwabuchi T: Importance of monitoring the circulating blood volume in patients with cerebral vasospasm after subarachnoid hemorrhage, **Neurosurgery 9(5):**514-520, 1981.
70. Kuroiwa T, Morita H, Tanabe H, et al: Significance of ST segment elevation in electrocardiograms in patients with ruptured cerebral aneurysms, **Acta Neurochir 133(3-4):**141-146, 1995.
71. Leipzig TJ, Redelman K, Horner TG: Reducing the risk of rebleeding before early aneurysm surgery: a possible role for antifibrinolytic therapy [see comments], **J Neurosurg 86(2):**220-225, 1997.
72. Lennihan L, Mayer SA, Fink ME, et al: Effect of hypervolemic therapy on cerebral blood flow after subarachnoid hemorrhage: a randomized controlled trial, **Stroke 31(2):**383-391, 2000.
73. Lewis DH, Eskridge JM, Newell DW, et al: Brain SPECT and the effect of cerebral angioplasty in delayed ischemia due to vasospasm, **J Nucl Med 33(10):**1789-1796, 1992.
74. Lindegaard KF, Nornes H, Bakke SJ, et al: Cerebral vasospasm after subarachnoid haemorrhage investigated by means of transcranial Doppler ultrasound, **Acta Neurochir Suppl 42:**81-84, 1988.
75. Locksley HB: Natural history of subarachnoid hemorrhage, intracranial aneurysms and arteriovenous malformations. Based on 6368 cases in the cooperative study, **J Neurosurg 25(2):**219-239, 1966.
76. Locksley HB: Natural history of subarachnoid hemorrhage, intracranial aneurysms and arteriovenous malformations, **J Neurosurg 25(3):**321-368, 1966.
77. Maroon JC, Nelson PB: Hypovolemia in patients with subarachnoid hemorrhage: therapeutic implications, **Neurosurgery 4(3):**223-226, 1979.
78. Martin WR, Baker RP, Grubb RL, et al: Cerebral blood volume, blood flow, and oxygen metabolism in cerebral ischaemia and subarachnoid haemorrhage: an in-vivo study using positron emission tomography, **Acta Neurochir 70(1-2):**3-9, 1984.
79. Mayberg MR, Batjer HH, Dacey R, et al: Guidelines for the management of aneurysmal subarachnoid hemorrhage. A statement for healthcare professionals from a special writing group of the Stroke Council, American Heart Association, **Circulation 90(5):**2592-2605, 1994.
80. Mayberg MR: Cerebral vasospasm, **Neurosurg Clin N Am 9(3):**615-627, 1998.
81. Mayer SA, LiMandri G, Sherman D, et al: Electrocardiographic markers of abnormal left ventricular wall motion in acute subarachnoid hemorrhage, **J Neurosurg 83(5):**889-896, 1995.
82. McGillicuddy J, Kindt G, Giannotta S: Focal cerebral blood flow in cerebral vasospasm: the effect of intravascular volume expansion, **Acta Neurol Scand Suppl 60:**490, 1979.
83. McKhann GM II, Le Roux PD: Perioperative and intensive care unit care of patients with aneurysmal subarachnoid hemorrhage, **Neurosurg Clin N Am 9(3):** 595-613, 1998.
84. Milhorat TH: Acute hydrocephalus after aneurysmal subarachnoid hemorrhage, **Neurosurgery 20(1):**15-20, 1987.
85. Mizoi K, Yoshimoto T, Takahashi A, et al: Prospective study on the prevention of cerebral vasospasm by intrathecal fibrinolytic therapy with tissue-type plasminogen activator, **J Neurosurg 78(3):**430-437, 1993.
86. Muizelaar JP, Becker DP: Induced hypertension for the treatment of cerebral ischemia after subarachnoid hemorrhage. Direct effect on cerebral blood flow, **Surg Neurol 25(4):**317-325, 1986.
87. Muizelaar JP, Zwienenberg M, Rudisill NA, et al: The prophylactic use of transluminal balloon angioplasty in patients with Fisher Grade 3 subarachnoid hemorrhage: a pilot study [see comments], **J Neurosurg 91(1):**51-58, 1999.
88. Nelson PB, Seif SM, Maroon JC, et al: Hyponatremia in intracranial disease: perhaps not the syndrome of inap-

propriate secretion of antidiuretic hormone (SIADH), **J Neurosurg 55(6):**938-941, 1981.
89. Nornes H, Magnaes B: Intracranial pressure in patients with ruptured saccular aneurysm, **J Neurosurg 36(5):** 537-547, 1972.
90. O'Laoire SA: Epilepsy following neurosurgical intervention, **Acta Neurochir Suppl 50:**52-54, 1990.
91. Origitano TC, Wascher TM, Reichman OH, et al: Sustained increased cerebral blood flow with prophylactic hypertensive hypervolemic hemodilution ("triple-H" therapy) after subarachnoid hemorrhage, **Neurosurgery 27(5):**729-739, 739-740, 1990.
92. Otsubo H, Takemae T, Inoue T, et al: Normovolaemic induced hypertension therapy for cerebral vasospasm after subarachnoid haemorrhage, **Acta Neurochir 103 (1-2):**18-26, 1990.
93. Pakarinen S: Incidence, aetiology, and prognosis of primary subarachnoid haemorrhage. A study based on 589 cases diagnosed in a defined urban population during a defined period, **Acta Neurol Scand 43(Suppl):**1-28, 1967.
94. Petruk KC, West M, Mohr G, et al: Nimodipine treatment in poor-grade aneurysm patients. Results of a multicenter double-blind placebo-controlled trial, **J Neurosurg 68(4):**505-517, 1988.
95. Philippon J, Grob R, Dagreou F, et al: Prevention of vasospasm in subarachnoid haemorrhage. A controlled study with nimodipine, **Acta Neurochir 82(3-4):**110-114, 1986.
96. Pickard JD, Murray GD, Illingworth R, et al: Effect of oral nimodipine on cerebral infarction and outcome after subarachnoid haemorrhage: British aneurysm nimodipine trial, **Brit Med J 298(6674):**636-642, 1989.
97. Polin RS, Coenen VA, Hansen CA, et al: Efficacy of transluminal angioplasty for the management of symptomatic cerebral vasospasm following aneurysmal subarachnoid hemorrhage, **J Neurosurg 92(2):**284-290, 2000.
98. Powers WJ, Grubb RL Jr, Baker RP, et al: Regional cerebral blood flow and metabolism in reversible ischemia due to vasospasm. Determination by positron emission tomography, **J Neurosurg 62(4):**539-546, 1985.
99. Rosenwasser RH, Armonda RA, Thomas JE, et al: Therapeutic modalities for the management of cerebral vasospasm: timing of endovascular options, **Neurosurgery 44(5):**975-979, 979-980, 1999.
100. Rosenwasser RH, Delgado TE, Buchheit WA, et al: Control of hypertension and prophylaxis against vasospasm in cases of subarachnoid hemorrhage: a preliminary report, **Neurosurgery 12(6):**658-661, 1983.
101. Samuels MA: Neurogenic heart disease: a unifying hypothesis, **Am J Cardiol 60(18):**15J-19J, 1987.
102. Sasaki T, Ohta T, Kikuchi H, et al: A phase II clinical trial of recombinant human tissue-type plasminogen activator against cerebral vasospasm after aneurysmal subarachnoid hemorrhage, **Neurosurgery 35(4):**597-604, 604-605, 1994.
103. Seifert V, Stolke D, Zimmermann M, et al: Prevention of delayed ischaemic deficits after aneurysmal subarachnoid haemorrhage by intrathecal bolus injection of tissue plasminogen activator (rTPA). A prospective study, **Acta Neurochir 128(1-4):**137-143, 1994.
104. Simon RP: Neurogenic pulmonary edema, **Neurol Clin 11(2):**309-323, 1993.
105. Sloan MA, Haley EC Jr, Kassell NF, et al: Sensitivity and specificity of transcranial Doppler ultrasonography in the diagnosis of vasospasm following subarachnoid hemorrhage, **Neurology 39(11):**1514-1518, 1989.
106. Sokoll MD, Kassell NF, Gergis SD: Hemodynamic effects of N2O, O2 barbiturate anesthesia and induced hypotension in early versus late aneurysm clipping, **Neurosurgery 11(3):**352-355, 1982.
107. Solenski NJ, Haley EC Jr, Kassell NF, et al: Medical complications of aneurysmal subarachnoid hemorrhage: a report of the multicenter, cooperative aneurysm study. Participants of the Multicenter Cooperative Aneurysm Study [see comments], **Crit Care Med 23(6):**1007-1017, 1995.
108. Solomon RA, Fink ME, Lennihan L: Early aneurysm surgery and prophylactic hypervolemic hypertensive therapy for the treatment of aneurysmal subarachnoid hemorrhage, **Neurosurgery 23(6):**699-704, 1988.
109. Solomon RA, Post KD, McMurtry JGd: Depression of circulating blood volume in patients after subarachnoid hemorrhage: implications for the management of symptomatic vasospasm, **Neurosurgery 15(3):**354-361, 1984.
110. Sundaram MB, Chow F: Seizures associated with spontaneous subarachnoid hemorrhage, **Can J Neurol Sci 13(3):**229-231, 1986.
111. Takeuchi H, Handa Y, Kobayashi H, et al: Impairment of cerebral autoregulation during the development of chronic cerebral vasospasm after subarachnoid hemorrhage in primates, **Neurosurgery 28(1):**41-48, 1991.
112. Teasdale GM, Drake CG, Hunt W, et al: A universal subarachnoid hemorrhage scale: report of a committee of the World Federation of Neurosurgical Societies [letter], **J Neurol Neurosurg Psychiatry 51(11):**1457, 1988.
113. Tsementzis SA, Hitchcock ER, Meyer CH: Benefits and risks of antifibrinolytic therapy in the management of ruptured intracranial aneurysms. A double-blind placebo-controlled study, **Acta Neurochir 102(1-2):**1-10, 1990.
114. Ullman JS, Bederson JB: Hypertensive, hypervolemic, hemodilutional therapy for aneurysmal subarachnoid hemorrhage. Is it efficacious? Yes. **Crit Care Clin 12(3):** 697-707, 1996.
115. Usui M, Saito N, Hoya K, et al: Vasospasm prevention with postoperative intrathecal thrombolytic therapy: a retrospective comparison of urokinase, tissue plasminogen activator, and cisternal drainage alone, **Neurosurgery 34(2):**235-244, 244-245, 1994.
116. Vale FL, Bradley EL, Fisher WS III: The relationship of subarachnoid hemorrhage and the need for postoperative shunting [see comments], **J Neurosurg 86(3):** 462-466, 1997.
117. van Gijn, J, Hijdra A, Wijdicks EF, et al: Acute hydrocephalus after aneurysmal subarachnoid hemorrhage, **J Neurosurg 63(3):**355-362, 1985.
118. Velthuis BK, Van Leeuwen MS, Witkamp TD, et al: Computerized tomography angiography in patients with subarachnoid hemorrhage: from aneurysm detection to treatment without conventional angiography, **J Neurosurg 91(5):**761-767, 1999.

119. Vermeulen M, Lindsay KW, Murray GD, et al: Antifibrinolytic treatment in subarachnoid hemorrhage, **N Engl J Med 311(7):**432-437, 1984.
120. Vermeulen M, van Gijn J: The diagnosis of subarachnoid haemorrhage, **J Neurol Neurosurg Psychiatry 53(5):**365-372, 1990.
121. Voldby B, Enevoldsen EM, Jensen FT: Cerebrovascular reactivity in patients with ruptured intracranial aneurysms, **J Neurosurg 62(1):**59-67, 1985.
122. Voldby B, Enevoldsen EM: Intracranial pressure changes following aneurysm rupture. Part 1: Clinical and angiographic correlations, **J Neurosurg 56(2):**186-196, 1982.
123. Vollmer DG, Takayasu M, Dacey RG Jr: An in vitro comparative study of conducting vessels and penetrating arterioles after experimental subarachnoid hemorrhage in the rabbit, **J Neurosurg 77(1):**113-119, 1992.
124. Vora YY, Suarez-Almazor M, Steinke DE, et al: Role of transcranial Doppler monitoring in the diagnosis of cerebral vasospasm after subarachnoid hemorrhage [in process citation], **Neurosurgery 44(6):**1237-1247, 1247-1248, 1999.
125. Weir B: **Aneurysms Affecting the Nervous System.** Baltimore: Williams & Wilkins, 1987.
126. Weir B: Intracranial aneurysms and subarachnoid hemorrhage: an overview, in Wilkins RH, Rengachary SS (eds): **Neurosurgery**. New York: McGraw-Hill, 1985, pp 1308-1329.
127. Wijdicks EF, Hasan D, Lindsay KW, et al: Short-term tranexamic acid treatment in aneurysmal subarachnoid hemorrhage, **Stroke 20(12):**1674-1679, 1989.
128. Wijdicks EF, Ropper AH, Hunnicutt EJ, et al: Atrial natriuretic factor and salt wasting after aneurysmal subarachnoid hemorrhage, **Stroke 22(12):**1519-1524, 1991.
129. Wijdicks EF, Vermeulen M, Hijdra A, et al: Hyponatremia and cerebral infarction in patients with ruptured intracranial aneurysms: is fluid restriction harmful? **Ann Neurol 17(2):**137-140, 1985.
130. Wijdicks EF, Vermeulen M, Murray GD, et al: The effects of treating hypertension following aneurysmal subarachnoid hemorrhage, **Clin Neurol Neurosurg 92(2):**111-117, 1990.
131. Wijdicks EF, Vermeulen M, ten Haaf JA, et al: Volume depletion and natriuresis in patients with a ruptured intracranial aneurysm, **Ann Neurol 18(2):**211-216, 1985.
132. Wijdicks EF, Vermeulen M, Van Brummelen P, et al: The effect of fludrocortisone acetate on plasma volume and natriuresis in patients with aneurysmal subarachnoid hemorrhage, **Clin Neurol Neurosurg 90(3):**209-214, 1988.
133. Winn HR, Richardson AE, O'Brien W, et al: The long-term prognosis in untreated cerebral aneurysms: II. Late morbidity and mortality, **Ann Neurol 4(5):**418-426, 1978.
134. Wood JH, Simeone FA, Kron RE, et al: Experimental hypervolemic hemodilution: physiological correlations of cortical blood flow, cardiac output, and intracranial pressure with fresh blood viscosity and plasma volume, **Neurosurgery 14(6):**709-723, 1984.
135. Wood JH, Snyder LL, Simeone FA: Failure of intravascular volume expansion without hemodilution to elevate cortical blood flow in region of experimental focal ischemia, **J Neurosurg 56(1):**80-91, 1982.
136. Yamakami I, Isobe K, Yamaura A, et al: Vasospasm and regional cerebral blood flow (rCBF) in patients with ruptured intracranial aneurysm: serial rCBF studies with the xenon-133 inhalation method, **Neurosurgery 13(4):**394-401, 1983.
137. Yonas H: Cerebral blood measurements in vasospasm, **Neurosurg Clin N Am 1(2):**307-318, 1990.
138. Zabramski JM, Spetzler RF, Lee KS, et al: Phase I trial of tissue plasminogen activator for the prevention of vasospasm in patients with aneurysmal subarachnoid hemorrhage, **J Neurosurg 75(2):**189-196, 1991.
139. Zaroff JG, Rordorf GA, Newell JB, et al: Cardiac outcome in patients with subarachnoid hemorrhage and electrocardiographic abnormalities, **Neurosurgery 44(1):**34-9, 39-40, 1999.
140. Zondra B, Buresova J: Epileptic seizures following subarachnoideal haemorrhage, **Acta Univ Palacki Olomuc Fac Med 137:**61-63, 1994.
141. Zouaoui A, Sahel M, Marro B, et al: Three-dimensional computed tomographic angiography in detection of cerebral aneurysms in acute subarachnoid hemorrhage, **Neurosurgery 41(1):**125-130, 1997.

CHAPTER 13

Stroke and Nontraumatic Hemorrhage

DAVID C. BONOVICH
J. CLAUDE HEMPHILL, III

Stoke is the third leading cause of mortality and the leading cause of adult disability in the United States. As the overall population ages, estimates of annual stroke incidence have been revised upward from approximately 550,000 new cases per year to more than 700,000.[2] Between the two subtypes of stroke, approximately 80% are ischemic and 20% are hemorrhagic (approximately 14% intracerebral hemorrhage and 6% aneurysmal subarachnoid hemorrhage). Although strategies for prevention of both ischemic and hemorrhagic stroke remain a cornerstone of management, advances in the acute treatment of cerebrovascular disease have brought the intensive care management of these patients to the forefront. The goal of this chapter is to review causes, clinical presentation, and critical care management of patients with acute ischemic stroke (IS) or nontraumatic intracerebral hemorrhage (ICH). Although some new treatments (such as intravenous tissue-type plasminogen activator [tPA] for acute ischemic stroke) have been evaluated in large randomized studies, the indications for and efficacy of many treatments in cerebrovascular critical care are still being evaluated. Thus the intensive care management of these patients relies on integrating an understanding of the basic mechanisms of brain injury in IS and ICH with clinical interventions likely to limit these injury cascades and thereby improve outcomes.

ISCHEMIC STROKE

Background and Etiologies

The term *ischemia* is derived from the Greek word *ischo*, which means "to take back."[104] Ischemia to brain tissue results when substrate delivery, principally oxygen and glucose, decreases below critical thresholds necessary to sustain cellular function. Ischemia may be focal, as when a single arterial supply becomes occluded, or global, as in cardiac arrest with absence of blood flow to the entire brain.

Ischemic stroke results from the occlusion, usually acute, of an arterial supply to a portion of the brain. Mechanisms of ischemic stroke have been divided into two basic categories: thrombotic and embolic. Thrombotic stroke results from occlusion of an intracranial vessel that in most circumstances has underlying narrowing from atherosclerotic disease. Patients with hypercoagulable states may also develop thrombotic strokes without underlying atherosclerosis. There are a variety of sources of embolic material, which can generally be divided into cardioembolic and artery-to-artery sources. Examples of predisposing conditions include atrial fibrillation, dilated cardiomyopathy, aortic arch atheromas, carotid artery stenosis, and intracranial large vessel stenosis. Lacunar infarcts, or small vessel strokes, are usually the product of thrombotic mechanisms caused by chronic damage to small penetrating arteries as a result of hypertension or diabetes. Understanding the mechanism of an acute stroke is essential to determining risk factors and future preventive strategies for individual patients (Table 13-1). Additionally, in many circumstances the mechanism of ischemic stroke also influences the choice of therapies in the intensive care management of patients with these conditions; these therapies may include intraarterial thrombolysis, hypertensive-hypervolemic therapy, and acute antithrombotic treatment for progressing stroke.

The intensive care management of patients with ischemic stroke has changed dramatically within the last decade. Prior approaches have focused on determining the cause of stroke and preventing medical complications such as pneumonia and deep vein thrombosis. The current approach to treatment of ischemic

TABLE 13-1 ■ Mechanisms of Acute Ischemic Stroke/Mechanisms of Ischemic Brain Injury

Global	Focal
Cardiac Arrest	Thrombotic
Hypotension	• Atherosclerosis
• Syncope	• Lacunar
• Infection	Embolic
• Medications	• Cardioembolic
	• Artery to artery
	Intracranial stenosis
	Carotid stenosis
	Dissection
	Traumatic
	Spontaneous
	• Paradoxical (venous via patent PFO)

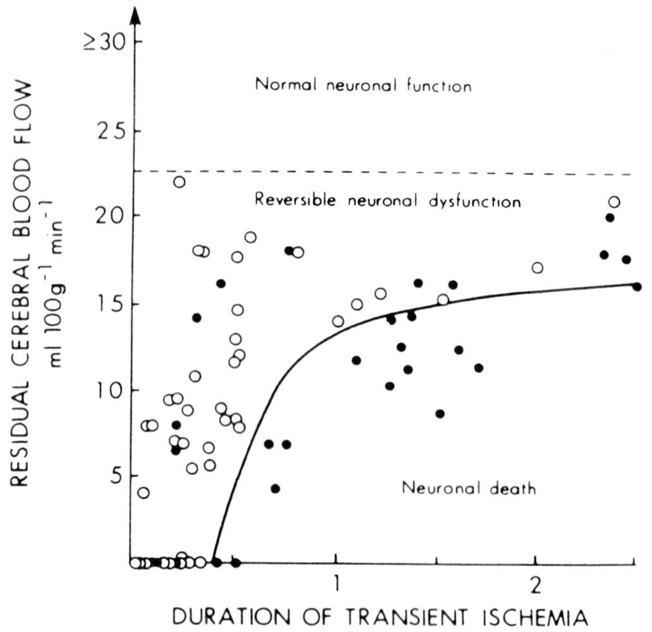

FIGURE 13-1 ■ The combined effects of the severity and duration of ischemia on neuronal viability. (From Powers WJ: Hemodynamics and metabolism in ischemic cerebrovascular disease, **Neurol Clin 10:**31-48, 1992.)

stroke focuses on attempting to *take back* (from the Greek term) brain tissue that is injured but not yet irreversibly infarcted. Understanding of the cellular cascade of ischemic injury demonstrates the possibilities, and the limitations, of current strategies of revascularization and neuroprotection. It also forms the basis for much of the neurological intensive care management of ischemic stroke.

Pathophysiology of Cerebral Ischemia

Resting cerebral blood flow (CBF) is approximately 50 ml/100 g of cerebral tissue/min; however, focal CBF is closely coupled to metabolism and may change depending on the particular local metabolic needs of the tissue. Decreases in CBF to approximately 18 ml/100 g of brain tissue are associated with attenuation or suppression of waveforms in the electroencephalogram (EEG), and at 12 ml/100 g of brain tissue/min, rapid depletion of adenosine triphosphate (ATP) may occur.[7,105] With the depletion of ATP, there is failure of the Na^+/K^+ pump, which is essential for maintaining cellular ionic gradients. In addition, the inadequate supply of oxygen and glucose causes cells to begin using anaerobic pathways to convert the residual glucose into ATP, resulting in lactic acidosis.[90] If reperfusion with restoration of adequate supplies of oxygen and glucose does not occur, cell death follows.

In ischemia the ability of neurons to survive depends on the severity and length of the ischemic period (Figure 13-1). When a vessel is occluded there is typically a core of severely ischemic tissue with insufficient blood supply to maintain energy metabolism. The ischemic core is surrounded by a larger area of progressively less ischemic tissue, where the degree of ischemia is related to the ability of collateral blood vessels to maintain blood flow. This zone of relative ischemia is referred to as the *ischemic penumbra.*[40] The penumbra is presumed to represent a dynamic tissue bed that may progress to further ischemia and cell death or, with sufficient collateral blood flow or restoration of blood flow, return to a normal functional state. Thus the penumbra represents the tissue at risk in cerebral ischemia. Reperfusion to recruit collateral flow via thrombolytic therapy, mechanical revascularization, or hypertensive therapy is designed to increase critical CBF to the penumbra before the ischemic cascade of cell injury has resulted in permanent cell death.

The *ischemic cascade* refers to a series of interrelated biochemical reactions that lead to cellular dysfunction and ultimately cell death. This cascade includes excitatory neurotransmitter effects, calcium influx into cells, free radical production, activation of certain proteases and lipases, and an inflammatory response. Other secondary effects include the activation of intracellular secondary messengers and the induction of genes that promote cell death via apoptotic injury.[47] *Neuroprotection* generally refers to approaches intended to limit ischemic brain injury by blocking individual or multiple pathways of this ischemic or apoptotic cell injury cascade.

Excitatory amino acids, especially glutamate, are strongly implicated in the biochemistry of ischemic brain injury.[23,44] The binding of glutamate to its membrane receptors results in membrane depolarization and increased cytosolic Ca^{++} levels. Under normal conditions glutamate is cleared from the synaptic cleft and Ca^{++} levels normalize. Under ischemic conditions the binding of glutamate to its receptors is prolonged and can lead to neuronal death.[23] Glutamate receptors include the *N*-methyl-D-aspartate (NMDA) receptor; kainic acid/α-amino-3-hydroxy-5-methyl-4-isoxazole propionic acid (KA/AMPA) receptor; and quisqualate receptor. Interaction with the NMDA receptor results in the influx of calcium and sodium into cells. Interaction of glutamate with the KA/AMPA receptor results in sodium influx into cells. Interaction at the quisqualate receptor helps modulate the activity of the NMDA and KA/AMPA receptors.[100] Normally the glutamate concentration in the extracellular space is kept at 1 to 5 μmol/L, and inside the cell at 5 to 10 μmol/L. The neurons and astrocytes using ATP-dependent membrane pumps maintain this difference.[8] A decrease in ATP availability as a result of ischemia may impair glutamate reuptake, leading to increased extracellular concentrations of glutamate. The decreased ATP may result in a decreased ability of the cells to maintain intracellular concentrations of glutamate, which move in reverse across cell membranes via the glutamate reuptake channels. Sodium influx into cells is followed by the influx of chloride ions (Cl^-) and water molecules. This may result in increased intracellular water content and ultimately cell lysis.[23] The sodium influx may take place via the KA/AMPA receptors or the quisqualate receptors. The influx of sodium is also a result of energy failure of the Na/K ATPase pump.[100]

Increases in intracellular Ca^{++} concentration may produce cellular injury via the activation of Ca^{++}-dependent proteases, lipases, and endonucleases and by the production of cytokines and other factors that can lead to cell injury and death. Ca^{++} enters the cell via voltage-dependent channels (VDCC). Depolarization of cell membranes may result in the opening of the VDCC, allowing an influx of Ca^{++}. Intracelluar Ca^{++} concentrations are maintained by ATP-dependent membrane pumps, and a loss of ATP as a result of ischemia impairs the ability of cells to maintain intracellular Ca^{++} concentrations at normal levels.[101]

The role of inflammatory mediators in ischemic injury is a subject of ongoing studies. Leukocytes may appear within 30 minutes of cerebral ischemia and reperfusion.[36] In experimental models, brain damage is reduced if leukocyte accumulation is attenuated after focal ischemia.[22] The mechanisms by which leukocytes may exacerbate ischemic injury are still being studied but appear to include the production of free radicals.[52]

Acidosis also plays a role in exacerbating cellular ischemic injury. When oxygen delivery falls to levels below thresholds of glucose delivery and tissue metabolism, the anaerobic metabolism of glucose occurs. This results in increases in tissue lactate levels and decreases in tissue pH.[38] Intracellular brain pH is normally 7.01 to 7.03. During focal ischemia in the setting of normal glucose levels, tissue pH may fall to 6.4 to 6.6, and in the setting of hyperglycemia it can fall to 6 to 6.1. The precise mechanism by which acidosis causes injury is not clear; however, it may involve the denaturing of proteins and increases in glial edema and may create a milieu that promotes free radical formation and inhibits the regeneration of NADH. Conversely, mild acidosis may actually be beneficial because once the pH falls below 6.8, the NMDA receptor no longer allows Ca^{++} influx.[1-4]

Although these various biochemical cascades may seem esoteric when contemplating acute intervention for cerebral ischemia, they form the basis for the understanding that cerebral ischemia may indeed be reversible and acute ischemic stroke may be treatable. Interventions for the treatment of acute ischemic stroke are generally focused on reperfusion or neuroprotection. Additionally, appreciation for the biochemistry of the ischemic cascade has also demonstrated the narrow therapeutic time window in which these interventions may be applied with any reasonable chance of success. Because "time is brain," current and emerging protocols for intensive care of acute cerebral ischemia emphasize coordinated approaches involving rapid assessment and treatment.

Clinical Presentation: Evaluation and Treatment

Until the publication of the National Institute of Neurological Disorders and Stroke's (NINDS) tissue Plasminogen Activator (tPA) Stroke Study in 1995, there was no direct treatment that had demonstrated benefit in terms of improved outcome after acute ischemic stroke.[108] To date only three treatments, intravenous (IV) tPA, intraarterial prourokinase (IA Proaqua), and ancrod (an intravenous defibrinogenating agent), have been shown in large, prospective randomized studies to improve outcome after acute ischemic stroke.[34,99,108] All must be administered within a narrow time window after stroke onset (3 hours for IV tPA and ancrod; 6 hours for IA pro-UK), and IV tPA has been approved for use by the U.S. Food and Drug Administration. In addition, although the benefits of these therapies are real, only a minority of patients demonstrated improvement with treatment. For example, in the NINDS IV tPA study, 39% of patients treated with IV tPA were essentially normal at 3 months, compared with 26% of the placebo group. In this study approximately 6% of the tPA patients suffered a symptomatic intracranial hemorrhage and mortality in the two groups was no different.[108] Efficacy of IA pro-UK and ancrod were somewhat less, but these studies are not directly comparable because different enrollment criteria were used and there was no direct comparison with IV tPA.[34,99]

As a result of these beneficial studies, current evaluation and management of acute stroke emphasizes rapid identification, neuroimaging, and triage to determine whether patients meet eligibility criteria for acute treatment (current principally with IV tPA). Eligibility criteria and protocol for IV tPA administration are summarized in Table 13-3. All patients with acute stroke, regardless of eligibility for acute intervention, should undergo urgent head imaging, usually a noncontrast computed tomography (CT) scan. The purpose of this scan is not to identify the stroke but rather to rule out hemorrhage, which may be indistinguishable. Electrocardiogram (ECG) should be performed on arrival in the emergency department and basic laboratory studies such as a complete blood count; basic chemistries, including sodium, glucose, and renal functions studies; and coagulation parameters (prothrombin and partial thromboplastin times) should also be obtained immediately. All patients with acute ischemic stroke should undergo a thorough evaluation for cause to define future preventative strategies. In addition, all stroke patients require attention to basic issues of nutrition, prevention of complications such as pneumonia and deep vein thrombosis, and consideration of appropriate acute and long-term antithrombotic therapy.

Primarily because of the narrow time window, only a small minority of ischemic stroke patients may be eligible to receive IV tPA. In addition, the majority of acute ischemic stroke patients do not require management in an intensive care unit. Thus it is appropriate for this chapter to focus on issues that lead to intensive care unit (ICU) admission of a patient with acute ischemic stroke and management issues pertinent primarily to the ICU (Tables 13-2 and 13-3).

TABLE 13-2 ■ Management Strategies for Patients Suffering from Acute Ischemic Stroke in the ICU

Clinical Principles of Ischemic Stroke Therapy

Treatment of Primary Injury

Reperfusion Therapy

- Intravenous thrombolytic therapy
- Intraarterial thrombolysis
- GIIb/IIIa inhibitors*
- Anticoagulation with heparin

Maintenance of Adequate Intravascular Volume

- Vasopressor therapy

Neuroprotective Agents*

Prevention of Secondary Ischemic Injury

Prevention of Secondary Clot Formation or Reembolization

- Anticoagulation with heparin
- Antiplatelet therapy
- Aspirin
- GIIb/IIIa inhibitors*

Treatment of Brain Edema

- Hyperosmotic therapy (mannitol, hypertonic saline)
- Hemicraniectomy
- Vasopressor therapy

*A potentially beneficial therapy.

Management Issues in the Neurological Intensive Care Unit

Indications for admissions of acute ischemic stroke patients to an ICU may fall into neurological, hemodynamic, and respiratory categories. Patients who have undergone IV or intraarterial (IA) thrombolysis should be admitted to the ICU for at least 24 hours after treatment. The purpose of this is twofold: close neurologi-

TABLE 13-3 ■ Thrombolytic Therapy in Acute Stroke with Intravenous t-PA

Clinical

- Symptoms are consistent with an ischemic stroke.
- Treatment must be initiated within 3 hours of symptom onset.
- Thrombolytic treatment with IV t-PA is not recommended when time of onset of symptoms cannot be reliably ascertained.
- Treatment should be reconsidered in patients with rapidly improving neurological symptoms.
- Pretreatment systolic blood pressure must be less than 185 mm Hg and diastolic pressure must be less than 110 mm Hg.
- No history of prior intracranial hemorrhage.
- No history of stroke or prior closed head injury in the previous 3 months.
- No history of gastrointestinal or urinary bleeding within the preceding 21 days.
- No history of recent myocardial infarction.
- No history of major surgery within the preceding 14 days.
- No history of heparin use within the preceding 48 hours.

Head CT

- No evidence of intracranial hemorrhage.
- No signs of major infarction: sulcal effacement, mass effect, and edema.

Laboratory evaluation

- Prothrombin time less than 15 seconds or international normalized ratio (INR) less than 1.7.
- Normal partial thromboplastin time.
- Platelet count greater than 100,000.
- Blood glucose greater than 50mg/dl and less than 400 mg/dl.

Treatment Protocol

- 0.9 mg/kg t-PA IV with 10% of total dose administered within the first minute and the remainder infused over 1 hour.

Emergency Ancillary Care

- Patients should be admitted to either an intensive care unit or to an acute stroke unit during t-PA administration and for at least 24 hours thereafter.

cal observation, which can lead to urgent CT scanning for identification of intracranial hemorrhagic complications, and tight control of blood pressure (usually below 185/110) with intravenous agents such as labetalol, nitroprusside, or nicardipine to decrease the risk of thrombolysis-associated intracranial hemorrhage. In addition, patients at high risk of acute deterioration, such as those with fluctuating large-vessel ischemic deficits or cerebellar infarct at risk for swelling and herniation, should be admitted for close neurological observation. Certainly patients who have concurrent myocardial infarction, who require hemodynamic support with vasopressors, or who cannot protect their airways because of obtundation or lower cranial neuropathies should be admitted to an ICU as well.

Management of systemic blood pressure after acute ischemic stroke remains controversial. Arterial hypertension is common after ischemic stroke, but in general it has a tendency to decline to preexisting levels within the first 48 hours after stroke.[13] In most cases blood pressure should not be lowered because it may lead to neurological deterioration, presumably by decreasing blood flow to the ischemic penumbra.[2,64,89,114] However, the use of medications to control or lower blood pressure may be appropriate in patients who have received thrombolytic therapy (as previously discussed) or in patients with concurrent systemic medical problems such as congestive heart failure, acute renal failure, or thoracic aortic dissection, which necessitate aggressive blood pressure management. In the absence of these conditions, lowering of blood pressure is usually deferred unless the mean arterial pressure (MAP) exceeds 130 mm Hg or the systolic blood pressure exceeds 200 mm Hg.[2] The specific agent used for blood pressure lowering also remains a point of controversy; some have suggested that nitroprusside may interfere with cerebral autoregulation and increase intracranial pressure (ICP).[25,76] If blood pressure is to be lowered, it should be done gradually over the course of hours using intravenous agents that can be easily titrated.

Interestingly, the use of induced hypertension to improve ischemic deficits has shown promise in the past and has more recently been the subject of a pilot study by Rordorf and colleagues.[95,116] In 10 of 30 patients, neurological deficits improved after blood pressure was raised using a phenylephrine challenge and subsequently worsened when blood pressure returned to prior levels. Patients that seemed to benefit most were those with thrombotic stroke, possibly because they were more likely to harbor significantly stenotic large cerebral arteries.[95]

Hypotension is uncommon after acute ischemic stroke and should prompt a search for an underlying cause.[2] Volume depletion from dehydration is the most common cause, although patients who have received thrombolytic therapy or anticoagulation with heparin may develop hemodynamically significant systemic hemorrhage. Restoring volume and using vasopressor medications may be helpful in maintaining adequate perfusion of the collateral arterial beds in the penumbra region. However, it is important to ensure that patients are adequately volume resuscitated before the institution of vasopressor therapy.

Anticoagulation in acute ischemic stroke patients is a point of significant controversy as well. Although the rationale of anticoagulation to prevent progression or recurrence of stroke is intuitively appealing, no study has yet demonstrated a conclusive benefit of acute anticoagulation with either intravenous or low-molecular-weight heparin in acute ischemic stroke patients.[5] Despite this, heparin is commonly used in patients with cardioembolic stroke, large-vessel stroke in progression, and basilar artery thrombosis. Importantly, protocols for the use of IV tPA call for avoiding all antithrombotic therapy, including heparin and aspirin, for the first 24 hours after thrombolysis.[3,108]

Other factors that experimentally have been shown to worsen cerebral ischemic injury are hyperthermia and hyperglycemia.[92] Aggressive measures should be undertaken to treat fevers should they develop. Standard antipyretic medications may be used and early antibiotic treatment should be considered in patients with fever and radiographical evidence of aspiration. Moderate hypothermia (33° C) has been suggested as a neuroprotective strategy in patients with traumatic brain injury and ischemic stroke, especially for massive cerebral edema.[71,96] This remains investigational, and currently a strategy of "avoiding hyperthermia" seems most rational for the great majority of patients. Likewise, definitive data demonstrating that hyperglycemia worsens functional outcome after stroke are lacking. However, hyperglycemia is unlikely to be beneficial, and close control using an intravenous insulin infusion is appropriate for ischemic stroke patients in the ICU.

Renewed attention is now being paid to management of stroke-associated cerebral edema and large hemispheric infarction with tissue shifts and herniation. Although cerebral edema is a potentially fatal complication of stroke, only about 15% of patients develop sufficient edema to result in clinical deterioration. Edema usually peaks from 3 to 5 days after stroke.[94] Treatment of symptomatic cerebral edema consists of standard measures such as avoidance of hyposmolar fluids and the use of osmotic diuretics such as mannitol. There is currently no role for glucocorticoids in treatment of stroke-associated cerebral edema.[11,83]

In patients with clinical deterioration from tissue shifts associated with large hemispheric infarction, attention solely to ICP may be misleading. Frank[33] demonstrated that only 26% of patients with clinical deterioration in the setting of large hemispheric infarction had an ICP greater than 15 mm Hg at the time of monitor placement, suggesting that tissue shifts at the level of the diencephalons were not reflected as elevations in global ICP measurements. The recognition that patients with large hemispheric infarction, especially of the nondominant hemisphere, may be potentially salvageable has led to pilot studies of hemicraniectomy and moderate hypothermia for control of this potentially deadly complicating condition.[96,98] Additionally, in patients with cerebellar infarction, decompressive posterior fossa surgery may be lifesaving if done early enough.[84] For this reason, in patients with cerebellar infarction associated with declining level of consciousness, proceeding immediately to surgical evacuation is recommended, even if the presence of hydrocephalus makes expectant management with a ventriculostomy a consideration.

A

B

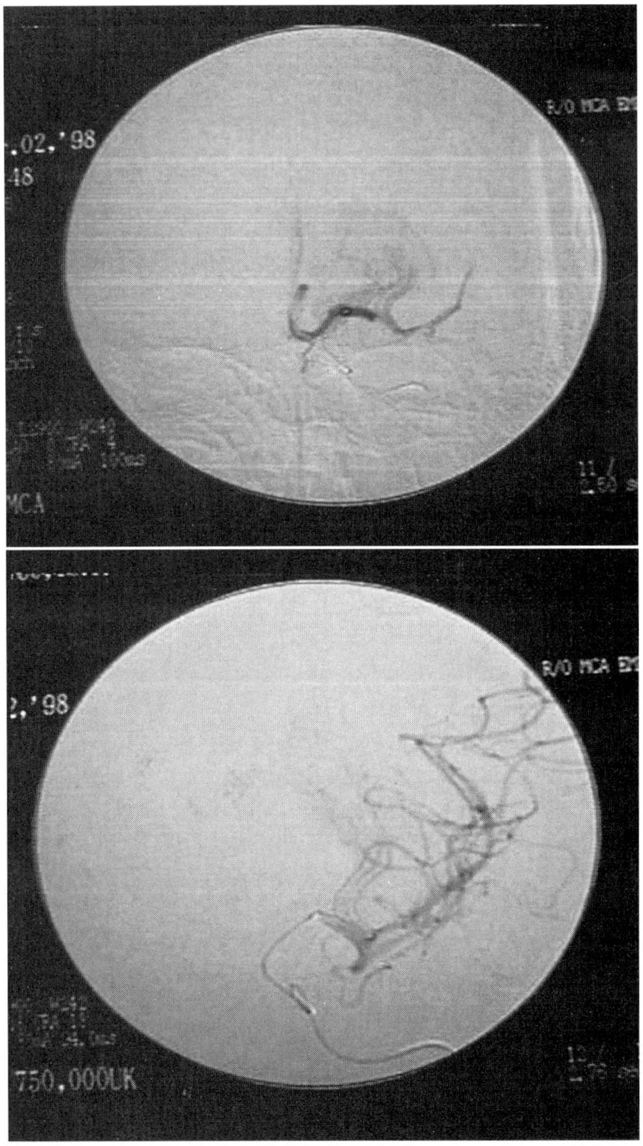

FIGURE 13-2 ■ Intracranial thrombolysis. A, Pretreatment angiogram showing a complete occlusion of the basilar artery. **B,** After treatment with intraarterial urokinase, the basilar artery is once again patent with normal anterograde flow.

Future Directions

Future directions in the intensive care management of patients with acute cerebral ischemia focus on three main areas: reperfusion, neuroprotection, and management of cerebral edema and tissue shifts. Intraarterial thrombolysis (Figure 13-2) for middle cerebral artery (MCA) occlusion was demonstrated to be beneficial in the PROACT II study.[34] Despite this, IA thrombolysis remains unapproved by the FDA and is used sparingly. There remains great interest in the appropriate use of this intervention, and it has also shown promise in basilar artery occlusion.[102] Because IA thrombolysis requires a neurointerventional team, its application is much more costly and labor intensive than IV tPA. Ongoing studies are investigating whether the use of combined IV and IA thrombolysis ("bridging therapy") offers benefit over either alone.[63] Additionally, new neuroimaging techniques such as diffusion- and perfusion-weighted magnetic resonance (MR) imaging (Figure 13-3) may allow improved selection of patients for acute reperfusion interventions.[4,57] At present there is essentially no role for emergency carotid endarterectomy or extracranial-intracranial (EC-IC) bypass surgery in treatment of acute ischemic stroke.

The promise of neuroprotective therapy for acute ischemic stroke has yet to be fulfilled. Despite multiple studies of different pharmacological agents, including NMDA antagonists, free radical scavengers, calcium channel blockers, and antiinflammatory antibodies, no neuroprotective agent has demonstrated conclusive benefit in a large, prospective, randomized efficacy study.[27] There is ongoing debate about whether this failure represents a biological difference between animal models of neuroprotection in cerebral ischemia (primarily rodents) and the human ischemic cascade or whether this failure is primarily a result of logistical issues related to clinical trial design (e.g., therapeutic time windows, heterogenous patient selection). There is interest in focusing future clinical studies on earlier treatment, perhaps even in the prehospital setting, to

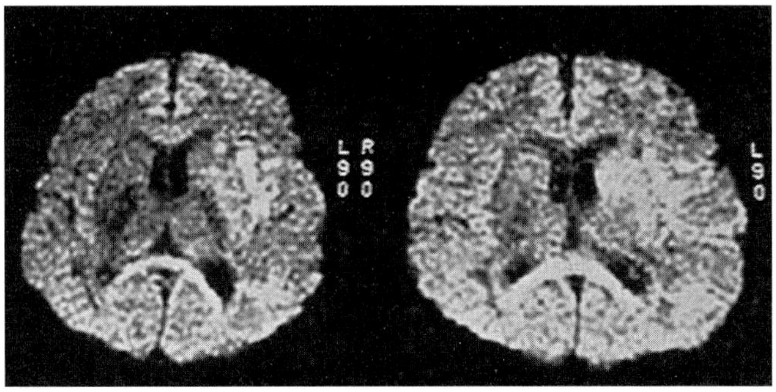

FIGURE 13-3 ■ MR diffusion scan demonstrating a diffusion abnormality in the left middle cerebral artery distribution in a patient with an acute left MCA stroke.

decrease the time to treatment and investigating combination therapy with neuroprotectants and thrombolytics.

Clinical trials are ongoing or in planning stages regarding treatment protocols for large hemispheric infarction. Interestingly, animal studies have suggested that early hemicraniectomy may actually decrease infarct size, perhaps by allowing improved pial arterial collateralization.[32,98] Initial results of hemicraniectomy (Figure 13-4) have been promising, with regard to both functional outcome and survivor satisfaction.[98] Given the recognition that both hemicraniectomy and hypothermia for large hemispheric infarction are "salvage therapies" that might allow patient survival but with significant neurological deficit, ongoing clinical trials of these therapies are evaluating both functional

A B C

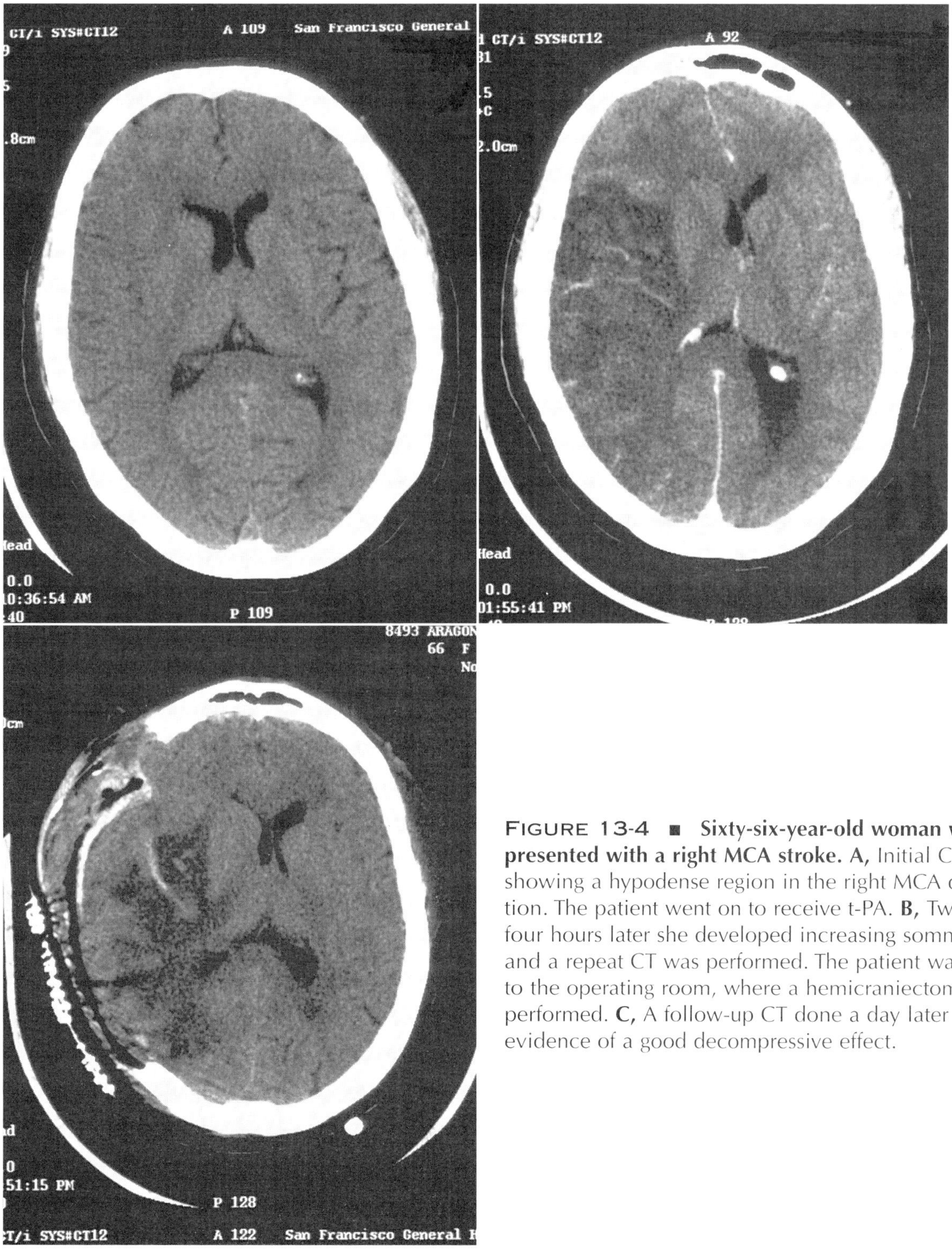

FIGURE 13-4 ■ **Sixty-six-year-old woman who presented with a right MCA stroke. A,** Initial CT scan showing a hypodense region in the right MCA distribution. The patient went on to receive t-PA. **B,** Twenty-four hours later she developed increasing somnolence and a repeat CT was performed. The patient was taken to the operating room, where a hemicraniectomy was performed. **C,** A follow-up CT done a day later shows evidence of a good decompressive effect.

and neuropsychological outcome, including focus on caregivers and cost. These approaches represent an important bridge between intensive care management and rehabilitation/recovery after massive stroke.

NONTRAUMATIC INTRACEREBRAL HEMORRHAGE

Background and Etiologies

Primary nontraumatic intracerebral hemorrhage (ICH) accounts for 10% to 15% of all strokes. The 30-day mortality rate from ICH is high, ranging from 35% to 52% across several series, with approximately half of all deaths occurring within the first 2 days.[14] In fact, ICH is more likely to result in death or major disability than cerebral infarction or subarachnoid hemorrhage (SAH).[15] Despite composing only 10% to 15% of all strokes, the societal burden of ICH is disproportionately high, with ICH accounting for 34% of years of potential life lost to strokes, which is comparable with that for ischemic stroke and SAH.[48] Current clinical care of patients with ICH is heterogenous. Despite important advances within the last decade in the care of patients with acute ischemic stroke and aneurysmal subarachnoid hemorrhage, ICH remains without a therapy of proven benefit in improving outcome.[14] Surgical hematoma removal is frequently undertaken, with an estimated 7000 such operations performed annually in the United States alone, although no randomized prospective study has demonstrated conclusive benefit for this procedure.[14] Medical therapy directed at controlling elevated intracranial pressure is also commonly instituted, again without clear evidence of benefit from clinical studies. Current approaches to the intensive care management of patients with ICH emphasize accurate diagnosis of the cause of the hemorrhage and management of complications related to elevated ICP, hydrocephalus, and brain herniation. Future approaches are focused on understanding the underlying mechanisms of ICH-related brain injury and improving methods of early hematoma evacuation.

TABLE 13-4 ▪ Intracerebral Hemorrhage

Causes	
Primary Intracerebral Hemorrhage	
Hypertension	
Amyloid angiopathy	
Secondary Intracerebral Hemorrhage	
Vascular	Coagulation Disorders
Aneurysm	Inherited
Saccular	Acquired
Mycotic	Drug induced
Vascular malformation	
Tumor	
Brain tumor	
Abscess	

Pathophysiology of Nontraumatic Intracerebral Hemorrhage

The pathophysiology of ICH has two principal components: (1) the nature of the vessel rupture that led to parenchymal hemorrhage and (2) the injury caused by the ICH to the brain itself. The underlying pathophysiology of vessel rupture relates to the etiology of the ICH (Table 13-4). Etiology is the principal determinant of risk of recurrent hemorrhage, which is the most feared complication of ICH. However, prognosis from the initial ICH is most influenced by volume of hemorrhage and clinical neurological status, which are determined primarily by the brain injury from the ICH itself regardless of etiology.[16,109] Thus both are important and interrelated aspects of ICH pathophysiology that influence long-term outcome.

Chronic hypertension is associated with approximately 70% of all ICH.[18,35,77] Hypertensive ICH occurs in typical locations, which include the putamen, thalamus, pons, and cerebellum.[35,51,56] Chronic hypertension may also be implicated in lobar hemorrhages, although this is often considered an atypical location that may suggest an alternative etiology. Figure 13-5 demonstrates CT findings in ICH of various locations. The majority of hypertensive ICHs are supratentorial, with cerebellar and brainstem sites composing approximately 10% to 15% of cases.[68] Hypertensive ICH in these typical locations results from rupture of small penetrating arteries. Hypertensive ICH is generally thought to result from the effects of chronic hypertension, not an acute hypertensive surge in an otherwise normal patient; however, the actual mechanism of vessel rupture in hypertensive hemorrhage is somewhat controversial. Bouchard and Charcot described "military aneurysms" in vessels of the brains of patients suffering from hypertension, which were different than the larger saccular aneurysms that predisposed to subarachnoid hemorrhage. Fisher felt that these microaneurysms were the result of a weakening of the vessel wall secondary to lipohyalinosis.[31] More recently, the association of military aneurysms with hypertensive hemorrhage has been called into question.[21]

Cerebral amyloid angiopathy (CAA) is a result of the deposition of amyloid protein in the media and intima of small to medium cortical and leptomeningeal blood vessels.[37,60,111] CAA may account for approximately 10% of ICHs and is not associated with systemic amyloidosis. Lobar sites are the most typical locations for amyloid-associated ICH. It is characteristically seen in the older population, and there may be an association with dementia. The amyloid protein itself is identical to that seen in the central cores of the neuritic plaques in patients with Alzheimer's disease.[86] The amyloid deposits are associated with arterial narrowing, fragmentation of the internal elastic lamina, and occasional fibrinoid necrosis.[85] The features most consistently associated with ICH are the presence of large deposits of amyloid in the vessel wall and fibrinoid necrosis.[112] Clinically, patients with CAA have a tendency toward recurrent hemorrhage or simultaneous

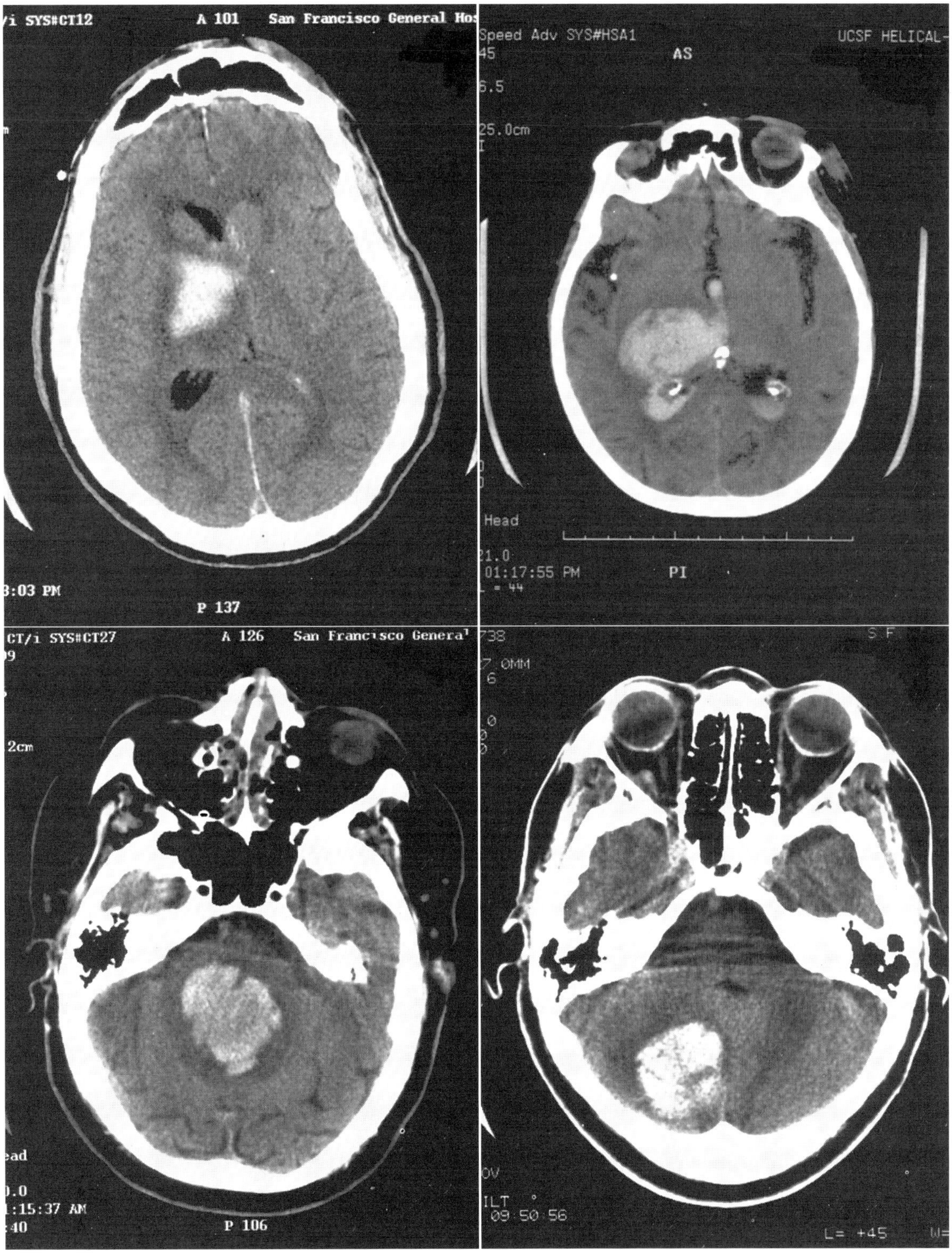

A B C D

FIGURE 13-5 ■ **A,** Basal ganglia hemorrhage. **B,** Thalamic hemorrhage with ventricular extension. **C,** Pontine hemorrhage. **D,** Cerebellar hemorrhage. *(Cont'd)*

E

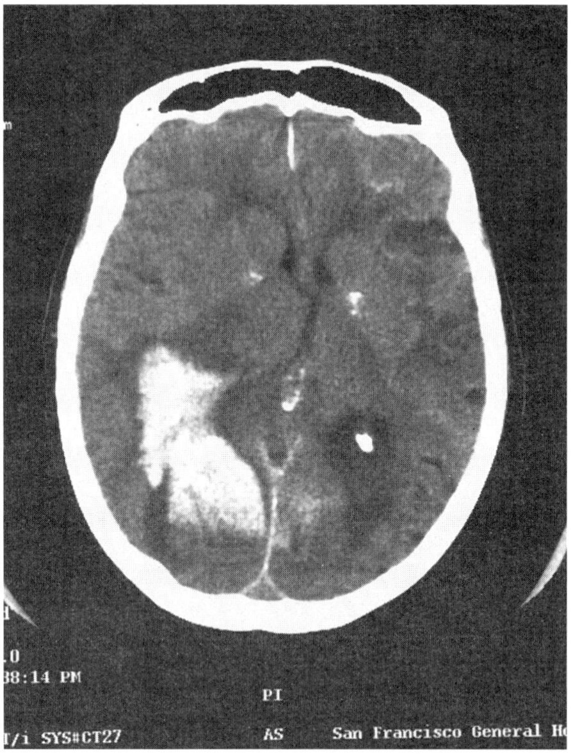

FIGURE 13-5—CONT'D ■ E, Lobar hemorrhage.

hemorrhage in different locations.[60] Vessels also tend to have difficulty constricting, a normal part of hemostasis, because the amyloid protein prevents efficient vasoconstriction at bleeding sites.[59] This may have relevance during surgical treatment of amyloid-related hemorrhages, and it has been suggested by some that patients with CAA-related ICH may be more prone to postoperative rehemorrhage.[58] Amyloid typically occurs as a sporadic illness, although some familial occurrences have been reported.[60,115]

ICH as a result of sympathomimetic drugs, such as amphetamine, cocaine, pseudoephedrine, and phenylpropanolamine, is well described.[1] Patients usually develop ICH within minutes to a few hours after using the drugs. Drug-related ICH may be associated with transient extremely high increases in blood pressure,[42,67] although other cases may be related to a reversible vasculitis that appears histologically similar to periarteritis nodosa. The vasculitis is felt to be a direct effect of the drugs on the blood vessels.[24] Rupture of an underlying aneurysm or vascular malformation may also be precipitated by use of sympathomimetic drugs.[53,69]

Coagulopathy may also be associated with spontaneous ICH. This coagulopathy may be iatrogenic, as in the case of warfarin-associated ICH, or related to an underlying disorder of coagulation such as hemophilia. Anticoagulation with warfarin has been reported to increase the risk of ICH up to tenfold, to approximately 1% per year in patients at risk for recurrent stroke.[43] Factors associated with warfarin-related ICH include older age (>70 years of age), hypertension, and concomitant use of antiplatelet agents, specifically aspirin.[43,46] Hemophilia and von Willebrand's disease account for up to 90% of hereditary bleeding abnormalities. Hemophilia is an X-linked recessive disorder of either factor VII (hemophilia A) or, more rarely, factor IX (hemophilia B), which results in a prolonged thromboplastin time. Von Willebrand's disease is an autosomal dominant disorder in which platelets fail to adhere to the subendothelium. ICH may arise spontaneously or after seemingly trivial head trauma in patients with hemophilia but is uncommon in patients with von Willebrand's disease.[72,84] Thrombocytopenia may occur in patients with aplastic anemia, idiopathic or thrombotic thrombocytopenic purpura, or disseminated intravascular coagulation. Platelet counts of greater than 50,000/mm^3 are usually not associated with severe hemorrhages, and spontaneous bleeding is rare with counts in excess of 20,000/mm^3.[1]

Rupture of vascular malformations of various categories may manifest as ICH. These include arteriovenous malformations (AVM), capillary telangiectasis, cavernous malformations, and venous malformations.[73] In AVMs there is direct communication between the arterial and venous beds; AVMS are composed of one or more feeding arteries, a nidus, and one or more draining veins. Hemorrhage may result from rupture of a feeding artery or nidal aneurysm or arterialized pressure in the venous drainage system, although often the specific cause of AVM rupture is not known. The risk of ICH from AVMs has been suggested to be approximately 3% to 4% per year,[26,55,87] although new approaches to understanding AVM rupture risks suggest that this may be an oversimplification.[107] Cavernous malformations tend to give rise to repeated episodes of small hemorrhage, although the risk of clinically significant hemorrhage has been felt to be small, in the range of 0.25% to 0.7% per year.[28,93] More recently, Kondziolka and colleagues have reported a risk of 0.6% per year in those without prior hemorrhage and as high as 4.5% in those with a history of prior hemorrhage.[54] Venous malformations and capillary telangiectasis are less commonly associated with ICH.

Spontaneous hemorrhage into brain tumors may occur and is most commonly associated with malignant glioma, melanoma, renal cell carcinoma, choriocarcinoma, and bronchogenic carcinoma.[66,70] The mechanism is felt to be secondary to tumor necrosis as a result of rapid growth in the setting of a rich but friable vascular supply.[50]

The mechanisms by which acute ICH injures the brain are incompletely understood. Acute ICH often causes massive tissue shifts and herniation, and this primary brain injury may result in significant neurological morbidity and early mortality. However, because current clinical trials have not shown benefit from surgical evacuation, other mechanisms of ICH-related brain injury are being explored. Initial animal models of ICH suggested an ischemic penumbra around an acute intracerebral hematoma, with neuroprotective pretreatment limiting the extent of injury.[19,75] Recently, however, Qureshi found no evidence for an ischemic penumbra in a dog model of massive ICH.[91] Other animal models have focused on perihematoma edema and the role of thrombin as a mediator of secondary brain injury.[113,117] Clinically, early hematoma enlargement and perihematoma edema are well described, but causes and preventive measures or treatments are poorly understood.[17,119] Additionally, initial human studies using positron emission tomography (PET) and MRI have not demonstrated extensive perihematoma ischemia in the limited numbers of patients studied.[20,45] Thus the role of ongoing perihematoma ischemia or other pathways of cellular injury in ICH are less well understood than in ischemic stroke or traumatic brain injury.

Clinical Presentation: Evaluation and Treatment

ICH typically presents as the sudden onset of a focal neurological abnormality that progresses over minutes to a few hours and is accompanied by increased blood pressure, depressed level of consciousness, and headache. Vomiting is an important diagnostic sign, especially in supratentorial ICH, because almost half of patients with supratentorial ICH in the Harvard Stroke Registry vomited, compared with only 2% of those with anterior circulation ischemia.[77] Importantly, however, no group of symptoms or signs has enough predictive power to clinically distinguish between ICH and ischemic stroke. Thus neuroimaging, usually with a noncontrast CT scan, is emergently indicated in all acute stroke patients. Essentially all acute intracerebral hemorrhages are identified on CT, and CT-demonstrated location of the hematoma is an important diagnostic clue to etiology. CT also demonstrates intraventricular extension of the hemorrhage and hydrocephalus, for which emergent external ventricular drain placement and cerebrospinal fluid (CSF) drainage may be indicated.[41]

Treatment of ICH is outlined in Table 13-5. Attention should first be given to airway, breathing, and circulation, as in any emergency. Those patients with altered consciousness who may not be able to protect their airways should be considered for emergency oral intubation. Oral intubation should be performed carefully, using established protocols to maximize preoxygenation, avoiding wide swings in blood pressure and cardiac rhythm disturbances. Placement of an arterial line and continuous cardiac monitoring facilitate close hemodynamic monitoring. All ICH patients should have a complete panel of laboratory studies performed, especially including prothrombin time and partial thromboplastin time (PT/PTT) and platelet count, because evidence of coagulopathy necessitates immediate transfusion with fresh frozen plasma (FFP) and platelets if indicated. An ECG and a chest x-ray study should also be performed to rule out concomitant myocardial injury or rhythm disturbance, as well as rule out the possibility of aspiration or the development of pulmonary edema. Rebleeding and enlargement of the hematoma in ICH were previously thought to be rare and highly suggestive of coagulopathy or an underlying lesion such as an AVM or aneurysm. However, it has now been demonstrated that rebleeding is common even in hypertensive ICH but usually occurs within the first 6 to 24 hours after onset.[17] Thus patients with ICH who clinically worsen should undergo urgent repeat head CT to determine if hematoma enlargement has occurred and to plan appropriate emergent management.

The role of surgical hematoma evacuation in the management of primary nontraumatic intracerebral hemorrhage remains controversial. In patients with cerebellar hematoma, early surgical evacuation can clearly be lifesaving. There is essentially no role for surgical evacuation of a pontine hematoma, although patients with underlying lesions, such as cavernous malformations, may benefit from surgical removal if they survive the initial hemorrhage.

TABLE 13-5 ■ Treatment Strategies for Patients Suffering from ICH

Treatment of Primary Injury

Treatment of mass effect
- Hyperosmotic agents
- Mannitol
- Hypertonic saline
- Ventricular drainage
- Surgical decompression
- Maintenance of cerebral perfusion
- Hypertensive therapy

Prevention of Secondary Injury

Avoidance of hypoxia
Avoidance of severe hypertension
Treatment of hypertension
- Infectious causes
- Central fever

Treatment/prevention of seizures
Identification/correction of underlying causes

A variety of surgical interventions for supratentorial ICH have been studied in clinical trials, with varying degrees of scientific rigor. No specific surgical intervention (and for that matter no specific medical intervention studied in other trials) has been shown to be of conclusive benefit in improving outcome after supratentorial ICH.[14] Despite this there is continued interest in the role of surgery for ICH, and prior treatment trials are instructive with regard to indications, timing, and outcome assessment.

McKissock and colleagues,[74] in the first truly randomized trial testing the efficacy of surgical evacuation in ICH, found worsened outcomes in the group of 180 patients randomized to craniotomy and evacuation. This study, published in 1961, was, however, in the pre-CT era and likely not representative of current approaches. Juvela and colleagues[49] randomized 52 patients to conservative or surgical management and found no statistically significant difference in outcome between the two groups. Auer and colleagues[9] studied endoscopic surgery for hematoma evacuation and found no difference in the outcomes of patients with basal ganglia and thalamic hemorrhages treated surgically or medically. However, surgically treated patients with subcortical ICH did do better than those treated medically, especially when hematoma volume was less than 50 ml. Finally, Batjer and colleagues[10] found no difference in outcomes in patients treated surgically for putaminal hemorrhages versus those managed medically, including patients who received ICP monitoring.

Despite the lack of benefit of surgery in these randomized studies, surgical evacuation for ICH is still advocated in certain circumstances. Surgical evacuation should always be considered for cerebellar ICH, although patients who are awake may be managed conservatively unless they deteriorate from hydrocephalus, edema, or rehemorrhage, and patients with profound brainstem dysfunction may not benefit from surgical evacuation. In supratentorial ICH, principally those originating in the putamen or lobar regions, surgery should be considered in the following two circumstances: (1) a relatively young individual with a nondominant hemisphere hemorrhage who deteriorates while under medical observation and (2) a patient with an ICH, especially lobar, that is suspicious for an underlying lesion such as tumor and for whom tissue is important for diagnostic purposes. If surgical evacuation is under consideration, an angiogram is often obtained to ensure adequate evaluation for an underlying AVM before surgical exploration. Future approaches to defining appropriate subsets of patients for surgical ICH removal, as well as investigations of less invasive methods of hematoma evacuation, are being investigated.

Management Issues in the Neurological Intensive Care Unit

In 1999 the Stroke Council of the American Heart Association (AHA) published "Guidelines for the Management of Spontaneous Intracerebral Hemorrhage."[14] These consensus-based guidelines provide a framework for the rational treatment of patients with ICH and address issues such as surgical hematoma evacuation (as discussed earlier) and various aspects of intensive care management and evaluation for underlying etiologies. They also emphasize that many of the approaches to ICH management are unproven and therefore a principal focus should be on future research into ICH mechanisms and treatments.

Management of elevated blood pressure in patients with ICH differs somewhat from that in ischemic stroke patients. There is concern that greatly elevated blood pressure may precipitate ongoing bleeding. On the other hand, if there is ischemia in the perihematoma region, then lowering blood pressure might decrease cerebral perfusion and create secondary ischemia. The target range of blood pressure in patients with ICH should take into account the cause of the hemorrhage, the ICP, and whether the patient has a history of hypertension. In general, maintaining a mean arterial pressure less than 130 mm Hg or, when ICP monitoring is used, maintaining the cerebral perfusion pressure (CPP) at greater than 70 mm Hg is reasonable.[14] Short-acting β-blockers such as labetalol, at a dose of 5 to 10 mg every 5 minutes, or an esmolol infusion may be useful in closely titrating blood pressure in an ICU setting.[14] Other effective agents for blood pressure control include nitroglycerin and nitroprusside, which are thought to relax smooth muscle through a nitric oxide–mediated mechanism, and nicardipine, a calcium channel blocker. It has been suggested that nitroprusside should be avoided because it may elevate ICP by increasing cerebral blood volume.[25,76] In the authors' practice this has not been a significant limiting issue.

Elevated intracranial pressure plays a major role in mortality after ICH.[14] Elevated ICP may be a result of mass effect exerted by the hematoma, local swelling related to the hematoma, or hydrocephalus. Although criteria for ICP monitoring may vary, the AHA guidelines support ICP monitoring in patients with a depressed level of consciousness (Glasgow Coma Scale [GCS] score <9) or neurological deterioration presumed to be due to elevated ICP.[14] If possible, ventriculostomy placement is preferred over an intraparenchymal monitor, because the former allows for CSF drainage as a therapeutic intervention for elevated ICP.

In general the goal of ICP therapy in patients with ICH is to maintain an ICP less than 20 to 25 mm Hg and a CPP greater than 70 mm Hg.[30] ICP management after ICH follows largely along the lines of ICP management for traumatic brain injury, for which ICP management protocols are more firmly established. A stepwise approach to ICP management after ICH has been suggested in the AHA guidelines.[14] This includes CSF drainage (if available), osmotherapy with intermittent mannitol dosing, mild hyperventilation, and use of sedatives and muscle relaxants if necessary. It is usually reasonable and appropriate to institute these therapies individually and maximize their individual efficacy before adding additional therapies, especially because some of these treatments may have deleterious side effects such as hyperventilation-induced cerebral ischemia and prolonged paralysis from overuse of nondepolarizing neuromuscular blocking agents.[39,118]

An important exception is seen in the patient with only mild mass effect from the hematoma but significant hydrocephalus from intraventricular hemorrhage (IVH). In this case aggressive CSF drainage is indicated as a primary therapy because CSF outflow obstruction is the complete mechanism of elevated ICP. As in head injury, the use of barbiturates is controversial and is usually reserved for patients deemed potentially salvageable and who have refractory intracranial hypertension despite other aggressive measures.[6,97] Corticosteroids are to be avoided, because two clinical trials found no benefit of steroid treatment after ICH and their use may increase infectious complications.[88,106] Steroid use in patients with ICH should be reserved for cases in which an underlying lesion, such as tumor or AVM, has profound associated vasogenic edema that creates significant mass effect.

Seizures may occur in 10% to 15% of patients with nontraumatic ICH.[12] If present, they typically occur at symptom onset in supratentorial ICH and rarely occur afterward.[12] Although some recommend the use of 1 month of prophylactic anticonvulsants in patients with supratentorial ICH, the authors' practice is to defer anticonvulsant treatment unless seizures occur.

Indications for mechanical ventilation in patients with ICH are similar to those for ischemic stroke and should be based on the ability of the patient to protect the airway, evidence of respiratory failure as determined by respiratory rate and tidal volume, or the presence of hypoxemia or hypercarbia. The choice of volume versus pressure cycled ventilation and the specific mode of ventilation should be determined by the patient's level of alertness, pulmonary compliance, and unique characteristics in terms of interfacing with the ventilator. A positive end−expiratory pressure (PEEP) of at least 5 cm H_2O should be considered in patients being mechanically ventilated; it is unlikely to clinically significantly elevate ICP.

The goal of fluid management is euvolemia. Hypervolemia is probably unnecessary and could conceivably exacerbate cerebral edema, especially if hypotonic fluids are used. Hypovolemia should be assiduously avoided. In general, maintaining a central venous pressure (CVP) above 5 mm Hg with isotonic fluids (e.g., normal saline or Ringer's lactate) is a reasonable approach, but the lack of studied comparisons allows great variation among physicians in the approach to fluid management (see Figure 13-5).

Future Directions

Current research is underway that addresses several aspects related to intracerebral hemorrhage, including basic mechanisms of disease in ICH, surgical and medical treatments for ICH, and improved patient selection and outcome prediction. Xi and colleagues[117] have postulated that thrombin is an important mediator of perihematoma edema in a pig model of lobar ICH and suggested that antithrombin therapies may have a role in ICH management. Wagner and colleagues[113] looked at ultra-early clot aspiration after lysis with tPA in a pig model of ICH and found decreased edema and protection of the blood-brain barrier.

Concurrently, new approaches to surgical hematoma evacuation are being investigated in human subjects. Both Zuccarello and colleagues[120] and Morgenstern and colleagues[79] reported results of preliminary studies of early clot evacuation (within 3 to 12 hours of presentation). Although there was no difference between surgical and medical arms in these small pilot studies, they did affirm that early ICH treatment is feasible, analogous to early thrombolytic therapy in acute ischemic stroke. Montes and colleagues[78] reported results of stereotactic CT-guided aspiration and thrombolysis of nontraumatic hematoma and suggested that this treatment is safe and can successfully reduce hematoma volume. Naff and colleagues[82] recently reported results of the use of intraventricular urokinase in the treatment of intraventricular hemorrhage, including that associated with ICH. Finally, Surgical Trial in Intracerebral Hemorrhage (STICH) is a study of outcome in surgically and medically treated ICH that is currently ongoing in Europe.

Several outcome prediction models have been previously developed for mortality and functional outcome after ICH.[16,65,109,110] Although numerous criteria have been suggested as affecting outcomes, GCS score and ICH volume on admission are most strongly associated with 30-day mortality and functional outcome, with supratentorial ICH patients with GCS less than 9 and ICH volume greater than 60 ml having a predicted 30-day mortality of greater than 90%.[16] Presence and degree of IVH can also be a useful predictor.[109,110] Although these models currently can provide some usefulness in prognostication, they may have future use in selecting patients most likely to benefit from specific surgical or medical interventions to improve outcome after ICH.[16]

SUMMARY

Acute ischemic stroke and intracerebral hemorrhage are common disorders with high morbidity and mortality. Current approaches to the intensive care management of these diseases derive from two principal sources: recent clinical studies of acute treatment protocols and basic science-derived understanding of the fundamental underlying mechanisms whereby these cerebrovascular diseases result in brain injury. The concept of an early therapeutic time window in which successful treatment can be delivered is common to both conditions and has yielded effective treatment for acute ischemic stroke. Additionally, approaches to limit secondary brain injury from cerebral ischemia and mass effect are fundamental to the intensive care management of patients with both ischemic stroke and ICH. Future approaches to the surgical and medical treatment of both these conditions rely on applying new understandings of the basic mechanisms of brain injury to well-selected patients most likely to benefit.

REFERENCES

1. Abbey E: Bleeding disorders, in Campbell J, Frisse M (eds): **Manual of Medical Therapeutics.** Boston: Little Brown, 1983, pp 285-296.
2. Adams HP, Jr., Brott TG, Crowell RM, et al: Guidelines for the management of patients with acute ischemic stroke. A statement for healthcare professionals from a special writing group of the Stroke Council, American Heart Association, **Stroke 25:**1901-1914, 1994.
3. Adams HP, Jr., Brott TG, Furlan AJ, et al: Guidelines for thrombolytic therapy for acute stroke: a supplement to the guidelines for the management of patients with acute ischemic stroke. A statement for healthcare professionals from a Special Writing Group of the Stoke Council, American Heart Association, **Stroke 27:**1711-1718, 1996.
4. Albers GW: Expanding the window for thrombolytic therapy in acute stroke. The potential role of acute MRI for patient selection, **Stroke 30:**2230-2237, 1999.
5. Albers GW, Easton JD, Sacco RL, et al: Antithrombotic and thrombolytic therapy for ischemic stroke, **Chest 114:**683S-698S, 1998.
6. Allen CH, Ward JD: An evidence-based approach to management of increased intracranial pressure, **Crit Care Clin 14:**485-493, 1998.
7. Astrup J, Symon L, Branston NM, et al: Cortical evoked potential and extracellular K+ and H+ at critical levels of brain ischemia, **Stroke 8:**51-57, 1977.
8. Attwell D, Barbour B, Szatkowski M: Nonvesicular release of neurotransmitter, **Neuron 11:**401-407, 1993.
9. Auer LM, Deinsberger W, Niederkorn K, et al: Endoscopic surgery versus medical treatment for spontaneous intracerebral hematoma: a randomized study, **J Neurosurg 70:**530-535, 1989.
10. Batjer HH, Reisch JS, Allen BC, et al: Failure of surgery to improve outcome in hypertensive putaminal hemorrhage. A prospective randomized trial, **Arch Neurol 47:**1103-1106, 1990.
11. Bauer RB, Tellez H: Dexamethasone as treatment in cerebrovascular disease. 2. A controlled study in acute cerebral infarction, **Stroke 4:**547-555, 1973.
12. Berger AR, Lipton RB, Lesser ML, et al: Early seizures following intracerebral hemorrhage: implications for therapy, **Neurology 38:**1363-1365, 1988.
13. Britton M, Carlsson A, de Faire U: Blood pressure course in patients with acute stroke and matched controls, **Stroke 17:**861-864, 1986.
14. Broderick JP, Adams HP, Jr., Barsan W, et al: Guidelines for the management of spontaneous intracerebral hemorrhage: a statement for healthcare professionals from a special writing group of the Stroke Council, American Heart Association, **Stroke 30:** 905-915, 1999.
15. Broderick JP, Brott T, Tomsick T, et al: Intracerebral hemorrhage more than twice as common as subarachnoid hemorrhage, **J Neurosurg 78:** 188-191, 1993.
16. Broderick JP, Brott TG, Duldner JE, et al: Volume of intracerebral hemorrhage. A powerful and easy-to-use predictor of 30-day mortality, **Stroke 24:**987-993, 1993.
17. Brott T, Broderick J, Kothari R, et al: Early hemorrhage growth in patients with intracerebral hemorrhage, **Stroke 28:**1-5, 1997.
18. Bruno A, Carter S, Qualls C, et al: Incidence of spontaneous intracerebral hemorrhage among Hispanics and non-Hispanic whites in New Mexico, **Neurology 47:**405-408, 1996.
19. Bullock R, Brock-Utne J, van Dellen J, et al: Intracerebral hemorrhage in a primate model: effect on regional cerebral blood flow, **Surg Neurol 29:**101-107, 1988.
20. Carhuapoma JR, Wang PY, Beauchamp NJ, et al: Diffusion-weighted MRI and proton MR spectroscopic imaging in the study of secondary neuronal injury after intracerebral hemorrhage, **Stroke 31:**726-732, 2000.
21. Challa VR, Moody DM, Bell MA: The Charcot-Bouchard aneurysm controversy: impact of a new histologic technique, **J Neuropathol Exp Neurol 51:**264-271, 1992.
22. Chen H, Chopp M, Zhang RL, et al: Anti-CD11b monoclonal antibody reduces ischemic cell damage after transient focal cerebral ischemia in rat, **Ann Neurol 35:**458-463, 1994.
23. Choi DW: Glutamate neurotoxicity and diseases of the nervous system, **Neuron 1:**623-634, 1988.
24. Citron BP, Halpern M, McCarron M, et al: Necrotizing angiitis associated with drug abuse, **N Engl J Med 283:**1003-1011, 1970.
25. Cottrell JE, Patel K, Turndorf H, et al: Intracranial pressure changes induced by sodium nitroprusside in patients with intracranial mass lesions, **J Neurosurg 48:**329-331, 1978.
26. Crawford PM, West CR, Chadwick DW, et al: Arteriovenous malformations of the brain: natural history in

unoperated patients, **J Neurol Neurosurg Psychiatry 49:**1-10, 1986.
27. DeGraba TJ, Pettigrew LC: Why do neuroprotective drugs work in animals but not humans? **Neurol Clin 18:**475-493, 2000.
28. Del Curling O, Jr., Kelly DL, Jr., Elster AD, et al: An analysis of the natural history of cavernous angiomas, **J Neurosurg 75:**702-708, 1991.
29. Delaney P, Estes M: Intracranial hemorrhage with amphetamine abuse, **Neurology 30:**1125-1128, 1980.
30. Diringer MN: Intracerebral hemorrhage: pathophysiology and management, **Crit Care Med 21:**1591-1603, 1993.
31. Fisher CM: Cerebral military aneurysms in hypertension, **Am J Pathol 66:**313-330, 1972.
32. Forsting M, Reith W, Schabitz WR, et al: Decompressive craniectomy for cerebral infarction. An experimental study in rats, **Stroke 26:**259-264, 1995.
33. Frank JI: Large hemispheric infarction, deterioration, and intracranial pressure, **Neurology 45:**1286-1290, 1995.
34. Furlan A, Higashida R, Wechsler L, et al: Intra-arterial prourokinase for acute ischemic stroke. The PROACT II study: a randomized controlled trial. Prolyse in acute cerebral thromboembolism, **JAMA 282:**2003-2011, 1999.
35. Furlan AJ, Whisnant JP, Elveback LR: The decreasing incidence of primary intracerebral hemorrhage: a population study, **Ann Neurol 5:**367-373, 1979.
36. Garcia JH, Liu KF, Yoshida Y, et al: Influx of leukocytes and platelets in an evolving brain infarct (Wiser rat), **Am J Pathol 144:**188-199, 1994.
37. Gilles C, Brucher JM, Khoubesserian P, et al: Cerebral amyloid angiopathy as a cause of multiple intracerebral hemorrhages, **Neurology 34:**730-735, 1984.
38. Ginsberg MD: Local metabolic responses to cerebral ischemia, **Cerebrovasc Brain Metabol Rev 2:**58-93, 1990.
39. Gooch JL: Prolonged paralysis after neuromuscular blockade, **J Toxicol Clin Toxicol 33:**419-426, 1995.
40. Hakim AM: The cerebral ischemic penumbra, **Can J Neurol Sci 14:**557-559, 1987.
41. Halpin SF, Britton JA, Byrne JV, et al: Prospective evaluation of cerebral angiography and computed tomography in cerebral hematoma, **J Neurol Neurosurg Psychiatry 57:**1180-1186, 1994.
42. Harrington H, Heller HA, Dawson D, et al: Intracerebral hemorrhage and oral amphetamine, **Arch Neurol 40:**503-507, 1983.
43. Hart RG, Boop BS, Anderson DC: Oral anticoagulants and intracranial hemorrhage. Facts and hypotheses, **Stroke 26:**1471-1477, 1995.
44. Heresco-Levy U, Javitt DC: The role of N-methyl-D-aspartate (NMDA) receptor-mediated neurotransmission in the pathophysiology and therapeutics of psychiatric syndromes, **Eur Neuropsychopharmacol 8:**141-152, 1988.
45. Hirano T, Read SJ, Abbott DF, et al: No evidence of hypoxic tissue on 18F-fluoromisonidazole PET after intracerebral hemorrhage, **Neurology 53:**2179-2182, 1999.
46. Hylek EM, Singer DE: Risk factors for intracranial hemorrhage in outpatients taking warfarin, **Ann Intern Med 120:**897-902, 1994.
47. Johnson EJ, Greenlund LJ, Akins PT, et al: Neuronal apoptosis: current understanding of molecular mechanisms and potential role in ischemic brain injury, **J Neurotrauma 12:**843-852, 1995.
48. Johnston SC, Selvin S, Gress DR: The burden, trends and demographics of mortality from subarachnoid hemorrhage, **Neurology 50:**1413-1418, 1998.
49. Juvela S, Heiskanen O, Poranen A, et al: The treatment of spontaneous intracerebral hemorrhage. A prospective randomized trial of surgical and conservative treatment, **J Neurosurg 70:**755-758, 1989.
50. Kase CS: Intracerebral hemorrhage: non-hypertensive causes, **Stroke 17:**590-595, 1986.
51. Kase CS, Williams JP, Wyatt DA, et al: Lobar intracerebral hematomas: clinical and CT analysis of 22 cases, **Neurology 32:**1146-1150, 1982.
52. Kirsch JR, Helfaer MA, Lange DG, et al: Evidence for free radical mechanisms of brain injury resulting from ischemia/reperfusion-induced events, **J Neurotrauma 9(Suppl 1):** S157-163, 1992.
53. Klonoff DC, Andrews BT, Obana WG: Stroke associated with cocaine use, **Arch Neurol 46:**989-993, 1989.
54. Kondziolka D, Lunsford LD, Kestle JR: The natural history of cerebral cavernous malformations, **J Neurosurg 83:**820-824, 1995.
55. Kondziolka D, McLaughlin MR, Kestle JR: Simple risk predictions for arteriovenous malformation hemorrhage, **Neurosurgery 37:**851-855, 1995.
56. Kunitz SC, Gross CR, Heyman A, et al: The pilot Stroke Data Bank: definition, design and data, **Stroke 15:**740-746, 1984.
57. Lansberg MG, Albers GW, Beaulieu C, et al: Comparison of diffusion-weighted MRI and CT in acute stroke, **Neurology 54:**1557-1561, 2000.
58. Leblanc R: Cerebral amyloid angiopathy and moyamoya disease, **Neurosurg Clin North Am 3:**625-636, 1992.
59. Leblanc R, Carpenter S, Stewart J, et al: Subacute enlarging cerebral hematoma from amyloid angiopathy: case report, **Neurosurgery 36:**403-406, 1995.
60. Leblanc R, Preul M, Robitaille Y, et al: Surgical considerations in cerebral amyloid angiopathy, **Neurosurgery 29:**712-718, 1991.
61. Levine SR, Brust JC, Futrell N, et al: A comparative study of the cerebrovascular complications of cocaine: alkaloidal versus hydrochloride—a review, **Neurology 41:**1173-1177, 1991.
62. Levine SR, Brust JC, Futrell N, et al: Cerebrovascular complications of the use of the "crack" form of alkaloidal cocaine [comment], **N Engl J Med 323:**699-704, 1990.
63. Lewandowski CA, Frankel M, Tomsick TA, et al: Combined intravenous and intraarterial r-TPA versus intraarterial therapy of acute ischemic stroke: Emergency Management of Stroke (EMS) Bridging Trial, **Stroke 30:**2598-2605, 1999.
64. Lisk DR, Grotta JC, Lamki LM, et al: Should hypertension be treated after acute stroke? A randomized controlled trial using single photon emission computed tomography, **Arch Neurol 50:**855-862, 1993.
65. Lisk DR, Pasteur W, Rhoades H, et al: Early presentation of hemispheric intracerebral hemorrhage: prediction of

outcome and guidelines for treatment allocation, **Neurology 44:**133-139, 1994.
66. Little JR, Dial B, Baelanger G, et al: Brain hemorrhage from intracranial tumor, **Stroke 10:**283-288, 1979.
67. Loizou LA, Hamilton JG, Tsementzis SA: Intracranial hemorrhage in association with pseudoephedrine overdose, **J Neurol Neurosurg Psychiatry 45:**471-472, 1982.
68. Lui TN, Fairholm DJ, Shu TF, et al: Surgical treatment of spontaneous cerebellar hemorrhage, **Surg Neurol 23:**555-558, 1985.
69. Lukes SA: Intracerebral hemorrhage from an arteriovenous malformation after amphetamine injection, **Arch Neurol 40:**60-61, 1983.
70. Mandybur TI: Intracranial hemorrhage caused by metastatic tumors, **Neurology 27:**650-655, 1977.
71. Marion DW, Penrod LE, Kelsey SF, et al: Treatment of traumatic brain injury with moderate hypothermia, **N Engl J Med 336:**540-546, 1997.
72. Martinowitz U, Heim M, Tadmor R, et al: Intracranial hemorrhage in patients with hemophilia, **Neurosurgery 18:**538-541, 1986.
73. McCormick WF: The pathology of vascular ("arteriovenous") malformations, **J Neurosurg 24:**807-816, 1966.
74. McKissock W, Richardson A, Taylor J: Primary intracerebral hemorrhage: a controlled trial of surgical and conservative treatment in 180 unselected cases, **Lancet 2:**222-226, 1961.
75. Mendelow AD: Mechanisms of ischemic brain damage with intracerebral hemorrhage, **Stroke 24:** I115-117, discussion I118-119, 1993.
76. Michenfelder JD, Milde JH: The interaction of sodium nitroprusside, hypotension, and isoflurane in determining cerebral vasculature effects, **Anesthesiology 69:**870-875, 1988.
77. Mohr JP, Caplan LR, Melski JW, et al: The Harvard Cooperative Stroke Registry: a prospective registry, **Neurology 28:**754-762, 1978.
78. Montes JM, Wong JH, Fayad PB, et al: Stereotactic computed tomographic-guided aspiration and thrombolysis of intracerebral hematoma: protocol and preliminary experience, **Stroke 31:**834-840, 2000.
79. Morgenstern LB, Frankowski RF, Shedden P, et al: Surgical treatment for intracerebral hemorrhage (STICH): a single-center, randomized clinical trial, **Neurology 51:**1359-1363, 1998.
80. Mueller SM: Neurologic complications of phenylpropanolamine use, **Neurology 33:**650-652, 1983.
81. Mueller SM, Muller J, Asdel SM: Cerebral hemorrhage associated with phenylpropanolamine in combination with caffeine, **Stroke 15:**119-123, 1984.
82. Naff NJ, Carhuapoma JR, Williams MA, et al: Treatment of intraventricular hemorrhage with urokinase: effects on 30-day survival, **Stroke 31:**841-847, 2000.
83. Norris JW, Hachinski VC: High dose steroid treatment in cerebral infarction, **Br Med J (Clin Res Ed) 292:**21-23, 1986.
84. Ojemann RG, Heros RC: Spontaneous brain hemorrhage, **Stroke 14:**468-475, 1983.
85. Okazaki H, Reagan TJ, Campbell RJ: Clinicopathologic studies of primary cerebral amyloid angiopathy, **Mayo Clin Proceed 54:**22-31, 1979.
86. Okoye MI, Watanabe I: Ultrastructural features of cerebral amyloid angiopathy, **Human Pathol 13:**1127-1132, 1982.
87. Ondra SL, Troupp H, George ED, et al: The natural history of symptomatic arteriovenous malformations of the brain: a 24-year follow-up assessment, **J Neurosurg 73:**387-391, 1990.
88. Poungvarin N, Bhoopat W, Viriyavejakul A, et al: Effects of dexamethasone in primary supratentorial intracerebral hemorrhage, **N Engl J Med 316:**1229-1233, 1987.
89. Powers WJ: Acute hypertension after stroke: the scientific basis for treatment decisions [editorial], **Neurology 43:**461-467, 1993.
90. Powers WJ: Hemodynamics and metabolism in ischemic cerebrovascular disease, **Neurol Clin 10:**31-48, 1992.
91. Qureshi AI, Wilson DA, Hanley DF, et al: No evidence for an ischemic penumbra in massive experimental intracerebral hemorrhage, **Neurology 52:**266-272, 1999.
92. Reith J, Jorgensen HS, Pederson PM, et al: Body temperature in acute stroke: relation to stroke severity, infarct size, mortality, and outcome, **Lancet 347:**422-425, 1996.
93. Robinson JR, Awad IA, Little JR: Natural history of the cavernous angioma, **J Neurosurg 75:**709-714, 1991.
94. Ropper AH, Shafran B: Brain edema after stroke. Clinical syndrome and intracranial pressure, **Arch Neurol 41:**26-29, 1984.
95. Rordorf G, Cramer SC, Efird JT, et al: Pharmacological elevation of blood pressure in acute stroke. Clinical effects and safety, **Stroke 28:**2133-2138, 1997.
96. Schwab S, Schwarz S, Spranger M, et al: Moderate hypothermia in the treatment of patients with severe middle cerebral artery infarction, **Stroke 29:**2461-2466, 1998.
97. Schwab S, Spranger M, Schwarz S, et al: Barbiturate coma in severe hemispheric stroke: useful or obsolete? **Neurology 48:**1608-1613, 1997.
98. Schwab S, Steiner T, Aschoff A, et al: Early hemicraniectomy in patients with complete middle cerebral artery infarction, **Stroke 29:**1888-1893, 1998.
99. Sherman DG, Atkinson RP, Chippendale T, et al: Intravenous ancrod for treatment of acute ischemic stroke: the STAT study: a randomized controlled trial. Stroke Treatment with Ancrod Trial, **JAMA 282:**2395-2403, 2000.
100. Siesjeo BK: Historical overview. Calcium, ischemia, and death of brain cells, **Ann N Y Acad Sci 522:**638-661, 1988.
101. Siesjeo BK, Bengtsson F: Calcium fluxes, calcium antag onists, and calcium-related pathology in brain ischemia, hypoglycemia, and spreading depression: a unifying hypothesis, **J Cereb Blood Flow Metab 9:**127-140, 1989.
102. Silver B, Weber J, Fisher M: Medical therapy for ischemic stroke, **Clin Neuropharmacol 19:**101-128, 1996.
103. Simon RP, Niro M, Gwinn R: Brain acidosis induced by hypercarbic ventilation attenuates focal ischemic injury, **J Pharmacol Exp Ther 267:**1428-1431, 1993.
104. *Stedman's Medical Dictionary*, 21st ed, Baltimore: Williams and Wilkins, 1966.
105. Symon L: The relationship between CBF, evoked potentials and the clinical features in cerebral ischemia, **Acta Neurol Scand Suppl 78:**175-190, 1980.

106. Tellez H, Bauer RB: Dexamethasone as treatment in cerebrovascular disease. 1. A controlled study in intracerebral hemorrhage, **Stroke 4:**541-546, 1973.
107. The Arteriovenous Malformation Study Group: Arteriovenous malformations of the brain in adults, **N Engl J Med 340:**1812-1818, 1999.
108. The National Institute of Neurological Disorders and Stroke t-PA Stroke Study Group: tissue plasminogen activator for acute ischemic stroke, **N Engl J Med 333:**1581-1587, 1995.
109. Tuhrim S, Dambrosia JM, Price TR, et al: Intracerebral hemorrhage: external validation and extension of a model for prediction of 30-day survival, **Ann Neurol 29:**658-663, 1991.
110. Tuhrim S, Horowitz DR, Sacher M, et al: Volume of ventricular blood is an important determinant of outcome in supratentorial intracerebral hemorrhage, **Crit Care Med 27:**617-621, 1999.
111. Vinters HV, Gilbert JJ: Cerebral amyloid angiopathy: incidence and complications in the aging brain. II. The distribution of amyloid vascular changes, **Stroke 14:**924-928, 1983.
112. Vonsattel JP, Myers RH, Hedley-Whyte ET, et al: Cerebral amyloid angiopathy without and with cerebral hemorrhages: a comparative histological study, **Ann Neurol 30:**637-649, 1991.
113. Wagner KR, Xi G, Hua Y, et al: Ultra-early clot aspiration after lysis with tissue plasminogen activator in a porcine model of intracerebral hemorrhage: edema reduction and blood-brain barrier protection, **J Neurosurg 90:**491-498, 1999.
114. Wallace JD, Levy LL: Blood pressure after stroke, **JAMA 246:**2177-2180, 1981.
115. Wattendorf AR, Bots GT, Went LN, et al: Familial cerebral amyloid angiopathy presenting as recurrent cerebral hemorrhage, **J Neurol Sci 55:**121-135, 1982.
116. Wise G, Sutter R, Burkhold J: The treatment of brain ischemia with vasopressor drugs, **Stroke 3:**135-140, 1972.
117. Xi G, Wagner KR, Keep RF, et al: Role of blood clot formation on early edema development after experimental intracerebral hemorrhage, **Stroke 29:**2580-2586, 1998.
118. Yundt KD, Diringer MN: The use of hyperventilation and its impact on cerebral ischemia in the treatment of traumatic brain injury, **Crit Care Clin 13:**163-184, 1997.
119. Azaulia AR, Diringer MN, Derdeyn CP, et al: Progression of mass effect after intracerebral hemorrhage, **Stroke 30:**1167-1173, 1999.
120. Zuccarello M, Brott T, Derex L, et al: Early surgical treatment for supratentorial intracerebral hemorrhage: a randomized feasibility study, **Stroke 30:**1833-1839, 1999.

CHAPTER 14

Management of Patients With Epilepsy

DAVID KING-STEPHENS
PETER WEBER

Seizures in the intensive care unit (ICU) setting complicate the management of critically ill patients. A seizure is a time-limited convulsive or nonconvulsive event that occurs as a result of excessive electrical discharges in archicortical or neocortical structures. Status epilepticus (SE) is the persistence of these abnormal electrical discharges. The principles employed in the management of isolated or recurrent seizures depend on the clinical setting. SE is a life-threatening emergent condition that requires aggressive sequential interventions to arrest the abnormal electrical activity, preserve function, and prevent mortality. This chapter presents a review of seizures and the management of abnormal electrical activity.

DIAGNOSIS AND CHARACTERIZATION OF SEIZURES

The currently accepted classification scheme of seizure type recognizes two major groups—partial and generalized onset seizures.[5] Partial onset seizures may secondarily generalize. Partial onset seizures are generally divided into simple partial (usually with motor or sensory signs or symptoms but without alteration of consciousness) and complex partial seizures (with alteration of consciousness). There are many categories of generalized epilepsy (atonic, myoclonic, clonic, absence, tonic, and tonic-clonic), few of which are seen in their pure form in the ICU setting. The most common seizure type in the ICU setting is a secondarily generalized seizure.[40] Epileptic syndromes (i.e., syndromes classified according to cause; presence of seizure types; presence or absence of risk factors for epilepsy; presence or absence of a family history of epilepsy; findings on the neurological exam, magnetic resonance imaging [MRI], and electroencephalogram [EEG] studies; and prognosis) such as juvenile myoclonic epilepsy, Lennox-Gastaut syndrome, and benign rolandic epilepsy, may be encountered on rare occasions in the ICU setting. Epilepsies with a known cause are classified as symptomatic localization-related epilepsy; when the cause is unknown, they are classified as idiopathic, or cryptogenic, epilepsy.

Most seizures encountered in the ICU fit into categories such posttraumatic, lesional, toxic/metabolic, perioperative, and infectious. Because these seizures occur as a result of acquired derangements of structure or function, they are referred to as provoked seizures and can be either focal or generalized in onset. The most commonly encountered seizures associated with nonneurological medical conditions include metabolic disorders, such as electrolyte disturbances, hyponatremia, hypoglycemia and nonketotic hyperglycemia, hypocalcemia, and hypomagnesemia, and uremia; anoxia, alcohol withdrawal; infections; and intoxication with recreational drugs (cocaine, amphetamines, heroin, and phencyclidine).[12] These conditions do not require long-term treatment with anticonvulsant medications. On the other hand, seizures that occur as a result of a developmental or inherited anomaly are usually partial onset seizures with secondary generalization, classified as unprovoked seizures, and usually treated with anticonvulsant medications.

SEIZURE TYPE AND THE CONDITIONS THAT CAUSE THESE SEIZURES TO ARISE

Posttraumatic seizures complicate the management of head-injured patients. Nearly 10% of the 400,000 patients treated for head injuries in the United States each year suffer early or late posttraumatic seizures.[2] Risk factors for seizures in these patients include cortical contusions; subdural, epidural, or intracerebral hematomas; depressed skull fracture; penetrating head wound; and Glasgow Coma Scale score of 10 or less. If any of these criteria are met, the incidence of seizures is 20% or more. Seizures occurring within 7 days after injury are classified as early posttraumatic seizures; those occurring more than 7 days after injury are classified as late posttraumatic. Phenytoin and valproate have been shown to reduce the incidence of early posttraumatic seizures.[32,33] Prophylactic administration of antiepileptic medications does not prevent the onset of late posttraumatic seizures or epilepsy.[28] Adverse effects, such as intravenous (IV) site reactions, occur in 18% and 25% of patients receiving valproate or phenytoin, respectively.[1] Therefore the data support coverage of high-risk head-injured patients with antiepileptic medications in the first week after injury, the discontinuation of these drugs after this first week (if no seizures have occurred), and the administration of appropriate medications at the time of onset of late seizures if they occur.

The choice of seizure medications for prophylaxis against early posttraumatic seizures should be based on ease of administration, availability of intravenous form, cost, and side effects. Phenytoin, phenobarbital, and valproate (although valproate is not approved in the United States for the treatment of SE) meet many of these criteria.[8] The loading dose for phenytoin is 20 mg/kg, administered no faster than 50 mg/min to avoid cardiac arrhythmia and hypotension. Phenytoin has substantial potential neurobehavioral side effects.[32] Phenytoin needs to be diluted with normal saline because solutions containing glucose precipitate the mixture. For valproate, the loading dose is 10 to 15 mg/kg/day, administered as a 60-minute infusion at no more than 20 mg/min, although faster infusion rates (up to 500 mg/min) have been used without complications.[37,38] Valproate has the advantage of not requiring cardiac or blood pressure monitoring. The most common adverse events reported with valproate include dizziness, headache, nausea, and injection site pain.

Intracranial lesions such as tumors, infections, and vascular malformations are associated with seizures. Lesional epilepsy is a frequent cause for admission to the ICU. Intracranial lesions vary in their epileptogenicity. Lesional epilepsy is most often focal in onset (partial epilepsy), and secondary generalization of these seizures is common. Management of patients with lesional epilepsy follows the guidelines of medication administration for other epileptic conditions. Phenytoin, carbamazepine, phenobarbital, and valproate all have a role in the therapy of lesional epilepsy. Treatment of the lesion results in control of seizures in 30% to 60% of patients.[40] Patients admitted with intractable medically resistant lesional epilepsy are more likely to be cured of seizures if the surgical procedure includes removal of the epileptogenic cortex at the time of excision of the lesion.

Postoperative seizures can occur after any craniotomy performed for supratentorial lesions. Use of anticonvulsants in elective supratentorial craniotomies will decrease the rate of seizures and sequelae from these seizures (mental status changes, focal deficits, brain edema, transient hypoxia, and increased intracranial pressure).[23] Despite its limitations, phenytoin is still the most common prophylactically administered perioperative anticonvulsant. A study comparing carbamazepine with phenytoin, used for 6 months after surgery, found no difference in the reduction of postoperative seizures.[10] Intravenous forms of valproate may change this. The authors support the use of anticonvulsants in elective supratentorial intracranial procedures that violate the pia arachnoid and enter the substance of the brain. These medications can be withdrawn after the patient's neurological condition stabilizes if no seizures occur.

TREATMENT OF STATUS EPILEPTICUS

Generalized tonic-clonic SE is a common neurological emergency. Although prolonged seizures are usually easily recognized, an understanding of the definition of SE is essential in guiding the prompt and aggressive management schemes that have proven efficacy for this dangerous condition. A modern working definition of SE (perhaps better termed *early* established SE[21]) is as follows: "Generalized status epilepticus in adults and older children (>5 years old) refers to ≥5 minutes of (a) continuous seizures *or* (b) two or more discrete seizures between which there is incomplete recovery of consciousness."[19]

SE may occur as often as 150,000 to 250,000 times a year in the United States.[7,35] Mortality rates from SE may be as high as 8% to 65%.[16] Prolonged abnormal electrical activity can cause irreversible brain damage.[14]

The EEG characteristics of SE vary. Generalized convulsive SE (GCSE) may be confused with toxic or hypoxic myoclonus, and nonconvulsive SE may manifest as subtle confusion or dysphasia, making necessary the use of EEG for adequate diagnosis in intractable cases. GCSE presents in 70% to 80% of patients with focal behavioral or electrographic features.[34] Recurrent generalized convulsions can evolve into continuous seizure activity, followed by gradual attenuation of motor manifestations.[36] The EEG sequence is that of discrete seizures; waxing and waning of ictal discharges; a continuous pattern of ictal activity, later interrupted by periods of relative flattening; and finally periodic epileptiform discharges (PEDs). The presence of PEDs seems to be the only EEG feature that predicts outcome in SE, with a poor prognosis for recovery when present.[22] If the seizures are allowed to persist, an condition of electromechanical dissociation may occur when there are no outward manifestations of abnormal brain activity.

Focal SE presents with a variety of motor, sensory, and psychic symptoms or without clinical manifestations. The most common manifestations are focal motor seizures, prolonged confusion, and decreased level of consciousness. The most common causes are acute vascular disease, epilepsy, and tumor.[9] Treatment guidelines for nonconvulsive SE are the same as for generalized convulsive SE.

New resuscitative strategies and the timely application of these new strategies have decreased morbidity and mortality rates from status epilepticus. The time frame for application of these strategies is measured in minutes, not hours. The initial step is a brief history and physical examination of the patient and the establishment of intravenous access. Clues such as external evidence of head trauma, anisocoria, and active cerebrospinal fluid (CSF) leakage may suggest a treatable underlying condition. Laboratory studies should be ordered to rule out hypoglycemia, hypernatremia/hyponatremia, and other metabolic derangements. The patient should be monitored in the intensive care unit if the more aggressive interventions are anticipated. Continuous EEG monitoring can be helpful. Antiepileptic drug treatment begins with administration of thiamine 100 mg, followed by 50 ml of 50% dextrose if updated laboratory reports on the patient are not available. Administer a slow intravenous infusion of lorazepam 0.1 mg/kg at a rate of 2 mg/min until seizures stop or the dose is completed (maximum dose of 8 mg). If seizures persist and the patient is not taking antiepileptic medications, administer phenytoin (20 mg/kg IV at a rate of 50 mg/min or fosphenytoin 20 mg/kg [phenytoin equivalents] at a rate of 150 mg/min). An additional dose of 5 to 10 mg/kg of phenytoin or fosphenytoin can be administered if seizures persist after the first loading dose. If the patient still suffers seizures at this point in the therapeutic plan, we prefer to intubate and ventilate the patient and add propofol.

Propofol has been used effectively in the treatment of refractory status epilepticus, defined as seizure activity persisting over 2 hours despite treatment with first-line antiepileptic drugs, such as IV phenytoin and lorazepam or phenobarbital, in both adult and pediatric patients.[3] Propofol is an intravenous anesthetic agent with short duration of action that has barbiturate- and benzodiazepine-like effects on the γ-aminobutyric acid (GABA A) receptor.[26] Cardiovascular adverse effects, such as hypotension and bradycardia, are reported to be significantly less than those associated with barbiturates.[4]

Propofol has favorable pharmacodynamic properties.[31] In a mixed group of patients in status epilepticus with multiple medical problems (associated with structural lesions such as subdural hematomas or primary brain tumors) the mean time to seizure control was 2.6 minutes with propofol compared with the mean time to seizure control of 122 minutes with phenobarbital, a statistically significant difference.

The end point of propofol administration is the cessation of clinical seizure activity, the elimination of electrographic spikes on the EEG, or a burst suppression pattern on EEG. Propofol is administered as a loading dose of 1 to 2 mg/kg, followed by 2 to 10 mg/kg/hr thereafter as a maintenance infusion. This infusion can be maintained for 24 hours. Withdrawal of the propofol can begin at that time. Maintenance dosages for phenytoin or fosphenytoin should be continued. Continuous EEG monitoring is recommended during withdrawal of propofol in guiding interventions or restoring the propofol infusion.

Refractory generalized status epilepticus may require additional interventions.[20] Intravenous carbamazepine and valproic acid may soon be available as adjuncts to the above regimen. Alternative treatment options include continuous infusion of midazolam (0.2 mg/kg slow IV push, followed by 0.75 to 10 μg/kg/min infusion) or barbiturates such as pentobarbital given 10 to 15 mg/kg bolus over 1 hour, followed by 0.5 to 3 mg/kg/hr infusion (may require pressor support).

Newer Anticonvulsant Medications

Although seven new anticonvulsant medications have been approved in the United States since 1993, none of these have favorable pharmacokinetic profiles suitable for IV administration or for a rapid oral loading dose (to achieve rapid therapeutic concentrations) because of the high incidence of adverse effects. Levetiracetam, a broad-spectrum anticonvulsant approved for the adjunctive treatment of partial seizures, has a volume of distribution close to the volume of intracellular and extracellular water, with the potential for IV preparation and administration.[27]

TABLE 14-1 ■ IV Formulation of AEDs

Anticonvulsant Agent	Loading Dose	Maintenance Dose
Diazepam	0.2 mg/kg/dose	
Lorazepam	0.1 mg/kg/dose	
Phenytoin	20 mg/kg (<50 mg/min)	5-10 mg/kg
Fosphenytoin	20 mg/kg (150 mg/min)	
Phenobarbital	20 mg/kg (100 mg/min)	1-3 mg/kg
Pentobarbital	5 mg/kg followed by 0.5-3 mg/kg/hr with EEG monitoring	
Valproate*	30-555 mg/min[20,30]	
Midazolam	0.2 mg/kg followed by 0.75-10 μg/kg/min infusion	
Propofol	1-2 mg/kg followed by 2-10 mg/kg/hr	

*Not approved by the Food and Drug Administration for treatment of status epilepticus.

SEIZURE PROPHYLAXIS

Prophylactic administration of anticonvulsant medications in the setting of trauma, newly diagnosed primary and metastatic brain tumors, and intracranial hemorrhages and for postcraniotomy patients has been a common practice in the past. Seizure prophylaxis in the setting of head trauma is reviewed in Chapter 9. In a recent meta-analysis, 43% of patients undergoing craniotomy for primary brain tumors received prophylaxis.[13] This practice does not seem unreasonable if 20% of patients with newly diagnosed tumors have already had a seizure and a further 19% will suffer a seizure after the diagnosis. However, administration of prophylactic seizure medications may not be efficacious. The metaanalysis by Glantz and colleagues reviewed Class I and Class II data that showed no significant reduction in first seizures in patients undergoing intracranial surgery for brain tumors.[13] In addition, administration of prophylactic anticonvulsants was associated with a 20% to 40% complication rate. Similar data show lack of efficacy for the broader category of postcraniotomy anticonvulsant prophylaxis in patients without preexisting seizures.[15]

These findings suggest that long-term anticonvulsant prophylaxis is not necessary in all patients undergoing surgery for brain tumors.[29] Subcategory analysis of more specific scenarios (such as patients undergoing craniotomy with cortical stimulation) is not available in most cases. Perioperative anticonvulsants should be continued and levels checked postoperatively in patients with a history of epilepsy (recurrent seizures).

Various intracranial insults are associated with a high risk of developing epilepsy. Subarachnoid hemorrhage is associated with a 25% chance of developing epilepsy.[24] Traumatic brain injury is associated with a 20% to 50% risk of developing epilepsy.[32] Hemorrhagic strokes and ischemic strokes are associated with a 3% to 8% incidence of late poststroke seizures.[17,25] Recurrent seizures from these various intracranial pathologies require long-term use of anticonvulsant medications.

Patients undergoing resective surgery for intractable seizures (e.g., temporal lobectomy) may require close monitoring of antiepileptic drug levels because these levels may fluctuate widely after surgery. These fluctuations may be caused by steroid and antibiotic administration, use of inhalational anesthetics, and stress. Phenytoin and carbamazepine levels tend to fall in the first day after surgery, with carbamazepine levels increasing up to 27% in subsequent days.[6,11] Although surgery is designed to eradicate seizures, it is not uncommon for seizures to occur in the early postoperative interval. These seizures should be managed by the methods outlined earlier and by optimizing antiepileptic drug levels. These seizures, in the first week after surgery, have no prognostic implications for long-term seizure outcome.

REFERENCES

1. Anderson GD, Lin Y, Temkin NR, et al: Incidence of intravenous site reactions in neurotrauma patients receiving valproate or phenytoin, **Ann Pharmacother 34(6):**697-702, 2000.
2. Annegers JF, Grabow JD, Groover RV, et al: Seizures after head trauma: a population study, **Neurology 30:**683-689, 1980.
3. Begemann M, Rowan AJ, Tuhrim S: Treatment of refractory complex-partial status epilepticus with propofol: case report, **Epilepsia 41(1):**105-109, 2000.
4. Bryson HM, Fulton BR, Faulds D: Propofol: an update of its use in anesthesia and conscious sedation, **Drugs 21:**955-957, 1993.
5 Commission on Classification and Terminology of the International League Against Epilepsy: Proposal for revised clinical and electrographic classification of epileptic seizures, **Epilepsia 22:**489-501, 1981.
6. Cruz RF, Graves NM, Leppik IE, et al: Carbamazepine toxicity after epilepsy surgery, **Epilepsia 30:**640, 1989.
7. DeLorenzo RJ, Pellock JM, Towne AR, et al: Epidemiology of status epilepticus, **Clin Neurophysiol 12(4):**316-325, 1995.
8. Devinsky O, Leppik I, Willmore LJ, et al: Safety of intravenous valproate, **Ann Neurol 38:**670-674, 1995.
9. Drislane FW, Blum AS, Schomer DL: Focal status epilepticus: clinical features and significance of different EEG patterns, **Epilepsia 40(9):**1254-1260, 1999.
10. Foy PM, Chadwick DW, Rajgopalaln N, et al: Do prophylactic anticonvulsant drugs alter the pattern of seizures after craniotomy? **J Neurol Neurosurg Psychiatry 55:**753-757, 1992.
11. Friel P, Clarke H, Ojemann G, et al: Decreased serum anticonvulsant levels after epilepsy surgery, **Epilepsia 28:**588, 1997.
12. Gilmore R: Seizures associated with nonneurologic medical conditions, in Wyllie E (ed): **The Treatment of Epilepsy: Principles and Practice.** Philadelphia: Lea & Febiger, 1993, pp 667-677.
13. Glantz MJ, Cole BF, Forsyth PA, et al: Practice parameter: anticonvulsant prophylaxis in patients with newly diagnosed brain tumors. Report of the Quality Standards Subcommittee of the American Academy of Neurology, **Neurology 54(10):**1886-1893, 2000.
14. Knopman D, Margolis G, Reeves AG: Prolonged focal epilepsy and hypoxemia as a cause of focal brain damage: a case study, **Ann Neurol 1:**195-198, 1977.
15. Kuijlen JM, Teernstra OP, Kessels AG, et al: Effectiveness of antiepileptic prophylaxis used with supratentorial craniotomies: a meta-analysis, **Seizure 5:**291-298, 1996.
16. Leppik IE, Derivan AT, Homan RW, et al: Double blind study of lorazepam and diazepam in status epilepticus, **JAMA 249:**1452-1454, 1983.
17. Lesser RP, Luders H, Dinner DS, et al: Epileptic seizures due to thrombotic and embolic cardiovascular disease in older patients, **Epilepsia 26:**622-630, 1985.
18. Limdi N, Faught E: Safety of rapid infusions of valproate sodium, **Epilepsia 41(10):**1342-1345, 2000.

19. Lowenstein DH: Status epilepticus: an overview of the clinical problem, **Epilepsia 40(Suppl 1):**S3-8, S21-22, 1999.
20. Lowenstein DH, Alldredge BK: Current concepts—status epilepticus, **N Engl J Med 338:**970-976, 1998.
21. Meldrum B: The revised operational definition of generalised tonic-clonic (TC) status epilepticus in adults, **Epilepsia 40:**123-124, 1999.
22. Nei M, Lee JM, Shankar VL, et al: The EEG and prognosis in status epilepticus, **Epilepsia 40(2):**157-163, 1999.
23. North JB, Penhall RK, Hanieh A, et al: Phenytoin and postoperative epilepsy: a double-blind study, **J Neurosurg 58(5):**672-677, 1983.
24. Olafsson E, Gudmundsson G, Hauser WA: Risk of epilepsy in long-term survivors of surgery for aneurysmal subarachnoid hemorrhage: a population-based study in Iceland, **Epilepsia 41(9):**1201-1205, 2000.
25. Olsen TS, Hagenhaven H, Thage O: Epilepsy after stroke, **Neurology 37:**1209-1211, 1987.
26. Orser BA, Wang LY, Pennefather PS, et al: Propofol modulates activation and desensitization of GABA A receptors in cultured murine hippocampal neurons, **J Neurosci 14(12):**7747-7760, 1994.
27. Radtke R: Pharmacokinetics of levetiracetam, **Epilepsia 42(Suppl 4):**24-27, 2001.
28. Schierhout G, Roberts I: Prophylactic antiepileptic agents after head injury: a systematic review, **J Neurol Neurosurg Psychiatry 64(1):**108-112, 1998.
29. Shaw EG, Scheithauer BW, O'Fallon JR: Management of supratentorial low-grade gliomas, **Oncology 7(7):**10, 97-104, 1993.
30. Sinha S, Naritoku D: Intravenous valproate is well tolerated in unstable patients with status epilepticus, **Neurology 55:**722-724, 2000.
31. Stecker MM, Kramer TH, Raps EC, et al: Treatment of refractory status epilepticus with propofol: clinical and pharmacokinetic findings, **Epilepsia 39(1):**18-26, 1998.
32. Temkin NR, Dikmen SS, Anderson GD, et al: Valproate therapy for prevention of posttraumatic seizures: a randomized trial, **J Neurosurg 91:**593-600, 1999.
33. Temkin NR, Dikmen SS, Wilensky AJ, et al: A randomized double blind study of phenytoin for the prevention of posttraumatic seizures, **N Engl J Med 323:**497-502, 1990.
34. Treiman DM: Electroclinical features of status epilepticus, **J Clin Neurophysiol 12(40):**343-362, 1995.
35. Treiman DM, Meyers PD, Walton NY, et al: A comparison of four treatments for generalized convulsive status epilepticus, **N Engl J Med 339:**792-798, 1998.
36. Treiman DM, Walton NY, Kendrick C: A progressive sequence of EEG changes during generalized convulsive status epilepticus, **Epilepsy Res 5:**49-60, 1990.
37. Uberall MA, Trollmann R, Wunsiedler U, et al: Intravenous valproate in pediatric epilepsy patients with refractory status epilepticus, **Neurology 54(11):**2188-2189, 2000.
38. Venkataraman V, Wheless JW: Safety of rapid intravenous infusion of valproate loading doses in epilepsy patients, **Epilepsy Res 35:**147-153, 1999.
39. Vespa PM, Nenov V, Nuwer MR: Continuous EEG monitoring in the intensive care unit: early findings and clinical efficacy, **J Clin Neurophysiol 16(1):**1-13, 1994.
40. Weber JP, Silbergeld DL, Winn HR: Surgical resection of epileptogenic cortex associated with structural lesions, **Neurosurg Clin N Am 4(2):**327-336, 1993.

CHAPTER 15

Management of Patients with Brain Tumors

GUY LIN
G. EVREN KELES
MITCHEL S. BERGER

The goal of the intensive care management of patients with brain tumors is to anticipate and recognize potentially harmful problems both preoperatively and postoperatively. The management of these problems often requires medical or surgical manipulation of various organ systems to facilitate stabilization and recovery. This chapter reviews relevant central nervous system (CNS) physiology, perioperative systemic and neurological issues, and complications that may be encountered in the neurosurgical intensive care unit (ICU).

PHYSIOLOGY

A detailed understanding of the anatomy and pathophysiology of the CNS is essential to effectively manage patients with brain tumors in the ICU. After the closure of fontanels and sutures, which is normally completed by the second year of life, the skull may be considered as a rigid container of fixed volume. The intracranial contents are the brain bulk, blood, and cerebrospinal fluid (CSF), which respectively constitute 87%, 4%, and 9% of the total intracranial volume.[41] In brain tumor patients, in addition to the volume of these three components, the tumor volume becomes a part of the total intracranial volume. A significant increase in the volume of any intracranial component or a separate mass may result in an increased intracranial pressure (ICP) and subsequently reduced cerebral perfusion pressure (CPP) and cerebral blood flow (CBF). In addition to its effect on CPP and CBF, increased ICP may also cause damage through brain shifts causing distortion and herniation of the neural tissue. Supratentorial tumors may cause subfalcine or transtentorial herniation. Depending on the supratentorial distribution of the elevated pressure, downward transtentorial herniation may be unilateral (i.e., uncal) or bilateral (i.e., central). Posterior fossa tumors, however, may cause transforaminal or upward transtentorial herniation.

CSF volume appears to be the major compensatory mechanism, with the majority in the cerebrospinal subarachnoid spaces and only 10% in the ventricular system. The majority of CSF is secreted by active transport from the choroid plexus and absorbed passively by a hydrostatic gradient mainly through the arachnoid granulations into the venous circulation. The average total CSF volume in an adult is 150 ml, with a secretion rate of about 20 ml/hr. The rate of CSF production, 0.35 to 0.40 ml/min, is almost constant within the normal physiological range of intracranial pressures. CSF production rate decreases with increased ICP as a result of decreased CBF and CPP.[6,51] Its absorption rate, however, is linearly related to ICP.

CPP, which is the pressure gradient between arterial inflow and venous outflow, may be calculated as the difference between mean arterial pressure (MAP) and ICP. CPP is the driving force in maintaining adequate CBF. Normal autoregulation of CBF maintains adequate perfusion at approximately 50 ml/100g/min at mean arterial blood pressures ranging from 50 to 150 mm Hg. Patients with a history of arterial hypertension shift the autoregulatory curve to the right, so that a higher pressure is required to maintain adequate perfusion of brain parenchyma.[25] Although neurological symptoms may be present at CBF levels above 20 ml/100g/min, cerebral function is critically compromised at CBF less than 20 ml/100g/min, first by electrical impairment, followed by ionic pump failure at the 10 to 12 ml/100g/min level. A CPP of more than 55 mm Hg (adult average, 80 mm Hg) is adequate as long as clinical signs of cerebral dysfunction are absent.[10] Two additional hemodynamic alterations that should be considered in the postoperative care of a brain tumor patient include impaired blood-brain barrier and pressure limitations associated with blood vessels that were electrosurgically ablated during the operation.

In cases of brain edema the additional water content causes an increase in brain mass, adding to the mass effect of the tumor and resulting in an elevated ICP. Cerebral edema can be classified into five different theoretical types: vasogenic, cytotoxic, interstitial, hydrostatic, and osmotic. Each is caused by a different pathophysiological mechanism on which each specific therapy is based. Briefly, vasogenic edema results from a physical disruption of brain tissue with impairment of the blood-brain barrier. The pathophysiology involves an increase in capillary permeability and transmural capillary pressure together with retention of extravasated fluid in interstitial spaces. Damage to endothelial membranes, activation of transendothelial pinocytosis, and disruption of tight endothelial junctions may result in increased capillary permeability. Vasogenic edema occurs adjacent to brain tumors, traumatic lesions, intracerebral hemorrhages, inflammatory foci, and chronic subdural hematomas. Cytotoxic edema is caused by impairment of the sodium-potassium (Na-K) ATPase pump as a result of reduction of CBF below critical threshold levels. The ischemic process leads to a cascade of biochemical reactions, which result in high extracellular potassium and high intracellular calcium levels, leading to irreversible cell damage from membrane dysfunction. This type of edema occurs adjacent to areas of focal or global ischemia and hypoxia. Interstitial edema is caused by high-pressure obstructive hydrocephalus. Perifocal edema may lead to brain ischemia and neuronal dysfunction. A representative example is the patient with a posterior fossa tumor who presents with obstructive hydrocephalus causing neurological impairment secondary to hydrocephalus and increased interstitial edema. Hydrostatic edema is caused by an increase in transmural vascular pressure. An increased hydrostatic pressure gradient between the intravascular and extravascular spaces leads to an accumulation of extracellular fluid. Loss of cerebral autoregulation may lead to abruptly increased transmural pressure at the capillary bed.[23] Osmotic edema results from a critical fall in serum osmolality and hyponatremia.[3] Serum sodium levels less the 125 mEq/L may tip osmotic balance, causing cerebral edema.[4]

PREOPERATIVE MANAGEMENT

The neurological or medical condition of some patients with brain tumors may necessitate preoperative intensive care management. Brain tumor patients may require ICU management before surgery when they present with acute neurological deterioration secondary to status epilepticus, hemorrhage, increased ICP caused by hydrocephalus or cerebral edema, and, less frequently, endocrine insufficiency emergencies. Admission to the ICU allows stabilization of the clinical condition and recognition of potential additional problems while a detailed preoperative evaluation is performed.

In brain tumor patients, status epilepticus may be precipitated by increased surrounding vasogenic edema, tumor progression, low antiepileptic drug levels, electrolyte imbalance, or a recent hemorrhage. Immediate management should include maintenance of a patent airway and adequate blood pressure in addition to seizure control The acute pharmacologic management of status epilepticus in a patient with brain tumor is similar to that of status epilepticus of any other cause. However, after the patient is medically and neurologically stabilized, an imaging study with and without contrast is indicated to rule out an immediate need for surgical intervention.

Some intracranial tumors may present with intratumoral hemorrhage, leading to increased ICP and neurological compromise. Examples of these primary brain tumors are glioblastoma multiforme, oligodendroglioma, mixed glioma, ependymoma, medulloblastoma, germ cell tumor, and pituitary adenoma. In addition, metastatic melanomas have a high hemorrhage rate.[20] Approximately 2% of patients with brain tumors have acute neurological deterioration caused by an intratumoral hemorrhage.[20,49] In these cases, emergent measures to stabilize the patient medically must be undertaken and should include maintenance of respiratory and circulatory status, ICP management by medical or surgical treatment, and seizure control if necessary. If the patient is not on antiepileptic drugs at the time of the hemorrhage, prophylaxis is also indicated.

Neurological deterioration associated with acute hydrocephalus may be seen in patients with tumors involving the posterior fossa, pineal region, optic chiasm, or third ventricle. Although the initial management is administration of glucocorticoid steroids, ventricular drainage is indicated if the patient becomes stuporous. In patients with third ventricle masses that cause bilateral obstruction of the CSF flow, bilateral drainage may be necessary. External ventricular drainage may increase the risk of infection, intratumoral hemorrhage, parenchymal injury, and upward herniation.[48,55] Despite associated risks, emergent ventriculostomy placement is essential in life-threatening situations. In addition to direct treatment of hydrocephalus through CSF drainage, it enables ICP monitoring.

POSTOPERATIVE MANAGEMENT

The intensive care management of patients with brain tumors is aimed at prompt recognition and anticipation of potentially harmful postoperative systemic complications. The causes of postoperative clinical deterioration included increased ICP, intracranial hemorrhage, hydrocephalus, hypotension, hypoxemia, electrolyte disturbances, coagulation abnormalities, gastrointestinal bleeding, seizure, hyperthermia, vasospasm, cerebral infarct, and aspiration. Postoperative ICU management of brain tumor patients requires a systems-oriented approach to the pathophysiology and interventional therapy that includes assessing and monitoring the physical, neurological, cardiovascular, respiratory, renal, hematological, and gastrointestinal systems. A team approach and close communication must be maintained between all consulting services and the nursing staff to clearly define each patient's condition. Patients are usually monitored in the ICU for 24 hours after uneventful tumor surgery, and longer if systemic or neurological problems arise.

Neurological Evaluation

Initial neurological documentation upon emergence of the patient from general anesthesia, as well as frequent postoperative neurological assessment, are of critical importance to detect signs and symptoms of neurological deterioration. Neurological assessment should include the patient's level of consciousness as determined by the Glasgow Coma Scale (GCS), examination of papillary size and reactivity to light, monitoring of brainstem reflexes, and identification of new focal motor neurological signs. In fully conscious patients the examination should also assess the cranial nerves, as well as the motor, sensory, reflex, and cerebellar functions of the extremities. Signs and symptoms of neurological dysfunction related to the area of operative intervention should be documented.

If emergence from anesthesia occurs with new neurological deficits or a decreased level of consciousness, potential causes include residual effect of anesthetic agents, fluid and electrolyte imbalances, intracranial surgical complications, seizures, hypoxia, hypotension, and hypothermia. Transient papillary sluggishness, hyperreflexia, ankle clonus, and upgoing plantar responses may be associated with slow awakening or persistent somnolence. An emergent imaging study is indicated in case of any uncertainty. Under normal circumstances, a postoperative magnetic resonance (MR) scan is generally obtained 24 to 48 hours postoperatively to assess residual tumor and other intracranial complications.

Postoperative Seizures

Patients with a brain tumor who have a history of preoperative seizures are at a higher risk for ictal activity in the postoperative period.[15] Extraaxial lesions, such as meningiomas, carry a greater risk of postoperative seizure activity.[21] In a recent series including 1028 glioma patients treated in the computed tomography (CT) era, the incidence of epilepsy was 49% in patients with glioblastoma, 69% in patients with anaplastic gliomas, and 85% in patients with low-grade gliomas.[28] Postoperative metabolic problems, such as hypoxia, hypernatremia or hyponatremia, and hyperglycemia or acidosis, may increase the risk for seizures. Inadequate phenytoin levels are another major cause of postoperative seizures.[36] Specific tumor histologies, slow-growing lesions in particular, are associated with an increased risk of postoperative seizures.[13] Fifty percent to 81% of oligodendrogliomas are shown to be associated with perioperative seizures.[29] The location of the tumor is also a critical factor because supratentorial tumors are associated with a higher degree of seizure activity, with those tumors located in or adjacent to the motor cortex being especially prone to epileptogenic activity.[13] In a study evaluating the role of anticonvulsant medications in the management of patients with anaplastic gliomas, frontal, temporal, and parietal lesions all had a seizure incidence of 40%, whereas occipital lesions had a seizure incidence of 14%.[31]

Clinical characteristics of the seizure activity are similar both preoperatively and postoperatively.[21,26,37] Postoperative seizures usually occur in the early postoperative period, within the first 24 hours.[21,26] In a study by North and colleagues, which did not include patients with preoperative seizures, 45% of seizures occurred within the first week and 64% within first postoperative month.[36] In this double-blind randomized study evaluating the prophylactic use of phenytoin, a significant reduction in the frequency of postoperative epilepsy was observed in the group receiving the active drug up to the tenth postoperative week. Although phenytoin takes 7 to 10 days to reach steady-state kinetics, in this study the initial dose (15 mg/kg) was administered at the recovery stage.[36]

Seizure may affect the airway or cause secondary injuries resulting from uncontrolled movements during the ictal episode. Seizures also may put the postoperative patient at increased risk of cerebral acidosis, cerebral edema, or increased ICP. It is also known that seizures may cause structural brain injury, thus predisposing the patient to further delayed seizure activity.[13] For patients with supratentorial brain tumors, the standard approach is to start prophylaxis preoperatively and to continue with 5 to 6 mg/kg/day, with serum levels monitored.[13,27] Usually the prophylaxis is given for 3 to 6 months postoperatively, and longer if patient presented with epilepsy or developed postoperative seizures.

Increased Intracranial Pressure

The aim of ICP monitoring in patients with brain tumors is to detect and treat excessive elevation in ICP, which may occur postoperatively as a result of intracranial hematoma, cerebral edema, and hydrocephalus. Although these causes are all potentially remediable, they require prompt identification and early intervention to achieve an optimal outcome. Routine monitoring of ICP is not performed after uneventful brain tumor surgery. Indications for ICP monitoring include a GCS score less than 8, rapid deterioration of the patient's status on neurological examination, pharmacologically paralyzed or heavily sedated patients, patients ventilated with high airway pressures or positive end–expiratory pressure (PEEP), and after a limited resection or biopsy of a brain tumor, which may result in increasing mass effect and cerebral swelling. Devices that can be used to monitor ICP include a fiberoptic intraparenchymal monitor, subarachnoid screw, epidural transducer, subdural catheter, and intraventricular catheter.

Intraventricular catheterization is the most widely used method of recording ICP and considered the most accurate. It can be placed during the craniotomy and left for subsequent monitoring and CSF drainage, or it can be placed while the patient is in the ICU and under local anesthesia. In addition, it allows treatment of increased pressure through CSF drainage. This is the preferred method to use in patients with hydrocephalus. Disadvantages include a relatively higher rate of CNS infection, with increased risk at 5 to 7 days; risk of parenchymal hematoma with catheter placement; and the potential difficulty caused by slit ventricles or shifted intracranial contents.[45,54]

The fiberoptic catheter monitoring system that includes the transducer in the tip is most commonly used intraparenchymally. The system is routinely placed on the same side as the intracranial pathological condition, because a pressure differential may exist between the ipsilateral and contralateral sides.[50] This approach does not require the patient to remain in a constant position relative to an external transducer.

The subdural bolt measures ICP by creating fluid coupling between the CSF and the fluid-filled catheter. It can easily be placed at the time of surgery and left for subsequent monitoring. A fluid-filled catheter with multiple side holes can be used to transduce ICP readings with an accuracy comparable with that of ventriculostomy.[33] This method may have a lower infection risk than ventriculostomy and does not require cortical puncture.[35] The main advantage is simplicity. Disadvantages include less accuracy, the need to recalibrate with movement, and the tendency of the system to dampen out in patients with severely elevated ICP.

Regarding the prevention of neurosurgical infection, a metaanalysis concluded that there was a significant advantage of antimicrobial prophylaxis over placebo. However, there was no significant difference between regimens that did or did not cover gram-negative organisms or between single- and multiple-dose regimens.[17]

TABLE 15-1 ■ Treatment of Increased ICP

1. To decrease cerebral blood volume:
   Head elevation
   Hyperventilation
   Barbiturates, sedatives, and paralytic agents
   Prevention of hyperthermia
2. To decrease CSF and brain bulk:
   Osmotic and loop diuretics
   Glucocorticoid steroids
   Acetazolamide
   CSF drainage
   Surgical resection
3. To increase intracranial volume:
   Surgical decompression of adjacent brain
   Craniectomy and dural expansion

ICP monitoring is essential in patients with elevated ICP, so that appropriate treatment may be tailored to prevent brain herniation and secondary ischemia. Clinical signs of increased ICP may include decreased level of consciousness, Cushing's triad (bradycardia, hypertension, irregular breathing pattern), and papilledema. Treatment should be initiated when the ICP is above 20 mm Hg[22] (Table 15-1).

Cerebral blood volume can be rapidly altered. Hyperventilation of a patient with a Pa_{CO_2} of 25 to 30 mm Hg leads to cerebral arteriolar vasoconstriction and subsequent reduction in CBV and brain volume. Chronic hyperventilation should be avoided.[32] Cerebral lactic acidosis is also associated with poor outcome, and hyperventilation can transiently raise cerebral pH.[9] The patient's head should be elevated approximately 30 degrees above the heart to avoid cerebral venous outflow obstruction and an increased CBV. Cerebral vasoconstricting anesthetic agents that decrease CBF and CBV include thiopental, pentobarbital, and propofol. Mannitol may reduce CBV by reflex compensatory vasoconstriction resulting from the transient increase in CBF.

Analgesic, sedative, and paralytic agents lower ICP by decreasing agitation, somatic stimulation, and preventing breathing against the ventilator. Sedation is usually preferred before neuromuscular blockade because the former can usually be quickly and completely reversed and yet allows for sequential neurological evaluation. Propofol beginning at 10 μg/kg/min is an excellent agent for this purpose because it is a short-acting and powerful sedative.[2,43] If the patient cannot be controlled with sedatives, use of a neuromuscular blocking agent in addition to a sedative is indicated. Elective interventions that are painful or excessively stimulating should be avoided. Use of antipyretics is indicated for hyperthermia, which increases the rate of brain metabolism and level of carbon dioxide.

Mannitol and furosemide are used for rapid reduction of ICP. Mannitol (25%) at a dose of 0.25 to 1 g/kg administered intravenously is effective within 10 to 15 minutes and lasts up to 8 hours. Hyperosmolar agents and diuretics decrease brain swelling by increasing serum osmolarity and causing an osmolar gradient that forces water from the extracellular compartment. Adverse effects include hypotension secondary to hypovolemia, fluid and electrolyte disturbances, hyperosmolarity, and a rebound increase in ICP. Serum osmolarity and electrolytes should be closely monitored, and if the serum osmolarity exceeds 320 mOsm/L, diuretics should be discontinued to prevent potential complications such as hypernatremia, hyperkalemia, low bicarbonate level, metabolic acidosis, altered mental status, fluid overload, congestive heart failure, and acute renal failure. Mannitol also prevents water movement from the vascular to the intracellular space during membrane pump failure. In addition, mannitol decreases blood viscosity, decreases vascular resistance, and acts as an oxygen free radical scavenger.[34] Furosemide causes systemic diuresis and decreased CSF production without producing significant changes in serum osmolarity. Combined treatment with mannitol has a synergistic action and prolongs the effect of lower doses of mannitol but may lead to more electrolyte abnormalities and severe dehydration.

Acetazolamide is a carbonic anhydrase inhibitor that decreases CSF production both acutely and chronically. It can decrease CSF production by 16% to 66% in humans, and the effect of an intravenous dose appears to last for less than 2 hours.[42] A rapid intravenous dose of acetazolamide, however, may have a cerebral vasodilative effect and therefore cause a transient increase in ICP.

ICP can also be decreased by glucocorticoid steroid administration. Glucocorticoid steroids are used for the treatment of vasogenic peritumoral edema by reducing cerebral capillary permeability. Side effects include hyperglycemia, gastrointestinal bleeding, poor wound healing, impaired immune response, adrenocortical insufficiency, insomnia, psychosis, and hallucinations. Generally used at a dose of 8 to 32 mg/day, dexamethasone decreases capillary permeability as early as 1 hour after a single dose and lasts approximately 12 hours.

ICP can also be decreased by CSF drainage, surgical resection of the residual tumor or a selected portion of the brain adjacent to the tumor, or decompressive craniectomy with dural expansion.

Cardiovascular System

In patients without a history of hypertension, blood pressure is maintained in the normal range. In the first 6 to 8 postoperative hours, blood pressure control can be maintained using continuous infusion of nitroprusside.

Increasing blood pressure and decreasing heart rate are two cardiovascular clinical situations that are important to recognize from a neurosurgical perspective. Decreasing heart rate may be secondary to an increasing ICP but can also be precipitated by vagal stimulation, hypoxemia, or acidosis. Increasing blood pressure may indicate increasing postoperative ICP secondary to postoperative hemorrhage or swelling. When treating arterial hypertension, ICP should be monitored as well, because the elevated blood pressure can be critical to maintaining adequate cerebral perfusion pressure.

Patients who suffer nonfocal neurological deterioration while blood pressure is not controlled are more aggressively treated if blood pressure is still elevated when deterioration occurs. If deterioration occurs while blood pressure is lower than desired, it should be allowed to increase to highest acceptable value within the controlled range. If either of these solutions does not result in rapid correction of the problem, further clinical and radiological evaluation is required.

Respiratory System

Respiratory function monitoring involves monitoring adequate oxygenation with an oxygen saturation monitor and monitoring adequate ventilation via blood gases. Continuous end-tidal CO_2 monitoring may help titrate the degree of hyperventilation during intubation. Use of sedative and paralytic agents, as well as an altered level of consciousness, contribute to loss of airway protective reflexes and an increased incidence of atelectasis, aspiration, and pneumonia. Treatment consists of incentive spirometry, pulmonary toilet, use of bronchodilators, encouragement of deep coughing and breathing, and administration of appropriate antibiotics.

Hypercarbia is a contributing factor to postoperative morbidity in patients undergoing intracranial surgery because of the development of cerebral swelling. In a study conducted on patients undergoing craniotomy, 64 patients were monitored in the first 36 postoperative hours using transcutaneous CO_2 monitoring. Statistically significant differences were observed between the severely hypercarbic group (>60 mm Hg) and the rest of the patients with respect to higher incidence of seizures, lower average postoperative GCS score, and higher incidences of reintubation and ventilation. It was suggested that the subgroup of patients who have a higher risk of developing hypercarbia may be detected by routine postoperative transcutaneous CO_2 monitoring.[12]

Pulmonary embolus and deep venous thrombosis are covered later in this chapter.

Fluid and Electrolytes

Routine fluid and electrolyte monitoring is essential in the ICU and should include accurate monitoring of fluid intake and output to maintain a euvolemic state and a steady urine output. Fluid intake is limited in patients with significant brain swelling during surgery. In addition, monitoring of serum electrolytes, such as sodium, potassium, bicarbonate, and chloride, as well as serum osmolarity, blood urea nitrogen, creatinine, and glucose is routinely performed.

The use of 5% dextrose is known to result in cerebral edema in patients with a damaged blood-brain barrier. It has also been shown that hyperglycemia increases the risk of cerebral infarction caused by ischemic injury.[24,39,40] Continued glucose monitoring and treatment with short-acting insulin preparations if necessary are important to prevent secondary ischemic injury. It is generally appreciated that isotonic electrolyte solutions provide the most physiological replacement for adult patients who undergo surgery for a brain tumor.

The most common and clinically important electrolyte abnormality in patients with brain tumors is sodium imbalance, either in the form of hyponatremia or hypernatremia. Hyponatremia, defined as a serum sodium level of less than 135 mEq/L, should be carefully evaluated along with the patient's volume status because serum sodium is a marker for disturbances in free-water balance and an associated decrease in extracellular osmolality may increase cerebral edema. Common clinical symptoms of hyponatremia related to the rate of change in serum sodium level range from anorexia, headache, nausea, vomiting, and muscle weakness to irritability, confusion, seizures, lethargy, coma, and death.

Hyponatremia is commonly caused by increased antidiuretic hormone (ADH) secretion after administration of hypotonic replacement fluids, which results in increased absorption of free water and decreased serum sodium levels. Isovolumic hyponatremia may be secondary to hypothyroidism; polydipsia; iatrogenic water intoxication; drugs (e.g., carbamazepine and thiazide diuretics); hyperosmolar states (e.g., hyperglycemia or mannitol treatment); or syndrome of inappropriate ADH (SIADH) secondary to intracranial hypertension, hypoxia, stress, pain, hypercapnia, medications (e.g., barbiturates, halothane, morphine), CNS tumors, infections, or trauma. SIADH results in an expanded or normal intravascular volume; hypoosmolar hyponatremia; and continuing ADH secretion, causing inappropriately concentrated urine (urine osm > 100 mOsm/L) with a urinary sodium level of more than 25 mEq/L and hypotonic plasma (<280 mOsm/L) in the absence of adrenal, renal, thyroid, and pituitary dysfunction. Restriction of free-water intake using isotonic intravenous fluid is the treatment for mildly to moderately symptomatic SIADH, and serum sodium can be safely corrected over a 48-hour period. In severe hyponatremia (<120 mEq/L), rapid correction can lead to central pontine myelinosis and osmotic demyelination syndrome. The treatment consists of administration of hypertonic saline solutions together with intravenous diuretics to increase free water diuresis relative to sodium retention.

Hypovolemic hyponatremia occurs secondary to iatrogenic replacement of salt and water losses with hyponatremic fluids; diuretic use; mineralocorticoid deficiency; vomiting; diarrhea; or cerebral salt wasting (CSW). CSW is characterized by inappropriate natriuresis (renal sodium wasting, urine sodium concentration <80 mEq/L) and increased urine volume and results in hyponatremia and hypoosmolality with depleted intravascular and extracellular compartments. Restricted fluid intake results in further hypovolemia without correction of hyponatremia because there is continued urinary loss of sodium. Treatment of CSW involves volume-for-volume replacement of urine losses with isotonic saline, use of hypertonic saline for severe cases, oral salt supplementation, and mineralocorticoid administration.

Hypernatremia is defined as a serum sodium level greater than 145 mEq/L, which may be secondary to diabetes insipidus or iatrogenic causes. Therapeutic causes may include the use of diuretics for cerebral swelling and an excess of sodium intake in patients who are under fluid restriction; hypernatremia also occurs in patients who are febrile. Common clinical symptoms are dehydration, polydipsia, confusion, lethargy, tremors, and seizures. Central diabetes insipidus presents with polyuria, polydipsia, hypernatremia, high serum osmolarity, and diluted urine. If not recognized and treated, diabetes insipidus can rapidly cause hemodynamic instability as a result of dehydration. It is important to quickly recognize this condition, especially in uncommunicative patients. The diagnosis is confirmed with a rapid response to the ADH and analog desmopressin acetate (DDAVP) by decreased urinary output at a higher concentration. Treatment involves close monitoring of urinary output and electrolytes, replacement of free water in mild cases, and administration of vasopressin or desmopressin.

Hematological System

Routine monitoring in the ICU of white blood cell, hematocrit, and platelet counts in addition to a full coagulation profile is essential to direct transfusion therapy. Criteria for blood transfusion are based on hematocrit levels, clinical condition, and operative loss.

After brain injury or operative manipulation, disseminated intravascular coagulopathy may occur as a consequence of activation of the intrinsic or extrinsic cascades of the coagulation system. It is not uncommon after a brain tumor operation to note an elevated prothrombin time, which reflects activation of the extrinsic cascade by released thromboplastin. Disseminated intravascular coagulopathy is characterized by elevated prothrombin time, partial thromboplastin time, and fibrin degradation products and decreased plasma fibrinogen levels and platelet counts. Therapeutic management consists of early detection and treatment of the underlying pathophysiological process, in addition to supportive treatment and replacement of clotting factors with fresh frozen plasma, cryoprecipitate, platelet concentrates, and blood if required.

Despite decreasing perioperative morbidity and mortality rates for brain tumor surgery, deep venous thrombosis (DVT) and pulmonary embolism (PE) remain significant causes of morbidity and mortality after brain tumor operations. DVT is reported to occur in 29% to 43% of neurosurgical patients.[18,47] In an earlier series, 3% of all perioperative deaths among patients undergoing elective intracranial surgery were attributable to PE.[52] Mortality from pulmonary embolus ranges from 9% to 50%.[1] Brain tumor patients are particularly prone to thromboembolic complications because of long operation times, glucocorticoid therapy, dehydrating osmotic therapy, and relatively prolonged immobilization, which may be aggravated by neurological deficit. The question of whether the presence of a brain tumor increases the risk of DVT when compared with other malignancies remains largely unanswered. Clinical evaluation alone is unreliable for the detection of DVT because up to 83% of patients with DVT may remain asymptomatic.[47] The detection of DVT includes 125-I fibrinogen scanning, impedance plethysmography, Doppler ultrasonography, and venography. If PE is suspected clinically, the diagnosis and treatment should be aggressively pursued irrespective of evidence of DVT.

In addition to early mobilization, prevention of DVT includes mechanical methods, such as external pneumatic compression, compression stockings, and electrical stimulation of the calf muscles, and pharmacological methods, such as administration of heparin or low-molecular-weight heparin. There are randomized prospective studies that have shown that intermittent external pneumatic compression reduces the risk of DVT in neurosurgical patients.[44,46] Both methods of mechanical prevention, external pneumatic compression and compression stockings, are similarly effective in preventing DVT.[7] Concerns regarding potential intracranial hemorrhage have limited the use of pharmacological measures in neurosurgery patients. It has been shown that perioperative mini-dose heparin (5000 U subcutaneously q12h) decreases the incidence of DVT from 34% to 6% in neurosurgical patients.[8] However, even though the safety of medical prophylactic measures has been demonstrated in some studies, considerable concern remains about exacerbating problems with intraoperative hemostasis and postoperative intracranial hemorrhage.[5,8,30]

The standard therapy for DVT has been full anticoagulation with heparin, followed by oral anticoagulation with warfarin for 6 months. The safety of anticoagulation in patients with brain tumors is not well described. Recent intracranial surgery increases the risk of hemorrhage caused by anticoagulants. In one study, 9 of 21 neurosurgical patients suffered hemorrhagic complications.[11] To reduce the risk of hemorrhage, systemic anticoagulants should not be administered for at least 2 weeks postoperatively. There are, however, contradictory personal opinions favoring full anticoagulation with heparin as early as 48 hours postoperatively if there is no evidence of intracranial bleeding.[53] Because of the high risk of hemorrhagic complications with anticoagulation for the first several weeks after surgery and because of the danger of untreated DVT, an inferior vena cava interruption device is the best means of preventing PE. The safety and efficacy of the Greenfield filter without anticoagulation as primary therapy for DVT has been reported in the literature.[14,16] Patients with a documented PE after surgery for brain tumors receive supportive care, supplemental oxygen, intravenous hydration, vasopressors, and invasive intravascular monitoring if needed, as well as presumptive treatment for DVT. Anticoagulation or inferior vena cava interruption is used to prevent further embolism. Fibrinolytics, which are used to lyse the pulmonary clot in cases of PE, are contraindicated in postoperative neurosurgical patients.

Gastrointestinal System

The incidence of gastritis and peptic ulcer disease (PUD) is increased in ICU patients with brain tumors. An intracranial pathological condition by itself is a risk factor for gastritis, and at autopsy the incidence of hemorrhagic ulceration of the upper gastrointestinal tract is 2 times higher (12.5% versus 6%) in patients who died of intracranial causes than in those who died of other causes.[19] In addition, the risk is increased for patients receiving glucocorticoids. Protection against stress ulcers and gastrointestinal bleeding is essential in the care of patients who receive dexamethasone. Histamine type 2 blockers (e.g., ranitidine or cimetidine) and sucralfate are commonly used. If significant gastrointestinal bleeding occurs, urgent endoscopy and intervention is indicated.

Before initiating oral intake, an evaluation of the patient's swallowing ability is needed if the patient has undergone resection of a posterior fossa or brainstem tumor, which can affect cranial nerves IX, X, XI, and XII. Dietary consultation for the assessment of calorie counts, nitrogen balance, and other nutritional mineral and vitamin needs are essential in long-term ICU management.

REFERENCES

1. Agnelli G, Piovella F, Buoncristiani P, et al: Enoxaparin plus compression stockings compared with compression stockings alone in the prevention of venous thromboembolism after elective neurosurgery, **N Engl J Med 339:**80-85, 1998.
2. Albanes J, Martin C, Lacarelle B, et al: Pharmacokinetics of long-term propofol infusion used for sedation in ICU patients, **Anesthesiology 73:**214-217, 1990.
3. Arieff AL: Hyponatremia associated with permanent brain damage, **Adv Intern Med 32:**325-344, 1987.
4. Avellino AM, Winn HR: Management of acute head injury, in Albin MS (ed): **Textbook of Neuroanesthesia: With Neurosurgical and Neuroscience Perspectives.** New York: McGraw-Hill, 1997, pp 1137-1175.
5. Barnett HG, Clifford JR, Llewellyn RC: Safety of minidose heparin administration for neurosurgical patients, **J Neurosurg 47:**27-30, 1977.
6. Bruce DA: Concepts of intracranial volume and pressure, in James HE, Anas NG, Perkin RM (eds): **Brain Insults in Infants and Children: Pathophysiology and Management.** Orlando: Grune & Stratton, 1985, pp 19-23.
7. Bucci MN, Papadopoulos SM, Chen JC, et al: Mechanical prophylaxis of venous thrombosis in patients undergoing craniotomy: a randomized trial, **Surg Neurol 32:**285-288, 1989.
8. Cerrato D, Ariano C, Fiacchino F: Deep vein thrombosis and low-dose heparin prophylaxis in neurosurgical patients, **J Neurosurg 49:**378-381, 1978.
9. Cold G, Enevoldsen E, Malmros R: Ventricular fluid lactate, pyruvate, bicarbonate and pH in unconscious brain-injured patients subjected to controlled ventilation, **Acta Neurol Scand 52:**187-195, 1975.
10. Cucchiara RF, Black S, Stachniak J, et al: Anesthesia and intensive care management of patients with brain tumors, in Kaye AH, Laws ER (eds): **Brain Tumors: An Encyclopedic Approach.** Edinburgh: Churchill Livingstone, 1995, pp 263-292.
11. DiRicco G, Marini C, Rindi M, et al: Pulmonary embolism in neurosurgical patients: diagnosis and treatment, **J Neurosurg 60:**972-975, 1984.
12. Drummond KJ, Fearnside MR, Chee A: Transcutaneous carbon dioxide measurement after craniotomy in spontaneously breathing patients, **Neurosurgery 41:**365-367, 1997.
13. Duestschman CS, Haines SJ: Anticonvulsant prophylaxis in neurological surgery, **Neurosurgery 17:**510-517, 1985.
14. Fink JA, Jones BT: The Greenfield filter as the primary means of therapy in venous thromboembolic disease, **Surg Gynecol Obstet 172:**253-256, 1991.
15. Fukamachi A, Koizumi H, Nukui H: Immediate postoperative seizures: incidence and computed tomographic findings, **Surg Neurol 24:**671-676, 1985.
16. Greenfield L, McCurdy JR, Brown PP, et al: A new intracaval filter permitting continued flow and resolution of emboli, **Surgery 73:**599-606, 1973.
17. Hosein IK, Hill DW, Hatfield RH: Controversies in the prevention of neurosurgical infection, **J Hosp Infect 43:**5-11, 1999.
18. Joffe SN: Incidence of post operative deep vein thrombosis in neurosurgical patients, **J Neurosurg 42:**201-203, 1975.
19. Karch SB: Upper gastrointestinal bleeding as a complication of intracranial disease, **J Neurosurg 37:**27-29, 1972.
20. Kondziolka D, Bernstein M, Resch L, et al: Significance of hemorrhage into brain tumors: clinicopathological study, **J Neurosurg 67:**852-857, 1987.
21. Kvam DA, Loftus CM, Copeland B, et al: Seizures during the immediate postoperative period, **Neurosurgery 12:**14-17, 1983.
22. Lang EW, Chesnut RM: Intracranial pressure: monitoring and management, **Neurosurg Clin N Am 5:**573-605, 1994.
23. Langfitt TW, Weinstein JD, Kassell NF: Cerebral vasomotor paralysis produced by intracranial hypertension, **Neurology 15:**622-641, 1965.
24. Lanier WL, Stangland KJ, Scheithauer BW, et al: The effects of dextrose infusion and head position on neurologic outcome after complete cerebral ischemia in primates: examination of a model, **Anesthesiology 66:**39-48, 1987.
25. Lassen NA: Control of cerebral circulation in health and disease, **Circ Res 34:**749-760, 1974.
26. Lee ST, Lui TN, Chang CN, et al: Early postoperative seizures after posterior fossa surgery, **J Neurosurg 73:**541-544, 1990.
27. Lee ST, Lui TN, Chang CN, et al: Prophylactic anticonvulsants for prevention of immediate and early postcraniotomy seizures, **Surg Neurol 31:**361-364, 1989.
28. Lote K, Stenwig AE, Skullerud K, et al: Prevalence and prognostic significance of epilepsy in patients with gliomas, **Eur J Cancer 34:**98-102, 1998.
29. Lund M: Epilepsy in association with intracranial tumors, **Acta Psychiatr Neurol Scand 8:**1-149, 1952.
30. Macdonald RL, Amidei C, Lin G, et al: Safety of perioperative subcutaneous heparin for prophylaxis of venous thromboembolism in patients undergoing craniotomy, **Neurosurgery 45:**245-252, 1999.
31. Mahaley MS, Dudka L: The role of anticonvulsant medications in the management of patients with anaplastic gliomas, **Surg Neurol 16:**399-401, 1981.
32. Marsh ML, Marshall LF, Shapiro HM: Neurosurgical intensive care, **Anesthesiology 47:**149-163, 1977.
33. Mollman HD, Rockswold GL, Ford SE: A clinical comparison of subarachnoid catheters to ventriculostomy and subarachnoid bolts: a prospective study, **J Neurosurg 68:**737-741, 1988.
34. Muizelaar JP, Wei EP, Kontos HA, et al: Mannitol causes compensatory cerebral vasoconstriction and vasodilation in response to blood viscosity changes, **J Neurosurg 59:**822-828, 1983.
35. North B, Reilly P: Comparison among three methods of intracranial pressure recording, **Neurosurgery 18:**730-782, 1986.

36. North JB, Penhall RK, Hanieh A, et al: Phenytoin and postoperative epilepsy. A double-blind study, **J Neurosurg 58:**672-677, 1983.
37. Ramamurthi B, Rami B, Ramanchandran V: Convulsions with meningiomas: incidence and significance, **Surg Neurol 14:**415-416, 1980.
38. Rehncrona S, Rosen I, Siesjo BK: Brain lactic acidosis and ischemic cell damage. 1. Biochemistry and neurophysiology, **J Cereb Blood Flow Metab 1:**297-311, 1981.
39. Rehncrona S, Rosen I, Siesjo BK: Excessive cellular acidosis: an important mediator of neuronal damage in the brain, **Acta Physiol Scand 110:**435-437, 1980.
40. Rosenburg H, Clofine R, Bialik O: Neurologic changes during awakening from anesthesia, **Anesthesiology 54:**125-130, 1981.
41. Rosomoff HL: Methods for simultaneous quantitative estimation of intracranial contents, **J Appl Physiol 16:**395-396, 1953.
42. Rubin RC, Henderson ES, Ommaya AK, et al: The production of cerebrospinal fluid in man and its modification by acetazolamide, **J Neurosurg 25:**430-436, 1966.
43. Sebel PS, Lowdon JD: Propofol: a new intravenous anesthetic, **Anesthesiology 71:**260-277, 1989.
44. Skillman JJ, Collins RE, Coe NP, et al: Prevention of deep vein thrombosis in neurosurgical patients: a controlled, randomized trial of external pneumatic compression boots, **Surgery 83:**354-358, 1978.
45. Smith RW, Alksne JF: Infections complicating the use of external ventriculostomy, **J Neurosurgery 44:**567-570, 1976.
46. Turpie AGG, Gallus AS, Beattie WS, et al: Prevention of venous thrombosis in patients with intracranial disease by intermittent pneumatic compression of the calf, **Neurology 27:**435-438, 1977.
47. Valladares JB, Hankinson J: Incidence of lower extremity deep vein thrombosis in neurosurgical patients, **Neurosurgery 6:**138-141, 1980.
48. Vaquero J, Cabezudo JM, de Sola RG, et al: Intratumoral hemorrhage in posterior fossa tumors after ventricular drainage. Report of two cases, **J Neurosurg 54:**406-408, 1981.
49. Wakai S, Yamakawa K, Manaka S, et al: Spontaneous intracranial hemorrhage caused by brain tumor: its incidence and clinical significance, **Neurosurgery 10:**437-444, 1982.
50. Weaver DD, Winn HR, Jane JA: Differential intracranial pressure in patients with unilaterial mass lesions, **J Neurosurg 56:**660-665, 1982.
51. Weiss MH, Wertman N: Modulation of CSF production by alterations in cerebral perfusion pressure, **Arch Neurol 35:**527-529, 1978.
52. Wetzel N, Anderson MC, Shield TW: Pulmonary embolism as a cause of death in the neurosurgical patient, **J Neurosurg 17:**664-668, 1960.
53. Wilson CB: General considerations, in **Brain Surgery: Complication Avoidance and Management.** New York: Churchill Livingstone, 1993, pp 177-185.
54. Wyler AR, Kelly WA: Use of antibiotics with external ventriculostomies, **J Neurosurg 37:**185-187, 1972.
55. Zuccarello M, Dollo C, Carollo C: Spontaneous intratumoral hemorrhage after ventriculoperitoneal shunting, **Neurosurgery 16:**246-246, 1985.

CHAPTER 16

The Pediatric Neurosurgical Patient

DANIEL FALCO
GREGORY B. HAMMER

INTRODUCTION

Since the development of specialized pediatric intensive care units in the 1970s, the field of pediatric intensive care has matured into a distinct specialty. It is now standard care for hospitals in which significant numbers of critically ill children are managed to have a multidisciplinary pediatric intensive care unit. Such a unit offers care provided by a variety of pediatric surgeons and other pediatric subspecialists in conjunction with pediatric critical care physicians. In addition, care is provided by specially trained pediatric nurses, respiratory therapists, pharmacists, and social workers in a highly coordinated effort. However, critically ill infants and children may also be cared for in adult intensive care units as a result of trauma center designation or limited access to a pediatric facility.

Management of the pediatric neurosurgical patient demands a broad-based knowledge of general neurological intensive care as well as an understanding of pediatric anatomy and physiology. Principles of adult neurological intensive care are covered extensively in other chapters of this text. The focus of this chapter, therefore, is to review pediatric anatomy and physiology pertinent to neurological intensive care, followed by discussion of important differences between adult and pediatric pathophysiology and management.

RESPIRATORY SYSTEM

The purpose of the respiratory system is to exchange oxygen and carbon dioxide across the alveolar-capillary membrane. Respiratory failure is associated with hypoxemia and/or hypercarbia. The causes of respiratory failure in pediatric neurosurgical patients are shown in Table 16-1.

From the naris to the terminal bronchiole, the caliber of the airways in infants and children is small. Because the resistance to gas flow through airways is inversely proportional to the fourth power of their

TABLE 16-1 ■ **Causes of Respiratory Failure in Pediatric Neurosurgical Patients**

Impaired Control of Ventilation
Head trauma
Intracranial hemorrhage
Intracranial hypertension
Meningitis
Status epilepticus
Drug effect
Neuromuscular Disorders
Spinal cord injury
Phrenic nerve injury
Chest Trauma
Pneumothorax
Hemothorax
Multiple rib fractures ("flail chest")
Airway Obstruction
Trauma (edema, hemorrhage)
Nasopharynx, tongue, glottis
Inhalation injury
Postintubation tracheal edema
Foreign body aspiration
Alveolar Disease
Pulmonary edema
"Neurogenic," ARDS
Pulmonary aspiration
Pulmonary contusion, hemorrhage

radius,[1] there is an inherently elevated resistance to gas flow in the airways of infants and children. Any lesion that causes further airway narrowing may raise gas flow resistance to a critical level. This may limit gas flow such that adequate alveolar gas exchange cannot occur, thereby causing respiratory failure. Patients with normal central nervous system (CNS) function will increase their effort of breathing in response to airway obstruction in an attempt to overcome elevated resistance to gas flow. Patients with CNS impairment may have limited ability to increase their respiratory effort and are therefore at increased risk of respiratory failure. The resulting hypoxia and hypercarbia may exacerbate existing CNS damage.

Infants are predisposed to respiratory failure because of their increased metabolic requirements as compared with adults. Infants normally consume approximately 6 to 8 ml of O_2/kg/min and produce about an equal amount of CO_2, compared with a normal adult minute O_2 consumption and CO_2 production of 2 to 3 ml/kg/min.[11] Conditions that cause reduced alveolar gas exchange in infants therefore produce a more precipitous drop in arterial oxygen saturation and elevation of arterial CO_2 tension. Infants are therefore at increased risk of the "secondary injury" of hypoxia and/or hypercarbia during recovery from a primary CNS injury. The appearance of tachypnea, nasal flaring, exhalatory grunting, and intercostal retractions signal the need for immediate intervention in the infant or child with CNS injury. Alternatively, signs of respiratory depression, including somnolence with decreased respiratory rate for age, merit urgent treatment. Respiratory failure may be accompanied by tachycardia or bradycardia, hypertension or hypotension, depending on the underlying condition and age of the patient. In the hypoxic neonate and infant, limited sympathetic neural tone often results in bradycardia.

Monitoring of the neurologically impaired patient with respiratory compromise should include continuous electrocardiography (EKG), respiratory rate, pulse oximetry, and frequent blood pressure measurements by automated cuff or continuous intraarterial monitoring. Arterial CO_2 tension may be estimated with transcutaneous CO_2 monitoring or nasal capnometry.[7,19] Supplemental oxygen should be continuously administered to achieve oxygen saturation of 98% to 100%. Indications for tracheal intubation and mechanical ventilation include the inability to maintain oxygen saturation in this range (or PaO_2 >80-100 mm Hg) despite an FiO_2 of more than 0.60 or respiratory acidemia. Mechanical ventilation should also be instituted regardless of oxygenation or ventilation status, with signs of impending or existing unconsciousness, absent protective airway reflexes, intracranial hypertension, or severe neuromuscular weakness.

TRACHEAL INTUBATION

The purposes of tracheal intubation in infants and children include maintenance of alveolar gas exchange and oxygenation, prevention of pulmonary aspiration of gastric contents, and control of intracranial pressure (ICP).

Before tracheal intubation, bag-and-mask ventilation should be performed with 100% oxygen. A continuous oxygen source and bag-and-mask system with the appropriate size face mask for positive pressure ventilation should be maintained for this purpose at each patient's bedside. Circuits employing self-inflating bags or "anesthesia bags" may be used safely and effectively during controlled ventilation as long as the operator is familiar with the system in use. Self-inflating bags do not allow adequate gas exchange during spontaneous ventilation in infants and children. A range of oropharyngeal and nasopharyngeal airways should be readily available to maintain extrathoracic airway patency during bag-and-mask ventilation. As with adult patients, nasopharyngeal airways should not be used in the presence of basilar skull fracture with possible discontinuity of the nasopharyngeal mucosa, nor in patients with bleeding diatheses.

All patients with CNS injury and respiratory failure should be considered as having a "full stomach," because these conditions are associated with increased gastric acidity and volume. Bag-and-mask ventilation may result in gaseous distension of the stomach, increasing this risk. The appropriate application of cricoid pressure during bag-and-mask ventilation and laryngoscopy reduces the likelihood of this potentially catastrophic event by occluding the esophagus. Cricoid pressure should be initiated after neuromuscular blockade is obtained and maintained until correct placement of the tracheal tube has been confirmed by auscultation.

Equipment for performing tracheal intubation in infants and children includes appropriately-sized laryngoscope blades and tracheal tubes. Anatomic features of the infant's airway may render tracheal intubation more difficult than in the adult patient. These features include large head size relative to neck, shoulders, and thorax; small mandibular size; relatively large tongue; and a glottis that is displaced cephalad and anteriorly (Figure 16-1). In neonates and infants, a straight laryngoscope blade (e.g., Miller, Wis-Hipple) may be most efficacious. Such a blade is designed to directly elevate the epiglottis, which is relatively large, soft, and floppy in the first 12 months of life. After this age, a curved

[1]Poiseuille's law: $R = 8nl/\Pi r^4$, in which R = resistance, *n* = viscosity, *l* = length of airway, and r = radius.

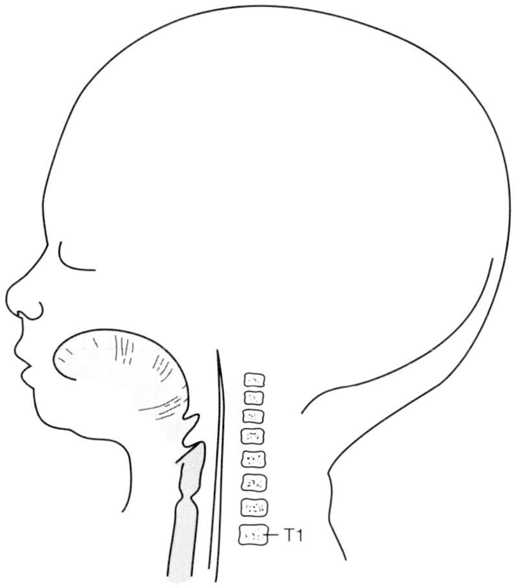

FIGURE 16-1 ■ Infant airway. Note the large tongue and the larynx, which is anterior and cephalad. The airway is most narrow at the level of the cricoid cartilage, not the vocal cords as in the adult.

blade (e.g., Macintosh), designed to indirectly elevate the epiglottis by displacing the valecula anteriorly, is preferred by some operators. Suggested laryngoscope blades and tracheal tubes are listed in Table 16-2.

Because the subglottic trachea is the narrowest portion of the extrathoracic airway in children younger than 7 or 8 years of age, uncuffed tracheal tubes are generally employed in this age group. If the indwelling tracheal tube is too small, leakage of inspired gas around the tube may preclude maintenance of adequate lung volumes and alveolar ventilation. If the tracheal tube is too large, pressure exerted against the tracheal mucosa may cause ischemic injury leading to subglottic scarring and stenosis. Therefore, after confirmation of correct positioning of the tracheal tube, appropriate size must also be confirmed. During slow positive pressure inspiration, the anterior neck overlying the trachea is auscultated. The inflating pressure at which a gas leak around the tracheal tube is first auscultated is noted. If the initial leak is auscultated at a pressure of up to 10 cm H_2O, the indwelling tube should be replaced with the next larger size (e.g., a no. 4 tube is replaced with a no. 4.5 tube). If no leak is auscultated at an inflating pressure of 35 cm H_2O, a smaller tube should be inserted if the patient's clinical status permits.

PHARMACOLOGICAL THERAPY

Pharmacological therapy is often essential to provide the best possible conditions for tracheal intubation while preventing or minimizing elevation of ICP during laryngoscopy and tracheal intubation. Hypnotic agents, opioids, muscle relaxants, and local anesthetics may be used in combination for this purpose.

Barbiturates and propofol produce sedation/hypnosis, a decrease in cerebral oxygen consumption, and a diminution in cerebral blood flow. These agents may also cause an increase in venous capacitance, myocardial depression, and a decrease in systemic arteriolar tone, resulting in inadequate cerebral perfusion. These effects may be especially pronounced in patients with diminished intravascular volume and/or myocardial dysfunction. Thiopental is the barbiturate most commonly used before tracheal intubation, in a dose of 4 to 7 mg/kg intravenously (IV). The induction dose of propofol in children is 2 to 3 mg/kg IV. These doses

TABLE 16-2 ■ Tracheal Tube and Laryngoscope Blade Sizes By Age

Age	Tube Size (mmID)	Laryngoscope Blade
Preterm newborn		
weight <1500 g	2.5	Miller 0
weight >1500 g	2.5-3.0	Miller 0
Term newborn-2 months	3.0-3.5	Miller 0 or 1
3-8 months	3.5	Miller 1
9-15 months	4.0	Miller 1, Wis-Hipple 1.5
16-24 months	4.5	Wis-Hipple 1.5, Macintosh 2
2-3 years	4.5-5.0	Wis-Hipple 1.5, Macintosh 2
4-5 years	5.0-5.5	Miller 2* or Macintosh 3
6-7 years	5.5-6.0	Miller 21 or Macintosh 3
8-11 years	6.0 cuffed	Miller 21 or Macintosh 3
12-15 years	6.5-7.0 cuffed	Miller 21 or Macintosh 3
>15 years (male)	8.0 cuffed	Miller 21 or Macintosh 3
>15 years (female)	7.0 cuffed	Miller 21 or Macintosh 3

For children over the age of 2 years, ETT size (mmID) = age (yr) ÷4 +4.
*May substitute Wisconsin or other straight blade.

should be reduced in patients with diminished intravascular volumes and/or myocardial dysfunction, and these agents should be not be given to patients with very low cardiac output. The circulatory and neurological effects of a single dose of thiopental generally dissipate after 10 to 15 minutes, whereas the offset of propofol is 20% to 30% more rapid.

Etomidate is a nonbarbiturate hypnotic agent that has a minimal effect on circulatory function. Like thiopental and propofol, etomidate lowers cerebral oxygen consumption, cerebral blood flow, and ICP. Because of its limited effects on systemic blood pressure, it maintains cerebral perfusion pressure to a greater extent than thiopental or propofol. Potential adverse effects of etomidate include myoclonic movements and adrenocortical suppression, which may last for 4 to 8 hours after a single dose. The intravenous induction dose of etomidate is 0.3 to 0.4 mg/kg.

Ketamine is a phencyclidine derivative that produces hypnosis as well as analgesia. In this regard, ketamine is unlike thiopental, propofol, and etomidate, which do not produce analgesia. Ketamine causes central sympathetic stimulation and thereby may cause an elevation in heart rate and blood pressure. Like etomidate, ketamine may be useful in patients with hemodynamic compromise. Ketamine may cause an increase in cerebral metabolism and blood flow as well as ICP in patients with normocapnia. Concomitant hyperventilation probably attenuates the increase in cerebral blood flow and ICP. Nevertheless, ketamine should generally be avoided in patients with ICP elevation. The intravenous induction dose of ketamine in children is 1 to 2 mg/kg, or 3 to 5 mg/kg intramuscularly (IM).

Opioids cause a diminution in sympathetic neural response (e.g., tachycardia and hypertension) to laryngoscopy, tracheal intubation, and pharyngeal or tracheal suctioning. Fentanyl, as compared with morphine or meperidine, has a more rapid onset and does not provoke histamine release.[16] All opioids, however, may cause decreased cardiac output and hypotension in patients with diminished intravascular volume and/or severe myocardial dysfunction and should be used in reduced doses or avoided in this setting. The administration of fentanyl in a dose of 8 to 10 μg/kg in combination with thiopental usually prevents sympathetic neural response to laryngoscopy and tracheal intubation.[24] Chest wall rigidity may result from this dose of fentanyl and is prevented by the antecedent administration of muscle relaxants.

Sympathetic neural stimulation produced by laryngoscopy and tracheal intubation may be also be modulated by the use of local anesthetics. Lidocaine may be delivered via aerosol as a 4% solution to topically anesthetize the tongue, pharynx, vocal cords, and trachea. Intravenous lidocaine in a dose of 1 to 1.5 mg/kg administered 60 to 90 seconds before laryngoscopy also diminishes untoward sympathetic response.[41] This dose may produce myocardial depression in the presence of preexisting myocardial dysfunction.

Muscle relaxants increase mandibular mobility and cause vocal cord paralysis, thereby facilitating tracheal intubation. These drugs also allow efficient mechanical ventilation and control of ICP by reducing muscular tone of the chest wall and diaphragm. Muscle relaxants commonly used in pediatric patients include succinylcholine, vecuronium, rocuronium, and pancuronium. Rapacuronium is a new, nondepolarizing muscle relaxant with a rapid onset and relatively short duration.

Of the muscle relaxants currently in use, succinylcholine has the most rapid onset, producing profound neuromuscular blockade within 60 seconds after a dose of 1 to 1.5 mg/kg IV. Its offset is also usually rapid because of metabolism by pseudocholinesterase, with return of neuromuscular function within 5 to 7 minutes. Succinylcholine may produce hyperkalemia and release of myoglobin in patients after burn or crush injuries, denervation (upper motor neuron) injuries, or renal failure. Rarely, succinylcholine may trigger malignant hyperthermia. In patients with pseudocholinesterase deficiency, muscle relaxation may persist for several hours. Succinylcholine may cause bradycardia, especially with repeated dosing and in infants. Because of these adverse effects, succinylcholine should be used only when rapid onset and offset of neuromuscular blockade are imperative. Rapacuronium, administered in an intravenous dose of 1.5 to 2.5 mg/kg, has an onset nearly as rapid as succinylcholine and a duration of 20 to 25 minutes.[28] The duration can be significantly decreased by the administration of reversal agents such as neostigmine.

Vecuronium and rocuronium are "intermediate-acting" nondepolarizing muscle relaxants. Although the usual intravenous intubating dose of vecuronium is 0.1 mg/kg, onset is hastened by the administration of doses 2 to 4 times this amount. The onset of profound muscle relaxation after the administration of 0.3 to 0.4 mg/kg of vecuronium is approximately 90 seconds, and in most cases tracheal intubation can be facilitated after approximately 60 seconds.[45] The duration of paralysis after a dose of 0.1 mg/kg IV is approximately 40 to 45 minutes and increases to approximately 115 minutes after 0.4 mg/kg IV is administered.[45] The usual intubating dose of rocuronium is 1.0 mg/kg; after approximately 60 seconds, tracheal intubation may be performed. Offset occurs within 45 minutes after this dose of rocuronium.

Pancuronium is a longer-acting muscle relaxant commonly used in the management of neurosurgical patients both in the operating room and the intensive care unit. Because of its vagolytic effect, pancuronium commonly causes tachycardia. Pancuronium is most often used in the patient who is expected to require long-term muscle relaxant therapy.

MECHANICAL VENTILATION

The goal of mechanical ventilation in the neurosurgical pediatric patient is to ensure optimal exchange of oxygen and carbon dioxide while causing minimal adverse effects on cerebral perfusion. Several important developmental aspects of respiratory mechanics impact the practice of mechanical ventilation of the pediatric patient. The normal respiratory rate of the newborn is 20 to 60 breaths per minute, as opposed to 12 to 16 in the adult. Inspiratory time in the infant is normally 0.4 to 0.5 seconds, compared with about 1.25 seconds in the adult.[30] Tidal volume remains relatively constant throughout childhood at approximately 6 to 8 ml/kg.[1,13] The static and dynamic differences in the developing respiratory system dictate the technical requirements of respiratory support in infants and children.[29]

In the neonate and infant, ventilators that are pressure limited and/or time limited are most commonly employed. These ventilators offer the advantages of avoiding excessive inflating pressures and, presumably, decreased risk of barotrauma. However, a decrease in the compliance (or conductance) of the patient's respiratory system (or ventilator circuit) will cause a reduction in delivered tidal volume. Conversely, an increase in compliance will result in an increased tidal volume. Volume-limited ventilators, on the other hand, deliver a relatively constant volume of gas despite changes in the patient's chest compliance. The presence of high inflating pressures signal decreased compliance or conductance of the breathing circuit (e.g., occluded tracheal tube) or the patient (e.g., offset of neuromuscular blockade, bronchospasm). Disadvantages of these ventilators include the potential generation of very high inflating pressures and the possibly increased risk of barotrauma. With proper monitoring of inspiratory pressure, however, changes in the patient's pulmonary mechanics can be observed and the risk of excessive barotrauma minimized. Because of technical difficulties in accurately delivering very small tidal volumes (e.g., less than 100 ml), pressure-limited ventilators have been primarily used in patients weighing less than 10 kg. Recently, volume-limited ventilators have been used in these patients because of improvements in delivery and measurement of very small tidal volumes.

Gas leaks around uncuffed tracheal tubes represent an important source of "volume loss" during mechanical ventilation. The magnitude of such gas leaks may vary with the patient's head position. As a result, there may be a variable discrepancy between inspiratory and expiratory tidal volumes related to head position. It is important, then, to monitor both inspired and exhaled tidal volumes closely in pediatric patients with indwelling uncuffed tracheal tubes to facilitate appropriate alveolar ventilation.

Positive end–expiratory pressure (PEEP) is used to maintain alveolar patency during mechanical ventilation. Caution must be used to avoid excessive levels of PEEP, which may impede cerebral venous return.

Vigilance is essential to prevent secondary CNS injury caused by complications associated with mechanical ventilation, including hypoxemia, hypercarbia, excessive PEEP, and barotrauma. Ventilator alarms, pulse oximetry, and capnography or transcutaneous CO_2 monitoring should be used at all times.

THE CIRCULATORY SYSTEM

There are differences in heart rate, systemic blood pressure, and cardiac output between infants, children, and adults. The normal heart rate in infants is 120 to 160 beats per minute (bpm). The systemic arterial blood pressure is lower in the infant and increases to adult values by adolescence. In the infant, stroke volume is relatively limited so that increased cardiac output is largely mediated by increased heart rate.

Infants and children have a larger intravascular volume per kilogram of body weight than adults. A premature infant has an intravascular volume of nearly 100 ml/kg. This decreases to 90 ml/kg in the term newborn, 80 ml/kg in the 3 to 24 month old, and 70 ml/kg in the older child. Infants and smaller children, however, have a smaller absolute volume than older children and adults. A 60-ml hemorrhage represents approximately 10% of the total blood volume of an 8-kg infant. Therefore, an infant can have scalp and/or intracranial hemorrhages that cause anemia, decreased cardiac output, and even hypotension.

After birth, oxygen consumption in the term neonate rises from approximately 4.5 ml to 8 ml O_2/kg body weight/min at the age of 1 month. Oxygen consumption increases further with exposure to a cold environment and as body temperature deviates either above or below normal. The infant has a diminished ability to maintain neutral body temperature in the presence of variations in environmental temperature. This may precipitate systemic lactic acidemia as O_2 consumption exceeds the ability of cardiac output to meet such demands. It is therefore of critical importance that infants be maintained in a thermoneutral environment at all times, with appropriate use of warming devices such as radiant heating beds and heat lamps.

Acute hypoxia, like hypothermia or hyperthermia, is a potent stimulus for an increase in cardiac output. This increase in cardiac output is mediated in part by increased sympathetic efferent stimulation.[14] The developing heart is better able to tolerate acute hypoxia than the adult heart. This is, at least in part, related to the increased capacity of the immature myocardium to maintain anaerobic metabolism as a result of improved glycolytic activity.[12] Unfortunately the infant brain does not appear to be similarly protected against hypoxic injury.

Autonomic control of circulation is less well developed in the infant than in the adult. The infant appears to have a relative predominance of parasympathetic neural tone, with a diminution of generalized sympathetic innervation. The infant may, for example, exhibit an exaggerated vagotonic response to hypoxemia, laryngoscopy, or gastroesophageal reflux, leading to bradycardia. Conversely, the infant may demonstrate increased sensitivity to exogenous catecholamines. For example, norepinephrine dose-response curves in fetal, newborn, and adult lambs show that fetal heart muscle is three times more sensitive to norepinephrine than the adult myocardium.[17] Physicians should be aware that pharmacological manipulation of the circulation in critically ill pediatric patients may differ from adult patients.

As with adult patients, recognition of impending or existing circulatory failure in children is largely dependent on physical examination.[37] Dyspnea, tachycardia, cardiomegaly, and hepatomegaly are the hallmarks of congestive heart failure. Because of the infant's relatively soft, incompletely calcified thoracic cage, dyspnea is often accompanied by suprasternal, intercostal, and subcostal retractions. Tachycardia may be seen relatively early in the course of cardiac failure in the infant because cardiac output is more dependent on heart rate than increased stroke volume. Hepatomegaly may also appear early because of the increased distensibility of the liver. Distension of neck veins, however, is relatively difficult to appreciate in infants and young children. Chest radiography may be useful in differentiating cardiac from pulmonary disease and to aid in assessment of cardiomegaly. Interpretation of other diagnostic studies in pediatric patients also demands familiarity with age- and size-related differences between these and adult patients. Accurate noninvasive measurement of blood pressure requires appropriate selection of cuff size. A cuff that is too small may overestimate the blood pressure, whereas a cuff that is too large may underestimate the blood pressure. During the first months to years of life, significant electrocardiographic changes occur with which the interpreter must be familiar.

Primary hypertension is uncommon in infancy and early childhood. In infants with secondary hypertension as a manifestation of brain injury, the primary cause of blood pressure elevation (such as elevated ICP) should be aggressively treated before antihypertensive agents are invoked. Beta-blockers should be used with extreme caution in infants. These agents may precipitously cause a fall in cardiac output given the infant heart's relative dependency on heart rate to increase cardiac output. Calcium channel blockers should not be used in infants. The infant myocardium is dependent on extracellular calcium because of an immature endoplasmic reticulum.

NERVOUS SYSTEM

Pediatric Neurological Examination

The neurological exam is different for the newborn, infant, toddler, and older child. Detailed descriptions of the normal child's neurological examination have been published.[42,43] A list of normal developmental milestones is found in Table 16-3.

The child's general appearance, level of alertness, and spontaneous motor activity may be revealing, as well as response to sound, touch, and light stimuli. An examination of the child's muscle tone is best performed when the child is relaxed, with special attention to symmetry. Infants normally exhibit dominance of flexor muscles, even during sleep. Hypotonia or flaccidity is abnormal at all ages. In the infant, flaccidity or lack of movement of one or more limbs is often the result of a lesion involving the spinal cord or peripheral nerve rather than the cerebrum.

Peripheral nerves are not myelinated at birth. Evaluation of both gross and fine motor activity is dependent on the child's age. The motor developmental milestones provide a reference against which to evaluate an individual infant or child. Hand preference is rare before 18 months and may suggest an abnormality when present. A formal sensory exam requires cooperation and is difficult to perform in the child less than 5 years of age.

Cranial nerves are myelinated at birth and can be examined at all ages; however, certain cranial nerve findings that are abnormal in adults may be normal in children. Young infants may have an asymmetric

TABLE 16-3 ■ Motor Developmental Milestones[42]

Age	Motor Activity
1 week	Extends head in prone position
3-4 months	Has head control
5-6 months	Rolls over prone to supine
6-7 months	Rolls over supine to prone
7-8 months	Sits alone; transfers objects hand-to-hand
9-11 months	Stands with support (holding on)
11-12 months	Walks with assistance
13-15 months	Walks unassisted
18 months	Climbs stairs with assistance
24 months	Runs

blink. Disconjugate gaze occurs occasionally in infancy but should resolve by 4 to 6 months of age. Strabismus is common in 3- to 6-year-old children. Infants may have irregular movements of the tongue both on protrusion and at rest.

Infants have normal reflexes that disappear with age. The newborn's Moro reflex (extremity extension, then flexion, followed by crying in response to a stimulus) disappears at approximately 6 months. Bilateral extensor plantar reflex can be normal up to 1 year of age. The normal infant's deep tendon reflexes may be absent but more commonly are brisk, and ankle clonus can often be elicited.

The assessment of increased ICP is similar in the child and adult, although an infant's head circumference can rapidly enlarge in the setting of increased ICP and should be regularly measured. In the infant the anterior fontanel is usually flat when sitting and may pulsate and expand in size during crying. A tense fontanel suggests raised ICP. Vomiting as a sign of increased ICP is seen more commonly in children than in adults. Papilledema is not an acute sign of increased ICP in children and indicates a longer period of elevated ICP than in adults.

The normal infant's optic disc margins are often indistinct and slightly elevated. A unilateral retinal hemorrhage may have no significance, but bilateral retinal hemorrhages suggest a dramatic and rapid increase in ICP and are often associated with a subdural hemorrhage.[34] Combined subdural and retinal hemorrhages are associated with nonaccidental trauma that occurs with a shaking injury.

The pediatric neurosurgical patient may have an abnormal level of consciousness for a variety of reasons, including increased ICP, metabolic abnormalities, and/or the effects of drugs and toxins. The physicians and nurses must, in a consistent and objective manner, document this exam at hourly intervals. Rather than relying on subjective descriptions such as "lethargic" or "stuporous," the adult Glasgow Coma Scale (GCS) is often used. However, it is difficult to use the GCS on preverbal children who at best would only score 2 on the verbal score (for nonspecific sounds) and 5 on the motor score (for localized pain), for a maximum total of 11 out of 15.

There is no consensus on how to score the younger pediatric patient. Some authors prefer to adapt the GCS by making a modified coma scale for infants, for example, a verbal score of 5 if the infant coos or babbles (Table 16-4). The maximum score is similar to the GCS. Another alternative is to use the children's coma scale (Table 16-5). This scale is designed for infants and young children, has a range of scores from 3 to 11, and may be useful in evaluating subcortical and brainstem function. The proponents of this scoring system feel that it offers prognostic outcome value for the head-injured patient under 36 months of age. Neither of these two modified coma scales has been proven to be a predictor of outcome for closed head injuries in infants or children.

TABLE 16-4 ■ Modified Coma Scale for Infants[42,43]

Response	Score
Eye opening	
Spontaneous	4
To speech	3
To pain	2
None	1
Verbal	
Coos, babbles	5
Irritable cry	4
Cries to pain only	3
Moans to pain	2
None	1
Motor	
Normal spontaneous movements	6
Withdraws to touch	5
Withdraws to pain	4
Abnormal flexion	3
Abnormal extension	2
None	1

TABLE 16-5 ■ Children's Coma Scale[34]

Response	Score
Ocular	
Pursuit	4
Extraocular muscles (EOM) intact, reactive pupils	3
EOM impaired	2
EOM paralyzed, fixed pupils	1
Verbal	
Cries	3
Spontaneous respirations	2
Apneic	1
Motor	
Flexes and extends	4
Withdraws from painful stimuli	3
Hypertonic	2
Flaccid	1

The Skull

The infant skull, with its open fontanel, soft calvaria, and open, moveable sutures, is considerably different from the adult's skull. One advantage to the open fontanel is that it allows a visual and tactile assessment of the infant's ICP. Further, the infant's skull can expand somewhat and partially compensate for the slowly developing increases in ICP that can accompany hydrocephalus, hematomas, or other intracranial mass lesions. However, the open fontanel does not fully protect the child against elevated ICP. The presence of split sutures and a bulging fontanel denotes elevated ICP and suggests that compensatory mechanisms have been exhausted.[4] The anterior fontanel normally closes at about 1 year of age, with a range of 7 to 19 months in 90% of children.[21]

Because an infant's skull is elastic, it can absorb some of the energy associated with trauma instead of transmitting the energy to the brain. However, rather than protecting the brain, the soft skull may also allow more brain compression and distortion than in the adult. The compliant skull, relatively large infant head compared to body, and poorly developed neck musculature allow more to-and-fro motion of the brain with a shaking injury; this may result in tearing of the bridging veins and may produce a subdural hematoma. Additionally, the floor of the anterior and middle fossa is smooth, with few convolutional markings compared with the adult, which provides for less resistance to brain movement.[34]

The infant's skull may be fractured in a different manner than the adult's skull. A depressed skull fracture may occur without an associated scalp laceration.[20] Skull fractures in infants tend to have a larger separation than in the adult or occur with diastasis of the sutures.[27] Occasionally an infant with an unrecognized skull fracture and underlying laceration of the dura may develop a delayed growing skull fracture as a result of the entrapment of an arachnoid cyst.[40] All pediatric skull fractures warrant neurosurgical consultation.

The Brain

The newborn's brain is poorly developed and functions mainly at a subcortical level. Brainstem reflexes are present but cortical functions are less well developed. The autonomic nervous system exists in an immature form and is more responsive to parasympathetic stimuli than to sympathetic stimuli.

At birth the brain has already reached 25% of the weight of the adult brain. Intrauterine growth results in rapid cell division, and most neuronal cell division is complete by 20 weeks gestation. Rapid growth of the brain continues postnatally, with a doubling in size in the first 6 months of age. The brain reaches 75% of adult size by 2 years of age (Figure 16-2). This postnatal growth consists of proliferation of glial cells, dendritic arborization, and myelination (Figure 16-3). The postnatal growth and differentiation of the brain results in increases in its volume, weight, and complexity.

Because of its rapid growth and differentiation, the newborn and infant brain is particularly vulnerable to injury during the first few months of life. Although neurons do not regenerate, they do respond to injury by forming new synaptic connections. Additional connections may either decrease the amount of permanent neurological damage or may result in increasing disability and spasticity.

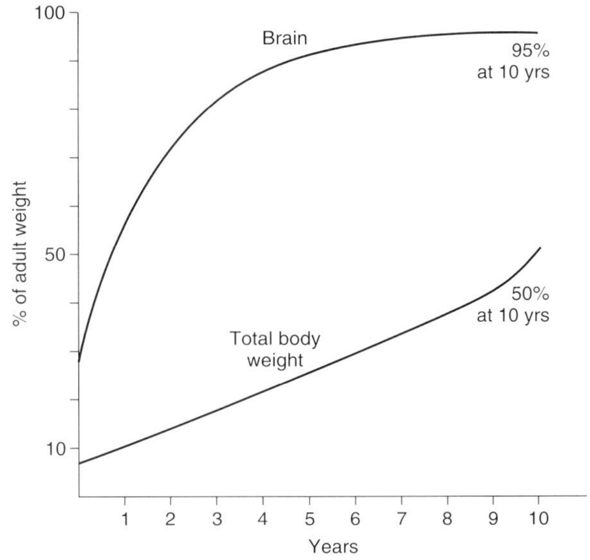

FIGURE 16-2 ■ Brain growth compared with that of the body.[33]

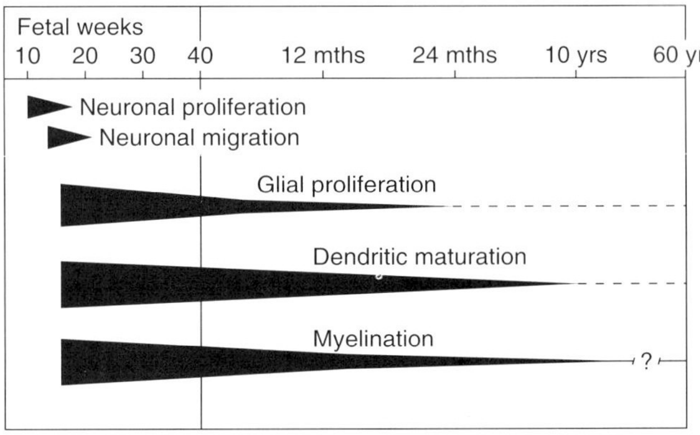

FIGURE 16-3 ■ Postnatal brain growth.[33]

The type and pattern of traumatic injuries to the brain reflect the structural development of the brain and skull at different ages. Epidural hematomas provide one example of the relationship between brain development and pattern of injury. Children under 2 years of age have a close and strong attachment between the skull and dura, which makes bleeding into the epidural space less likely than in adults.[22] Epidural hematomas are uncommon in children, especially those younger than 2 years of age. Subdural hematomas are more common following severe, traumatic head injury in infancy.

The infant's brain has more mobility within the skull, resulting in stretching and tearing of cortical veins. The absence of arachnoidal adhesions to the dura in infancy may also result in venous bleeding. With slow bleeding and no documented history of trauma, these infants may present many hours after their injury with seizures, depressed level of consciousness, and elevated ICP.

Some injuries that are common in adults are uncommon in infancy and vice-versa. The contrecoup lesion seen in nearly 90% of all fatal, traumatic adult brain injuries is extremely rare in infancy.[26] Brain lacerations, however, are more prevalent in traumatically injured infants than older children and adults. This might be explained by the thin and mobile skull, which may be fractured or depressed into the brain, or by the lack of myelination, resulting in a gelatinous consistency of the brain that increases its risk of shearing. Injuries to the basal ganglia after blunt head trauma are more common in infants and may be the only injury present. This may be explained as a vascular injury with stretching of the lenticular perforating vessels of the middle cerebral artery, leading to infarction.[25]

In addition to a different pattern of injury, children have a distinct physiological response to traumatic brain injury. The usual adult findings of decreased cerebral blood flow and metabolism can be seen in children with severe subarachnoid hemorrhage or diffuse axonal injury. An alternative response, however, consisting of increases in cerebral blood flow and metabolism, can also been seen in children but is uncommon in adults. This second pediatric response has been described by Bruce and colleagues[6] as diffuse cerebral swelling. In fatal pediatric closed head injury, the most common findings on computed tomography (CT) are absence of significant hemorrhage, a diffusely swollen brain with small ventricles, and loss of the perimesencephalic cisterns and subarachnoid space.[36] Bruce[6] suggests that the brain swelling is caused by increased cerebral blood flow, as opposed to increased brain water, because the swelling occurs rapidly and the CT scan resembles hyperemia more than edema. Explanations for this diffuse brain swelling include increased cerebral blood flow caused by a loss of autoregulation and/or increased brain metabolism resulting in increased cerebral blood flow. More recently, a different explanation has been postulated by Clasen and colleagues[9] to account for the cerebral swelling. Clasen argues that diffuse traumatic edema, rather than cerebral congestion, is the cause of cerebral swelling.

CEREBRAL BLOOD FLOW AND CEREBRAL HEMODYNAMICS

Cerebral blood flow (CBF) and cerebral oxygen consumption ($CMRO_2$) are relatively low in the neonate, increase during the first year of life, and subsequently decrease during childhood to adult values (Table 16-6). Cerebral function is compromised at a CBF of 15 to 20 ml/min/100 g of brain. Infarction in the infant's brain does not occur until CBF is less than 10 ml/min/100 g of brain, a lower level than in the adult.[20]

TABLE 16-6 ■ Cerebral Blood Flow (CBF) and Cerebral Metabolic Rate for Oxygen ($CMRO_2$) in the Neonate, Infant, and Adult[3]

	CBF (ml O_2/100 g brain/min)	$CMRO_2$ (ml O_2/100 g brain/min)
Neonate	40	2.3
Infant	90-100	5.0
Adult	53	3.0

Although hyperventilation below a $PaCO_2$ of 20 mm Hg does not further decrease CBF in adults, it can decrease CBF in children.[5] In newborn animal models, CBF continued to decrease until the $PaCO_2$ was 12 to 15.[3] The use of jugular venous catheterization to measure arterial-jugular oxygen differences ($AJDO_2$) has been advocated as a means of comparing CBF with cerebral metabolism.

The neonate is adapted to a lower intrauterine oxygen tension and the newborn's hemoglobin F has a higher affinity for oxygen. CBF in the older child increases in response to hypoxia with a PaO_2 of less than 50 mm Hg, but this does not occur in infants until the PaO_2 is less than 25 mm Hg.[3]

Autoregulation occurs at much lower systemic arterial blood pressures in infants compared with adults. The normal mean arterial blood pressure of the newborn is approximately 40 mm Hg, much less than the normal adult cerebral perfusion pressure. CBF is decreased and autoregulation may be lost in the critically ill infant with respiratory distress syndrome or asphyxia. In these cases, CBF is pressure dependent and may result in ischemia or hemorrhage.

Control of Intracranial Pressure

There are a number of pediatric neurosurgical conditions that may have an associated increase in ICP, including head trauma, infections, tumors, and congenital lesions.[38] Although the basic mechanisms that result in increased ICP in the adult apply to the child, the previously noted differences in control of CBF and arterial blood pressure require that caution be used when applying adult management strategies to the child or infant.

The normal neonate has an ICP of 2 mm Hg or less, the 1 year old has an ICP of 2 to 6, and the older child has an ICP of 3 to 13.[44] The cerebral compliance in infants has been noted to be different than in older

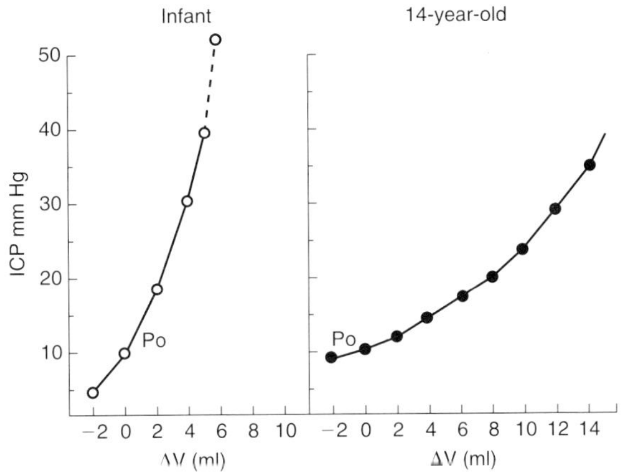

FIGURE 16-4 ■ Intracranial pressure-volume curves in the normal infant and adolescent. Note the decreased compliance in the infant.[38]

children and adults. The slope of the infant's pressure-volume curve is steeper for any given change in intracranial volume. Even small changes in an infant's intracranial volume can lead to potentially catastrophic increases in ICP (Figure 16-4). In contrast, if ICP rises slowly and the infant's sutures have separated, the infant brain can tolerate larger increases in intracranial volume than the adult brain can endure.

Control of elevated ICP in the child follows similar guidelines as in the adult. General measures of head elevation, sedation, and avoidance of noxious stimuli are observed. Hyperventilation is used to manage acute increases in ICP until the underlying cause is determined. Extremes of hyperventilation, down to a $Pa{CO_2}$ of 12 to 15, may be effective in lowering ICP in the infant or young child, but the risk of ischemia is considerable unless $AJDO_2$ is monitored and jugular venous oxygen tension is kept over 20 mm Hg.[5]

CENTRAL NERVOUS SYSTEM MONITORING

CT scans of the head are often obtained initially to help provide diagnostic and prognostic information. Any deterioration in the neurological status warrants an emergent repeat of the head CT scan. Infants with an open fontanel can be imaged by ultrasound. The ultrasound confers the advantage of portability, although resolution in certain areas of the brain is less than with CT scans. Continuous EEG monitoring is useful in detecting seizures in children when subclinical seizures are suspected or the neurological exam is confounded by neuromuscular blockade.

Electrophysiological monitoring is becoming more common in the pediatric patient to help assess outcome after head trauma or hypoxic-ischemic encephalopathy. Brainstem auditory evoked responses (BAER) can provide a means of evaluating the brainstem function in a comatose child. The auditory-evoked potential is virtually unaffected by medications, including high-dose barbiturate therapy, that may influence the results of an EEG.[8] Lutsch and colleagues[23] studied 43 consecutive comatose children after head trauma or asphyxia and found that a loss of auditory evoked potential components was associated with a poor outcome. Fisher and colleagues[15] studied 89 children after cardiac arrest from submersion accidents and found that auditory evoked potentials had a prognostic value for predicting outcome.

Cervical Spine

Although only 1% to 3% of all cervical spine injuries occur in young children, the pattern of injury is different in young children and can result in distinct radiological findings. The newborn spine is elastic, and the laxity of ligaments allows longitudinal distraction of up to 2 inches. However, the newborn spinal cord is relatively inelastic, and injuries to the spinal cord can occur during delivery. Developmental differences of the spine in children under 8 years of age predispose them to upper cervical injuries. More horizontal orientation of the facet joints of the upper cervical vertebrae and anterior wedging of the vertebral bodies allow increased forward movement of the upper cervical spine with flexion. The child with a large, heavy head and less well-developed neck musculature can develop increased angular momentum, with flexion and extension resulting in cervical spine injury.

Radiographic diagnosis of cervical spine injuries in children is complicated by a number of pediatric normal variants. The distance between the anterior arch of C1 and the dens can be up to 5 mm in children, whereas in adults it is never more than 3 mm. Pseudosubluxation, a normal variant of C2 displacement on C3, occurs in up to 40% of children, with more than 50% of these children having a 3 mm or greater degree of shift. Pseudosubluxation of C3 on C4 is a less common normal variant, occurring 15% of the time. Epiphyseal plates in the spine close between 2 and 10 years of age and can resemble fractures. Unless the physician is aware of these normal variants, an incorrect diagnosis can easily be made.

Of more concern are the false-negative cervical spine films. Although the syndrome of spinal cord injury without radiological abnormality (SCIWORA) is reported in adults, it is much more common in children.[32] It is thought that either transient dislocation of the spine occurs followed by spontaneous reduction or that a flexion-extension injury results in a vascular insult to the cord. In a series of pediatric cervical spine injuries reported by Pang and Wilberger,[32] two thirds of the children had normal cervical spine films. Half of the patients in this series presented with delayed symptoms up to 96 hours after injury. Some of the injuries were severe, including cases of complete quadriplegia as a result of spinal cord transection.

FLUID AND ELECTROLYTE REQUIREMENTS

The maintenance fluid requirement per kilogram is higher in children than adults. The absolute fluid requirement can, however, be quite small. This necessitates accurate monitoring of all fluid sources to avoid overhydration. In addition, the body fluid compartments vary in their percentages with age, as do electrolyte requirements. Infants have a limited ability to self-regulate intravascular volume because of their diminished renal concentrating ability.

The relationship of fluid compartments to age is shown in Figure 17-5. Total body water and extracellular fluid decrease until approximately 1 year of age and then remain fairly constant until puberty. Intracellular fluid increases until 1 year and then levels off until puberty. Intravascular volume as a percentage of weight also decreases with age, as shown in Table 16-7.

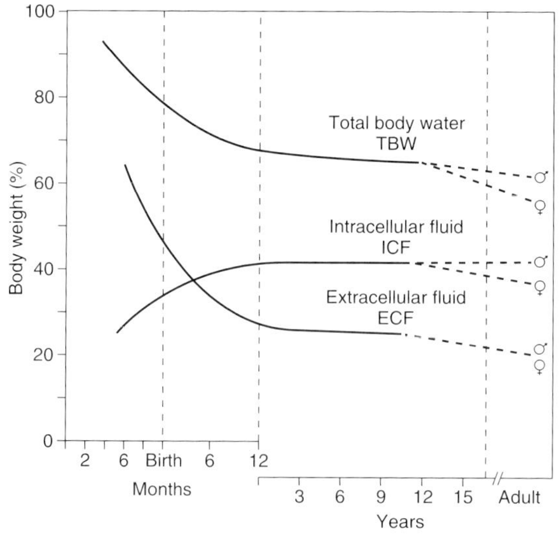

FIGURE 16-5 ■ Distribution of body water as a percentage of body weight. Adult values are approached by 1 year of age. (Adapted from Fris-Hansen BJ, Holiday MA, Stapleton T: Total body water in children, **Pediatrics 7**:321-326, 1951.)

TABLE 16-7 ■ Blood Volume Related to Age[20]

Age	Intravascular Volume (ml/kg)
Premature	100
Term newborn	90
3-24 months	80
>24 months	70

The child's maintenance fluid requirement is usually approximated on the basis of weight. Maintenance fluid requirements (ml) and caloric requirements (kcal) are equivalent (Table 16-8). For example, for a 10-kg infant, the maintenance requirements are 100 ml/kg/day and 100 kcal/kg/day for fluids and calories, respectively. Urinary losses account for 50 to 55 ml/kg/day, skin losses approximately 30 ml/kg/day, respiratory losses about 15 ml/kg/day, and stool losses 0 to 5 ml/kg/day. The clinician needs to adjust the maintenance fluids when losses from any of these systems are excessive or diminished. If not accounted for, excessive losses from hyperthermia, diarrhea, nasogastric suction, rapid respiratory rate, or indwelling drains will result in dehydration.

The primary object of fluid management is to maintain normal intravascular volume. If osmotherapy is used to control elevated ICP, the goal should be euvolemic dehydration with elevation of serum osmolality to 300 to 320 mOsm/L while maintaining normal intravascular volume. If diuresis from mannitol or furosemide results in hypovolemia, physiological blood volume can be maintained by replacing urinary losses with packed red blood cells, fresh frozen plasma, or other isotonic fluids such as lactated Ringer's solution or normal saline.[46]

Signs of dehydration in the infant include a sunken anterior fontanel, decrease or absence of tears with crying, and decreased skin turgor with tenting of the skin. A dehydrated infant should receive an initial bolus of 10 to 20 ml/kg of isotonic crystalloid such as lactated Ringer's solution or normal saline and then be reevaluated.

Maintenance fluid should contain 3 mEq of sodium/kg/day and 2 mEq of potassium/kg/day. Adjustments will be needed based on the patient's serum electrolyte values and ongoing electrolyte losses. Regulation of serum calcium, phosphorous, and magnesium in children is similar to that in adults. Serum phosphorous levels are maintained higher in infants (4.5-8.5 mg/dl) and in children (3.7-5.9 mg/dl) than in adults. This is thought to be due to increased growth hormone level

TABLE 16-8 ■ Fluid, Calorie, and Protein Requirements By Age[35]

Requirements Per Day	Fluid	Calories	Protein
Infant (0-1 yr, 0-10 kg)	100 ml/kg	100-110/kg	2 g/kg
Child (1-5 yr, 10-20 kg)	1000 ml +50 ml/kg over 10 kg	80/kg	1.5 g/kg
Child (5-10 yr, 20-40 kg)	1500 ml +20 ml/kg over 20 kg	55/kg	1 g/kg
Adolescent >10 yr, >40 kg)	1900 ml + 20 m/kg over 40 kg	2000-2500	1 g/kg

TABLE 16-9 ■ Fluid and Calorie Requirements on Basis of Weight[35]

Weight (kg)	Fluid Requirement	Caloric Requirement
0-10 kg	100 ml/kg	100 cal/kg
10-20 kg	1000 ml + 50 ml/kg for weight over 10 kg	1000 cal + 50 cal/kg for weight over 10 kg
>20 kg	1500 ml + 20 ml/kg for weight over 20 kg	1500 cal + 20 cal/kg for weight over 20 kg

and decreased gonadal hormone levels of children compared with adults.[10]

Hyponatremia

As in the adult neurosurgical patient, hyponatremia needs to be evaluated and treated promptly. The differential diagnosis in the pediatric neurosurgical patient includes excessive free water administration, syndrome of inappropriate antidiuretic hormone (SIADH), and cerebral salt wasting.[31] Serum sodium should be measured frequently to detect hyponatremia and to assess the efficacy of its treatment. Unappreciated hyponatremia may result in significant morbidity in the pediatric neurosurgical patient. Hyponatremic seizures may occur with a serum sodium below 125 mEq/L and are difficult to control without partial correction of the serum sodium concentration. Rapid increases in serum sodium can be achieved using 3% saline infusion with a goal of increasing the serum sodium above 125 mEq/L in the patient with seizures caused by hyponatremia. A 3% sodium chloride solution in a dose of 5 ml/kg will raise serum sodium by 5 mEq/L. A number of reports have described fatal cerebral edema caused by hyponatremia in the pediatric patient recovering from head injury.[2,21] It is therefore reasonable to start maintenance fluid in the head-injured patient with lactated Ringer's solution or normal saline with or without 5% dextrose rather than using hypotonic saline solutions.

RENAL MATURITY

The kidneys continue to mature after birth. The newborn's glomerular filtration rate is only 2.5 ml/min, increases to 15 ml/min at 6 months of age, up to 50 ml/min in the preschooler, and finally reaches the adult value of 130 ml/min in early adolescence.[18] The newborn has limited renal concentrating ability and is able to concentrate urine to only 700 mOsm/kg, compared with the adult value of 1400 mOsm/kg.

NUTRITIONAL REQUIREMENTS

Infants have the highest caloric requirement per kilogram because of their rapid growth, increased activity, and larger heat losses as a result of their proportionately higher body surface area. Early nutritional support is needed in infants because infants have decreased energy stores and an increased basal metabolic rate (BMR) compared with adults. The BMR of infants is 40 to 50 kcal/kg/day compared with the BMR in adults of 25 to 30 kcal/kg/day.[35] An estimated 50% of children in pediatric ICUs have protein-calorie malnutrition,[39] which leads to breakdown of protein stores and loss of muscle mass. Caloric requirements are increased by the same factors in children and adults, including fever, trauma, increased respiratory rate, and sepsis. Caloric requirements for infants and children are outlined in Table 16-9. A pediatric dietician can assist in the assessment of baseline nutritional status by anthropometry of height, weight, and head circumference as well as in calculating caloric and protein requirements.

SUMMARY

Care of infants and children with neurosurgical diseases remains one of the greatest challenges in intensive care medicine. Anatomic and physiological changes in these patients occur during maturation and impact profoundly on their medical and surgical management. An understanding of such developmental changes in addition to an in-depth knowledge of general neurological intensive care is essential to the appropriate care of critically ill pediatric patients.

This chapter has outlined fundamentals of pediatric anatomy and physiology that pertain to care of the neurosurgical pediatric patient. The principles described in this chapter should be integrated with essential information contained within the other chapters in this text. As a result, an improved understanding of the problems of infants and children with neurosurgical diseases may facilitate optimal care of these challenging patients.

REFERENCES

1. Auld PAM: Pulmonary physiology of the newborn infant, in Scarpelli EM (ed): **Pulmonary Physiology of the Fetus and Newborn Child.** Philadelphia: Lea and Febiger, 1975, p 140.

2. Berger MS, Pitts LH, Lovely M: Outcome from severe head injury in children and adolescents, **J Neurosurg 62:**194, 1985.
3. Bruce DA: Cerebrovascular dynamics, in James HE, Anas NG, Perkin RM (eds): **Brain Insults in Infants and Children: Pathophysiology and Management.** Orlando: Grune and Stratton, 1985, pp 53-60.
4. Bruce DA: Concepts of intracranial volume and pressure, in Hames HE, Anas NG, Perkin RM (eds): **Brain Insults in Infants and Children: Pathophysiology and Management.** Orlando: Grune and Stratton, 1985, pp 19.
5. Bruce DA: Ventilation, hyperventilation, megaventilation, and cerebral blood flow, in James HE, Anas NG, Perkin RM (eds): **Brain Insults in Infants and Children: Pathophysiology and Management.** Orlando: Grune and Stratton, 1985, pp 257-262.
6. Bruce DA, Alavi A, Bilaniuk L: Diffuse cerebral swelling following head injuries in children, **J Neurosurg 54:**170, 1981.
7. Bucher HU, Fanconi S, Fallenstein F, et al: Transcutaneous carbon dioxide tension in newborn infants: reliability and safety of continuous 24-hour measurement at 42oC, **Pediatrics 78:**631, 1986.
8. Chiappa KH: Electrophysiologic monitoring, in Ropper AH, Kennedy SK: **Neurological and Neurosurgical Intensive Care.** Rockville: Aspen Publishers, 1988, pp 129-156.
9. Clasen RA, Penn RD: Traumatic swelling and edema, in Cooper PR (ed): **Head Injury,** 2nd ed. Baltimore: Williams and Wilkins, 1987, pp 285-312.
10. Dabbagh S, Ellis D: Regulations of fluids and electrolytes in infants and children, in Motoama EK, Davis PJ (eds): **Smith's Anesthesia for Infants and Children.** St. Louis: Mosby, 1990, pp 105-142.
11. Dawes GS: **Fetal and Neonatal Physiology.** Chicago: Yearbook Medical, 1973, p 191.
12. Dawes GS, Mott JC, Shelley HJ: The importance of cardiac glycogen for the maintenance of life in foetal lambs and newborn animals during anoxia, **J Physiol 146:**516, 1959.
13. Doershuk CF, Fisher BJ, Matthews LW: Pulmonary physiology of the young child, in Scarpelli EM (ed): **Pulmonary Physiology of the Fetus, Newborn, and Child.** Philadelphia: Lea and Febiger, 1975, p 166.
14. Downing SE: Neural regulation of circulation during hypoxia and acidosis with special reference to the newborn, **Fed Proceed 31:**1209, 1972.
15. Fisher B, Peterson B, Hicks G: Use of brainstem auditory-evoked response testing to assess neurologic outcome following near drowning in children, **Crit Care Med 20(5):**578-585, 1992.
16. Flacke JW, Flacke WE, Bloor BC, et al: Histamine release by four narcotics: a double-blind study in humans, **Anesth Analg 66:**723, 1987.
17. Friedman WF: The intrinsic physiologic properties of the developing heart, in Friedman WF, Lesch M, Sonnenblick E (eds): **Neonatal Heart Disease.** New York: Grune and Stratton, 1973, p 21.
18. Hazinski MF, van Stralen D: Physiologic and anatomic differences between children and adults, in Levin DL, Morriss FC (eds): **Essentials of Pediatric Intensive Care.** St. Louis: Quality Medical, 1989, pp 5-17.
19. Hess D: Capnometry and capnometry: technical aspects, physiologic aspects, and clinical applications, **Respir Care 35:**557, 1990.
20. Hollinger IB, Goodrich JT: Pediatric neuroanesthesia, in Frost EAM (ed): **Clinical Anesthesia in Neurosurgery,** 2nd ed. Boston: Butterworth, 1991, pp 287-333.
21. Humphrys RP, Hendrick EB, Hoffman HJ: The head-injured child who "talks and dies." **Childs Nerv Syst 6:**139, 1990.
22. James HE: Head injury in infants, children, and adolescents, in Nussbaum E (ed): **Pediatric Intensive Care,** 2nd ed. New York: Futura, 1989, pp 39-54.
23. Lutsch J, Pfenninger J, Ludin HP: Brain-stem auditory evoked potentials and early somatosensory evoked potentials in neurointensively treated comatose children, **Am J Dis Child 137:**421, 1983.
24. Martin DE, Rosenberg H, Aukburg SJ, et al: Low-dose fentanyl blunts circulatory responses to tracheal intubation, **Anesth Analg 61:**680, 1982.
25. McLaurin RL, Towbin R: Cerebral damage, in Raimondi AJ, Choux M, Rocco CD (eds): **Head Injuries in the Newborn and Infant.** New York: Springer Verlag, 1986, pp 183-202.
26. McLaurin RL, Towbin R: Diagnosis and treatment of head injury in infants and children, in Youmans JR (ed): **Neurological Surgery,** 3rd ed. Philadelphia: W.B. Saunders, 1990, p 2149.
27. Mealey J: Skull fractures, in McLaurin RL, Schut L, Venes JL, et al (eds): **Pediatric Neurosurgery,** 2nd ed. Philadelphia: W.B. Saunders, 1989, p 263.
28. Miguel R, Witkowski T, Nagashima H, et al: Evaluation of neuromuscular and cardiovascular effects of two doses of rapacuronium (ORG 9487) versus mivacurium and succinylcholine, **Anesthesiology 91:**1648-1654, 1999.
29. Mushin WW, Rendell-Baker L, Thompson PW, et al (eds): Clinical aspects of controlled respiration, in **Automatic Ventilation of the Lungs.** Oxford: Blackwell Scientific, 1980, p 33.
30. Nelson NM: Neonatal pulmonary function, **Pediatr Clin North Am 13:**769,1966.
31. Nelson PB, Seif SM, Maroon JC: Hyponatremia in intracranial disease, **J Neurosurg 55:**938, 1981.
32. Pang D, Wilberger JE: Spinal cord injury without radiographic abnormalities in children, **J Neurosurg 57:**114, 1982.
33. Peacock WJ: The postnatal development of the brain and its coverings, in Raimondi AJ, Choux M, Rocco CD (eds): **Head injuries in the Newborn and Infant.** New York: Springer Verlag, 1986, pp 53-66.
34. Raimondi AJ, Hirschauer J: Clinical criteria—children's coma score and outcome scale for decision making in managing head injured infants and toddlers, in Raimondi AJ, Choux M, Rocco CD (eds): **Head Injuries in the Newborn and Infant.** New York: Springer Verlag, 1986, pp 141-150.
35. Reed MD: Principles of total parenteral nutrition, in Blumer JL (ed): **A Practical Guide to Pediatric Intensive Care.** St. Louis: Mosby, 1990, pp 582-591.
36. Rockoff, MA, Kennedy SK: Physiology and clinical aspects of raised intracranial pressure, in Ropper AH, Kennedy SF (eds): **Neurological and Neurosurgical Intensive Care,** 2nd ed. Rockville: Aspen Publishers, 1988, pp 9-22.

37. Schieber RA: Noninvasive recognition and assessment of the failing circulation, in Swedlow DB, Raphaely RC (eds): **Cardiovascular Problems in Pediatric Critical Care.** New York: Churchill Livingstone, 1986, p 90.
38. Shapiro K, Marmarou A: Mechanisms of intracranial hypertension in children, in McLaurin RL, Schut L, Venes JL, et al (eds): **Pediatric Neurosurgery,** 2nd ed. Philadelphia: W.B. Saunders, 1989, p 238.
39. Smith BC, Hickman RO, Morray JP: Nutritional support, in Morray JP (ed): **Pediatric Intensive Care.** 1989, pp 21-42.
40. Stein B, Tenner ST: Enlargement of skull fracture in childhood due to cerebral herniation, **Arch Neurol 26:**137, 1972.
41. Stoelting RK. Circulatory changes during direct laryngoscopy and tracheal intubation: Influence of duration of laryngoscopy with or without prior lidocaine, **Anesthesiology 47:**381, 1977.
42. Swaiman KF: Neurologic examination after the newborn period until 2 years of age, in Swaiman KF (ed): **Pediatric Neurology: Principles and Practice.** St. Louis: Mosby, 1989, pp 35-44.
43. Swaiman KF: Neurologic examination of the older child, in Swaiman KF (ed): **Pediatric Neurology: Principles and Practice.** St. Louis: Mosby, 1989, pp 15-34.
44. Trauner DA: Increased intracranial pressure, in Swaiman KF (ed): **Pediatric Neurology: Principles and Practice.** St. Louis: Mosby, 1989, pp 169-176.
45. Tullock WC, Diana P, Cook DR, et al: High-dose vecuronium: onset and duration, **Anesth Analg 67:**S235, 1988.
46. Walker ML, Storrs BB: Medical management of head injuries in neonates and infants, in Raimondi AJ, Choux M, Rocco CD (eds): **Head Injuries in the Newborn and Infant.** New York: Springer Verlag, 1986, pp 151-162.

CHAPTER 17

Withholding and Withdrawal of Life Support in the Intensive Care Unit

John M. Luce

THE COMPLEXITY OF WITHHOLDING AND WITHDRAWING LIFE SUPPORT

The withholding and withdrawal of life support are processes by which various medical interventions either are not given to or are taken away from patients with the expectation that they will die as a result. These processes are carried out in many medical settings but are especially common in the intensive care unit (ICU), where an array of therapies capable of sustaining life are employed. An example of withholding life support is not providing mechanical ventilation to a patient who, if not placed on a ventilator, will probably die. An example of withdrawing life support is removing mechanical ventilation from a patient with the provision that the patient will neither be ventilated again nor resuscitated if he or she decompensates. This second patient is different from a third patient who is being weaned from mechanical ventilation and will be ventilated again or resuscitated if he or she deteriorates during the weaning process.

Strictly speaking, all patients who die while receiving close medical attention in an ICU or elsewhere do so as a direct result of the withholding or withdrawal of life support. This is either because a decision has been made in advance of decompensation not to resuscitate the patient or because vigorous resuscitation will not be provided indefinitely if decompensation occurs. For example, the third patient described earlier would receive cardiopulmonary resuscitation (CPR) if he or she were to suffer an unexpected cardiopulmonary arrest during weaning, but CPR would be discontinued if a viable cardiac rhythm could not be restored in a reasonable amount of time. The withdrawal of life support from this third patient is comparable to the withholding of CPR from the second patient, except for that in the case of the second patient deliberate planning has taken place before cardiopulmonary arrest. This chapter focuses on this more deliberate form of withholding and withdrawal.

ETHICAL ASPECTS OF WITHHOLDING AND WITHDRAWING LIFE SUPPORT

Position Statements by Professional Societies

Physicians who care for critically ill adults and who are considering withholding or withdrawing life support can draw from several summaries of the ethical propriety of limiting care.[1,4,7,20,27] One of the most succinct group statements is the "Consensus Report on the Ethics of Forgoing Life-sustaining Treatments in the Critically Ill," which was prepared by the Task Force on Ethics of the Society of Critical Care Medicine and published in 1990.[29] In this report it was noted that it is ethically appropriate to withhold or withdraw therapy either because a patient or surrogate decides to forgo treatment or because a physician judges that the major goals of therapy are unachievable. A decision to withdraw a treatment should not be more problematic than a decision not to initiate a treatment, particularly because starting therapy may be necessary to adequately evaluate a patient's condition. Any treatment derives its medical justification from the benefits that a patient and physician hope to achieve by employing it. When the treatment has achieved those benefits or can no longer be expected to do so, it loses its justification and may be withdrawn.

The task force's consensus statement also noted that there are no intrinsic moral differences between categories of treatment, such as CPR, ventilatory support, medications such as vasopressors and antibiotics, and the provision of hydration and nutrition by artificial means. Each treatment should be considered from a patient's perspective in light of the overall benefit that it may offer and the burdens it may entail, as well as the professional duties that are involved. Because treatment choices must be considered in relation to a patient's overall condition, a treatment offering a reasonable expectation of physiological benefits may be withheld from terminally ill patients. Treatments that serve only to prolong the dying process should not be used, and indefinitely maintaining patients in a persistent vegetative state raises ethical concerns both for the dignity of the patient and for the inappropriate use of health care resources.

A basic provision of the consensus statement was that the wishes of an informed adult patient with decision-making capacity should be the primary consideration in almost all decisions regarding treatment. When a patient (or surrogate in the case of a patient who is incapable of making decisions) and a physician (and other members of the health care team) agree that therapy should be limited, it usually should be. Treatments rejected by a patient or surrogate generally should not be imposed by a physician. When a patient or surrogate requests therapy that a physician considers futile, the physician should clarify the goals of treatment with the patient and may accede to the patient's wishes. The physician is not ethically obligated to provide therapy, however, and may elect to transfer the patient's care.

The Society of Critical Care Medicine's consensus report did not discuss situations in which patients or their surrogates disagree with physicians but care cannot be transferred. Nor did it describe the role of ethics committees in resolving conflicts or the place of health care institutions in developing policies regarding the withholding or withdrawal of futile care. Furthermore, presumably because of when it was written, the report did not deal with the issue of how the physician-patient relationship has been affected by the growth of managed care, cost containment, and concern with limited medical resources. In this regard, some physicians think that their traditional duty to individual patients increasingly is being compromised by the desire of health care organizations to restrict access to certain services, including those of uncertain benefit. An alternative view is that physicians properly should broaden their advocacy of individual patients with a proportioned advocacy whereby more patients can receive treatment by limiting the provision of nonbeneficial care to a few.

LEGAL ASPECTS OF WITHHOLDING AND WITHDRAWING LIFE SUPPORT

Physicians clearly are influenced by real or perceived legal requirements in their attitudes regarding the withholding or withdrawing of life support. A few of these requirements have come in the form of statutes in areas such as brain death and organ transplantation, but most have been expressed through case law. As a result, it is important to understand how in recent years the courts have underscored the right of patients to refuse treatment, affirmed the concept that human life is more than a biologic process that must be continued in all circumstances, defined how therapies may or may not benefit patients, argued against a distinction between the withholding and withdrawing of life support, established guidelines for limiting life-sustaining treatment, and approached the resolution of disagreements among physicians and patients or their surrogates.

The Quinlan Case

The first major judicial decision regarding the withholding and withdrawing of life support occurred in the case of Karen Ann Quinlan (1976), in which the father of a girl who was in a persistent vegetative state petitioned the court to be appointed guardian with the power to remove her from mechanical ventilation.[15] The lower court denied the petition, but the New Jersey Supreme Court reversed that decision. In doing so the court reasoned that patients generally would accept or refuse medical treatment on the basis of its ability to support sentient life over mere biologic existence. Having concluded that Ms. Quinlan, if she had been capable of making decisions herself, would have foregone therapy that could only prolong biologic life but not sentient life, the court decided that her right to privacy would be abrogated if it prevented the exercise of that right on her behalf. The court therefore granted the father's petition, allowing him to exercise "substituted judgment" for his daughter, and stated that life support could be withdrawn if her physicians and a hospital ethics committee agreed that such support did not alter Ms. Quinlan's underlying condition.

The Barber Case

The case of *Barber v. Superior Court* (1983) involved two California physicians who performed surgical closure of an ileostomy on a Mr. Herbert, who subsequently suffered cardiopulmonary arrest.[3] Five days later, determining that Mr. Herbert's coma was irreversible and with the consent of his family, the physicians withdrew not only mechanical ventilation but also intravenous fluids and nutrition. Although the family found no fault with this at the time, the physicians were accused of murder by a district attorney. After the case was heard by several courts, the California Court of Appeals ruled that because the physicians had considered it medically futile to continue treatment because sentient life could not be restored, they had not failed to perform their duty. The court did not distinguish between removing mechanical ventilation and removing fluids or nutrition because all were interventions that could either benefit or burden. Finally, the court held that, without evidence of malevolence, family members are the proper surrogate for patients who cannot make decisions and that prior judicial approval is not necessary if surrogates and physicians decide to limit care.

The Cruzan Case

The only case involving withholding and withdrawing of life support to be heard by the U.S. Supreme Court was *Cruzan v. Director, Missouri Department of Health* (1990).[8] This case involved Nancy Cruzan, a young woman in a persistent vegetative state who required tube feeding rather than mechanical ventilation. Believing that she would not want to live in such a state, her parents asked to have tube feedings discontinued and were authorized to do so by a trial judge in Missouri. The Missouri Supreme Court reversed this decision, however, arguing that no one could exercise Ms. Cruzan's right to refuse treatment on her behalf. The court also said that because the state had an interest in preserving life regardless of its quality, support could be terminated only if it could be shown by "clear and convincing evidence" that Ms. Cruzan had rejected such treatment. The U.S. Supreme Court, although acknowledging that patients had a constitutional right to refuse any form of life-sustaining treatment, also concluded that the constitution did not prohibit Missouri or other states from requiring evidence of a patient's wishes regarding life support. The court did not require that other states follow Missouri's lead, however, and its decision does not affect the laws, ethical principles, or clinical practices elsewhere. In effect, the decision highlighted the desirability of all persons filling out advance directives, including living wills and durable powers of attorney for health care, to facilitate medical decision making if and when they become critically ill.

The Wanglie Case

The case of Helen Wanglie (1991) involved an 85-year-old woman who had a cardiopulmonary arrest during an attempt at weaning from mechanical ventilation at a long-term care facility.[14] She was returned to Hennepin County Medical Center (Minneapolis, Minnesota) in a persistent vegetative state. Mrs. Wanglie's physician recommended to her husband and children that life-sustaining therapy be withdrawn, but the family insisted that therapy be continued because they valued biologic life. Eventually a new physician told the family that he did not wish to continue mechanical ventilation because it was not beneficial, because it could not heal Mrs. Wanglie's lungs or end her unconsciousness; because mechanical ventilation could prolong life, it was not described as being physiologically futile. After the family tried and failed to find another facility willing to care for the patient, the medical center asked the district court first to appoint a conservator other than Mr. Wanglie to decide if ventilation was beneficial and, second, for a hearing to determine whether ventilation was required if the conservator held that it was not beneficial. The court refused to replace Mr. Wanglie on the grounds that he could best represent his wife's interests. Because Mr. Wanglie died before a hearing could be held, the issues of whether ventilation was beneficial and whether physicians could override family wishes were not resolved.

The Gilgunn Case

The most recent case to explore the issue of whether physicians can override family wishes involved a 72-year-old woman named Catherine Gilgunn who was being cared for at Massachusetts General Hospital (Boston).[5] Mrs. Gilgunn was comatose with irreversible brain damage and had congestive heart failure and gastrointestinal bleeding. Although Mrs. Gilgunn's husband and two of her daughters agreed to physician recommendations for a do not resuscitate (DNR) order, another daughter disagreed, and the DNR order was discontinued. At a subsequent meeting to discuss the DNR order, this daughter stormed out without confronting the issue. The other two daughters agreed to reinstate the DNR order, and Mrs. Gilgunn was removed from the ventilator. The daughter who had refused the DNR order brought action against her mother's physicians and the hospital. Subsequently, the jury in Suffolk Superior Court absolved the physicians and hospital of liability, apparently because they believed that further care was futile despite the possibility that Mrs. Gilgunn might have wanted to be kept alive. Thus, for the first time, a U.S. jury determined that life-sustaining therapy may be discontinued despite the objections of a patient or his or her surrogate.

CLINICAL ASPECTS OF WITHHOLDING AND WITHDRAWING LIFE SUPPORT

Incidence of Withholding and Withdrawing Life Support from the Critically Ill

Information about the clinical aspects of withholding and withdrawing life support has come primarily from surveys of physicians and other health professionals and from observational studies of the limiting of life-sustaining care. For example, several surveys[2,10,30] have suggested that the great majority of critical care physicians have withheld or withdrawn life support at one time or another and that many have done so frequently. Similarly, retrospective studies[17,24,31] have found that about half the patients who die in ICUs do so during the withholding or withdrawing of life-sustaining therapy. Prospective studies[10,32] the authors conducted in two ICUs in hospitals (Moffitt-Long Hospital and San Francisco General Hospital) affiliated with the University of California, San Francisco (UCSF) revealed that the withholding and withdrawal of life support preceded 90% of deaths in 1992 and 1993, compared with 51% of deaths in 1988 and 1989. Many of the patients whose care was limited had neurological illnesses, including head trauma, and some were brain dead.

Withholding and Withdrawal of Life Support from Patients with Severe Head Trauma

Although the author was able to determine from the two studies at UCSF that severe head trauma was a common underlying condition in patients from whom life support was withheld or withdrawn, the author was not able to determine how frequently life support was withheld or withdrawn from such patients because not all head-injured patients admitted to the ICU were followed. Earlier findings also provided little information about the accuracy of physicians' prognosticating in cases of severe cranial trauma, or about many aspects of the process through which physicians and patients' families make decisions about limiting treatment.

To overcome these limitations, the author collected data and subsequently reported[23] on all patients admitted to the medical-surgical ICU at San Francisco General Hospital (SFGH) during 1990 with severe head trauma and a Glasgow Coma Scale score of 7 or less. All such patients routinely had an endotracheal tube placed and were mechanically ventilated on or immediately before their admission to the ICU, either because they could not protect their airway or breathe for themselves or because they were hyperventilated to reduce intracranial pressure (ICP). Most, but not all, received other forms of life support, such as ICP monitoring, hemodynamic monitoring, and infusions of vasoactive drugs. As in our other studies from UCSF, patients who were declared brain dead on or after admission were included in this investigation because the process through which life support is withheld or withdrawn is similar, especially from the surrogates' standpoint, whether the patients are brain dead or irrevocably neurologically impaired.

During the 12-month study period, 47 patients with severe head trauma were included in the study. A total of 436 patients were admitted to the neurosurgery service during the same period, 113 of whom had head injuries. Thus the study patients represented approximately half the head-injured patients cared for at SFGH. Motor vehicle accidents and falls accounted for most of the injuries; the next most frequent cause was violent assault. Of the 47 patients with severe head trauma, 24 (51%) had life support withheld or withdrawn during the study period and 23 did not. Of the 24 patients from whom life support was withheld or withdrawn, 22 died (14 in the ICU, 6 during hospitalization, and 2 after discharge to a chronic care center). Of the 22 patients from whom life support was withheld or withdrawn and who died, 11 were found to be brain dead at the time of ICU admission or shortly thereafter; of these patients, 7 became organ donors. None of the 23 patients for whom care was limited died.

Life support was restored at the request of the family for 2 of the 24 patients from whom support was initially withheld or withdrawn because their prognosis changed from "likely death" to "vegetative" during their hospitalization at SFGH. These were the two patients from whom care was limited who actually survived. One of these patients already had been transferred from the ICU, where his prognosis improved, and the other did not require further ICU care because he was not ventilator dependent. Both these patients remained vegetative 6 months after admission to SFGH and discharge to chronic care facilities.

Families were available to participate in medical decisions for 45 (96%) of the 47 patients studied and for 23 (96%) of the 24 patients from whom life support was withheld or withdrawn. Data on prognosis as assessed by families at various intervals during hospitalization, beginning with the patients' admission to the ICU, were available for 42 patients, including all those who had life support withheld or withdrawn. For 31 patients (73%), including 22 of the 24 patients from whom life support was withheld or withdrawn, the prognosis as assessed by the family was completely congruent with the prognosis projected by physicians from the time of the patients' admission to the ICU. In the other two cases, the families' assessment of prognosis was more optimistic than the physicians'; these were the patients whose prognosis ultimately improved from likely death to vegetative.

Physicians recommended limiting treatment for the same reasons that families gave for accepting their recommendations. The most frequent reasons cited by both physicians and families were brain death, poor prognosis, futility, and an unacceptable quality of life for the patient. In four cases the families' requests to forgo further care for the patients coincided with the physicians' recommendations of that course of action. In another four cases the physicians complied with the families' requests to honor the patients' previously expressed wishes to limit terminal care. No formal prognostic scoring systems were used in evaluating the patients, and the SFGH ethics committee was never involved (it was not involved in the first two studies either).

Life support initially was withdrawn from patients in more cases than it was withheld in the ICU, largely because mechanical ventilation was used only in that setting. In fact, ventilators were removed from a total of ten patients, seven of whom remained intubated until they died. The endotracheal tube was removed from an additional three of the ten previously ventilated patients, and oxygen was removed from another three patients. Vasopressors were discontinued from one additional patient; two patients had fluids and feedings removed. Medications, including antibiotics, were withdrawn from three patients, all of whom were outside the ICU. Fluids and feedings were withheld from another two patients who died elsewhere in the hospital.

At 6 months after the patient's admission to SFGH, we located 33 families, 21 of whom agreed to be interviewed. Of these 21 families, most expressed thanks for the manner in which their relatives were cared for, including management of their death. Six families stated that the physician's frequent and clear communication had been of great value to them during the patient's hospitalization. Only one family felt they had received inadequate information from the physicians. Three families considered it helpful in their decision to limit care to know that the patient became an organ donor. Belief in miracles was of permanent concern for another three families, one of which was the family of a patient for whom life support was resumed after the prognosis changed from likely death to vegetative. The family of the other patient for whom life support was resumed after the prognosis changed, a family that also believed in miracles, commented on the difficulty of dealing with the patient in a vegetative state.

Our study showed that life support was withheld or withdrawn from slightly more than half of patients with severe cranial trauma admitted to the medical-surgical ICU at SFGH in 1990. Physicians based their recommendation to limit care, and families made their decision to accept the recommendation, primarily on the basis of pain prognosis, including brain death. Because all but two of the patients from whom life support was withheld or withdrawn died, and because the two who did not die remained in a persistent vegetative state, it appeared that the physicians' prognostications were reasonably accurate.

Furthermore, because the overall mortality for patients with severe head trauma (51%) was similar to that observed for similarly injured patients in other studies, such prognostication probably was not self-fulfilling; that is, care was not limited for patients who might have lived and regained consciousness were it prolonged. The general agreement of families with physicians regarding prognosis observed in our study presumably was attributable primarily to the physicians' ability to convey the prognosis and the reasons on which it was based. At the same time, the general satisfaction of families probably resulted from the adequacy of their communication with physicians.

National Survey of Withholding and Withdrawal of Life Support

To determine whether limiting care is as commonplace as suggested by the aforementioned studies from UCSF, a prospective survey[25] was conducted in 1994 and 1995 of 167 ICUs associated with all U.S. training programs in critical care medicine or pulmonary and critical care medicine. Data from 6110 deaths of 71,513 admissions (8.5% mortality) in the 107 sites responding to the survey revealed that 1517 (25%) deaths followed full ICU care and failed CPR; 1407 (23%) deaths occurred in patients who received full ICU care excluding attempted resuscitation; 768 patients (13%) had some form of life support withheld before death; 2032 (33%) deaths followed the withdrawal of life support; and 386 patients (6%) were brain dead and had therapy withdrawn, in some cases after their organs were transplanted. If patients who did not receive CPR, who had life support withheld or withdrawn, and who were brain dead are considered as a group, 75% of the patients in this study had treatment limited in some manner. This suggests that withholding and withdrawing life support are now common practices in most American ICUs.

Despite the fact that life support was commonly withheld or withdrawn in this study, substantial variability was noted among ICUs with regard to mortality (from 2% to 45%), failed CPR (from 4% to 79% of deaths), and willingness to withdraw life support (from 6% to 71%). Clearly, considerable heterogeneity exists in the processes of withholding and withdrawing life-sustaining treatment within the United States. Presumably this heterogeneity also occurs on an international basis, although this issue has not been explored from a research standpoint. Because of the heterogeneity, there is no precise standard of care in the practice of withholding and withdrawing life support, even though the practice is more common than ever before.

Why and How Life Support is Withheld or Withdrawn

Most surveys[2,10,18,30] and studies[1] have indicated that physicians recommend that life support be withheld or withdrawn either because patients or surrogates request this action or because physicians think that further care is futile. Physicians vary in their definitions of futility, but the term generally conveys the ideas that a patient cannot benefit from treatment, that the patient's acute disorder is not reversible, that the patient will not survive the current hospital stay, or that the quality of the patient's life following discharge will be poor. These ideas clearly stem from prognostication on the physicians' part. They generally arrive at estimates of prognosis through their personal experience and knowledge of the medical literature, although prognostic scoring systems such as the Acute Physiology and Chronic Health Evaluation system are used in some ICUs. If present, persistent coma, other unacceptable neurological prognoses, and multiple organ system failure are important rationales for withdrawing care. The need for ICU beds, patients' social worth, and financial cost-benefit analyses are not important rationales.

Most patients have not prepared medical directives in advance of suffering a critical illness, and most patients are too neurologically depressed by their disease or by therapeutic drugs to make medical decisions when they become critically ill. Surrogates were available and willing to take part in the decision-making process in the prospective studies[26,28] from UCSF of withholding and withdrawing life support. When surrogates were not available, physicians were willing to make decisions for the patients. Although consultation from other physicians often was sought before deciding to limit care, hospital ethics committees were infrequently involved.

The surrogates that were available in these studies[26,28] either recommended by themselves that support be withheld or withdrawn when patients were not improving or accepted physicians' recommendations to that effect. These recommendations were not always accepted immediately but, in most cases, the surrogates agreed within a few days. Only rarely did surrogates insist on continued care against the advice of physicians and, in all cases, care was continued. In certain instances, however, the physicians stopped short of providing CPR in patients who were otherwise supported.

Although differences between physicians and surrogates do occur over the issue of limiting care, their incidence is uncertain. In a survey[2] of self-identified members of the critical care section of the American Thoracic Society, 34% of respondents reported that they had refused surrogate requests to withdraw care either because they thought that the patient had a reasonable chance of recovery or that the surrogates might not be acting in the best interest of the patient. At the same time, 83% of physicians reported that they had unilaterally withheld life-sustaining treatment on the basis of futility, often without patient or surrogate knowledge or consent, and 82% had withdrawn treatment on the same basis.

Cardiopulmonary resuscitation probably is the therapy most often withheld from ICU patients, as suggested by the finding that DNR orders preceded 60% of all in-unit deaths between 1980 and 1990 in a large observational study[33] in 40 U.S. hospitals, compared with only 39% of all in-unit deaths from 1979 to 1982 in a similar study.[16] Antibiotics, vasoactive drugs, renal dialysis, and mechanical ventilation were commonly withheld in the two studies[26,28] from ICUs in hospitals affiliated with UCSF. Mechanical ventilation was the therapy most commonly withdrawn in these studies, followed by vasoactive drugs. In the survey[2] of American Thoracic Society members, 89% of the respondents had withdrawn mechanical ventilation, 88% had withdrawn vasoactive drugs, and 80% had stopped blood or blood products.

A survey[11] of randomly selected U.S. members of the Society of Critical Care Medicine in 1991 and 1992 revealed that 15% of respondents almost never withdrew mechanical ventilators from patients who were expected to die, 15% almost always did so, and the remainder withdrew ventilators some or most of the time. Of physicians who withdrew ventilators, 33% preferred the gradual withdrawal of supplemental oxygen and positive end–expiratory pressure treatment before removing the ventilator, a process called terminal weaning[12]; 13% preferred rapid extubation; and the remainder used both methods. Reasons for preferring terminal weaning included patient comfort (65%), family perceptions (63%), and the belief that terminal weaning was less active (49%). Reasons for preferring extubation included the directness of the action (72%), family perceptions (34%), and patient comfort (34%).

In this survey[11] of Society of Critical Care Medicine members, morphine sulfate and other opiate analgesics were used by 74% and diazepam and other benzodiazepines by 53% of physicians who withdrew ventilators; 6% used muscle relaxants at least occasionally. In a study[32] conducted in 1988 and 1989 in the two ICUs at hospitals affiliated with UCSF, analgesics and sedatives were given to 75% of non−brain dead patients during the withholding and withdrawal of life support. Patients who did not receive medication were comatose and considered incapable of benefiting from the drugs. Physicians ordered analgesics and sedatives to decrease pain in 88% of patients, to decrease anxiety in 85%, to comfort families in 82%, to decrease air hunger in 76%, and to hasten death in 39%; in no instance was hastening death the only reason cited. The amounts of opiates and benzodiazepines averaged 3.3 mg/hr of morphine and 2.2 mg/hr of diazepam in the 24 hours before withholding and withdrawing life support and 11.2 mg/hr and 9.8 mg/hr, respectively, in the 24 hours thereafter. The median time until death following the initiation of withholding and withdrawing life support was 3.5 hours in the patients who received drugs and 1.3 hours in those patients who did not. Thus the administration of sedatives and analgesics did not appear to hasten death in this study.

It would appear from these surveys and studies that the withholding and withdrawal of life support from adults occurs frequently in most ICUs in the United States and that these processes commonly follow a similar course. Furthermore, professional attitudes and behaviors on the part of physicians are consistent with ethical pronouncements and judicial decisions regarding the withholding and withdrawing of life support. The only major area in which consistency may be lacking concerns physicians' refusal to follow surrogate demands either to limit care in certain circumstances or, more commonly, to provide care that the physicians consider futile. This finding is not surprising given the lack of legal clarification of the issue and the frequent conflicts over ethical principles such as patient autonomy and distributive justice in ICUs.[19,32]

RESOLVING CONFLICTS BETWEEN PATIENTS AND HEALTH CARE PROFESSIONALS

Although physicians' refusal to provide care has not been legally clarified, the medical profession cannot wait for case law to develop before defining its own values and describing methods for resolving conflicts between patients and their physicians. The Ethics Committee of the Society of Critical Care Medicine[9] recently developed a Consensus Statement Regarding Futile and Other Possibly Inadvisable Treatments to assist in such a resolution. Because of the wide variation in physician definitions of futility, the ethics committee decided to define as futile only those treatments that cannot accomplish their intended physiological goal. Treatments that are extremely unlikely to be beneficial, are extremely costly, or are of uncertain benefit they considered inappropriate and hence inadvisable.

Although physicians do not have a responsibility to provide futile or inadvisable care,[22] they should not withhold or withdraw life support based solely on their research notions of futility, but instead should rely on institutional or multi-institutional policies.[21] Such a policy has been developed by representatives of major hospitals in Houston, Texas.[13] Under that policy, when a physician determines that an intervention is inadvisable but a patient or surrogate insists that it be provided, the physician first must discuss the reason for his or her judgment, the possibility of transferring care without abandoning the patient, and alternative treatments such as palliative care. If agreement is not reached at this point, the physician must obtain a second opinion from another physician who has examined the patient and must present the case before an institutional review body. If the review body affirms that a treatment is inappropriate, the treatment is terminated, a plan for alternative care is established, and intrainstitutional transfer to another physician to provide the treatment that has been deemed inadvisable is not allowed. On the other hand, if the review body finds that the intervention is appropriate, orders to terminate the treatment are not recognized as valid without patient or surrogate assent.

The Houston collaborative policy is limited in that it was developed by institutional representatives without explicit community involvement. The legal standing of the policy remains uncertain, and it is not clear whether the policy is workable in ICUs or that physicians will follow it rather than openly or surreptitiously limiting care on their own. Nevertheless, the policy represents a commendable approach in balancing patient autonomy and professional and institutional integrity, and its presence seems to have prompted dispute resolution before institutional review bodies are required. Ideally, policies such as this should move society closer to a consensus on which treatments are truly beneficial and how limited resources should be allocated.

REFERENCES

1. American Thoracic Society: Withholding and withdrawing life-sustaining therapy, **Am Rev Respir Dis 144:**726-731, 1991.
2. Asch DA, Hansen-Flaschen J, Lanken PN: Decisions to limit or continue life-sustaining treatment by critical care physicians in the United States: conflicts between physicians' practices and patients' wishes. **Am J Respir Crit Care Med 151:**288-292, 1995.
3. **Barber v. Superior Court,** 195 Cab RPTR, 147 Col. App. 3d 1054 (1983).
4. Butler P, Carton RW, Elpern E, et al: Ethical and moral guidelines for the initiation, continuation, and withdrawal of intensive care, **Chest 97:**949-958, 1990.
5. Civetta JM: Futile care or caregiver frustration? A practical approach, **Crit Care Med 24:**346-351, 1996.
6. Cook DJ, Guyatt GH, Jaeschke R, et al: Determinants in Canadian health care workers of the decision to withdraw life support from the critically ill, **JAMA 273:**703-708, 1995.
7. Council on Ethical and Judicial Affairs, American Medical Association: Decisions near the end of life, **JAMA 267:**2229-2233, 1992.
8. **Cruzan v. Director, Missouri Department of Health,** 497 U.S. 261 (1990).
9. Ethics Committee of the Society of Critical Care Medicine: consensus statement of the Society of Critical Care Medicine's Ethics Committee regarding futile and other possibly inadvisable treatments, **Crit Care Med 25:**887-891, 1997.

10. Faber-Langendoen K: The clinical management of dying patients receiving mechanical ventilation: a survey of physician practice, **Chest 106:**880-888, 1994.
11. Faber-Langendoen K, Bartels DM: Process of forgoing life-sustaining treatment in a university hospital: an empirical study, **Crit Care Med 20:**570-577, 1992.
12. Grenvik A: "Terminal weaning": discontinuance of life-support therapy in the terminally ill patient, **Crit Care Med 11:**394-395, 1983.
13. Halevy A, Brody BA: A multi-institutional collaboration policy on medical futility, **JAMA 276:**571-574, 1996.
14. **In re: Helen Wanglie,** Fourth Judicial District (Dist. Ct. Probates Ct. Div.) PX-91-280, Hennipin County, Minnesota.
15. **In re: Quinlan,** 70 N.J. 10 (1970).
16. Jayes RL, Zimmerman JE, Wagner DP, et al: Do-not-resuscitate orders in intensive care units, **JAMA 270:**2213-2217, 1993.
17. Koch KA, Rodeffer HD, Wears RL: Changing patterns of terminal care management in an intensive care unit, **Crit Care Med 22:**233-243, 1994.
18. Lee DKP, Swinburne AJ, Fedullo AJ, et al: Withdrawing care: experience in a medical intensive care unit, **JAMA 271:**1358-1361, 1994.
19. Luce JM: Conflicts over ethical principles in the intensive care unit, **Crit Care Med 20:**313-315, 1992.
20. Luce JM: Ethical principles in critical care, **JAMA 263:**696-700, 1990.
21. Luce JM: Making decisions about the forgoing of life-sustaining therapy, **Am J Respir Crit Care Med 156:**1715-1718, 1997.
22. Luce JM: Physicians do not have a responsibility to provide futile or unreasonable care if a patient or family insists, **Crit Care Med 23:**760-766, 1995.
23. O'Callahan J, Fink C, Pitts LH, et al: Withholding and withdrawal of life support from patients with severe head injury, **Crit Care Med 23:**1567-1575, 1995.
24. Parker JM, Landry FJ, Phillips YY: Use of do-not-resuscitate orders in an intensive care setting, **Chest 104:**1592-1596, 1993.
25. Prendergast TJ, Luce JM: A national survey of withdrawal of life support from critically ill patients, **Am J Respir Crit Care Med 153:**A360, 1996.
26. Prendergast TJ, Luce JM: Increasing incidence of withholding and withdrawal of life support from the critically ill, **Am J Respir Crit Care Med 155:**15-20, 1997.
27. Ruark JE, Raffin TA: Stanford University Medical Center Committee on Ethics: Initiating and withdrawing life support: principles and practice in adult medicine. **N Engl J Med 318:**25-30, 1988.
28. Smedira NG, Evans BH, Grais LS, et al: Withholding and withdrawal of life support from the critically ill, **N Engl J Med 322:**309-315, 1990.
29. Task Force on Ethics of the Society of Critical Care Medicine: Consensus report on the ethics of forgoing life-sustaining treatments in the critically ill, **Crit Care Med 18:**1435-1439, 1990.
30. The Society of Critical Care Medicine Ethics Committee: Attitudes of critical care medicine professionals concerning forgoing life-sustaining treatments, **Crit Care Med 20:**320-326, 1992.
31. Vincent JL, Parquier JN, Preiser JC, et al: Terminal events in the intensive care unit: review of 258 fatal cases in one year, **Crit Care Med 17:**530-533, 1989.
32. Wilson WC, Smedira NG, Fink C, et al: Ordering and administration of sedatives and analgesics during the withholding and withdrawal of life support from critically ill patients, **JAMA 267:**949-953, 1992.
33. Zimmerman JE, Knaus WA, Sharpe SM, et al: The use and implications of do-not-resuscitate orders in intensive care units, **JAMA 255:**351-356, 1986.

CHAPTER 18

Declaration of Brain Death

GRANT E. GAUGER

Although the functions of the heart and lungs have been recognized for centuries as essential to human survival, it is the activity of the brain that progressively has come to define the life and death of the individual.

Two practical benefits have emerged from such a definition: the ability to focus resources on the care of patients whose brains are not irretrievably damaged and who might recover from illness or injury, and organ donation on behalf of others suffering from advanced disease of any of several organ systems. Intelligent responses to these subjects requires some understanding of the concept of brain death, including its neurological and laboratory features. The clinical applications of such understanding are still evolving.

THE CONCEPT OF BRAIN DEATH

C. Miller Fisher has noted that "human life is best defined in terms of preservation of the brain and mind. Brain function is the final determinant of life, not the beat of the heart. The brain and mind are the essence of mankind; they constitute meaningful life and their absence defines human death."[14] These comments reflect the fact that the heart can continue to act, for a time, when brain activity has been irretrievably lost. Although cardiac death produces brain death, the reverse may not be true over the short term. The same scientific progress that has made modern technological support of critically ill or injured patients so successful has also elicited more careful thought concerning the definition of death.

As Fischer states, "It is one matter to speak of the death of the brain but quite another to use brain death determined critically and electrically as the determinant of death of a person, officially for legal purposes."[14] This recognizes not only the now-accepted identity of death of the brain with the death of the person, but the litigious "climate of general public unease about brain death . . . , partly engendered by sensational fiction," noted by Sweet.[38]

The unease may also be shared by physicians, because published criteria of brain death have provoked controversy and disagreement, and the proliferation of terminology has produced very serious semantic confusion.

The terms *whole brain death, brain death, brainstem death, cerebral death,* and *irreversible coma* have varying implications, as delineated by Pallis.[29] Confusion of the last term with *persistent vegetative state,*[21] clearly not synonymous with brain death, limits its usefulness. Whole brain death implies a presently nonexistent capacity to access activity in every brain area. Cerebral death suggests loss of hemispheric activity underlying higher functions (however, where defined as *total destruction of the brain,* it may be synonymous with brain death). Brain death was defined in the *Report of the President's Commission* (1981) as "the irreversible cessation of all functions of the entire brain, including the brainstem."[18] These definitions and their implications are not trivial, because they determine what conditions, findings, and test results establish brain death. It cannot be declared if it is not defined.

The use of irreversible loss of brain function as the major criterion of death is a modern phenomenon that follows several individual and organizational investigations of the subject. The widely known 1968 Harvard study considered that the comatose patient was dead when responsiveness to external stimuli and inner need was absent.[1] Two clinical examinations performed by a competent physician, with an interval of 24 hours or more between them, were recommended, with supplementation by electroencephalography (EEG) when possible.

In 1981, the President's Commission for the Study of Bioethics and Medicine suggested criteria for brain death that included time between examinations of

6 hours in those patients in whom irreversible injury was known.[18] In the case of anoxic injury, a waiting period of 24 hours was recommended. Ancillary tests were advised in the case of children under 5 and when less than 12 hours had elapsed before the repeat examination.

Although no single set of guidelines for the determination of brain death has been legally adopted by all states, the National Conference of Commissioners on Uniform State Laws was among several organizations endorsing the 1981 *Report of the President's Commission*. This included the statement that "an individual who has sustained either (1) irreversible cessation of circulatory and respiratory function, or (2) irreversible cessation of all functions of the entire brain, including the brainstem, is dead. A determination of death must be made in accordance with accepted medical standards."[18]

Thus the concept of total and irreversible loss of functioning of the whole brain as the determinant of death has received the endorsement of a presidential commission and progressive acceptance by students of the law. The complex sequence of studies of the factors associated with the declaration of brain death has been summarized in a comprehensive review by Black.[4]

Pallis' observation that brainstem death is the "physiological core of brain death" is highly useful in eliminating confusion. It is internally consistent and physiologically sound. As he notes, it "implies an irreversible unconscious patient with irreversible apnea and irreversible loss of brainstem reflexes." Further, "the crucial attribute of irreversibility can only be established by due attention to context. There must be a known and sufficient 'primary diagnosis' to account for the patient's condition, and all reversible causes of brainstem dysfunction must have been excluded. The passage of sufficient time and resort to all relevant therapeutic measures are also essential components of irreversibility."[29]

This emphasis on the brainstem can lead to a practical assessment of neurological findings and the selection of supplementary tests. It is also consistent with the conclusion that "death of the brain occurs when the organ irreversibly loses its capacity to maintain the vital integrative functions regulated by the vegetative and consciousness-mediating centers of the brainstem."[31]

CLINICAL CRITERIA

Criteria for the determination of brain death are concisely outlined in Table 18-1[9] and are more fully developed in the President's Commission study.[18] An outline of clinical tests of brain death is presented in modified form (Table 18-2).[9]

The patient must demonstrate unresponsive coma. Spontaneous movements are usually absent, although rare complex movement of spinal origin has been described.[25] Seizures, shivering (revealing hypothalamic activity), or decerebrate or decorticate posturing indicating brainstem function are not consistent with brain death.[32] By contrast, spinal activity, productive of muscle-stretch reflexes, plantar flexion, plantar withdrawal (triple flexion), or tonic neck and abdominal reflexes may be present and do not exclude brain death.[6]

TABLE 18-1 ■ Criteria for Determination of Brain Death

- Absent cerebral and brainstem function
- Well-defined, irreversible etiology
- Persistent absence of all brain function after observation and/or treatment
- Hypothermia, drug intoxication, metabolic encephalopathy, and shock excluded

TABLE 18-2 ■ Clinical Tests of Brain Death

- Cerebral unresponsiveness
- No spontaneous motor activity
- Absent papillary, corneal, and oculocephalic/oculovestibular reflexes
- Absent cough reflex with deep tracheal suctioning
- No increase in heart rate in response to intravenous administration of atropine
- No respiratory efforts on apnea testing (PA_{CO^2} > 60 mm Hg)

The pupils need not be dilated,[2] but they must be unreactive to light in the absence of major cataract, primary ocular trauma, or agents compromising the light response, including neuromuscular blocking compounds, glutethimide, opiates, scopolamine, dopamine, or atropine.

Absence of the corneal reflex may reflect facial paresis. There is a suggestion that its threshold is influenced by the duration of lid closure.[28]

The oculocephalic (doll's eye) reflex is tested by rotation of the patient's head. Movement of the eye within the orbit indicates retention of some brainstem function.

The oculovestibular (caloric) reflex may persist despite loss of the doll's eye response. It is tested by the infusion of cold water into each ear canal, bathing the tympanic membrane for 20 to 30 seconds, with the head elevated 30 degrees. Ocular motion as a response to this powerful labyrinthine stimulus is inconsistent with complete brainstem failure. Barbiturate or other intoxication and severe disease of the inner ear may compromise this test.

Presence of the cough or gag reflexes reveals function of glossopharyngeal and vagal mechanisms. The latter also may also be assessed by the administration of 1 mg of atropine sulfate intravenously. Absence of an acceleration of heart rate indicates that the vagus nerve was not moderating that rate before its pharmacological suppression.

The significance of respiratory action in the setting of hypercarbia has made the apnea test a widely discussed component of the diagnosis of brain death. Careless performance of the test may render it both invalid and a form of "self-fulfilling prophecy." Preoxygenation with 100% oxygen during mechanical ventilation and introduction of 4 to 6 L/min oxygen flow by intratracheal catheter will permit the development of a hypercarbic state (P_{CO_2} of 60 torr) without accompanying hypoxia.[30] The time required is a function of P_{CO_2} increase of approximately 3 to 6 torr/min and is influenced by several factors, including temperature.[10] The total interval of apneic oxygenation may be minimized by an adjustment of ventilation that permits a pretest rise to high normal level. Monitoring and documentation of oxygen and carbon dioxide levels are important in ensuring that organs are not placed at risk of hypoxia, leading to compromise of later transplantation when appropriate.

Several conditions may undermine or even fully invalidate both clinical and confirmatory testing in the determination of brain death. These include hypothermia, shock, drug intoxication, metabolic coma, and hypophosphatemia.[42] A body temperature lower than 32° C, especially in association with ingestion of alcohol, makes either ancillary testing or an extended period of observation desirable. Similarly, barbiturate intoxication or the presence of diazepam, methaqualone, trichloroethylene, meprobamate, or narcotic or other agents may make the study of brain blood flow advisable in certification of brain death.[18] Brain death simulation by succinylcholine sensitivity, with full recovery, has also been described.[39]

The value of a skillful neurological examination in the determination of brain death can scarcely be overstated. Accomplished in the context of full historical and general physical findings, it forms the basis of this process. It may be performed in any setting, independent of the availability of one or more supplementary tests. These may be helpful, but they do not supplant the clinical assessment of brain function, which remains the cornerstone of the determination. An underlying diagnosis that is reasonable, explains the important clinical facts, and withstands repeated questions is essential. A recent report and subsequent comment emphasize this requirement.[19,41]

CONFIRMATORY TEST

Powner has suggested an outline of confirmatory brain death tests (Table 18-3).[33] Additional, newer studies are in development. The absence of electrical activity on EEG study continues to be the most frequently cited ancillary observation in the establishment of brain death. A single EEG examination conducted with 2μV/mm or higher sensitivity that shows absence of waveform activity during a period of 30 minutes is highly supportive of brain death; however, this conclusion is not justified if hypothermia or drug intoxication is present.[34]

TABLE 18-3 ■ Confirmatory Brain Death Tests

Dependent on neuronal function:
• Clinical examination
• EEG and cerebral function monitors
• Evoked potentials
• Biochemical correlates
Dependent on intracranial blood flow:
• Angiography (contrast)
• Radioisotope angiography
• Ultrasonography
• Digital subtraction angiography/venography
• Computed tomography
• Intracranial pressure
• Echoencephalography
• Ophthalmic artery blood flow

The American EEG Society has specified that "electrocerebral silence (ECS) or electrocerebral inactivity is defined as no electrical activity over 2μV when recording from scalp or referential pairs 10 or more centimeters apart with interelectrode resistance under 10,000 ohms (or impedances under 6,000 ohms), but over 100 ohms."[7] Related technical requirements are important. These include identification of sources of artifact as influenced by the intensive care unit (ICU) environment and by amplification settings.

A repeat study should be considered when doubt about the character or significance of the recording exists. There is no uniform acceptance of the interval between examination. When the criteria of brain death have been met on clinical grounds, repeated testing may not contribute any further "objective" information and may compromise the success of organ transplantation through the further passage of time.

Clinicians should recall that the EEG reflects the activity of a small proportion of cortical neurons and is not a measure of activity in all centers. It does not indicate brainstem processes and cannot exclude the activity of scattered cellular clusters. Residual EEG activity in the presence of a nonfunctioning brainstem has been described.[20] It appears that the EEG only infrequently contributes predictive information not already derived from a thorough neurological examination.[35]

The pressure of electrical activity elicited by visual, auditory, or somatosensory stimulation excludes the diagnosis of brain death.[33] However, such evoked-potential study may provide helpful supplementary data.

The magnitude and character of intracranial blood flow may reflect in a parallel and indirect manner the viability of the brain. The absence of flow on four-vessel angiography has been considered diagnostic of brain death. The usefulness of this test may be greatest in patients whose assessment is complicated by metabolic or pharmacological factors, or hypothermia. A recent article has revealed the value of two-phase spiral computed tomography (CT) in documenting the absence of cerebral blood flow.[12]

Transcranial doppler (TCD) study permits detection of cerebral blood flow. A pattern suggesting an alternating intraluminal motion has been described in brain-dead patients.[36] In a series of 130 clinically brain-dead patients, only one showed a false-negative result, retaining TCD angiographic flow. There were no false-positive results.[11]

Radionuclide imaging can be a valuable indicator of cerebral blood flow. Activity confined to the sagittal sinus has been described in patients with angiographically demonstrated loss of the cerebral circulation.[37] The less invasive and portable nature of the radionuclide method contributes to its usefulness.[16]

Other confirmatory tests that are directly or indirectly reflective of intracranial blood flow include digital subtraction angiography, ultrasonography, ophthalmic artery flow, echoencephalography, and intracranial pressure (ICP) measurement. ICP monitoring may be useful in patients under treatment with large doses of barbiturates, which invalidates EEG findings. Cerebral perfusion pressure approaches zero as ICP reaches or exceeds mean systemic pressure. Loss of the pulsatile character of the ICP tracing usually follows. It has occasionally persisted even when angiography has documented absence of cerebral blood flow.[40]

Although data concerning the cerebral circulation may provide highly significant ancillary support, they are inferential with respect to neuronal activity. Evolving new approaches more directly address the location and extent of cerebral metabolism.

Positron emission tomography (PET) monitors chemical reactions of the brain in real time, providing valuable kinetic, and not simply structural, information; however, its use in this application is currently limited by significant radiopharmaceutical and equipment constraints.

Near infrared spectroscopy is a noninvasive means of assessment of regional cerebral oxygenation.[22] The limitations of its application to the clinical study of brain death have been documented.[23]

SPECT brain perfusion imaging may be used for bedside cerebral angiography employing a portable planar camera. Absence of perfusion on the angiographic phase and lack of cerebral activity on the subsequent static planar or SPECT images are confirmatory findings.[27] The absence of flow voids in magnetic resonance (MR) study can indicate cessation of intracranial blood flow.[26]

Diffusion-weighted magnetic resonance imaging (DWI) can contribute to diagnosis by indicating widespread ischemia, supplementing a T2-weighted demonstration of edema.[24] The combination of apparent diffusion coefficient (ADC) data and DWI can disclose the presence of cytotoxic, versus vasogenic, edema, strongly suggesting an extensive and severe ischemia inconsistent with continued brain function.

Finally, proton MR spectroscopy, when combined with serial MR study, permits the correlation of biochemical with clinical events, both of which can confirm an expected sequence of changes that follows very severe hypoxic-ischemic cerebral injury.[13] A marked decrease in cortical-N-acetylaspartate indicates severe neuronal damage in the acute phase and is followed by an increase in choline, reflecting white matter degeneration. This approach promises to provide more specific and reliable data for the noninvasive identification of the chemistry of neuronal death, including its spatial extent.

DIAGNOSIS OF BRAIN DEATH IN CHILDREN

The determination of brain death in pediatric patients is not fundamentally different from that in adults. It should, however, reflect recognition of the possibility of a greater potential for recovery of the child's brain, especially in infancy. The use of a method of blood flow determination in supplementing the clinical examination is advised when any question exists regarding cerebral function. A task force has specifically addressed these and other related aspects, including recommended observation periods.[17]

For infants of age 7 days to 2 months, two examinations and EEGs separated by at least 48 hours are advised. For ages 2 months to 1 year, two examinations and EEGs with a 24-hour interval, or an examination, EEG, and radionuclide angiographic study demonstrating no visualization of cerebral arteries, are recommended. For patients over 1 year with an "irreversible cause," an observation period of at least 24 hours, without a requirement for laboratory testing, is specified.

The task force noted the difficulty in interpretation of clinical and laboratory findings in infants, and especially in premature newborns. The special circumstances attendant on the determination of brain death in the newborn have been discussed in a recent review.[3] The prognosis associated with hypoxic-ischemic encephalopathy may be obscure in any pediatric age category. A longer observation period, with supplementary blood flow information, may be essential in some of these cases.

DISCUSSION

A clear understanding of the definitions and identification of brain death serves both the patient's family and the health professional interacting with them. Relatives and friends are able to recognize the reality of their loss and are spared the prolonged anguish that uncertainty promotes. They can see and understand the fact and its permanence and can more quickly begin to move past the first shock of death. They can be helped by nurses, social workers, and physicians in the process of acceptance and in handling decisions that cannot be deferred.

The health care team, including intensive care workers, can direct its energies to the care of patients who may benefit from therapy, thereby focusing and conserving human and material resources. Critical care beds and equipment such as ventilators can be made available to patients who urgently need them.

The potential sense of psychological abandonment of the brain-dead patient can be countered by explicit recognition and by the thoughtful explanation of the equivalence of brain death with the death of the individual.

As important as these benefits are, another may transcend them: the potential availability of organs and tissues on behalf of a large and growing number of patients whose lives depend on successful transplantation.

Although the number of patients awaiting organ transplantation far exceeds the number of donors, these in turn represent only a subset of the potential donor pool.[15] Several factors have been shown to influence organ availability. They include the early identification of brain death and its communication to the family in clear and unequivocal terms by a responsible member of the health care team caring for the patient. They also include the character of the request for consideration of organ donation. Such a request should be made only after brain death has been identified and explained to family members, with an interval permitting them to begin the process of acceptance. The request need not be made by those most directly involved in the patient's care at that point. What appears most important in determining the success of the process of organ donation is the skill and experience of the person who raises this question with the family. A representative of the appropriate organ procurement organization who is sensitive to range of personal, cultural, and ethical issues involved in each specific patient's circumstances may most effectively conduct this discussion. In fact, a disconnection or decoupling between the announcement of brain death and the request for organ donation, and between the persons performing these important functions, has been shown to be highly significant in the successful outcome of such requests.

Early identification of brain death can preserve both time and effort. Communication with families by persons best suited through training and temperament can further reduce stress and promote the efficiency of the process. Nevertheless, the application of concepts of brain death to the subjects of organ and tissue donation and transplantation is unavoidably associated with several intellectual and emotional demands on physicians, nurses, and allied health workers. These demands also include attention to the requirements of continuing physiological support of the organ donor following declaration of death.[8]

Currently there appear to be two principal potential remedies for the current critical dependence on human organ donation. They are the application of safe and practical xenotransplantation and the creation of fully artificial replacement organs. Both will demand the highest degree of imagination and persistence in surmounting current technological challenges. Both may have significant promise in addressing the current crisis in organ availability by circumventing it.

Meanwhile the clinical, psychological, and administrative difficulties associated with organ donation can only be minimized, not eliminated, but the final result can be the creation of new hope, often from tragedy, through the return to normal health of another person. And every such creation is, as Albert Camus expressed it, "a gift to the future."[5]

REFERENCES

1. A definition of irreversible coma. Report of the Ad Hoc Committee of the Harvard Medical School to examine the definition of brain death, **JAMA 205:**337, 1968.
2. An appraisal of the criteria of cerebral death: a summary statement: a collaborative study, **JAMA 237:**982, 1976.
3. Ashwal S: Brain death in the newborn. Current perspectives, **Clinics in Perinatology 24:**859-882, 1997.
4. Black P McL: Brain death (Parts 1 & 2). **N Engl J Med 299:**338, 393, 1978.
5. Camus A: **The Myth of Sisyphus.** New York: Vintage Books, 1959, p 151.
6. Caronna JJ: The neurological intensive care unit, in Parrillo JE, Ayres SM (eds): **Major Issues in Critical Care Medicine.** Baltimore: Williams & Wilkins, 1984, p 202.
7. Cohen RJ, Henry CE: The electroencephalogram in head injury, in Becker DP, Gudeman SK (eds): **Textbook of Head Injury.** Philadelphia: WB Saunders, 1989, p 273.
8. Darby JM, Powner DJ, Stein KL, et al: Management of the organ donor, in Rippe JM, Irwin RS, Alpert JS, et al (eds): **Intensive Care Medicine.** Boston: Little, Brown, 1991, pp 1657-1659.

9. Darby JM, Stein K, Grenvik A, et al: Approach to management of the heartbeating "brain dead" organ donor, **JAMA 261**:2224, 1989.
10. Dominguez-Roldan JM, Berrera-Chocon JM, Murillo-Cabezas F, et al: Clinical factors influencing the increment of blood carbon dioxide during the apnea test for the diagnosis of brain death, **Transplantation Proceedings 31**:2599-2600, 1999.
11. Ducrocq X, Braun M, Debrouverie M, et al: Brain death and trancranial Doppler: experience in 130 cases of brain dead paitents, **J Neurol Sci 160**:41-46, 1998.
12. Dupas B, Gayet-Delacroix M, Villers D, et al: Diagnosis of brain death using two-phase spiral CT, **AJNR Am J Neuroradiol 19**:641-647, 1998.
13. Falini A, Barkovich AJ, Calabrese G, et al: Progressive brain failure after diffuse hypoxic ischemic brain injury: a serial MR and proton MR spectroscopic study. **ANJR Am J Neuroradiol 19**:648-652, 1998.
14. Fischer CM: Brain death—a review of the concept, **J Neurosci Nurs 23**:330,1991.
15. Garrison RN, Bentley FR, Raque GH, et al: There is an answer to the shortage of organ donors, **SG&O 173**:391, 1991.
16. Goodman JM, Heck LL, Moore BD: Confirmation of brain death with portable isotope angiography: a review of 204 consecutive cases, **Neurosurgery 16**:492, 1985.
17. Guidelines for the determination of brain death in children, **Ann Neurol 21**:616, 1987.
18. Guidelines for the determination of death. Report of the medical consultants on the diagnosis of death to the president's commission for the study of ethical problems in medicine and biomedical and behavioral research, **JAMA 246**:338, 393, 1978.
19. Hughes R, McGuire G: Neurologic disease and the determination of brain death: the importance of a diagnosis, **Crit Care Med 25**:1923-1924, 1997.
20. Jennett B, Gleave J, Wilson P: Brain death in three neurosurgical units, **Br Med J 282**:533, 1981.
21. Jennett B, Plum, F: Persistent vegetative state after brain damage: a syndrome in search of a name, **Lancet 1**:734, 1972.
22. Kytta J, Ohman J, Tanskanen P, et al: Extracranial contribution to cerebral oximetry, **Anesthesiology 11**:252-254, 1999.
23. Lewis, S: Non concordance between near infra-red spectroscopy and cerebral oxygen saturation in brain death, in **Proceedings of the Tenth International ICP Symposium.** New York: Springer-Verlag, 1998.
24. Lovblad K-O, Bassetti C: Diffusion-weighted magnetic resonance imaging in brain death, **Stroke 31**:539-542, 2000.
25. Mandel S, Areanas A, Scasta D: Spinal automatism in cerebral death, **N Engl J Med 307**:501, 1982.
26. Matsumura A, Meguro K, Tsurushima H, et al: Magnetic resonance imaging of brain death, **Neurol Med Chir 36**: 166-171, 1996.
27. Mettler, FA Jr, Guilerteau J: **Essentials of Nuclear Medicine,** 4th ed. Philadelphia: WB Saunders, 1998, pp. 82-83.
28. O'Leary DJ, Millodot M: Brain death and the corneal reflex. **Lancet** 2:1379, 1980.
29. Pallis C: Brainstem death, in Vinken PJ, Bruyn GW, Klawans HL, et al (eds): **Head Injury. Handbook of Clinical Neurology,** vol 57. Amsterdam: Elsevier, 1990, pp 441-496.
30. Pitts LH, Kaktis J, Caronna J, et al: Brain death, apneic diffusion oxygenation, and organ transplantation, **J Trauma 18**:180, 1978.
31. Plum F, Posner JB: **The Diagnosis of Stupor and Coma**, 3rd ed. Philadelphia: FA Davis, 1982, p 322.
32. Polacek DJ, Grenvik A: Brain death, in Parrillo JE (ed): **Current Therapy in Critical Care Medicine**, Philadelphia: B.C. Decker, 1987, p 236.
33. Powner DJ: The diagnosis of brain death in the adult patient, **J Intesive Care Med 2**:184, 1987.
34. Powner, DJ: Drug-associated isoelectric EEGs: a hazard in brain-death certification. **JAMA 236**:1123, 1976.
35. Powner DJ, Fromm GH: The electroencephalogram in the determination of brain death, **N Engl J Med 300**:502, 1979.
36. Ropper AH, Hehne SM, Wechsler L: Transcranial Doppler in brain death, **Neurology 37**:1733, 1987.
37. Schwartz JA, Baxter J, Brill D, et al: Radionuclide cerebral imaging confirming brain death, **JAMA 249**:246, 1983.
38. Sweet WH: Brain death (editorial), **N Engl J Med 299**: 410, 1978.
39. Tyson RN: Simulation of cerebral death by succinylcholine sensitivity, **Arch Neurol 20**:409, 1974.
40. Wilkinson HA: Intracranial pressure monitoring: techniques and pitfalls, in Cooper, PR (ed): **Head Injury,** 2nd ed. Baltimore: Williams and Wilkins, 1987, pp 220-222.
41. William M, Suarez J: Brain death determination in adults: more than meets the eye, **Crit Care Med 25**:1787-1788, 1997.
42. Young GB, Amaker AL, Paulseth JE, et al: Hypophosphatemia versus brain death, **Lancet 1**:617, 1982.

Index

A

A-a (alveolar-arterial) gradient, 3
  in shunt, 4
A/C (assist control) ventilation, 4
Abdominal compartment syndrome, 152–153
Abscess
  cerebral, 104–105
    amebic, 115
  epidural, 100–101, 101t
  subgaleal, 100
Acalculous cholecystitis, 154
Acanthamoebae infection, 114
Acetazolamide, for elevated ICP, 201
Acid-base disorders, 72–74
  metabolic, 73–74
  respiratory, 72–73
Acidosis
  ischemic stroke and, 175
  metabolic, 73–74
  respiratory, 72–73
Acquired immunodeficiency syndrome, 96. *See also* Human immunodeficiency virus infection
  opportunistic CNS infections and neoplasms in, 109–110
ACTH (adrenocorticotropic hormone), 89
Actinomyces israelii infection, 114
Actinomycosis, 114
Acute hypoxia, in pediatric patient, 211–212
Acute lung injury, 149
Acute respiratory distress syndrome
  fluid restriction in, 150
  inflammatory modification in, 150–151
  management, 6–7
  PEEP in, 150
    effectiveness, 6
  phases, 149
  ventilator use in
    practices, 150
    weaning criteria, 150
Acute tubular necrosis, renal failure and, 156
Addisonian crisis, 89–90
Adenosine triphosphate level, in ischemic stroke, 175
ADH. *See* Antidiuretic hormone
Admittance, to ICU
  head injury, criteria for, 126–127
  stroke patients, criteria for, 176–177
Adrenal insufficiency, 89–90
Adrenocorticotropic hormone, 89
AIDS. *See* Acquired immunodeficiency syndrome
Airway
  in infant, 209f
    intubation, 208–209, 209t
  management
    in multisystem injury, 145–146
    in spinal cord injury, 137–138
Alkalosis
  metabolic, 73
  respiratory, 72
Alveolar-arterial gradient, 3
  in shunt, 4
Alveolar ventilation, 1
Amebic brain abscess, 115
Amino acids, excitatory, in ischemic stroke, 174–175
e-Aminocaproic acid, for subarachnoid rebleeding, 163
Aminosteroids
  for multisystem injury patient, 158
  pediatric use, 210–211
Analgesia
  in multisystem injury patient, 158–159
  in postoperative brain tumor patient, 200
Aneurysmal subarachnoid hemorrhage. *See* Subarachnoid hemorrhage
Angioplasty, for vasospasm, 164–165
Antacid therapy, in spinal cord injury patient, 140
Antibiotics
  for CNS bacterial infections, 103t
    in critically-ill patient, 106–107, 106t
    empiric, 101t, 102t
  prophylactic
    in critically-ill patient, 105–106
    in trauma patient, 156–157
Anticoagulation
  deep vein thrombosis and, 155
  intracerebral hemorrhage and, 182
  in stroke patient, 177
Anticonvulsants, 193
  in head injury patient, 133
  IV formulations, 193t
  prophylactic use, 194
Antidiuretic hormone, 56, 201
  inappropriate levels. *See* Syndrome of inappropriate ADH
Antiepileptic drugs, 193
  IV formulations, 193t
  prophylactic use, 194
Antifibrinolytic agents, for subarachnoid rebleeding, 163
Antigen-presenting cells, 96
Antiinflammatory therapy, for ARDS, 150
Antioxidant therapy, for ARDS, 150
APCs (antigen-presenting cells), 96
Apnea, postventilation, 23
Apneustic breathing, 23
ARDS. *See* Acute respiratory distress syndrome
Arginine vasopressin, 56–57, 89
Arterial blood gases, neurological status and, 26–27
Aspergillosis, 113–114
Aspergillus sp. infection, 113–114
Assist control ventilation, 4
Ataxic breathing, 23
ATP (adenosine triphosphate) level, in ischemic stroke, 175
Atrial natriuretic peptide, sodium regulation by, 58–59
Autonomic control, pediatric circulatory system and, 212
Autoregulation, cerebral. *See* Cerebral autoregulation
Autotransfusion, in multisystem injury, 148
AVP (arginine vasopressin), 56–57, 89
Axonal damage, 126

B

Bacterial infections
  in AIDS patients, 109–110
  central nervous system, 99–107. *See also* Central nervous system infections, bacterial
Bacteriuria, in spinal cord injury patient, 141
BAER (brainstem auditory evoked responses), in pediatric patient, 216
Barbiturate coma, 130
Barbiturates, for elevated ICP, 52
  in head injury patient, 130
  in pediatric patient, 209–210
Barotrauma, 5
Basal energy expenditure, 85
Basal metabolic expenditure, 84
BEE (basal energy expenditure), 85
Benzodiazepines
  for epileptic seizures, 193
    IV formulation, 193t
  for multisystem injury, 157–158
Bicarbonate therapy, for metabolic acidosis, 149
Blastomyces dermatitidis infection, 113
Blood
  oxygen content in, 1–3, 2f
    improving in head injury patient, 128
  and oxyhemoglobin dissociation curve, 1–2, 2f
  viscosity, 31
Blood flow
  cerebral. *See* Cerebral blood flow
  velocity, vessel radius and, 38
Blood pressure
  management
    in intracerebral hemorrhage, 184–185
    in spinal cord injury, 140
    in stroke patient, 177
  measuring, 22–23
Blood volume
  cerebral. *See* Cerebral blood volume
  cerebral blood flow and, 48, 48f
  in pediatric patient, 211

Bloodstream infections, in critically-ill patients, 99
BME (basal metabolic expenditure), 84
Body compartments, water and electrolyte distribution in, 55
Body temperature
  measuring, 22
  monitoring in intracranial hypertension, 50
Body water
  balance disorders, 64–72. *See also individual disorders*
  in critically-ill patient, 59–64
  distribution, 55, 56f
  in pediatric patient, 217, 217f
  regulation, 56–57
  transcapillary flux, 57–58
Brain. *See also* Cerebral *entries*
  abscess, 104–105, 115
  autoregulation and. *See* Cerebral autoregulation
  blood flow in. *See* Cerebral blood flow
  compliance/elastance, 48–49
  cytokine synthesis in, 97t
  edema. *See* Cerebral edema
  injury to. *See* Brain injury
  metabolism, 39–40
    metabolic coupling, 40–41
    monitoring techniques, 41–43
  in neonate, 214–215, 214f
  oxygen in, measuring. *See* Brain oximetry
  tumors. *See* Brain tumors
Brain death
  clinical criteria, 230–231, 230t
  concept, 229–230
  confirmatory tests, 231–232, 231t
  diagnosing in children, 232–233
  organ procurement and, 233
  psychological and practical sequelae, 233
  terminology, 229
  transcranial color Doppler tracing in, 38, 39f
Brain injury
  ischemic. *See also* Ischemic stroke
    mechanisms, 174t
    vasospasm and, 164
  in pediatric patient, 214–215
Brain oximetry
  in CBF measurement, 39
  in metabolic monitoring, 41
Brain tumors
  and CNS physiology, 197–198
  postoperative management, 198–203
    fluid and electrolytes, 201–202
    Increased ICP, 199–201, 200t
    respiratory system, 201
    seizures, 199
  preoperative management, 198
  spontaneous hemorrhage into, 182
Brainstem function, assessment of, 25–26. *See also* Neurological examination
Breathing
  in multisystem injury resuscitative phase, 145–146
  patterns, monitoring, 23
Bupivacaine, for multisystem injury, 159

C

CAA (cerebral amyloid angiopathy), in intracerebral hemorrhage, 180–182
Calcium-blocking drugs, for vasospasm prevention, 164
Calcium levels, in ischemic stroke, 175
Calorie requirements, in pediatric patient, 217, 217t–218t
Calpains, axonal damage and, 126
Candida albicans infection, 113
Carbamazepine
  for epileptic seizures, 193
  prophylactic, in head injury patients, 133
Carbon dioxide
  gas exchange and, 1–4, 2f, 3f
  monitoring in pediatric patient, 208
  partial pressure, 1
  vasoresponsivity, 33
Cardiac circuit, 11, 12f
Cardiac contractility
  defined, 13
  force of, factors determining, 13
  management, 18
  monitoring, 15
Cardiac output. *See also* Hemodynamics
  defined, 11
  monitoring, 15
Cardiogenic shock, in neurotrauma, 129
Cardiopulmonary resuscitation
  failed, 225
  life support and, 221, 226
Cardiorespiratory variables, 16f
Cardiovascular system
  in head injury patient, 127
  hemodynamic stability and. *See* Hemodynamics
  in postoperative brain tumor patient, 201
  in spinal cord injury patient, 139–140
  in subarachnoid hemorrhage, 166
CBF. *See* Cerebral blood flow
CBV (cerebral blood volume), in subarachnoid hemorrhage, 161
$CD4^+$ cells, 96
Central nervous system infections
  bacterial, 99–107
    antibiotic therapy for, 103t
      in critically-ill patients, 106–107, 106t
      empiric, 101t, 102t
      prophylactic, 105–106
    brain abscess, 104–105
    epidural abscess, 100–101
    meningitis, 101–104, 102t
    osteomyelitis, 100
    postoperative, 105
    subdural empyema, 104
    subgaleal abscess, 100
  fungal, 112–114
    actinomycosis, 114
    aspergillosis, 113–114
    blastomycosis, 113
    candidiasis, 113
    coccidiomycosis, 112–113
    cryptococcosis, 112
    histoplasmosis, 113
    nocardiosis, 114
    phycomycosis, 114
  in head injury patient, 133
  opportunistic, in AIDS, 109–110
  parasitic, 114–115
    amebic brain abscess, 115
    echinococcosis, 115
    meningoencephalitis, 115
    neurocysticercosis, 114–115
  prion, 111–112
  viral, 107–111
    herpes simplex encephalitis, 108–109
    human immunodeficiency virus, 109–110
    Reye's syndrome and, 110–111
Central venous pressure, 13, 14, 16, 61
  in head injury patient, 129
    monitoring, 127–128
  in intracerebral hemorrhage, 185
  in multisystem injury patient, 146, 147
Cerebral amyloid angiopathy, in intracerebral hemorrhage, 180–181
Cerebral artery spasm, TCD tracing in, 38, 38f
Cerebral autoregulation, 29, 31–34
  Cushing's response and, 34
  ischemic penumbra and thresholds, 33–34
  limits, 32–33, 32f
  theories, 33
  vasoresponsivity, 33
Cerebral blood flow, 29–31
  autoregulation and, 29, 31–34
  and blood volume, 48, 48f
  and cerebral metabolism, 39–40
  in CNS physiology, 197–198
  in ischemic stroke, 174
  measurement methods
    at bedside, 34
    continuous, 36–37
    in head injury patient, 131
    imaging modalities, 34–36
    indirect, 37–39
  normal values, 31f
  in pediatric patient, 215–216, 215t
  physiological formulas, 30f
  in subarachnoid hemorrhage, 161
  in vasospasm, 164
Cerebral blood flow/metabolic coupling, 40–41
Cerebral blood volume, in subarachnoid hemorrhage, 161
Cerebral edema, 48, 198
  in Reye's syndrome, 111
  stroke-associated, 177
Cerebral ischemia. *See* Ischemic stroke
Cerebral perfusion pressure, 31, 32f
  in CNS physiology, 197
  in head injury patient, 129
    management, 130
    monitoring, 127
  in subarachnoid hemorrhage, 161
Cerebral salt wasting syndrome, 65
  in head injury patient, 132
  in pediatric patient, 218
Cerebrospinal fluid, 47
  CNS bacterial infections and, 99
  in CNS physiology, 197
  drainage, 50
    in postoperative brain tumor patient, 201
Cerebrovascular system, pathophysiology and monitoring, 29–43
Cheyne-Stokes respirations, 23
Children's Coma Scale, 213, 213t
Cholecystitis, acalculous, 154
Cisatracurium, for multisystem injury, 158
CJD (Creutzfeldt-Jakob disease), 111

Closed head injury, admittance to ICU with, 126–127
CMV (cytomegalovirus) infection, in AIDS patients, 110
CNS. *See* Central nervous system
CO. *See* Cardiac output
Coagulopathy
  diffuse intravascular. *See* Disseminated intravascular coagulation
  intracerebral hemorrhage and, 182
  in multisystem injury, 148–149
Coccidioides immitis infection, 112–113
Colloid solutions, 62, 62t
  in multisystem injury resuscitative phase, 147–148
  vs. crystalloid solutions, 63
Colonic ileus, in multisystem injury patient, 153–154
Compliance
  cerebral, 48–49
  lung, 4–5, 5f
Computed tomography
  in brain death determination, 232
  in deep vein thrombosis diagnosis, 155
  in head injury, 127
  in intracerebral hemorrhage, 180, 181f–182f
  in ischemic stroke evaluation, 176
  of pediatric head, 216
  in subarachnoid hemorrhage, 162
  in vasospasm diagnosis, 164
Computed tomography angiography, in subarachnoid hemorrhage, 162
Consciousness level. *See also* Neurological examination
  abnormal, motor assessment in, 26
  assessment of, 24–25
  in pediatric patient, 213
Contractility. *See* Cardiac contractility
Core body temperature
  measuring, 22
  monitoring in intracranial hypertension, 50
Corneal reflex, in brainstem function assessment, 25
  brain death and, 230
Cough reflex, brain death and, 230–231
CPP. *See* Cerebral perfusion pressure
CPR. *See* Cardiopulmonary resuscitation
Creutzfeldt-Jakob disease, 111
Critically-ill patient
  acid-base disorders in, 72–74. *See also individual disorders*
  fluid and electrolytes in
    changes, 59
    disorders, 64–72. *See also individual disorders*
    requirements, 59–60
  infectious disease in
    bacterial, of CNS, antibiotic therapy for, 106–107, 106t
    of bloodstream, 99
    pneumonia, 98
    sinusitis, 98–99
    of urinary tract, 99
  volume resuscitation in, 60–61, 61t
    fluids for, 61–64, 62t
Cruzan v. *Director, Missouri Department of Health* (1990), 223
Cryptococcus neoformans infection, 112–113
  in AIDS patients, 110
Crystalloid solutions, 62, 62t
  in multisystem injury resuscitative phase, 147
  vs. colloid solutions, 63
CSF (cerebrospinal fluid), 47
CTA (computed tomography angiography), in subarachnoid hemorrhage, 162
Cushing's reflex, 23
Cushing's triad, autoregulation and, 34
CVP. *See* Central venous pressure
Cytokines, 96t
  synthesis in brain, 97t
Cytomegalovirus infection, in AIDS patients, 110
Cytotoxic edema, cerebral, 198

D

Dead space ventilation, 1
Decompressive craniectomy, for elevated ICP, 131
Decubitus ulcers, in spinal cord injury patient, 141
Deep vein thrombosis
  following spinal cord injury, 139
  in head injury patient, 133
  in postoperative brain tumor patient, 203
  prophylactic measures for, 155
  signs and symptoms, 155
  in subarachnoid hemorrhage, 166
Dehydration. *See* Cerebral salt wasting syndrome
Delayed axotomy, 126
Delayed ischemic deficits, in subarachnoid hemorrhage, 161, 164
Dextran solution, 62, 62t
Diabetes insipidus, 67–69
  in head injury patient, 132
Digital subtraction angiography, in subarachnoid hemorrhage, 162
Disseminated intravascular coagulation
  in head injury patient, 133
  in multisystem injury, 148–149
  in postoperative brain tumor patient, 202–203
Diuretic agents
  for intracranial hypertension, 50–51
  intravenous, 17, 17f
DNR (do not resuscitate) order, 223, 226
Doll's eye maneuver, 26
  brain death and, 230
DSA (digital subtraction angiography), in subarachnoid hemorrhage, 162
DVT. *See* Deep vein thrombosis
DWI (diffusion weighted MRI). *See* Magnetic resonance diffusion imaging

E

ECG. *See* Electrocardiography
Echinococcus granulosus infection, 115
Echinococcus multilocularis infection, 115
Edema
  cerebral, 48, 198
  neurogenic pulmonary, following spinal cord injury, 139
  pulmonary, in subarachnoid hemorrhage, 166
EEG. *See* Electroencephalography
EKG. *See* Electrocardiography
Electrocardiography
  in ischemic stroke evaluation, 176
  neurological status and, 27
  in pediatric patient, 208
Electrocerebral silence, 231
Electroencephalography
  in brain death determination, 229, 231
    in children, 232
  continuous, in pediatric patient, 216
  in status epilepticus, 192
Electrolytes. *See* Fluids and electrolytes
Embolism, pulmonary. *See* Pulmonary embolism
Empyema
  subdural, 104
  treatment, 101t
Encephalitis, herpes simplex, 108–109
Endocrine system, 89
  disturbances in, 89–91
Endotracheal intubation
  in head injury patient, 128
  in head injury patient, indications for, 128
  in multisystem injury, 146
Endovascular techniques, for vasospasm management, 164–165
Energy requirements
  calculation, 84–85, 85f
  predicting, in head-injured patient, 85, 85f
Enteral nutrition, 87
  in spinal cord injury patient, 140
  and stress gastritis prevention, 153
Epidural abscess, 100–101, 101t
Epidural analgesia, for multisystem injury, 159
Epilepsy
  diagnosis, 191
  seizures in
    characterization, 191
    conditions causing, 191–192
    lesional, 192
    postoperative, 192
    posttraumatic, 191–192
    precipitation in brain tumor patients, 198
    prophylactic measures, 192, 194
  treatment, 192–193
Ethics, life support and, 221–222
Etomidate, pediatric use, 210
Euvolemia, in intracerebral hemorrhage management, 185
Excitatory amino acids, in ischemic stroke, 174–175
Exotoxins, bacterial production of, 95–96
Extubation, indications for, 151

F

Fatal familial insomnia, 111
Feeding
  enteral. *See* Enteral nutrition
  oral, 88
  and overfeeding, complications of, 84, 84t
  parenteral. *See* Total parenteral nutrition
  timing, 88
Fentanyl, in multisystem injury patient, 159
FFP (fresh frozen plasma) transfusion, for intracerebral hemorrhage, 183
Flexion, abnormal, 26

Flowmetry, in CBF measurement
  laser Doppler, 37
  thermal diffusion, 37
Fluid restriction, in ARDS, 150
Fluids and electrolytes
  balance disorders, 64–72. *See also individual disorders*
  in critically-ill patient, 59–64
  distribution in body compartments, 55
  nutritional requirement and status, 86
  in pediatric patient, requirements, 217–218, 217f, 217t–218t, 218t
  in postoperative brain tumor patient, 201–202
  regulation, 56–57
  for resuscitation, 61–64, 61t, 62t, 64f
    in intracerebral hemorrhage, 185
  transcapillary flux, 57–58
Fosphenytoin, for epileptic seizures, 193
  IV formulation, 193t
Fracture, depressed skull, 126
Functional residual capacity, 4–5, 5f
Fungal infections
  in AIDS patients, 110
  central nervous system, 112–114. *See also* Central nervous system infections, fungal
Furosemide, for elevated ICP in postoperative brain tumor patients, 201

G
Gabapentin, prophylactic, in head injury patients, 133
Gag response, 26
  brain death and, 230–231
Gastritis
  in postoperative brain tumor patient, 203
  stress, in multisystem injury patient, 153
Gastrointestinal system
  in head injury patient, 133
  in postoperative brain tumor patient, 203
  in spinal cord injury patient, 140
  in subarachnoid hemorrhage, 167
GCS. *See* Glasgow Coma Scale
Generalized tonic-clonic status epilepticus, 192
Genitourinary system, in spinal cord injury, 141
Glasgow Coma Scale, 24, 24f. *See also* Neurological examination
  in head injury evaluation, 125
  modified, for pediatric use, 213, 213t
Glucocorticoid steroids, for elevated ICP in postoperative brain tumor patients, 201

H
Haloperidol, for multisystem injury patient, 158
Head injury
  cardiopulmonary monitoring and management in, 127–128
  circulatory dysfunction management in, 128–131
  energy requirements in, 85, 85f
  hyperventilation therapy in, 128
  ICU admittance criteria, 126–127
  mechanisms, 125–126
  metabolic consequences, 83–84, 84f
  metabolic management in, 131–132
  mild, 125
  moderate, 125
  neurological monitoring in, 127
  nutritional management in, 132
  respiratory failure management in, 127–128
  severe, 125
  withholding and withdrawal of life support in, 224–225
Heart rate, monitoring, 23. *See also* Cardiac *and* Cardio- *entries*
Hematological system, in postoperative brain tumor patient, 202–203
Hematoma evacuation, in intracerebral hemorrhage, 183
  new approaches in, 185
Hemodynamics
  cerebral, in pediatric patient, 215–216, 215t, 216f
  intracranial, of subarachnoid hemorrhage, 161
  monitoring, 14–15, 14f, 15f
  stabilized, maintaining, 15–18
Hemofiltration, continuous venovenous, 156
Hemorrhage
  gastrointestinal
    in head injury patient, 133
    in spinal cord injury patient, 140
  intraventricular, hydrocephalus from, 185
  nontraumatic intracerebral, 180–186. *See also* Nontraumatic intracerebral hemorrhage
  subarachnoid. *See* Subarachnoid hemorrhage
Herniation, in intracerebral hemorrhage, 183
Herpes simplex encephalitis, 108–109
Histamine receptor antagonists, spinal cord injury patient and, 140
Histoplasma capsulatum infection, 113
HIV infection. *See* Human immunodeficiency virus infection
Host defense system, infectious disease and, 95–96
Host-microorganism interaction, 95
HSV (herpes simplex) encephalitis, 108–109
Human immunodeficiency virus infection, 109–110. *See also* Acquired immunodeficiency syndrome
  primary neurological sequelae, 109
Hydatid cysts, 115
Hydrocephalus, 47–48
  in brain tumor patients, 198
  from intraventricular hemorrhage, 185
  in subarachnoid hemorrhage, 165
Hydroxyethylstarch solution, 62, 62t
Hypercapnia
  neurological status and, 27
  permissive, 7
Hyperglycemia, cerebral metabolism and, 40
  in head injury patient, 132
Hypermetabolic response, to multisystem injury, 154
Hypernatremia
  in head injury patient, 132
  and hyperosmolarity, 66–69, 68f
  in postoperative brain tumor patient, 202
Hyperosmolar therapy, for elevated ICP in head injury patient, 130
Hyperosmolarity, hypernatremia and, 66–69, 68f
Hypertension
  chronic, in intracerebral hemorrhage, 180
  intracranial. *See* Intracranial hypertension
  in pediatric patient, 212
  in stroke patient management, 177
Hyperthermia
  malignant, in multisystem injury, 158
  in stroke patient, 177
Hypertonic-hyperoncotic fluid resuscitation, 63
Hypocalcemia, 70
Hypoglycemia
  cerebral metabolism and, 40
  in stroke patient management, 177
Hypokalemia, 69–70
Hypomagnesemia, 71–72
Hyponatremia, 64–66
  causes, 64–65
  in head injury patient, 132
  in pediatric patient, 218
  in postoperative brain tumor patient, 202
  in subarachnoid hemorrhage, 165–166
  treatment, 65–66, 66t
Hypophosphatemia, 70–71
Hypotension
  neurological status and, 26–27
  in stroke patient management, 177
Hypotensive agents, 17, 18f
Hypothermia, in multisystem injury, 148
Hypothermia therapy, for elevated ICP, 52
  in head injury patient, 130–131
Hypothyroidism
  signs and symptoms, 90, 90t
  treatment, 90
Hypovolemia, 60
Hypovolemic hyponatremia, in postoperative brain tumor patient, 202
Hypovolemic shock
  in multisystem injury, 146–147
  in neurotrauma, 128–129
Hypoxia
  acute, in pediatric patient, 211–212
  neurological status and, 26, 27
  in severe head injury, 126

I
ICH (intracerebral hemorrhage), nontraumatic. *See* Nontraumatic intracerebral hemorrhage
ICP. *See* Intracranial pressure
Ileus, colonic, in multisystem injury patient, 153–154
IMV (intermittent mandatory ventilation), 4
Infant
  airway, 209f
    intubation, 208–209, 209t
  cerebral blood flow in, 215, 215t
  ICP control in, 216, 216f
  mechanical ventilation in, 211
  reflexes in, 213
  respiratory failure in, 208
  skull in, 213–214

Infections
  central nervous system. *See also* Central nervous system infections
    bacterial, 99–107
    fungal, 112–114
    parasitic, 114–115
    prion, 111–112
    viral, 107–111
  and host defense system, 95–96
  inflammatory response in, 96
  nosocomial. *See* Nosocomial infections
  opportunistic, in AIDS patients
    bacterial, 109–110
    fungal, 110
    parasitic, 110
    viral, 110
  pulmonary, in head injury patient, 133
  urinary tract
    in critically-ill patient, 99
    in head injury patient, 133
Inflammatory modification
  in ARDS, 150–151
  in ischemic stroke, 175
Inflammatory response, to infection, 96
Insomnia, fatal familial, 111
Intensive care unit
  neonatal, monitoring head injury in, 127
  patient in. *See* Critically-ill patient
Intermittent mandatory ventilation, 4
Intraabdominal organ perfusion, in abdominal compartment syndrome, 152
Intracellular volume, regulation of, 57
Intracerebral hemorrhage, nontraumatic. *See* Nontraumatic intracerebral hemorrhage
Intracranial pressure.
  in brain death determination, 232
  and cerebral perfusion pressure, 31, 32f, 129, 197
  CNS physiology and, 197–198
  Cushing's reflex and, 23
  elevated. *See* Intracranial hypertension
  in head injury patient
    monitoring, 129
    treatment, 129–131
  measuring, 21, 22
  in pediatric patient, 215–216, 216f
    assessment of, 213
  in postoperative brain tumor patients
    monitoring, 199–200
    treatment, 200–201, 200t
  in stroke patient, 177–178
  in subarachnoid hemorrhage, 161
    intravenous monitoring, 162
  volume resuscitation and, 61
Intracranial pressure volume curve, 47, 47f
Intravenous t-PA therapy, for ischemic stroke, 175–176, 176t
Intubation
  for airway management
    in multisystem injury, 146
    in spinal cord injury, 137–138
    tracheal, in infant, 208–209, 209t
  endotracheal
    in head injury patient, 128
    in multisystem injury, 146
Ischemic penumbra, 33–34
Ischemic stroke, 173–180
  background and etiologies, 173–174
  evaluation and treatment, 175–176, 176t
    management strategies, 176t
    thrombolytic therapy, 176t
  future directions in, 178–180
  management issues, 176–177
  mechanisms, 174t
  middle cerebral artery, 178, 178f
    treatment protocols, 179–180, 179f
  neuronal viability and, 174, 174f
  pathophysiology, 174–175
  severe head injury and, 126
IVH (intraventricular hemorrhage), hydrocephalus from, 185

J

JC virus infection, in AIDS patients, 110
Jugular desaturation, diagnosing and treating, 42, 43f
Jugular venous oxygen saturation, monitoring, 41–42
  in head injury patient, 131

K

Ketamine, pediatric use, 210
Kety-Schmidt technique, CBF measurement, 34
Kidney
  in abdominal compartment syndrome, 152
  in multisystem injury patient
    failure, 155–156
    renal replacement therapy, 156
  in pediatric patient, 218
Kuru, 111

L

Lidocaine, pediatric use, 210
Life support, withholding and withdrawing
  clinical aspects, 223–225
  complexity, 221
  conflict resolution in, 227
  ethical aspects, 221–222
  incidence, 223–224
  legal aspects, 222–223
  national survey on, 225
  reasons for, 225–227
  in severe head injury, 224–225
  techniques, 225–227
Lindegaard ratio, 38
Lorazepam
  for epileptic seizures, 193
    IV formulation, 193t
  for multisystem injury patient, 157–158
Lung compliance, 4–5, 5f
Lung injury
  acute, 149
  barotrauma, 5
  diffuse alveolar, 6
  ventilator-associated, 5
Lungs. *See also* Pulmonary *and* Respiratory *entries*
  infections, in head injury patient, 133
  injury to. *See* Lung injury
  physiology. *See also* Respiratory function
    gas exchange in, 1–4, 2f, 3f
    ventilation in, 1
  in subarachnoid hemorrhage, 166
Lysosomal inhibition proteins, viral, 95–96

M

Magnetic resonance angiography, in subarachnoid hemorrhage, 162
Magnetic resonance diffusion imaging
  in brain death determination, 232
  in CBF measurement, 34, 35f
Magnetic resonance imaging, in intracerebral hemorrhage, 183
Magnetic resonance perfusion imaging, in CBF measurement, 34–35
Magnetic resonance spectroscopy
  in brain death determination, 232
  in metabolic monitoring, 43
Malignant hyperthermia, in multisystem injury patient, 158
Mannitol, for elevated ICP
  in head injury patients, 130
  in postoperative brain tumor patients, 201
Marcus Gunn pupillary test, 25
Mean arterial pressure, 15, 15f
  in multisystem injury, 152
  in stroke management, 177
  in vasospasm, 164
Mechanical ventilation
  airway pressure in, 4–5
  indications for, 4
  in intracerebral hemorrhage, indications for, 185
  in pediatric patient, 211
  positive end-expiratory pressure in, 5–6
  in spinal cord injury patient, 138–139
  supplemental oxygen in, 5
  volume vs. pressure cycled modes, 4
  weaning from, 8
MEE (metabolic energy expenditure), 84
Meningitis, 101–104
  empiric therapy for, 102t
Meningoencephalitis, 115
Mental status, assessment of, 23–24
Meperidine, for multisystem injury, 159
Metabolic acidosis, 73–74
  bicarbonate therapy for, 149
Metabolic alkalosis, 73
Metabolic rate, manipulation of, 154
Metabolic theory, of autoregulation, 33
Metabolism
  cerebral, blood flow and, 39–40
    metabolic coupling, 40–41
    monitoring techniques, 41–43
  management in head injury patient, 131–132
  in multisystem injury patient, 154
  and nutrition, 83–89. *See also* Nutrition
  response to injury, 83–84, 84f
N-Methyl-D-aspartate receptor, in ischemic stroke, 175
Microdialysis, in metabolic monitoring, 42–43
Micronutrients, 86
Midazolam
  for epileptic seizures, 193
    IV formulation, 193t
  for multisystem injury, 157–158
Middle cerebral artery
  occlusion, 178, 178f
    intracranial thrombolysis for, 178, 178f
    treatment protocols, 179–180, 179f
  velocities, in vasospasm diagnosis, 163
Minute ventilation, 1

Moro reflex, 213
Motility, gastrointestinal, in spinal cord injury patient, 140
Motor function. *See also* Neurological examination
  assessment, 26
  developmental milestones, 212, 212t
MRA (magnetic resonance angiography), in subarachnoid hemorrhage, 162
Multisystem injury management
  complications, preventing and managing, 149–157
    abdominal compartment syndrome, 152–153
    acalculous cholecystitis, 154
    acute lung injury, 149
    acute respiratory distress syndrome, 149–151
    colonic ileus, 153–154
    deep venous thrombosis, 154–155
    hypermetabolic response, 154
    in pulmonary artery catheter use, 152
    pulmonary embolism, 154–155
    renal failure, 155–156
    stress gastritis, 153
    in ventilator weaning, 151
  pharmacological, 157–159
  resuscitative phase, 145–149
Muscle relaxants, pediatric use, 210–211
Myoclonus, 26
Myogenic theory, of autoregulation, 33

N

N-methyl-D-aspartate receptor, in ischemic stroke, 175
Near-infrared spectroscopy
  in brain death determination, 232
  in metabolic monitoring, 41
Neonatal intensive care unit, monitoring head injury in, 127
Neonate
  brain development in, 214–215.214f
  cerebral blood flow in, 215, 215t
  with head injury, monitoring of, 127
  ICP control in, 215–216, 216f
  mechanical ventilation in, 211
  oxygen consumption in, 211
  reflexes in, 213
Neoplasms, opportunistic CNS, in AIDS, 109
Neurocysticercosis, 114–115
Neurogenic pulmonary edema, following spinal cord injury, 139
Neurogenic theory, of autoregulation, 33
Neurological examination
  arterial blood gases and, 26–27
  brainstem function, 25–26
  consciousness level and mental status, 24–25
  electrocardiogram in, 27
  Glasgow Coma Scale, 24
  in head injury patient, 127
  motor function, 26
  patient history in, 21
  in pediatric patient, 212–213, 212t, 213t
  physical aspect, 23–24
  in postoperative brain tumor patients, 199
  vital signs in, 22–23
Neurological status, monitoring, 21–27
  in head injury patient, 131
Neuroprotective therapy, for ischemic stroke, 178–179
Neurotrauma, circulatory dysfunction in, 128–129
NIRS (near-infrared spectroscopy), in metabolic monitoring, 41
Nitrogen balance, evaluation of, 85–86, 86f
Nitrous oxide technique, CBF measurement, 34
NMDA (*N*-methyl-D-aspartate) receptor, in ischemic stroke, 175
Nocardiosis, 114
Nonsteroidal antiinflammatory drugs, in multisystem injury patient, 159
Nontraumatic intracerebral hemorrhage, 180–186, 183
  background and etiologies, 180, 180t
  evaluation and treatment, 183–184, 184t
    future directions in, 185–186
    management issues, 184–185
  outcome prediction models, 185–186
  pathophysiology, 180–183, 181f–182f
  primary injury
    causes, 180t
    treatment, 183t
  secondary injury
    causes, 180t
    treatment, 183t
  supratentorial, 184
Nosocomial infections
  bloodstream, 99
  in critically-ill patients, 96–99
    pathogenesis and prevention, 96–98
  pneumonia, 98
  sinusitis, 98–99
  urinary tract infection, 99
NSAIDs (nonsteroidal antiinflammatory drugs), in multisystem injury patient, 159
Nutrition
  advances in, 88–89
  electrolytes, 86
  energy, 84–85, 85f
  feeding methods and, 86–88
  for head injury patient, 132
  lipids, 86
  micronutrients, 86
  needs in multisystem injury patient, 154
  overfeeding complications, 85, 85t
  for pediatric patient, 218
  protein, 85–86, 86f, 86t
  timing of feeds and, 88

O

Obstructive shock, in neurotrauma, 129
Oculocephalic reflex, in brainstem function assessment, 25–26
  brain death and, 230
Oculovestibular reflex, brain death and, 230
Ogilvie's syndrome, in multisystem injury patient, 153–154
Ohm's law, 29
Opioid therapy
  for multisystem injury, 159
  in pediatric patient, 210
Opportunistic infections/neoplasms, of CNS, in AIDS patients, 109–110
Optic nerve function, assessment of, 25
Oral feeding, 88
Organ procurement, brain death and, 233
Osmolality, 55–56
  regulation, 56–57
Osmotic edema, cerebral, 198
Osteomyelitis, 100
Oxygen
  alveolar-arterial gradient, 3
  cerebral metabolism and, 39–40
  partial pressure, 1
    in alveolus, 3
    in arterial blood, 2, 3
  supplemental
    for head injury patient, 128
    in mechanical ventilation, 5
Oxygen consumption, in neonate, 211, 215, 215t
Oxygen content, in blood, 2, 2f
  in multisystem injury patient, 147
Oxyhemoglobin dissociation curve, 1–2, 2f

P

Pain control, in multisystem injury patient, 158–159
Pancuronium
  for multisystem injury patient, 158
  pediatric use, 210–211
PA_{O_2} (partial pressure of oxygen in alveolus), 3
Papaverine infusion, for vasospasm, 165
Paralytic agents
  for intracranial hypertension, in postoperative brain tumor patients, 200
  for intracranial hypertension control, 50, 51t
  for multisystem injury, 158
Parasitic infections
  in AIDS patients, 110
  of central nervous system, 114–115. *See also* Central nervous system infections, parasitic
Partial prothrombin time, 148
  intracerebral hemorrhage and, 183
  subarachnoid hemorrhage and, 166
Patient-controlled analgesia, for multisystem injury, 159
P_{CO_2} (partial pressure of carbon dioxide), 1
PCWP. *See* Pulmonary capillary wedge pressure
PE. *See* Pulmonary embolism
Peak inspiratory pressure, 4
Pediatric patient. *See also* Infant; Neonate
  brain death in, diagnosing, 232–233
  central nervous system monitoring in, 216
  cerebral hemodynamics and blood flow in, 215–216, 215t, 216f
  circulatory system in, 211–212
  coma scales for, 213, 213t
  fluid and electrolyte requirements in, 217–218, 217f, 218t–219t
  kidney in, 218
  mechanical ventilation in, 211
  nervous system in, 212–215, 212t, 213t, 214f
  neurological examination in, 212–213
  nutritional requirements in, 218
  pharmacological therapy in, 209–211

Pediatric patient—cont'd
renal maturity in, 218
respiratory system in, 207–208
causes of failure, 207t
tracheal intubation in, 208–209, 209t
PEEP. *See* Positive end-expiratory pressure
Penetrating trauma, to head, 126
Peptic ulcer disease, in postoperative brain tumor patient, 203
Periodic epileptiform discharges, treatment of, 192
Peripheral nerves, in pediatric patient, 212
Permissive hypercapnia, 7
PET. *See* Positron emission tomography
Phencyclidine, pediatric use, 210
Phenobarbital, prophylactic, in head injury patients, 133
Phenytoin
for epileptic seizures, 193
IV formulation, 193t
prophylactic, in head injury patients, 133
Phycomycosis, 114
Physiological dead space, 1
PIP (peak inspiratory pressure), 4
Pituitary tumors, 89
PML (progressive multifocal leukoencephalopathy), in AIDS patients, 110
Pneumonia
in critically-ill patients, 98
following spinal cord injury, 139
nosocomial, in spinal cord injury patient, 140
in subarachnoid hemorrhage, 166
ventilator-assisted, 7
Po_2 (partial pressure of oxygen), 1
Pao_2 (partial pressure of oxygen in arterial blood), 2, 3
in shunt, 3f, 4
Poiseuille's law, 29
components, 31
Positive end-expiratory pressure, 5–6
in ARDS, 150, 151
auto-PEEP, 6
Positron emission tomography
in brain death determination, 232
in CBF measurement, 35–36
in intracerebral hemorrhage, 183
in metabolic monitoring, 43
in vasospasm diagnosis, 164
Postventilation apnea, 23
PPT. *See* Partial prothrombin time
Preload, ventricular
defined, 11
management, 16–17
monitoring, 14
President's Commission for the Study of Bioethics and Medicine (1981), 229–230
Pressor agents, 17, 18f
Pressure control ventilation, 4
Pressure-cycled ventilator modes, 4
Pressure support ventilation, 4
Pressure volume index, 48, 49f
Prion infections, of central nervous system, 111–112
Prophylaxis
antibiotic therapy
for CNS bacterial infections, 105–106
in trauma patient, 156–157
anticonvulsant
in epileptic patients, 192, 194
in head injury patient, 133
calcium-blocking, for vasospasm prevention, 164
for deep vein thrombosis prevention, 155
in head injury patient
perioperative antibiotics, 133
postoperative anticonvulsants, 133
for stress ulcer prevention, 153
Propofol
for epileptic seizures, 193
IV formulation, 193t
for multisystem injury patient, 157
pediatric use, 209
Protein requirements
evaluation of, 85–86, 86t
in pediatric patient, 217, 217t
Prothrombin time, 148
intracerebral hemorrhage and, 183
Proton MR spectroscopy, in brain death determination, 232
PT. *See* Prothrombin time
Pulmonary artery catheters, 14, 14f
in head injury patient, 128
in multisystem artery management, 152
Pulmonary capillary wedge pressure, 13, 14, 14f, 16–17, 61
in multisystem injury patient, 146, 147
Pulmonary edema, in subarachnoid hemorrhage, 166
Pulmonary embolism
anticoagulation therapy for, 155
diagnostic tests, 155
following spinal cord injury, 139
in head injury patient, 133
in multisystem injury patient, 154–155
in postoperative brain tumor patient, 203
signs and symptoms, 155
in subarachnoid hemorrhage, 166
Pulmonary vascular resistance, 15, 17
Pupils, in brainstem function assessment, 25. *See also* Neurological examination
brain death and, 230
Purified protein fraction solution, 62, 62t
PVR (pulmonary vascular resistance), 15, 17

Q

Quinlan, Karen Ann (1976), life support and, 222

R

Radionuclide imaging, in brain death determination, 232
Rapacuronium
for multisystem injury patient, 158
pediatric use, 210
RAS (reticular activating system), 24, 25
Rebleeding, in subarachnoid hemorrhage, 162–163
REE (resting energy expenditure), 85
Refractory generalized status epilepticus, 193
Remifentanyl, for multisystem injury, 159
Renal failure, in multisystem injury patient, 155–156
Renal function, in abdominal compartment syndrome, 152
Renal replacement therapy, in multisystem injury patient, 156
Respiratory acidosis, 72–73
Respiratory alkalosis, 72
Respiratory dysfunction. *See* Respiratory function
Respiratory failure
classification, 146
management of, in head injury patient, 128
in pediatric patient, causes of, 207t, 208
spinal cord injury associated with, 7–8
Respiratory function
in abdominal compartment syndrome, 152–153
cardiorespiratory variables and, 16f
in head injury patient, 127–128
mechanical assistance. *See* Mechanical ventilation
monitoring, 1–8, 23
physiology, 1–4, 2f, 3f
in postoperative brain tumor patient, 201
problems specific to, management of, 6–8
in spinal cord injury, management of, 137–139
airway, 137–138
complications, 139
ventilation, 138–139
Resting energy expenditure, 85
Resting metabolic expenditure, 85
Resuscitation
epileptic patients, strategies for, 193
fluids for, 61–64, 61t, 62t, 64f
in intracerebral hemorrhage, 185
in multisystem injury
airway and breathing, 145–147
autotransfusion for, 148
coagulopathy and, 148–149
colloid solutions for, 147–148
crystalloid solutions for, 147
hypothermia and, 148
metabolic acidosis and, 149
ongoing, 145
transfusion for, 148
Reticular activating system, 24, 25
Reye's syndrome, 110–111
Rhabdomyolysis, renal failure and, 156
RME (resting metabolic expenditure), 85
Rocuronium
for multisystem injury patient, 158
pediatric use, 210

S

SAH. *See* Subarachnoid hemorrhage
SBP (systolic blood pressure), measuring, 22–23
SCI. *See* Spinal cord injury
SCIWORA syndrome, in pediatric patient, 216
Sedation
for elevated ICP, 50, 51t
in head injury patients, 130
in postoperative brain tumor patients, 200
in multisystem injury patient, 157–158
Seizures
in epileptic patients. *See* Epilepsy, seizures in
in intracerebral hemorrhage, 185
postoperative, in brain tumor patients, 199
in subarachnoid hemorrhage, 165

Shock
  in multisystem injury, 146–147
  in neurotrauma, 129
Shunt fraction, 4
SIADH. *See* Syndrome of inappropriate ADH
Single-photon emission computed tomography
  in brain death determination, 232
  in CBF measurement, 35, 36f
  in vasospasm diagnosis, 164
Sinusitis, in critically-ill patients, 98–99
$Sjvo_2$ (jugular venous oxygen saturation), monitoring, 41–42
Skull
  depressed fracture, 126
  in infant, 213–214
Society of Critical Care Medicine
  member survey results, 226–227
  task force on life support of critically ill, 221–222
Sodium
  imbalance. *See* Hypernatremia; Hyponatremia
  regulation, 58–59
SPECT. *See* Single-photon emission computed tomography
Spinal cord injury
  cervical, in pediatric patient, 216
  incidence, 137
  management
    cardiovascular, 139–140
    gastrointestinal, 140
    genitourinary, 141
    integumentary, 141
    protocol for, 137
    respiratory, 137–139
  metabolic response to, 83–84, 84f
  respiratory failure associated with, 7–8
Spiral computed tomography, in brain death determination, 232
Status epilepticus. *See* Epilepsy
Stepwise therapy, targeted therapy vs., for intracranial hypertension, 52–53
Stress gastritis, in multisystem injury patient, 153
Stress ulcers
  in multisystem injury patient, prevention of, 153
  in subarachnoid hemorrhage, 167
Stroke. *See* Ischemic stroke
Subarachnoid hemorrhage
  cause, 161
  consequences
    medical, 165–167
    neurological, 162–165
  diagnosis, 162
  intracranial hemodynamics, 161
  management, 162
Subdural empyema, 104
Subgaleal abscess, 100
Succinylcholine
  for multisystem injury patient, 158
  pediatric use, 210
Sucralfate therapy, for spinal cord injury patient, 140
Surfactant therapy, for ARDS, 150
Surgery, epileptic seizures after, 192
SVR. *See* Systemic vascular resistance
Swan-Ganz catheters. *See* Pulmonary artery catheters
Sympathomimetic drugs, intracerebral hemorrhage and, 182
Syndrome of inappropriate ADH, 64–65, 89
  in head injury patient, 132
  in pediatric patient, 218
  in postoperative brain tumor patient, 202
Systemic vascular resistance, 15
  in multisystem injury patient, 146, 147
Systolic blood pressure, measuring, 22–23

T

Taenia solium infection, 114–115
Tapeworm infection, 114–115
Targeted therapy, vs. stepwise therapy, for intracranial hypertension, 52–53
TBI (traumatic brain injury). *See* Brain injury
TBW (total body water), 55
TCD. *See* Transcranial Doppler sonography
Therapeutic hypothermia, for elevated ICP, 52
  in head injury patient, 130–131
Thermal diffusion flowmetry, in CBF measurement, 37
Thiamine, for epileptic seizures, 193
Thiopental, pediatric use, 209–210
Thromboembolism, in subarachnoid hemorrhage, 166
Thrombolysis, intracranial, for middle cerebral artery occlusion, 178, 178f
Thyroid disease, 90–91, 90t
Thyroid-stimulating hormone, 89
Thyrotoxicosis
  signs and symptoms, 90, 90t
  treatment, 90–91
Thyrotropin-releasing hormone, 89
Tidal volume, 1
Tissue plasminogen-activator therapy, for ischemic stroke, 175–176, 176t
Tissue shifts, in intracerebral hemorrhage, 183
Tonicity, 55–56
  regulation, 56–57
Total body water, 55, 56f
Total parenteral nutrition, 87–88
  bloodstream infections and, 99
  in head injury patient, 132
Toxoplasma gondii infection, in AIDS patients, 110
tPA (tissue plasminogen-activator) therapy, for ischemic stroke, 175–176, 176t
TPN. *See* Total parenteral nutrition
Trace elements, requirements and status, evaluation of, 86
Tracheal intubation, in pediatric patient, 208–209
  tube and blade sizes by age, 209t
Tracheostomy, in mechanical ventilation weaning process, 8
Transcapillary water flux, 57–58
Transcranial Doppler sonography
  in brain death determination, 38, 39f, 232
  in CBF measurement, 37–39, 37t, 38f, 39f
  in vasospasm diagnosis, 163–164
Transfusion
  for intracerebral hemorrhage, 183
  in multisystem injury, 148
  red blood cell, 63–64, 64f
Transluminal balloon angioplasty, for vasospasm, 164–165
Treponema pallidum infection, in AIDS patients, 110
TRH (thyrotropin-releasing hormone), 89
"Triple-H" therapy, for vasospasm, 164
TSH (thyroid-stimulating hormone), 89
Tube feedings, 87–88

U

Ulceration, in spinal cord injury patient
  decubitus ulcers, 141
  gastrointestinal, 140
Ultrafiltration, renal, in multisystem injury patient, 156
Ultrasound. *See* Transcranial Doppler sonography
Urinary tract infection
  in critically-ill patient, 99
  in head injury patient, 133

V

V/Q (ventilation/perfusion) mismatch, 3
V_A (alveolar ventilation), 1
Variant Creutzfeldt-Jakob disease, 111
Vascular malformation rupture, intracerebral hemorrhage and, 182
Vascular radius (r^4), 31, 32f
  blood flow velocity and, 38
Vasogenic edema, cerebral, 198
Vasoresponsivity, 33
Vasospasm, in subarachnoid hemorrhage, 163–165
  diagnosis, 163–164
  management, 164
  prevention, 164
  treatment, 164–165
VDCC (voltage-dependent channels), in ischemic stroke, 175
Vecuronium
  for multisystem injury patient, 158
  pediatric use, 210
VEDV (ventricular end diastolic volume), 11, 14, 16
Ventilation, 1
  alveolar, 1
  assist control, 4
  dead space, 1
  intermittent mandatory, 4
  inverse ratio, 7
  mechanical. *See* Mechanical ventilation
  minute, 1
  pressure control, 4
  pressure support, 4
  in spinal cord injury patient, 138–139
Ventilation/perfusion mismatch, 3
Ventilator
  in ARDS
    practices, 150
    weaning criteria, 151
  weaning from, 138–139
Ventilator-assisted pneumonia, 7
Ventilator-associated lung injury, 5
Ventilator modes, 4
  for spinal cord injury patient, 138
Ventricular end diastolic volume, 11, 14, 16
Viral infections
  in AIDS patients, 110

of central nervous system, 107–111. *See also* Central nervous system infections, viral
Virchow's triad, deep vein thrombosis and, 155
Vital signs, in neurological examination, 22–23
Voltage-dependent channels, in ischemic stroke, 175
Volume-cycled ventilator modes, 4
Volume resuscitation, 60–61
fluids for, 61–64, 62t, 64f
protocol for, 61, 61t

W

Water. *See* Body water
Water and electrolyte balance
in critically-ill patient, 59–64
disorders, 64–72. *See also individual disorders*
Weaning, from ventilator, 138–139
criteria for, 151
protocols for, 151

X

Xe-CT (xenon computed tomography), in CBF measurement, 35, 164
Xenon-133, in CBF measurement, 34, 164